ANNUAL PROGRESS
IN CHILD PSYCHIATRY AND
CHILD DEVELOPMENT

ANNUAL PROGRESS IN CHILD PSYCHIATRY AND CHILD DEVELOPMENT 1968

Edited by

STELLA CHESS, M.D.

Associate Professor of Psychiatry
New York University School
of Medicine

and

ALEXANDER THOMAS, M.D.

Professor of Psychiatry
New York University School
of Medicine

BRUNNER/MAZEL *Publishers* • New York

PREFACE

Keeping up with the literature in such a rapidly expanding field as child psychiatry and child development has become a task of herculean proportions. In addition to the older journals, which continue to grow in size and scope, a number of new publications have been launched in recent years. To help cope with the increasing volume of material, several abstracting services have proved useful. Inevitably, however, these are limited by their format to brief summaries of articles. All too often contributions of lasting interest are lost in the welter of current publication and are not readily available for later consultation.

For this reason we have long thought that it would be worthwhile to collect in an annual volume those articles that might be of most value to workers in this field both for immediate information and for long-term reference. The present volume attempts to achieve this aim for articles appearing in 1967. The contributions are reprinted without change, including all bibliographic references. Only articles in the English language published in a professional journal during the calendar year are included. We have omitted from consideration material that originally appeared in some other volume.

Naturally, there can be no easy formula for selection. We have tried to make our criteria as objective as possible, though we are of course aware that judgment of what is an outstanding contribution cannot avoid having some personal component. While we have searched the literature as extensively as we could, it is not unlikely that we have missed valuable articles. To minimize this possibility, we have informally consulted a number of leading workers in specialized areas, and we thank them for the time and thought they gave to suggesting material for our consideration.

The articles were chosen for their intrinsic merit rather than in terms of a quota of selections to fit a predetermined series of topics. Although the table of contents reflects a broad range of studies, it is not intended to represent all the major subdivisions of child psychiatry and child development.

In general, the articles are of two types: 1) original work that holds promise of making a contribution to progress in this field, and 2) review articles which, even though they report little or no new work, present a

v

clear, thoughtful, and systematic picture of the present state of knowledge in an important area.

The uniformly favorable response of the authors whom we approached was gratifying, and the publishers of various journals have also been most cooperative in working out agreements for reproducing material that first appeared in their pages. The project could not have been accomplished without the participation of our editorial associate, Dr. Samuel Sillen, in all phases of the work. We also extend our appreciation to the publisher, Mr. Bernard Mazel, whose consistent concern was to produce a volume on the highest possible professional level.

STELLA CHESS, M.D.
ALEXANDER THOMAS, M.D.

CONTENTS

1

THE ROLE OF BIOLOGICAL RHYTHMS IN EARLY PSYCHOLOGICAL DEVELOPMENT

Peter H. Wolff, M.D.

Harvard Medical School and Judge Baker Guidance Center (Boston)

INTRODUCTION

In a recent review of biological rhythms research, Sollberger[1] lists over 2000 references pertaining to the rhythmical features of animal behavior. Even in such an exhaustive survey, however, the empirical relations between intrinsic rhythms and the experience of time,[2] the development of a time concept,[3-4] and the acquisition of motor syntax and language[5] are barely considered although such relations imply many of the classical arguments in human psychology. As Sollberger's review indicates, the investigation of periodicities in human behavior has usually focused on cycles of motility, sexual activity, sleep and waking, work proficiency, psychopathology, and the like, and therefore on the analysis of macro-rhythms or temporal sequences with basic frequencies of hours, days, months or seasons. Others have worked out the adaptive significance of macro-rhythms in animals,[6-9] and clarified the extent to which these are endogenous, can be entrained on external synchronizers, or are "learned."

Rhythmical repetition, however, is also characteristic for reflex activities of the human neonate, although in this case the cycles have much higher basic frequencies of seconds and fractions of seconds. It has been

Reprinted from BULLETIN OF THE MENNINGER CLINIC, Vol. 31, No. 4, July, 1967 pp. 197-218. An earlier version of this paper was presented at The Menninger Foundation in October, 1966, upon the occasion of the 1966 Helen Sargent Memorial Award. Work for this study was carried out while the author was supported by the Career Development Program of the U.S.P.H.S.-N.I.M.H., Grant K-MH-3461.

proposed that such *micro-rhythms* may represent primitive controls for sensorimotor behavior in the human infant,[3] but the significance of this assertion is difficult to assess, since most references to high frequency rhythms in neonatal behavior are of a general descriptive nature without any quantification of their temporal features. The first section of this essay will attempt a formal analysis of two such high frequency rhythms in the human neonate, and will show that even apparently simple motor patterns are organized in complex time sequences.

As a corollary to the proposition that micro-rhythms have a controlling function in early motor activity, it has been assumed that the manifest rhythms are suppressed in development and replaced by qualitatively different regulations.[3] An alternative possibility — that the endogenous rhythms of neonatal behavior have their own rules of development, that they persist to give rise to more complex temporal sequences, and that as such they influence the sequential order of cognitive functions, as well as of motor habits, in the adult — has not been seriously explored. The intrinsic regulation of time-sequences in adult human behavior is, however, a question of theoretical interest for the psychology of cognition, language and logic. In his essay on the problem of serial order in behavior, for example, Lashley[5] presents cogent reasons why one must postulate the existence of endogenous high frequency oscillators, and why in the final analysis one can not account for the serial order of voluntary adult behaviors without assuming their presence at birth. To Lashley's exposition one could only add the suggestion that a developmental study of such rhythms would clarify important aspects of the problem which an investigation of their final forms alone cannot. Clinical examples of motor rhythms in older children, and their possible relevance for the development of micro-rhythms as regulators of adaptive behavior, will be considered in the second part of this essay.

Heart rate, respiration and "brain wave" activity are the instances of micro-rhythms which have been studied most carefully in man. While among these the electroencephalogram is most directly, or at least most obviously related to early psychological development, studies of EEG activity in humans have more often and more persuasively demonstrated the limitations imposed by neural rhythms on perceptual-motor performance than they have shown that neural pulses directly instigate rhythmical motor sequences.[10]

Such an inherent relation between central nervous system pulses and rhythmical motor action has been demonstrated for lower species by von Holst, [11, 12] and Paul Weiss,[13-15] who worked with deafferented nonmammalian vertebrates. Using a variety of experimental techniques these investigators showed that motor organs which are essential for locomotion under normal circumstances can also be activated in the absence of any peripheral feedback. From these studies one must conclude that the deafferented central nervous system generates stable high frequency rhythms, and that the corresponding autonomous oscillatory mechanisms interact reciprocally to instigate complex behavior sequences.

The studies mentioned above have been carried out only on the central nervous systems of lower species which have a capacity for extensive "repair" after derangement experiments. Totally deafferented yet viable human organisms do not occur as "experiments in nature," and even nonhuman primates become totally unresponsive when surgically deafferented. It might therefore seem to be only an academic exercise to invoke the adaptive role of high frequency oscillators in human behavior, were it not for Lashley's persuasive demonstration that there is a functional continuum from spontaneous rhythmical motor movements instigated by an isolated nervous system to the simple motor reflexes of human infants, to the violinist's rapid finger movements in playing an arpeggio, to the syntax of spoken language; and that whenever human behavior is arranged in temporal sequences of high frequency, central regulatory mechanisms come into play which cannot be reduced to experience alone, but must originate in intrinsic regulators of serial order.[5]

In this essay, I will present an account of only isolated studies and clinical cases, which pertain primarily to the repetition of simple reflexes. While I have not attempted to examine more complex phase interactions in behavior, it is to be expected that their analysis would provide answers of far greater relevance to the problem of serial order in voluntary behavior than any numerical analysis of simple repetitions alone.

CRYING

The first instance of high frequency rhythms in behavior to be considered is that of neonatal crying. To visualize the vocalizations pattern for a detailed analysis of their form and rhythms, samples of crying were recorded under natural conditions in the nursery, and the recorded samples analyzed by the sound spectrograph.[16] Under limited and specifiable conditions, neonatal crying is arranged in patterns of remarkably stable serial order that can be demonstrated visually with the sonogram (Figure 1). This pattern has sometimes been called the "hunger cry" because it is often heard when one might expect an infant to be hungry; but since most crying infants eventually vocalize in this pattern regard-

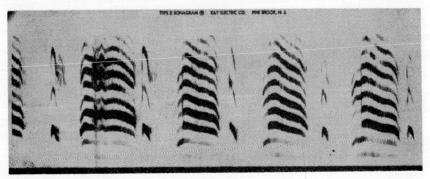

FIG. 1. Basic cry of 4-day-old full-term infant. Abscissa-time base (4.8 seconds); ordinate-frequency range (0-8000 cycles per second).

less of the offending cause unless they fall asleep or get exasperated, it has also been called the "basic cry."[17, 18] It is present in all normal four-day-old neonates, in older infants, and in many infants with minor cerebral dysfunction. In Table 1 the distinct features of one string of basic cries from a normal neonate were grouped as expiratory cries (mean duration 0.62 seconds), rest periods (mean duration 0.085 sec-

TABLE 1

RHYTHMICAL CRY—FOUR-DAY-OLD INFANT

Cry Expiratory	Rest Period	Inspiratory Whistle	Rest Period
.63 secs.	.08 secs.	.03 secs.	.17 secs.
.62	.05	.03	.15
.70	.06	.04	.26
.51	.08	.03	.15
.87	.10	—	—
.24	.05	—	—
.64	.02	.04	.17
—	—	.04	.28
.57	.04	.04	.17
.64	.03	.03	.27
.70	.09	.04	.09
.64	.16	.04	.14
.64	(?)	.05	.24
.61	.24	.04	.24
.79	.09	.04	.21
.59	.10	.04	.19
.56	.09	.05	.19
Mean .62	.09	.04	.20

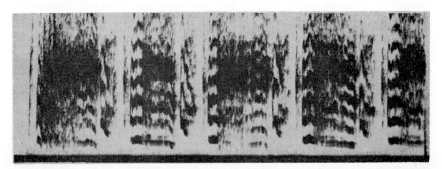

FIG. 2. "Mad" cry of a 4-day-old full-term neonate.

onds), inspiratory whistles (mean duration 0.039 seconds), and rest periods (mean duration 0.195 seconds), to demonstrate the stability of rhythmical features.

A vocalization pattern, which some mothers call the "angry" cry because of its strident character, is quite similar to that of the basic cry except for the greater turbulence which occurs when an excess amount of air is forced through the vocal cord, and which on the sonogram appears as diffuse black areas (see Figure 2).[17] Turbulence does not interfere with the basic rhythm demonstrated above, so that the "mad cry" has approximately the same rhythmical features as the basic cry (mean duration of expiratory cry 0.69 seconds; of rest periods 0.20 seconds; of inspiratory whistles 0.049 seconds; and of second rest periods 0.11 seconds — see Table 2).

Cries in response to other causes are organized in different sequences: The first response to a heel prick, for example, is a long vocal expiration which lasts five to six times as long as the expiratory vocalization of the basic cry, and is followed by a long silence in expiration that may last up to seven seconds. When the tape recording of a pain cry was played to mothers so that they did not know their child was not crying, they responded with great concern. But when the time sequence of the same recorded cry was altered by removing most of the long silent period, mothers uniformly responded with less distress. The temporal arrangement of vocalizations thus served an important signaling function even in the newborn period.[18]

A cry of different pattern is provoked by giving the infant a pacifier to suck, removing it, and giving it back, until he is exasperated. Cries recorded just after the pacifier has been removed a number of times are similar in most respects to the pain cry except that the long period of breath holding in expiration is not present (see Table 3). When the tape recordings of such cries are played to a mother who cannot see her baby, she reacts with far less anxiety than to the pain cry, and with about the same concern as to a pain cry from which the long silence in expiration has been removed.

In a preliminary experiment to observe whether the distortion of auditory feedback would alter the rhythm of crying, masking noise was played into the ears of seven infants while they are crying in the basic pattern. Although the noise itself often stopped the crying completely, the *rhythm* itself was not altered by the masking sound as long as the infants continued to cry. These preliminary findings, when considered in conjunction with the almost universal appearance of stable crying rhythms in healthy neonates,[17] were considered a circumstantial evidence that the vocalization rhythms of the neonate are partially controlled by autonomous central mechanisms.[22, 23]

SUCKING

A second motor rhythm of high frequency can be observed in the neonate's spontaneous mouthing activity and in his response to a pacifier. From an extensive study of pacifier sucking,[19] I will summarize here only details relevant to the proposition that central rhythms extrinsic to the motor act itself control the rhythms of non-nutritive sucking. During restful sleep shortly before a meal, many infants make spontaneous rapid movements with the lips, jaw and tongue that can be distinguished without difficulty from the sucking and chomping movements observed during lighter sleep.[19, 24] These movements are grouped in bursts of 4-12 distinct events separated by rest periods lasting from 2-10 seconds. The mean duration of bursts and rest periods may vary among infants, but remains the same for any one infant over several days. When the individual movements were counted and timed by stopwatch, and the length of bursts, the duration of rest periods, and the mean frequency of sucks per second in a burst were calculated, they constituted a regular pattern that was quite stable over time for each infant. For technical reasons, the method of direct observation, however, was not reliable, and it could not capture the finer details of the moment to moment changes in sucking (see below). To obtain more precise measures, the infant's mouthing activity was therefore recorded from a pacifier attached to a pressure transducer and polygraph writer, so that the changes of positive pressure in the pacifier could be recorded as the infant pressed on the pacifier with his lips and tongue. Since the sensorimotor components of pacifier

TABLE 2

"Mad" Cry—Three-Day-Old Infant

Cry Expiratory	Rest Period	Inspiratory Whistle	Rest Period
.78 secs.	.18 secs.	.04 secs.	.17 secs.
.69	.15	.04	.15
.69	.19	.04	.24
.77	.21	.06	.15
.74	.23	.04	.14
.68	.24	.04	.11
.65	.29	—	—
.60	.27	.04	.06
.70	.30	.06	.09
.62	.23	.06	.11
.62	.30	.07	.02
.62	.18	.10	.06
		.06	.09
		.08	.04
.90	.15	.03	.04
		.04	.12
.62	.09	.03	.15
.76	.21	.06	.12
.67	.06	.03	.15
.67	.04	.03	.12
.61	.24	.03	.09
—	—	—	—
Mean .69	.20	.05	.11

sucking were thought to be different from those of spontaneous mouthing, it was expected that the two types of rhythmical mouthing would have entirely different temporal patterns. Yet the serial order of pacifier sucking in sleep was exactly the same as that of spontaneous mouthing, and the two patterns were statistically indistinguishable.

Twenty full-term infants, who were delivered to healthy mothers after uncomplicated deliveries and tested on the fourth day after birth, all mouthed the pacifier at a mean frequency of about two sucks per second during regular sleep (range 1.9-2.3 sucks per second). Variation in mean frequency from burst to burst were extremely small for any one infant· and slight across individuals (for the twenty infants the standard deviations varied from 0.09 to 0.24 sucks per second).* The mean frequency

---

* Mean frequency of sucks was calculated by dividing the number of sucks in a burst by the total duration of that burst; standard deviations were calculated from mean frequencies per burst, rather than from individual sucks, for reasons to be indicated below.

TABLE 3

CRY IN RESPONSE TO PAIN AND TO BEING TEASED

| | Cry in Response to Pain (Mean Value for 5 Infants at 4 Days) | | | |
	Cry Proper	Rest	Inspiratory Whistle	Rest
First Sequence After Pain Stimulus	3.83 secs.	3.99	0.18	0.16
Mean of Subsequent Sequences	0.78	0.25	0.08	0.25

| | Cry in Response to Being Teased (Mean Value for 7 Infants, 3-4 Days Old) | | | |
	Cry Proper	Rest	Inspiratory Whistle	Rest
First Sequence After Pacifier Removed	2.67	0.07	0.13	0.13
Mean of Subsequent Cry Sequences	0.59	0.02	0.07	0.12

per second in a burst was the most constant feature of the sucking rhythm but the mean number of sucks in a burst, and the mean duration of rest periods were also stable values which constituted a second rhythm of lower frequency superimposed on basic rate.

Despite the invariance of mean values per burst, the individual sucks of a burst were not all equal in length, and varied systematically around the mean for that burst. Peak times (*i.e.,* the distance between two adjacent sucks in a burst — see Figure 3) at the start of the burst were invariably shorter than those near the end, whether the recording was taken from a normal full-term neonate, a premature, or an older infant. This rise in peak time was shown by graphing intervals between successive sucks within the burst as continuous function and plotting each burst as a separate line (Figure 4). The same rise was demonstrated

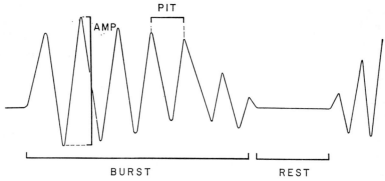

FIGURE 3. Diagrammatic representation of sucking pattern on pacifier—peak time (PIT), amplitude, burst length, and rest period.

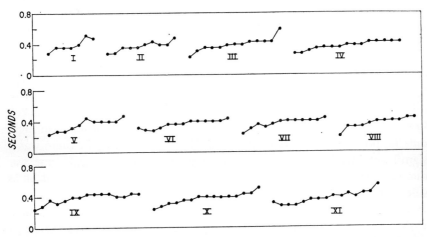

FIGURE 4. Progressive rise of peak times in a burst. Each of 11 consecutive bursts is represented by a line, every peak time between 2 consecutive sucks in a burst by a point on that line; distance between lines does not indicate length of rest periods.

by dividing all bursts of a record, regardless of their lengths, into three equal segments and comparing the mean frequency of the first, second and third segments. In all twenty infants (and in other normal infants tested subsequently) the sucks at the end of a burst were consistently slower than those near the start ($p = .001$ by Friedman 2-Way Analysis of Variance). One might, of course, attribute this rise in peak time to muscle fatigue, and assume that during the rest period the infant recovered from fatigue. The sucking performance of premature infants, however, indicated that this interpretation was unsatisfactory. During the early portion of a record, very young prematures of 31-32 weeks gestation who sucked for only 10 or 15 bursts, and then either stopped sucking altogether or else sucked in unanalyzable patterns, showed the *same* rather than a *greater* rise in peak time from the start to the end of a burst as normal infants, even though their sucking was clearly susceptible to fatigue. Full-term infants who sucked for one-half hour or more without any signs of tiring, showed the same relative rise in peak times as prematures, whereas the rise in peak time after one-half hour of continuous recording was the same as at the beginning in the babies born at term.

Further support for the conclusion that fatigue was not responsible for the rise in peak time came from the performance of infants with chronic or progressive brain disease. One infant who had received four intrauterine transfusions and another three exchange transfusions after birth, because of an Rh incompatibility, was brought to the hospital at two months of age because he had failed to gain weight. This infant sucked on the pacifier in unusually long bursts of 30-40 sucks, yet the peak times remained relatively *constant* throughout the burst until the last three or four sucks when it rose significantly. Other infants with diffuse brain damage, leukodystrophy, subacute encephalitis, also sucked in excessively long bursts and the peak times remained constant throughout the burst until the last three to four sucks, when again there was a significant increase. Were one to assume that a rise in peak time was due to fatigue, patients with central nervous system disease should be as susceptible as normal children and should show its effects after at least 10-15 continuous sucks. Yet the rise in peak time was always associated with the approaching *end,* rather than with the length of the burst. A more satisfactory explanation for the rise seemed to be the assumption that there is one mechanism which is responsible for both the increase of peak times and the termination of a burst; that this mechanism is central in origin (since it can be altered by central nervous system disease); and that it first slows down, and eventually arrests rhythmical sucking in the manner of a positively dampened oscillator. Acquired disease of the central nervous system may destroy this inhibitory mechanism selectively, and leave the basic pacemaker for sucking intact. In other diseases of the central nervous system, such as Down's Syndrome, the pacemaker itself may be altered without destroying the mechanisms responsible for the rise in peak times of the grouping of sucks in bursts.[21]

The sucking performance of infants with congenital defects of the face, jaw and mouth represented an "experiment in nature," with which to test the role of sensory feedback in controlling the basic sucking frequency and the segmentation of sucking in bursts and rest periods. If the feedback from motor end organs were a significant determinant of serial order in sucking, one would expect that sucking pattern of infants with cleft palates and hare lips, or of infants with Pierre Robin's Syndrome, should differ from that of normal children. All such children who were at all capable of sucking, however, sucked at the *same* rate, in the *same* pattern of bursts and rest periods, and with the *same* rise in peak time from the start to the end of a burst, as normal infants.

The infant's performance on the pacifier during deep sleep also suggested that the pulses which trigger bursts of sucking at regular intervals were central in origin. One can, for example, calculate the mean number of sucks per burst for a particular infant, and predict with reasonable accuracy when a new burst is likely to start, and how long it will last.

When such an infant is allowed to suck on the pacifier for as long as he will in regular sleep with the pacifier tied in place, he usually stops sucking altogether 10-15 minutes after an episode of restful sleep starts, although he can be made to resume sucking at any point by an arousing stimulus. Once sleep has inhibited mouthing proper, the infant may continue to show rapid tremors of the tongue and jaw, which have a frequency of seven to eight per second, and are organized in bursts of 5-15 separate movements. Such tremors appear in many normal infants after they have sucked for at least ten minutes, and much more frequently in children with presumptive minor cerebral dysfunction or gross neurological damage, where the tremors may start as soon as the infant begins to suck. Tremors may precede or follow a burst of sucking or, in pathological cases, may be imposed on the sucking movement itself. Their only relevance to this discussion is that they involve motor coordination patterns which are entirely different than those for mouthing activity proper, and that they, too, may appear at regular intervals. In deep sleep, bursts of tremors appeared at intervals which corresponded exactly to the moment when a burst of sucking would have started in lighter sleep. It would seem, therefore, that the appearance of activity bursts at regular intervals was not specific to spontaneous and pacifier-provoked rhythmical mouthing, but that some central pacemaker which has a lower frequency than that for the basic sucking rate activates a variety of different peripheral motor patterns at the same rate. Which motor pattern is activated depends on the level of arousal, but the pacemaker for episodic bursts of activity is extrinsic to, or autonomous of, sucking itself.

When the pacifier was removed right after the start of a burst of sucking, the infant often continued to make empty mouthing movements as if the pacifier were still in his mouth. In such an experiment, the number of empty mouthing movements after the pacifier was removed, plus the number of sucks before the pacifier was removed, usually equalled the mean number of pacifier sucks in a burst for that infant. Once a burst had been triggered, it therefore ran its course regardless of changes in peripheral feedback, as if the length of a burst represented a finite potential for activity that was independent of sensory feedback from the pacifier.

Clinical evidence and *ad hoc* experiments suggest that the temporal organization of non-nutritive sucking is to a large extent regulated by central mechanisms which determine or co-determine (1) the basic rate of sucking; (2) the rise of peak time in the burst; (3) the onset and termination of bursts, and (4) the duration of rest periods.

Graduating by one step to a higher level of integration, one finds that the rhythms which are characteristic for the activity of one motor end *organ* can spread to control the rhythmical organization of other reflexes at the same time. Peiper[26] has shown, for example, that *nutritive sucking* "drives" swallowing and breathing whenever all three reflexes are simultaneously active, as they must be during feeding. When nutritive sucking begins, the rate of respiration changes until a 1-1 or a 1-2 ratio is established.[26]

Both Prechtl[25] and Peiper[26] have observed a phase-relation between sucking and kneading movements of the front paws in nursing kittens, as well as between sucking and grasping in premature human infants. In two-month-old human infants with suspected minor cerebral dysfunction, I have found a one-to-one correspondence between nutritive sucking and blinking that is constant at the start of a feeding, but breaks down as the infant's hunger is satisfied. The rhythm of sucking thus controls not only the physiologically dependent functions of swallowing and breathing, but can spread to anatomically and physiologically unrelated reflexes which have their own natural rhythm when acting alone, but under special motivational conditions are locked in phase with nutritive sucking.

STEREOTYPIES

Several neonatal motor patterns have been described so far whose stable and relatively fixed rhythms were compatible with the hypothesis that the rhythms observed in reflex behavior are intrinsic, and do not depend either on experience or specific sensory inputs. From the simple reflex rhythms of the neonate it is, however, a big jump to the stereotypic mannerisms of older children, since the latter involve more complex motor coordinations, and are more easily influenced by experience, perceptual input, and motivational disposition than congenital reflexes. Since stereotypies are nevertheless stable and relatively simple motor rhythms whose temporal sequences can be analyzed directly, their relation to personality development was relegated to a secondary position for the purposes of this essay, and the rhythmical features were stressed.

Dynamic psychology defines stereotypies as autoerotic activities, with the implications that their primary function is the discharge of instinctual drive tension, and that their aim of tension reduction is fused with the means for achieving it. In specific clinical contexts, sterotypies are also called autisms when they occur in autistic children, and blindisms when they appear in blind children. The neutral term *mannerism* seemed more appropriate than any clinical designation because the behavior patterns to be described were not pathological formations as such, but could occur among normal adequately cared for children, children with *acquired* central nervous system lesions, and retarded children raised in good homes, as well as among institutionalized mongoloid children.

Both the relatively high incidence of stereotypies among institutional children, and the successful inhibition of mannerisms by social-therapeutic interventions, point to a causal relation between mannerisms and social deprivation.[27-30] This relation, however, can not account for the frequent occurrence of mannerisms among blind and feeble-minded children who have been properly cared for, or for the emergence of mannerisms in children who showed no stereotypic activity until the onset of progressive neurological signs and symptoms, or for the instrumental (adaptive) function of mannerisms at particular stages in sensorimotor development.

The observations to follow were selected from a collaborative study, in which Dr. Sadako Imamura and I studied the development of stereotypic mannerisms in a homogeneous population of institutionalized mongoloid children. We traced the transformation of different stereotypic motor patterns over time; investigated the changing relation of form and function in the mannerisms; and compared the forms of mannerism in one diagnostic group with those in normal children and children with other organic illnesses. The primary population for the study was a group of infants with Down's Syndrome, all residing in the same institution. We did not attempt to define mannerisms precisely at the outset, but with certain qualifications scored as mannerisms all movements involving the head or the face, one or more limbs, or one of its parts, the entire body, or any combination among these that were repeated in approximately the same form at regular, short intervals.* The abnormality or uniqueness of a mannerism was not a defining criterion for its inclusion in the tabulation since almost every type observed among the mongoloid children also occurred either as a transient phenomenon in normal children, or as a persisting preoccupation in children with organic or functional pathology. With the exception of the intricate rhythmical behavior patterns invented by older autistic children which most of us could not imitate without a great deal of practice, the stereotypies were in no way unusual in form.

---

* The tabulation also included a group of repetitive motor patterns like intermittent hyperextension and relaxation of the entire body, even though they had no discernible rhythmical pattern; repetitive reflex actions like eye-blinking and respiration, which could be observed in any normal child or adult under the most varied conditions, were not included.

Although the specific rates of mannerisms was the primary issue for this essay, our preliminary impressions concerning the functional significance of mannerisms will be summarized briefly before turning to the quantitative data, in order to give some substance to the otherwise sterile numbers, and in order to indicate the range of different functions which these motor patterns can assume.

Early in the observations it became clear that new stereotypies did not appear in the child's motor repertory at random, but that the sequence of their emergence closely paralleled the overall sequence in motor development.

The development of mannerisms adhered closely to Werner's heuristic ordering principle (the "orthogenetic law") which made it possible to arrange the sequential changes of mannerisms in a rational order.[31] Most of the mongoloid children began between the sixth and the twelfth month with an intermittent stiffening and relaxation of the entire body that was not rhythmical beyond a global activation and relaxation of variable length. As the extensor rigidity abated, the infants began to move the separate body parts independently in simple stable rhythms. Eventually the component parts were reintegrated as articulated patterns and in complex temporal sequences.

Mannerisms were also not simply modes of self-gratification, or goals in their own right. Some infants used a particular rhythmic pattern as long as they were content, but stopped as soon as they became unhappy or began to cry; others used the same motor repetition when they first encountered a familiar person; another group started the mannerism at the moment when they were abandoned; and still others started rocking only after they had been alone and "bored" for some time. To the degree that the meaning of the mannerisms could be inferred from the context by direct observation, stereotypies were used as motor expressions of affect and modes of social encounter as often as they represented executive actions for tension discharge.

A child often used the same mannerisms in distinctly different ways at different stages in development, and the form-function relation of stereotypic mannerisms changed systematically over time. Mannerisms which at first were simple empty repetitions with no apparent relation to external objects, might become not only the instrument but also the target of the activity. An empty grasping movement, for example, was transformed into a movement of hitting the face; empty kicking was replaced by kicking one leg with the other. At a more advanced stage, the infants directed their motor activities away from their own bodies and toward objects in the environment. A child who had been rubbing his body began to rub the sheet of the bed in the same repetitive manner; the child who had kicked one leg with the other now kicked the bars of his crib in the same way and at the same rate. Some children eventually incorporated the bodies of other persons as an essential part of the total configuration. A child who had previously hit her mouth with her hand while opening and closing the mouth rhythmically, now banged Dr. Imamura's hand against her own mouth in the same form and at about the same frequency as she had previously used her own hand. An infant who had persistently rubbed his ear back and forth against the sheet as he lay on his side, now used Dr. Imamura's body as the adequate surface, and while being held rubbed himself repetitively against Dr. Imamura's chest.

The mannerisms thus went through systematic structural and functional changes. At first they might serve as channels for drive tension discharge, but eventually they were often used as motor means toward a concrete goal. To the extent that mannerisms became the means for exploring the physical environment, and for contacting the people in it, they reflected not only a child's social condition, motor and postural development, but also his intellectual performance.[32]

A quantitative assessment of *rates* revealed that different mongoloid children performed a particular mannerism consistently at the same frequency. The similarity between these rates and rates of pacifier sucking in normal neonates suggested to me that the basic rhythm of spontaneous mouthing observed in infancy might be preserved even after the motor patterns themselves have undergone structural modifications.

When hand and mouth movements were coordinated, the new mannerisms (*e.g.,* tapping the chin with the dorsal surface of the hand) usually took twice as long as mouthing alone (range 1.0-1.4 movements per second). Similarly, children who previously had kicked their legs by extending and flexing them at the rate of one full kick per second, later kicked their legs against an object, and then mean rate was 0.5-0.7 movements per second.

One of the common mannerisms seen among mongoloid children, which I have called "rocking proper," was also observed in normal children and children with other organic illnesses. To perform it the child supported himself on his hands and knees facing the mattress, and rocked back and forth on his haunches in a continuous back and forth motion. All mongoloid children who engaged in "rocking proper" did so at a rate of 1.0 complete movements per second, with no variation from day to day, or from child to child. When children assumed this posture but kept their bodies at rest and nodded their heads up and down, the rate varied from 1.8-2.2 movements per second.

Children with other illnesses rocked at about the same rate as those with Down's Syndrome. Three autistic children, who rocked in this fashion, did so at the same constant rate of 1.0 movements per second. At other times two of them also nodded their heads at the rate of two movements per second while at rest in this position. Several normal infants between 9-12 months, and one child of 18 months with suggestive signs of minor cerebral dysfunction, rocked in the same pattern and at the same rate except at the start or end of a period of rocking.

For three normal infants who were starting to crawl, "rocking proper" was clearly a point of transition from sitting to physical displacement. For these infants rocking was an end in itself during the early weeks after onset. Eventually, however, it became the child's means for propelling his body forward. Once he was in motion he crawled in the usual fashion; but when an obstacle arrested his progress he briefly resumed rocking back and forth before moving in a new direction.

There would be little point in reporting the rate for each type of mannerism, or in extending the list of their possible functions. So far I have found no children in whom the rate of a familiar mannerism deviated significantly from the rates reported above. The findings converge on the tentative conclusion that every mannerism has its own rate, regardless of individual experience or diagnostic category. From isolated clinical instances it would, of course, be specious to argue for a discrete endogeneous oscillator specific to each stereotypy of a particular frequency which is immune to external influences. Children who rock habitually can be started off by music, and the musical rhythm may modify, even if it does not control their rates. Mechanical factors related to body structure, muscle tension, elasticity, fatigue and level of excitation, as well as external synochronizers and other environmental distractions thus influence the manifest rhythm of stereotypic mannerisms to a significant degree, and it would be misleading to assume that motor rhythms are the direct expression of endogenous central pacemakers. They may nevertheless represent "natural" frequencies instigated by central oscillator of a fixed frequency and modified by environmental and physiological factors. Barring opportunities for experimental stimulation during neurosurgical procedures, one must rely on the comparison of minor variations in frequency among many instances of the same stereotypy, to derive the natural frequency of particular forms.

Earlier I mentioned that the patterns and manifest rhythm of mannerisms did not differ significantly in normal and pathological children.

What did distinguish the mannerisms was their persistence in the pathological children, and the gradual transformation into more complex rhythms in the normal children. Normal infants eventually stopped repeating a particular mannerism after they had acquired the new locomotor pattern or posture for which the mannerism seemed to be a prelude. Pathological children either continued the repetitive motor rhythm at the expense of developing the corresponding motor skill, or else they continued to rock in the archaic pattern despite the acquisition of the new motor skill. Except in the case of the elaborate mannerisms invented by some autistic children (which may well be qualitatively novel forms), stereotypic repetitions were nothing more than perseverations of the usual sensory motor schemata, long after repetition for the sake of practice or "cumulative assimilation" had lost its adaptive function.[33]

The behavior of individuals in a state of neurological regression provided circumstantial evidence for the assumption that the rhythms associated with particular mannerisms were preserved as potential regulators of serial order after the motor patterns themselves had been integrated in more complex sequences. At the most primitive level this became apparent in the behavior of an adult patient with chronic encephalitis and a total loss of voluntary motor functions. When given a pacifier, she *chewed* it rhythmically at exactly the same rate and in the same pattern of alternating bursts and rest periods as the young infant sucks on the pacifier. For the sake of comparison, I asked normal adults to suck on the pacifier, but they were totally incapable of reproducing the typical infantile pattern. In the same vein, children between the ages of four and six years with severe obstructive hydrocephalus sucked in stable infantile patterns, while age mates with a mild form of the disease responded to the pacifier exactly like their normal peers, and either refused altogether to suck or produced erratic patterns.

At a more complex level, children with diagnoses varying from suspected third ventricle tumors, to demyelinizing diseases, to "nonspecific" chronic encephalitis, who had as one of their presenting symptoms the onset of stereotypic mannerisms, showed the same forms of motor repetition as normal, mongoloid and autistic children — rocking back and forth in sitting position, "rocking proper," head nodding, mouthing, leg kicking, and the like. Whenever mannerisms associated with the onset of the neurological disease resembled those observed in normal home reared or institutionalized mongoloid children, the rates of performance were the same. In most cases, the parents of children with acquired neurological lesions reported that their children had shown no mannerisms for several years before the onset of other neurological symptoms.

Thus, the clinical evidence on patients with acquired neurological lesions also favors the interpretation that a specific motor mannerism is associated with a particular rhythm, regardless of age or diagnosis.

Motor development may then be viewed as the transformation of simple rhythmical repetition or "circular reaction" into integrated actions,[33] whose rhythmical origins are no longer apparent exactly because the component motor parts have been integrated and the associated rhythms have been submerged in complex phase sequences. In keeping with Lashley's thesis, but unprejudiced by fact, I have assumed that the simple rhythms of neonatal behavior are not *replaced* by qualitatively different regulations of serial order, but that the endogenous rhythms are dissociated from their manifest reflex patterns, and enter into complex phase relations with other dissociated rhythms which can then control the sequence of internalized actions and thought patterns. Empirical support for these assertions is hard to come by from the study of humans alone. One would not expect the resultant complex rhythms in behavior to be obvious to direct observations, but with refined instrumentation designed to detect subtle phase interactions, and by developmental studies focusing on the transformation of simple rhythms, it should be possible to investigate the problem empirically.

CONCLUSIONS

The systematic observation of neonates has shown that some reflex activities of the young infant are organized in remarkably stable, high frequency rhythms. Circumstantial evidence was presented which admits, even if it does not prove, the proposition that the human central nervous system instigates motor rhythms analogous to the endogenous automatisms described by von Holst and Weiss for lower species, and that the influence of these rhythms is not limited to one motor end organ alone, but can influence anatomically unrelated motor activities as well. At a primitive level of integration, motor rhythms of different frequencies are known to interact so that one drives the other by a "magnet effect." Two rhythms may also interact to generate rhythms whose temporal properties differ entirely from those of either component rhythm, although no instances for such phase interactions in human behavior have yet been described. The interaction of *more* than two distinct rhythms should give rise to a complexity of sequences in behavior which could only be detected with the use of refined experimental techniques, but would nevertheless be rhythmical in its organization.

From the comparative study of normal and neurologically damaged individuals, it was concluded that a regression in neurological function is associated with the reemergence of simple motor rhythms and mannerisms. Stereotypic motor rhythms may thus be viewed as segments of the behavior repertory which have either not been integrated with other motor patterns, or else have "de-differentiated" in the course of neurological regression. Extrapolating from the disintegration of complex behavior patterns and the parallel reappearance of simple rhythms, it was proposed that the apparent suppression of rhythms in behavior is achieved by a phase interaction of two or more discrete rhythms as these motor patterns are coordinated. Finally it was speculated that after appropriate developmental transformation, about which nothing is known at present, the derivatives of simple high frequency rhythms may regulate the serial order of thought patterns and voluntary movements in the adult.

Preliminary results from the study of mannerisms in mongoloid children also suggested that rhythmical repetition may function not only as a consumatory behavior (in the sense of tension discharge) but also as the motor means by which the retarded child explores his surroundings. Especially among blind, and probably among autistic children, stereotypic mannerisms may dominate the child's motor repertory so completely that they interfere with lawful cognitive and social development.

These speculations about the developmental significance of high frequency rhythms may have some peripheral implication for the treatment of stereotypic mannerisms in disturbed and defective children. Techniques of negative reinforcements for the suppression of mannerisms have the advantage that they yield concrete results and rapid success; and wherever the intensity of mannerisms makes their persistence incompatible with physical health or life, such suppressive techniques must be considered an essential clinical tool. In less dramatic instances, however, it might be more fruitful to recognize the biological substrate of motor mannerisms, and to devise methods for converting stereotypic mannerisms from global ends into motor means. This seems to be what Dr. Bruno Bettelheim has accomplished in his treatment of autistic children at the Orthogenic School in Chicago; it is the method by which Dr. Lukas Kamp successfully treated an autistic twin; and it is the method by which Dr. Bibace and his students at the Worcester State Hospital have sought to establish social contact with their juvenile and young adult schizophrenic patients. In each instance it seems to the outsider that the therapist has entered into the apparently aimless self-sufficient stereotypy with the patient, and has then converted the mannerism into a behavior that can be entrained on external synchronizers (for example, music), or related to concrete events and persons in the environment. While I must assume responsibility for this interpretation of the therapeutic endeavors, it offers a developmentally consistent formulation about the significance of stereotypic mannerisms wherever they may occur, and it may provide guidelines for an organismic approach to their treatment when their preponderance interferes with normal developmental differentiation.

REFERENCES

1. SOLLBERGER, A.: *Biological Rhythm Research.* New York, Elsevier, 1965.
2. UEXKULL, JACOB VON: *Umwelt und Innenwelt der Tiere.* Berlin, Springer, 1909.
3. PIAGET, JEAN: Les Trois Structures Fondamentales de la vie Psychique: Rhythme, Regulation et Groupement. *Revue Suisse de Psychologie* 1:9-21, 1942.
4. FRAISSE, PAUL: *Les Structures Rhythmiques.* Louvain, Nauwelaerts, 1956.
5. LASHLEY, K. S.: The Problem of Serial Order in Behavior. In *The Neuropsychology of Lashley,* F. A. Beach and others, eds. New York, McGraw-Hill, 1960, pp. 506-528.
6. PITTENDRIGH, C. S. and BRUCE, V. G.: An Oscillator Model for Biological Clocks. In *Rhythmic and Synthetic Processes in Growth,* Dorothea Rudnick, ed. Princeton, Princeton University, 1957.
7. CLOUDSLEY-THOMPSON, J. L.: *Rhythmic Activity in Animal Physiology and Behavior.* New York, Academic Press, 1961.
8. BUNNING, ERWIN: *The Physiological Clock.* New York, Academic Press, 1964.
9. RICHTER, C.P.: *Biological Clocks in Medicine and Psychiatry.* Springfield, Ill., Charles C Thomas, 1965.
10. ANLIKER, JAMES: Simultaneous Changes in Visual Separation Threshold and Voltage of Cortical Alpha Rhythm. *Science* 153:316-318, 1966.
11. HOLST, E. VON: Versuche zur Theorie der Relativen Koordination. *Pfluger's Archiv.* 237:93-121, 1936.
12. ————: Bausteine zu einer Vergleichenden Physiologie der Lokomotorischen Reflexe bei Fischen: II. Mitteilungen. *Z. Vergl. Physiol.* 24:532-565, 1937.
13. WEISS, P. A.: Autonomous versus Reflexogenous Activity of the Central Nervous System. *Proc. Amer. Phil. Soc.* 84:53-64, 1941.
14. ————: Further Experiments with Deplanted and Deranged Nerve Centers in Amphibians. *Proc. Soc. Exp. Biol. Med.* 46:14-15, 1941.
15. ————: Specificity in the Neurosciences. *Neurosciences Research Program Bulletin,* Vol. 3, No. 5, 1965.
16. POTTER, R. K. and others: *Visible Speech.* New York, Van Nostrand, 1947.
17. TRUBY, H. M. and LIND, J.: Cry Sounds of the Newborn Infant. *Acta Paediatrica Scandinavica,* Suppl. 163, 1965, pp. 7-59.
18. WOLFF, P. H.: The Natural History of Crying and Other Vocalizations in Early Infancy. In *Determinants of Infant Behavior,* B. M. Foss, ed. London, Methuen, In Press.
19. ————: The Causes, Controls and Organization of Behavior in the Neonate. Psychological Issues, Vol. 5, No. 1, Monograph No. 17, 1966.
20. ————: La Theorie Sensori-Montorie de L'intelligence et la Psychologie du Development General. In *Psychologie et Epistemologie Genetiques: Themes Piagentiens.* Paris, Dunod, 1966, pp. 235-250.
21. ————: The Serial Organization of Sucking in the Young Infant. In Preparation.
22. LENNEBERG, E. H.: *Biological Foundations of Language.* New York, Wiley, 1967.

23. LIEBERMAN, PHILIP: *Intonation, Perception and Language.* Cambridge, M.I.T., 1967.
24. PRECHTL, H. F. R. and others: Polygraphic Studies of the Full-term Newborn Infant: I. Technical Aspects and Qualitative Analysis. *Developmental Med. and Child Neurol.* In Press.
25. PRECHTL, H. F. R.: Angeborene Bewegungsweisen Junger Katzen. *Experientia,* Vol. 8, 1952.
26. PEIPER, ALBRECHT: *Cerebral Function in Infancy and Childhood.* New York, Consultants Bureau, 1964.
27. BAKWIN, HARRY: Emotional Deprivation in Infants. *J. Pediat.* 35:512-521, 1949.
28. BOWLBY, JOHN: *Maternal Care and Mental Health,* Monograph #2. Geneva, World Health Organization, 1951.
29. PROVENCE, SALLY ANN and LIPTON, R. C.: *Infants in Institutions.* New York, International Universities, 1962.
30. SPITZ, R. A.: *The First Year of Life.* New York, International Universities, 1965.
31. WERNER, HEINZ: The Concept of Development from a Comparative and Organismic Point of View. In *The Concept of Development,* D. B. Harris, ed. Minneapolis, University of Minnesota, 1957, pp. 125-147.
32. SPITZ, R. A. and WOLF, K. M.: Auto-erotism: Some Empirical Findings and Hypothesis on Three of Its Manifestations in the First Year of Life. *Psychoanal. Study of the Child* 3&4:85-120, 1949.
33. PIAGET, JEAN: *The Origins of Intelligence of Children.* New York, International Universities, 1952.

2

PATTERN PREFERENCES AND PERCEPTUAL-COGNITIVE DEVELOPMENT IN EARLY INFANCY

Robert L. Fantz

and

Sonia Nevis

Western Reserve University

From birth the infant is receptive and responsive to environmental stimulation. This is a fact for which evidence has been accumulating at an accelerating rate during the past decade. But the implications of this fact for theories and practices of infant development are largely unknown. Presumably the young infant has the opportunity for experiencing and learning about objects and places in his surroundings. But to what extent can he use this opportunity to prepare for later adaptive responses to those objects and places? And how can we make use of our knowledge in this area to facilitate the psychological development of the infant, as well as to assess the progress of that development? Questions such as these need to be answered before the significance of the recent findings can be evaluated.

Reprinted from Merrill-Palmer Quarterly of Behavior and Development, Volume 13, No. 1, 1967, pp. 77-108. Copyright by The Merrill-Palmer Institute.

Presented at The Merrill-Palmer Institute Conference on Research and Teaching of Infant Development, February 10-12, 1966, directed by Irving E. Sigel, chairman of research. The research reported in this paper was supported by Grant HD 00314 from the National Institute of Child Health and Human Development, USPHS. The authors wish to acknowledge the assistance of Mrs. Mary Parker in the gathering and analysis of the data.

Recent data on the infant, obtained by a variety of methods, concern auditory and other modalities as well as vision. But this paper will be restricted to information on visual perception obtained by the visual preference method, with emphasis on some findings of an intensive longitudinal study, just completed and presented here for the first time.

It has long been known that the newborn infant can respond to light stimulation and probably to color. But it is patterned visual stimulation for which the vertebrate eye evolved, and from which derives almost all of the useful information taken in through the eye. Spatial orientation, object recognition, and social responsiveness in the child and adult are based largely on the perception of subtle variations in form and texture. Without pattern vision a person is blind for most practical purposes, even though light and color are received. Pattern vision is therefore of critical importance in studying perceptual development in the infant.

The traditional theory was that pattern vision and form perception were acquired through an associational process, acting upon the "primary sensory elements" of brightness and color. But it is now proven that even in the early weeks the young infant can resolve and discriminate patterns and other configurational aspects; also, that the young infant spends most of his time looking at these behaviorally important parts of the environment. The selectivity for patterns is just as important as the discrimination of patterns. The infant or adult who concentrated his attention on uniformly colored surfaces or spaces could make little use of his pattern-vision capacities. The behavioral evidence illustrated below is well supported by neurological evidence showing that the vertebrate visual system from retina to cortex is, predominantly and inherently, receptive and responsive to patterned input, rather than to unpatterned light (e.g., Hubel and Wiesel, 1963; Sackett, 1963).

VISUAL PREFERENCE METHOD

The visual preference method was chosen—following preliminary work with infant chimpanzees (Fantz, 1956, 1958a)—because it appeared to be the only procedure adaptable to the helpless young infant that could yield information on pattern discrimination (as distinct from a reflex following of a moving pattern). This early evaluation has turned out to be wrong in two respects. First, other feasible testing procedures, based on conditioning of head-turning (Bower, 1965) or on various measures of arousal have been, or show promise of being, worked out (Haith, 1966; Kagan and Lewis, 1965; Stechler, Bradford, and Levy, 1966; Wolff, 1963). Second, the findings have brought to light a special value of the visual preference method: it shows perceptual selectivities as well as perceptual capacities. And it is the selectivity of the early visual responses—it will be argued below—which is particularly revealing of early perceptual-cognitive development.

In brief, the procedure is to observe and record the infant's direction of gaze under controlled conditions so as to give a reliable indication of the relative attention value of various stimulus attributes. The technical requirements for doing this are fairly simple: a form-fitting crib or other means of holding the baby comfortably in a certain orientation; a test chamber covering the infant's field of view and giving a uniform and contrasting background for one or two stimulus targets; a mechanism for exposing the targets close to the infant for repeated short periods and for quickly changing the targets between exposures; a means for unobserved observation of the eyes of the infant; an objective criterion of target fixation; and equipment for quick and accurate recording of fixation times. Most of the studies have used a supine posture of the subject with targets exposed directly overhead. The test chambers have varied from a small structure of cardboard and orange crates for use on the kitchen table of the infant's home (Fantz, 1958b) to a felt-lined, stainless steel model used in the newborn nursery of a hospital (Fantz, 1963). Targets can be exposed and then hidden by movable shields or window shades, by projection on a screen, or by other devices. There are certain advantages to both the simultaneous presentation of pairs of targets with varied right and left positions, and the successive exposure of a number of targets, repeatedly, in the same location. The paired comparison procedure has recently appeared to be most effective in eliciting differential responsiveness. A small peephole in the chamber ceiling has proved a simple way of observing, with a minimum of distraction to the infant, the fixation of a particular target—as indicated by centering of the corneal reflection of that target over the pupillary opening. This or a similar criterion is essential even for reading photographic recordings of the responses, as was done in the preliminary studies (Fantz, 1956, 1958a). But we have since obtained accurate records more simply by direct observation, sensitive finger switches, and either electric timers or event recorders (Fantz, Ordy, and Udelf, 1962).

Most of the testing problems we have encountered are attributable to lack of cooperation of the subjects rather than to technical difficulties. Various changes in the apparatus and procedure have been directed toward reducing position preferences, keeping the infant's attention on the targets, and, especially, keeping the infant awake yet quiet throughout a testing session. One of the best ways of facilitating the testing has been simply to give the subjects the kind of a "show" they like—complex patterns and objects, changed at frequent intervals, rather than plain or colored surfaces or the same target for a long period. Even a 10-second period of "looking at nothing" between exposures can bring on a fussy or drowsy state, while it is not unusual to find that a baby initially in a seemingly untestable state becomes alert and cooperative as soon as the show starts.

The salient findings from a decade of research using the visual preference method will be illustrated by two experiments. One brings out the selectivity for patterns; the other, the ability to distinguish fine patterns.

Six circular discs were repeatedly presented, one at a time and in varied sequence, for the duration of the first fixation in each case (Fantz, 1963). The results were similar for newborn infants and for infants 2-6 months old. Three black-and-white patterns (schematic face, bull's eye, and newsprint) were highly preferred over three plain discs. None of the subjects looked longest at either red, fluorescent yellow, or white.

This strong visual attraction of the patterned over a plain surface gave the basis for testing the limits of pattern vision in young infants. By reducing the size of details in the pattern until this differential response was no longer shown, it was possible to estimate the acuity of the infant. Vertical black-and-white stripes were used, paired with gray of equal reflectance. It was found as expected that the infant, as he grows older and as his visual system matures, is able to see finer patterns (Fantz, Ordy, and Udelf, 1962). But even the newborn infant can discriminate ⅛-inch stripes from plain gray (Fantz, 1966) and probably could see still finer patterns under optimal conditions of illumination, distance, etc., if these were known. Since pattern vision requires the functioning of the visual cortex, this functioning then can be assumed to be present at birth.

The two complementary facts of pattern-vision capacity and pattern selectivity in the young infant have provided the foundation for numerous visual preference studies, involving thousands of tests and hundreds of subjects and targets. In retrospect, most of these studies seem to have been concerned with one or both of two aims: to determine the stimulus dimensions underlying the visual preferences at various ages, and to determine the effects of experience and learning of the preferences. While it is difficult to completely separate the two experimentally, this can be approximated by using abstract patterns or unfamiliar objects for the first aim (keeping in mind that non-specific effects of experience still are likely to be involved in all but newborn infants), and by using familiar patterns or objects for the second aim (keeping in mind that these also have intrinsic stimulus properties to influence their attention value). The distinction emphasizes two different classes of variables determining the development of visual preferences; it is not meant to imply that the preferences are "innate" in one case and "learned" in the other.

DETERMINING IMPORTANT DIMENSIONS OF PATTERN

What stimulus attribute of a pattern causes it to be looked at longer than a plain surface? A simple and appealing answer is *complexity,* which can be defined quantitatively in various ways—length of contour, number of elements or redundancy—and which can be varied systematically. But ease of measurement of a dimension does not assure its relevance to perception and behavior. After all, the young infant is not as adept at counting or measuring as we are. In view of the earlier, erroneous assumption of the importance of the dimensions of brightness and color, it is advisable to verify empirically the importance of complexity.

Starting with the simplest comparison, most any pattern seems to be preferred to a plain unpatterned surface by infants from birth to six months of age. In our studies the fixation time for various patterns has ranged from two to six times longer than for homogeneous surfaces, colored or not. Other investigators have obtained similar results (Spears, 1964; Stechler, 1964; Stirnimann, 1944).

The only exception we have found to this generalization is the absence of a consistent preference for a red checkerboard pattern over a red square by infants during the early weeks of age, observed during the longitudinal study discussed later in this paper. But this was probably due in part to the larger *area* of bright color in the square, the two targets being of equal overall size, since the same study showed marked size and brightness preferences during this early period. In a prior study (Fantz, 1958b), the checkerboard was paired on half of the exposures with a smaller square (equal in area of color to the checkerboard). On these exposures the checkerboard tended to be preferred even at less than one month of age. And in yet another study (Fantz, 1965a, fig. 6), a black-and-white checkerboard elicited considerably longer attention from newborn infants than did a gray square of equal reflectance.

Another plausible explanation is that the particular checkerboard used was too complex to be of high attention value to very young infants, as suggested by the results of Hershenson (1964) and those of Brennan, Ames, and Moore (1966). This brings us beyond the pattern vs. plain to the comparison among patterns of different complexity. Here the findings have been diverse. Infants have often shown a preference

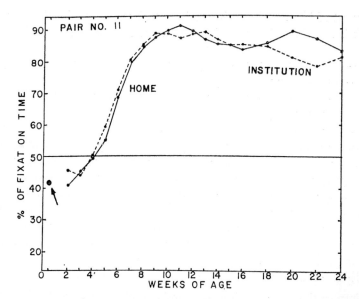

Fig. 1. Age-preference curves showing the relative amount of attention given to a bull's eye pattern when paired with horizontal stripes (see Pair 11 in Fig. 4), as part of the longitudinal study described in the text. Initial point (indicated by arrow) is for 20 unselected newborn infants.

for the most complex of several patterns (Berlyne, 1958; Fantz, 1966, table 2; Graefe, 1963; Lewis, Meyers, Kagan, and Grossberg, 1963; Spears, 1964; Stechler, 1964). But in other cases, they have preferred an intermediate degree of complexity (Hershenson, Munsinger, and Kessen, 1965; Thomas, 1965) or even the least complex (Hershenson, 1964). In still other cases, they have failed to show any consistent differential response to patterns or outline form of differing complexity (Berlyne, 1958; Fantz, 1958b; Graefe, 1963; Saayman, Ames, and Moffett, 1964).

One explanation for these divergent results lies in variations in the age of the subjects as well as in the type and range of complexities of stimulus targets. It might be hypothesized that if a sufficiently broad spectrum of complexities is tested, an optimal level will be discovered, with decreasing response on either side; also, that this optimal level will increase with age or experience. In support of this idea, Brennan, Ames, and Moore (1966) found that the preferred checkerboard pattern contained 4 squares for 3-week infants; 64 squares for 8-week infants; and 576 squares for 14-week infants.

It is clear beyond doubt that the complexity of a pattern is one determinant of its attention value to infants. But many other findings show that it is not the only determinant and perhaps not the most important one.

Spears (1964) found that none of three measures—length of contour, number of "turns," and the degree of symmetry or redundancy—could adequately account for the preferential ordering of stimulus patterns by 4-month-old infants. And yet preferences among the patterns were present and were dominant over color preferences. It is interesting to note that his most preferred target, a "bull's eye," has brought out the most consistent preferences and most marked age changes found in all of our studies, from the earliest (Fantz, 1958b) to the most recent (Nevis and Fantz, in prep.). In both of these studies there was a shift from preference for a horizontal striped pattern to a very consistent bull's eye preference by 2 months of age. In recent results (Fig. 1), infants during the third month of age looked *eight times as long* at the bull's eye as at the stripes, on the average. The early preference for stripes was not as marked as in earlier studies, perhaps because the new bull's eye pattern was simpler than the previous one and therefore more attractive to very young infants. Two experiments attempted to pin down the stimulus basis of these results by the use of various linear, circular, and other pattern arrangements.

In one study (Fantz, in press), 12 line segments of equal area were arranged into four different patterns that were exposed in all permutations to infants of varying ages. The average fixation times (Fig. 2) showed a slight preference for the linear arrangement (similar to horizontal stripes) by infants between 1 and 4 weeks of age, while at later ages the circular arrangement (similar to a bull's eye) became highly preferred over the other three patterns. A subsequent replication of the study with infants under 5 days of age showed no differentiation among the four patterns, thus bringing into question the initial linear preference suggested in Fig. 2. But it is supported by results from the recent longitudinal study of the same linear vs. circular patterns (see below, Fig. 6) showing the development of a reliable linear preference during the early weeks, before the development of a strong circular preference.

Non-form differences were still better controlled in the other experiment, using four arrangements of twenty-five $3/4$-inch white squares on the blue felt-covered stimulus plaques (matching the chamber lining). Three of the patterns were derived from a 5-by-5 matrix by rotating the squares into upright, diagonal, or random orientations; the fourth (circular) arrangement approximated the lattice in area covered (Fig.3).

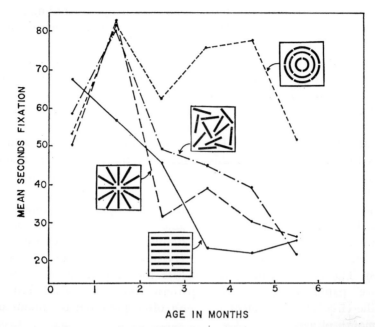

Fig. 2. Relative visual attention to four patterns at varying ages. Number of subjects at successive month intervals were 14, 11, 5, 8, 7, and 4 infants. Data are mean seconds of fixation time during 6 minutes of testing, including six 30-second exposures of each pattern. (From Fantz, in press.)

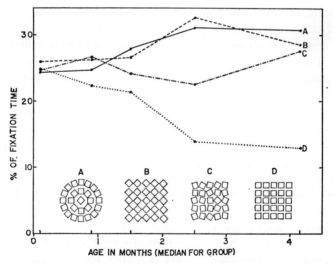

Fig. 3. Relative visual attention to four arrangements of white squares, averaged for infants in five age groups.

The patterns were again presented in all 12 pairings (including reversed right and left positions) for 20-second exposures, the sequence varying among the subjects. Testing chamber and general procedures were the same as in the recent longitudinal study (see below). The available subjects were divided for analysis into five groups, covering different ranges of age. The first included 19 infants from 1 day old to 10 days old (median 3 days), obtained at a hospital newborn ward. The remaining infants were all from a foundling home; they were sometimes given two tests at different age levels. The second group included 11 infants, 3 weeks to 1 month old; the third group, 13 infants between 1 and 2 months; the fourth, 11 infants between 2 and 3 months; and the last, 12 infants between 3 and 6 months.

The results (Fig. 3) indicated equal fixation by newborn infants, followed by increasing differentiation among the four patterns up to 3 months of age. The differences were significant at the .05 level or better for each of the three older groups (Friedman analysis of variance by ranks). The most consistent change was the drop in attention to the "lattice" pattern. The other three patterns showed a variable ordering, but the circular arrangement was most often preferred by infants over one month of age.

It is interesting that circular patterns were preferred in these experiments and that, to the adult at least, these patterns resemble the bull's eye preferred in other studies. But the main point is that, in these two experiments, infants by at least the second month of age have shown differential visual attention to patterns equated in length of contour, in number and size of elements, in overall area, and in light reflectance and contrast. They were not responding to "complexity" as defined by any of these variables. Of course, other dimensions might be found to vary among the patterns and might be designated as measures of complexity. But if all the variables which have been or might be proposed as measures of complexity were controlled, all form and pattern differences might thereby be eliminated, leaving us with a set of identical patterns. Whether the pattern preferences of infants are reduced to "response to stimulus complexity" or are considered to be an early type of "form perception" is a question of definition and experimenters' preference, not of fact. The terms "form perception" and "pattern discrimination and selection" appear to us to have definite advantages. First, such descriptions do not imply a single stimulus dimension of importance or a single underlying process, but leave this open for investigation. Second, they do not imply a minimal "reflex" level of visual or neural function before we know what the capabilities of the young infant are. In this connection, it would seem that complexity has begun to replace color and brightness as the "primary visual attribute" out of which all visual perception is built; thus providing a final line of defense against the admission of perceptual experience during the early months of life, now that the early importance of pattern can no longer be denied. Finally, "form perception" *does* imply a developmental continuity between the earliest and most primitive functioning of pattern vision and the most intricate and subtle visual performance of the adult, rather than postulating an emergent function at some point in infancy. And it *does* encourage the search for possible effects of early visual experiences on this developmental process.

DETERMINING EFFECTS OF EXPERIENCE

To qualify as a "stimulus variable," any dimension of patterns must ultimately be shown to be related to behavioral variables. This is easily forgotten when the dimension is derived from physics, geometry, information theory, or neurology. (It is ironical that the dependence upon *a priori,* nonbehaviorally based dimensions is especially prevalent among those most insistent upon being called behaviorists; e.g., see Fantz, in press; Hayek, 1952.) But some stimulus variables are derived from and perhaps definable only in reference to behavior and the behavioral environment, social stimulation providing perhaps the best example. This type of variable was the starting place for pursuing the second primary aim—that of determining the effects of experience and learning upon visual preferences and perceptual development.

The ability to distinguish the solidity or depth of objects is of consequence for behavior, at least by the time the infant is able to actively approach and manipulate such objects. Throughout the preceding months the infant has the opportunity to visually explore and learn about solid objects—especially since solid objects tend to stand out from background stimulation and attract more than their share of attention due to such factors as movement, parallax, figure-ground contrast, and spatial proximity. An effect of this perceptual experience might be evident from increased visual discrimination and selection of solid objects.

Several early studies showed the appearance of a consistent preference for a solid over a comparable flat object at around 2 months of age (Fantz, 1966). This was verified in the recent longitudinal study (described in the next section) by the development during the third month of a preference for a textured sphere over a textured disc, for a solid head model over an outline form, both painted white, and for a pat-

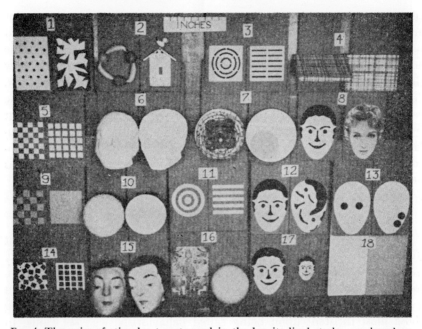

FIG. 4. The pairs of stimulus targets used in the longitudinal study, numbered according to order of presentation during each weekly test. In each pair, the target on the left is the one for which percentages were calculated in graphs of the results (except for familiarization tests). All of the targets were attached to blue felt plaques which matched the chamber lining. With the exception of eight of the pairs, the targets were made from cardboard or non-glossy photographic prints glued to the felt and were either, white, black-and-white, or a shade of gray. The eighth other pairs were as follows: Pair 2, brightly colored plastic fruit vs. red, blue, and white nursery light-switch plaque; Pair 4, boards covered with colored patterned plastic, one board slanting out and the other vertical; Pair 6, solid model of a head and flat outline of the same head; Pair 7, wire-mesh attached to wood with holes, partly painted white, vs. fluorescent red-and-yellow disc, rotating at 4 r.p.m.; Pair 9, fluorescent red checks and square; Pair 10, sphere and disc, each covered with pebble-textured white paint; Pair 15, solid head model with achromatic painted features vs. photograph of the same; Pair 16, an Egyptian art reproduction vs. translucent globe with a 40-watt orange light, flashing 48 times a minute.

terned board slanting down and towards the infant over a vertical patterned board. (The stimulus objects can be seen in Fig. 4). An earlier preference, starting at birth but disappearing during the second month, was present in the case of the slanting board. This was likely due to that object extending closer to the infant than the vertical board, and therefore being in better focus before the development of accommodation for distance (Haynes, White, and Held, 1965). The subsequent reappearance of the solidity preference cannot, however, be attributed to development of accommodation. Nor can it be attributed to development of binocular coordination, since similar results were obtained from infants who viewed the targets with one eye only (Fantz, 1966). Since dark-reared monkey infants failed to show a similar preference for solid objects until after several weeks of unrestricted visual experience (Fantz, 1965b), it is probable that effects of visual experience are involved for human infants as well.

It would be expected that the effects of early experience of visual preferences might be most evident relative to face-like stimuli, the human face being one of the most prominent and important objects in the world of the young infant. Actually, such has not been the case so far: the findings have been more variable and less conclusive than those for object solidity. This is especially true relative to the discrimination between more and less realistic face-like configurations without variations in either pattern complexity or solidity. These findings will be discussed later. Relative to the general attention value of face-like targets, on the other hand, targets with certain configurational aspects of a face have repeatedly been among the best elicitors of attention. But the fact that this has been true for newborn as well as for older infants makes one wonder what it means.

A test of this phenomenon was made by pairing a solid model of a female head (with achromatic painted figures) with each of five unfamiliar comparison targets. These five were selected from those available from previous experiments (primarily the recent longitudinal study) for their high attention value and for their similarity to the head model in complexity, size, and solidity. In addition, three were brightly-colored and one included a flickering light source. And yet the head model was preferred to each of the comparison objects by at least two-thirds of the subjects under 2 months of age (Fantz, in press). For infants between 2 and 5 months old, the head model preference was reduced for three of the pairings and reversed for a fourth, although it was still consistently preferred overall. The effect of social experiences was not evident in these results.

In the same experiment another familiar and reinforcing object—a nursing bottle containing milk—was also paired with each of five unfamiliar comparison targets. In this case smaller, simpler objects were chosen which had been of least attention value in previous tests (excluding unpatterned surfaces), in the attempt to give the basically unattractive nursing bottle a better chance. The attempt did not succeed, for each of the five comparison objects was significantly preferred over the nursing bottle by the infants of each age group. There was no indication of more interest in the bottle by infants with several additional months of reinforcing experiences. Nor was the bottle of more attention value within one hour of a scheduled feeding than it was within one hour after a feeding.

It would be very rash to conclude that the infant under 5 months of age cannot recognize or respond differentially to people or to the familiar source of nourishment, or that the early months of almost continual visual exploration of the environment during the waking hours have had no lasting effect. The results are more likely explained by certain limitations of the experimental conditions. Because of the use of artificial stimuli (in the case of the social stimulus) and an artificial, unfamiliar situation, the responses may not have been representative of those that would occur to the familiar object under familiar circumstances. Limitation to the use of a single response indicator may likewise have been a factor—one which comes under the category of exploratory behavior rather than appetitive behavior, and which is probably determined more by novelty and intrinsic stimulus properties than by familiarity and conditioning. At least in retrospect this seems the obvious answer.

Partial support for this explanation comes from one additional approach to finding the effects of early perceptual experiences. This is the direct approach of experimentally varying specific visual experiences. A certain complex visual stimulus (a magazine advertisement or photograph) was exposed to the infant repeatedly, and was paired with another "novel" stimulus that was changed nine times during the session (Fantz, 1964). Infants over 2 months of age showed a consistent decrease in fixation of the repeated stimulus as it became more "familiar." The novel stimulus brought out a corresponding increase in fixation so that the total response time remained about the same (Fantz, 1966, fig. 6). This short-term effect of experience is in the opposite direction to the long-term increase in attention which was expected in the other approaches given above, and which was apparently found in the case of object solidity. Further analysis of the data from the head model experiment (Fantz, in press) indicated a similar short-term satiation of visual interest from repeated exposures of the head model for the infants over 2 months. The younger infants, however, showed a short-term *increase* in response to the head model. This suggested that these opposite short-term effects were responsible for the apparent long-term decrease (that is, from the younger to the older group) in overall attention to the head model, thus obscuring any actual long-term experience effect. Clearly a confusing state of affairs!

But again, in retrospect, why should we expect that "the effects of experience" which include such a vast variety of phenomena in the child and adult, could be—even for the young infant with more restricted opportunities and abilities—encompassed by a single equation or paradigm of learning? Conversely, the discovery of such complexities and unknowns in the perceptual, motivational, and learning processes of young infants should remind us of the humorous side of our presumptuous, though necessary, attempts as experimental psychologists to reduce to a few scientifically elegant statements the behavior of adults, who presumably have not become less complex with age and experience.

But to return to the business of trying to give some order to the chaos that often appears in the response recordings, in spite of the best laid plans of the experimenter, it is a pleasure to report some data that have surpassed in orderliness our most optimistic expectations.

DETERMINING SIGNIFICANCE OF PREFERENCE CHANGES

This experiment represented a departure from the previous aims of pinning down the relevant stimulus variables for, and the effects of experience on, visual preferences. Here the primary aim was to determine whether the various changes in visual preferences that had appeared previously were indicative of basic perceptual-cognitive development. If this could be demonstrated, then the age-of-occurrence of these changes might be useful for the purposes for which the various developmental scales or "baby tests" had been devised but have failed to serve satisfactorily (Bayley, 1955). The failure of such tests to predict later behavior or intelligence might be due to the absence during the early months or years of individual differences correlated with later differences. But the failure might also be due to the fact that those tests primarily measured motor development, sensory-motor coordination, and other overt performances, rather than more strictly perceptual-cognitive functions such as discrimination and selectivity. If so, this gap might be filled in part by measures of the early development of pattern discrimination and selection.

The success of the present project in obtaining some clear-cut results may be attributed to the selection of subjects, stimulus targets, and testing procedures. In order to avoid waiting five years or so to see if infant visual preferences were predictive of later performance, the traditional representative-sample paradigm of longitudinal studies was reversed. Two samples were selected which could be expected to represent the upper and lower reaches of the intellectual continuum, to the degree that this might be possible on the basis of parentage and environ-

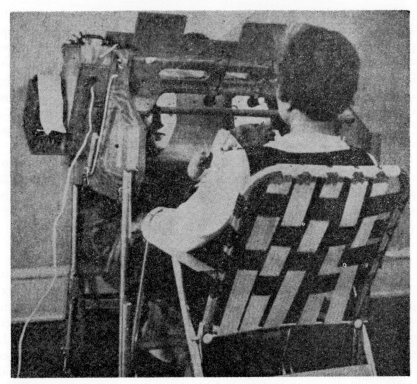

Fig. 5. Visual-preference testing apparatus in operation. Assistant (back toward camera) supports the infant on her lap in a canvas baby-seat with foam head-holder. Observer, barely visible behind the apparatus, looks through the peephole between the two targets and records fixations by pressing switch levers (upper left) to cause marks on the moving tape. The plaques to which the targets are attached extend up past the top of the stage.

mental beginnings. During the course of the study ten infants of the university faculty, reared in private homes, were compared with ten foundlings, reared in an institution. All of the institution-reared infants were presumably of caucasian parents and all were healthy; the Apgar scores available for eight of them were all in the normal range (either 9 or 10).

The stimulus pairs were selected partly on the basis of early data indicating a change in preference during the first 6 months, partly on the basis of results of a pilot study of a wide variety of stimulus variations, and partly on "experimental intuition." The final 18 pairs (Fig. 4) all had some promise of bringing out developmental changes in selective attention, and thereby revealing individual or group differences in rate of development.

Such a large battery of visual-preference tests required more effective techniques for obtaining the undivided attention of the subjects than had been used in the past. Such techniques were perfected in the pilot study, after being initially tried out on any available captive subject (this being, on most occasions, the senior author's infant daughter). The improved testing procedure (Fig. 5) was designed to keep the subject both comfortable and alert. The infant was held in a semi-reclining orientation in an adjustable canvas "baby seat" on the lap of an assistant seated in a rocking chair. Exposures were limited to 20 seconds and the contiguous presentations of the same pair of targets limited to two (with reversed positions of the pair). The infant was allowed to look at an interesting pattern during the between-exposure periods, which were made as brief as possible by an event recorder (to eliminate the manual recording of responses from timers), by a simple movable stage for exposing targets and by an electric-plug arrangement for quickly attaching and removing stimulus targets. Any stratagems were allowed (rocking, talking, moving the arms, etc.) between exposures for arousing or quieting the infant as needed. Finally, and probably most essentially, the assistant was allowed to administer *ad libitum* a pacifier.

Such manipulations of the subject's state did not constitute lack of experimental control. To the contrary, they tended to maintain, as much as was possible, a constant state of alertness for the successive stimulus pairs and for different subjects and ages. Moreover, the response measured was the direction of gaze, not the degree of arousal or other intensive aspects of attention. If there was any bias in the control of alertness between groups, it favored the institutionalized infants, who were more readily available for starting or for finishing the testing later in the day or on another day at a more auspicious time.

A final essential ingredient in the experiment was the fortitude and perseverance shown by the investigator, Mrs. Nevis, and her assistant, Mrs. Parker. It often fell to their lot, after carrying a station wagon full of equipment through sleet and snow or up several flights of stairs to the residence of each subject for the weekly test, to politely concur when the subject decided the test had been scheduled at the wrong time or on the wrong day, pacifier or no, and however interesting the show!

The results are presented in detail elsewhere (Nevis and Fantz, in prep.). As an indication of the overall consistency of the results, a significant visual preference (.05 level, two-tailed sign test) was shown among the 20 infants on more than half of the 19 testing sessions (given weekly from 2 to 16 weeks and then biweekly through 24 weeks) for ten of the stimulus pairs. In one case (Pair 11), the bull's eye pattern was looked at

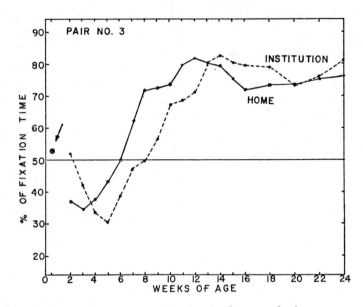

Fig. 6. Age-preference curves for the circular over the linear arrangement of line segments, for two samples of 10 infants on successive weeks of age. Initial point (indicated by arrow) is for 20 unselected newborn infants.

longer than the stripes by each of the 20 infants on seven of the testing weeks. Only two of the stimulus pairs (16 and 18)—showing a significant differential on only two or three testing weeks—failed to meet the criterion for significance of a series of related results. Definite age changes in the direction of the preference—either from one to the other target, or from no preference to a consistent preference (or the reverse)—were shown by both groups for all but Pairs 13 and 18. A preference change of 40% or more was shown for Pairs 3, 6, 7, 8 and 11. This does not imply necessarily that such strong differential visual responses and such marked age changes are frequent among everyday objects of the infant's environment (an interesting question requiring a different manner of choosing targets), but only that we succeeded in choosing stimulus pairs revealing of early developmental changes.

The questions of most interest here are the differences in development for the two highly selected samples of infants, and the type of stimulus variables showing the most change and the most difference between samples.

GROUP DIFFERENCES IN PREFERENCE DEVELOPMENT

Starting with the fixation time for 40-second exposure of each pair (with reversed positions after 20 seconds), the percentage for a particular target of the pair (the one pictured on the left in Fig. 4) was obtained for each testing week. Successive percentage scores for a single infant were sometimes quite variable. To reduce the random part of the variation and accentuate any developmental changes, the individual response curves were smoothed by making a running average (one-half of a given point combined with one-quarter of the preceding and following points), rather than by averaging several weeks and thereby losing the advantage of the weekly tests. The resulting curves were averaged for each sample. To fill in the age gap prior to the first test at 2 weeks, 20 unselected infants from a hospital newborn ward, less than one week of age, were tested with 12 of the stimulus pairs. The average scores for these infants are indicated on the same graphs.

The most consistent difference between samples was for Pair 3—linear vs. circular line arrangements—as shown in Fig. 6. The two curves are almost identical, except that the home curve is shifted about 2 weeks to the left, as if a basic developmental process was involved but was speeded up slightly for the home sample.

To determine the statistical significance of such a difference, the preference scores for the two groups were compared at each week of age by a one-tailed Mann-Whitney U test (.05 level) of ranked percentages. The hypothesis was for higher percentages to be shown by the home sample for each of the pairs—except for Pairs 8, 17, and 18, where the change was downward and lower percentages were thus expected. For Pair 3 the hypothesized difference was shown at 7, 8, 9, and 11 weeks of age.

To determine the developmental significance of the between-sample difference, visual-preference results were related to results from a traditional type of infant performance test, in which was determined the age of first occurrence of postural, locomotor, sensory-motor, vocal, social, or other responses. For this purpose, we used the Griffiths Mental Development Scale (Griffiths, 1954) but omitted those items which seemed to be ambiguous in preliminary trials with infants of varying ages, or which may have been biased against institution-reared infants—e.g., those based on the mother's report, those involving reactions to the mother, or those requiring experiences or training more likely present in a private home. This performance scale was given weekly, usually following the preference testing. The average scores for the two samples (Fig. 7)

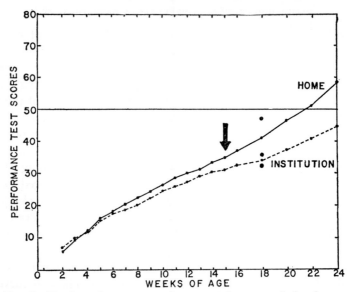

Fig. 7. Number of items passed on an infant mental development scale (performance test) at successive weeks of age. The heavy arrow indicates the first significant difference between the two samples. The separate points at 18 weeks of age are the average scores for the top-5-home, middle-10, and bottom-5-institution subsamples.

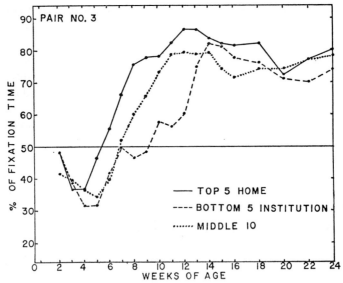

Fig. 8. Age preference curves for the circular over the linear line-arrangements, for subsamples based on performance test scores (compare with Fig. 6).

showed increasing differentiation during the 6 months, but the difference was not significant until 15 weeks of age and thereafter. This in itself provided substantiation for the expected difference between the two samples in rate of behavior development, even though it was not until the fourth month of age. To gain further information, the 20 infants were redivided into three subsamples based on performance scores at 18 weeks, the last test for which all the institution infants were still available. These three subsamples consisted of the top 5 of the home sample (which were above any of the institution sample), the bottom 5 of the institution sample (which overlapped the home sample), and the remaining 10 (which clustered closely together).

The visual-preference results for the three subsamples were then compared. The rationale was this: if the visual-preference changes were related to and predictive of the later rate of psychological development (as measured by the performance test), then the top-home and bottom-institution subsamples might show a wider separation in preference curves than the original home and institution samples. This was the case for Pair 3 (Fig. 8), showing about a 5-week difference between the "top 5" and the "bottom 5" curves in the age of development of a strong preference for the circular pattern.

The hypothesized group difference was supported by the overall results for the 17 pairs (this excluded Pair 2; see below, page 48). Considering all tests during the first three months of life—the period of development of most of the preferences—21 significant differences favored the home sample, while 4 favored the institution sample. Pairs 1, 3, 4, 5, 7, 13, and 17 favored the home sample on two or more of the testing weeks. For all of these except Pair 13, more difference was shown between the top and bottom subsample curves than between the total home and institution samples. Pair 6 and 9 alone showed differences favoring the institution sample on two of the testing weeks, and for both pairs less difference was shown between the subsamples.

Furthermore, the findings were clearly related to the stimulus variables. Three of the seven pairs that brought out a significant earlier or more marked preference change for the home sample consisted of two complex, flat, unfamiliar, achromatic patterns. In addition, Pair 14, which showed increased differentiation for the subsamples, was in this stimulus category. The only pair which could be placed in this category and which did not show a group difference was Pair 11 (see Fig. 1), the only patterns with simple, unbroken contours. This and the other four pairs of patterns all brought out a marked change in preference during the

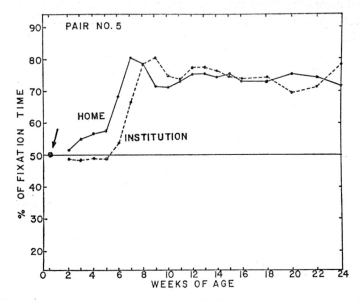

Fig. 9. Age-preference curves for the checkerboard over the lattice arrangement of white squares. Initial point (indicated by arrow) is for the unselected newborn infants.

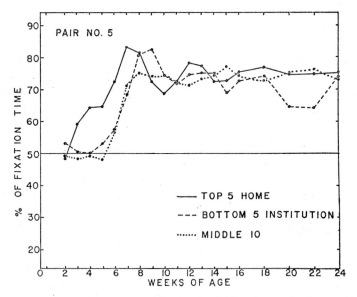

Fig. 10. Age-preference curves for the checkerboard over the lattice arrangement of squares, for the performance test subsamples (compare with Fig. 9).

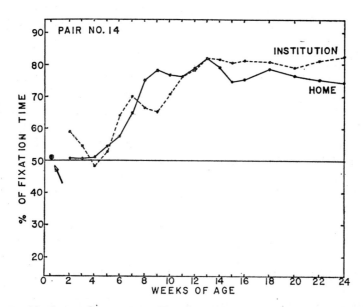

Fig. 11. Age-preference curves for the random over the lattice arrangement of black squares on white background. Initial point (indicated by light arrow) is for unselected newborn infants.

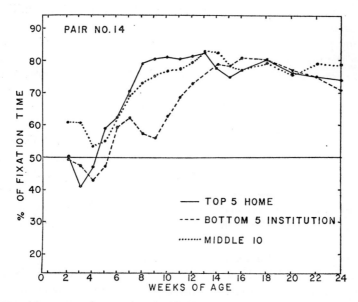

Fig. 12. Age-preference curves for the random over the lattice arrangments, for the performance test subsamples (compare with Fig. 11).

second month of life, followed by a consistent differential response to one of the patterns through the remainder of the first six months.

The results for two of the five pairs of patterns (Pairs 3 and 11) have been given. For Pair 5 (Fig. 9), the checkerboard arrangement was preferred to the lattice arrangement a week or so sooner for the home sample (reliably so); and the top-home subsample was a little earlier in this development (Fig. 10). For Pair 14 (Fig. 11), the suggested difference in the development of preference for a random over a regular arrangement of squares was not reliable; however, the curves for the top-home and bottom-institution subsamples were separated much further (Fig. 12). For Pair 1 (Fig. 13), there was a change in predominant visual attention from the irregular, angular pattern to the "polka dot" pattern; the change occurred earlier and more markedly for the home infants (the difference being reliable between samples and given some support by the subsample results). This pair differed in more stimulus dimensions than the other four. It had been included in the study not as a variation in intrinsic pattern properties, but to bring out the effect of repeated exposures of one of two patterns of expected equal initial attention value (see below). It is interesting that this pair nevertheless elicited preference changes and group differences comparable to those of the other pairs of abstract patterns.

Three other pairs were similar in that they included unfamiliar patterns or objects, but the physical stimulus difference was much greater. A strong preference for red checks over a red square (Pair 9) developed during the first two months; a small but significant developmental difference between the two samples favored the institution sample. For Pair 7 there was a shift in predominant attention during the first 3 months from a bright red spot rotating slowly on a bright yellow field to a dull, complex, stationary object. More advanced development was suggested for the home than for the institution sample (Fig. 14). This was supported by the subsample curves, showing little initial preference for the bright-colored-moving object by the top-home subsample. Pair 16 presented perhaps the grossest stimulus variations of all, but was one of the few pairs which did *not* bring out a reliable preference throughout the testing! In spite of the high variability in direction of preference, the trend was from an early low preference for the flashing orange light to a stronger preference for Egyptian art during the third month, then back to equal response. The home sample appeared to be a little ahead in this development. On balance, these three pairs suggest a higher preference for highly complex targets over plain, brightly colored, and moving or flashing targets by the home-reared infants. But this high degree of

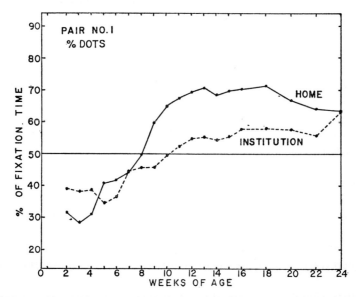

Fig. 13. Age-preference curves for the polka-dot pattern over the irregular-angular pattern on first presentation of this pair, before familiarization exposures.

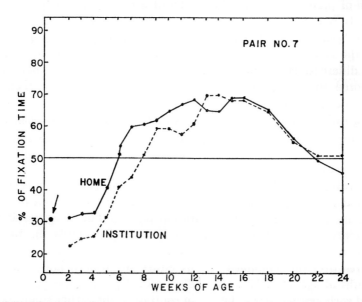

Fig. 14. Age-preference curves for the complex wire-mesh and wood object over the rotating bright red spot. Initial point (indicated by arrow) is for the unselected newborn infants.

stimulus difference elicited less differential attention and less group differentiation than some relatively subtle differences between patterns.

The remaining stimulus variations are for the most part similar to those used in the earlier attempts (see above) to determine the effects of experience. A number of pairs were representations of social stimuli, with variation in the degree of resemblance to a face. The most easily interpreted result was for Pair 17: an early preference for a life-size schematic face pattern over the same pattern reduced in size dropped to the chance level during the third month (Fig. 15). This change occurred earlier for the home sample (reaching statistical significance) and still earlier for the top-home subsample. Since the change was in the wrong direction to be an experimental preference for the more realistic facelike stimulus, it must instead be attributed to a decrease in the intrinsic attention value of size— at least, the size of an interesting pattern (other results have indicated a continuing size preference with unpatterned targets). That the change is earlier for the home infants is in keeping with their earlier or more marked attention to configurational differences.

Another significant group difference relative to face-like targets was for Pair 6 (Fig. 16), showing an earlier development by the institution sample of preference for a solid model of a head (without painted features). It is not at all clear that this was a "social preference" rather than a "solidity preference," since a solidity preference appeared at about the same age for two other target pairs. Nor is the meaning of the group difference clear, since one of the other solid-versus-flat pairs (Pair 4) favored the home sample significantly, while the other (Pair 10) showed little difference. To further confuse the matter, for another pair varying in both solidity and facial resemblance (Pair 15), a head model with painted features was not reliably preferred to a photograph of the model until 20 weeks of age, and even then the degree of differential was not great.

The correct location of "eye spots" on an oval (Pair 13) was slightly preferred throughout the age range by the home infants, but not until after 2 months of age by the institution infants. The latter result is in fair accord with earlier studies (see Fantz, 1966, table 3). But the correct arrangement of schematic features (Pair 12) was not reliably preferred over the scrambled face by either group until late in the first 6 months of age (Fig. 17), and the scrambled pattern was preferred on several early testing weeks. This is in contrast to the earlier studies which had varying results but, taken together, showed the most consistent preference between 2 and 3 months of age. Aside from this discrepancy,

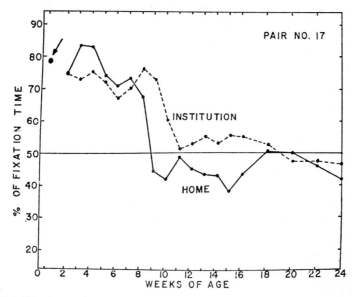

Fig. 15. Age-preference curves for the natural-size over the small schematic face. Initial point (indicated by arrow) is for the unselected newborn infants.

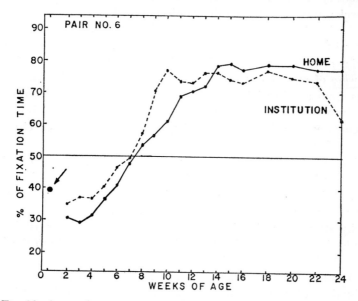

Fig. 16. Age-preference curves for the solid head model, painted white, over the white outline form. Initial point (indicated by arrow) is for the unselected newborn infants.

which we cannot account for, all results from these two pairs have agreed in the high variability and low degree of differential attention, in contrast to the frequent strong and consistent preferences found for pairs varying in intrinsic stimulus properties. Similarly, it would appear that the strongest preference elicited by a pair of face-like stimuli in this study (Pair 8, Fig. 18) can be accounted for only by attraction to intrinsic stimulus properties, since the schematic face pattern, with high contrast and low complexity, was initially preferred to the more realistic face photograph.

One class of stimulus variation remains: experimental variation in visual exposure, either on a long-term or short-term basis. Long-term exposure was provided by hanging one of the toys of Pair 2 above the home crib of each infant from the third week of age until the end of the experiment. The results (Fig. 19) were the biggest disappointment of the study. We expected attachment and increased attention to the familiar object from the familiar environment, and were encouraged in this by repeated reports from mothers and attendants of high attraction to the mobile from an early age. As it turned out, this was one of the pairs giving least evidence of a consistent differential response or of a consistent age change. Moreover, the slight change suggested was towards the novel, *not* towards the familiar object. The difference between groups suggested by the curves did not reach significance. One explanation—supported by the consistent choice by many infants for the "fruit" object (familiar or not) throughout the testing—is that intrinsic visual preferences were of more effect on the visual responsiveness than familiarity. Results from another laboratory have also been inconclusive on visual responsiveness to a familiar mobile, and have shown interference from preferences among the objects used (Greenberg, Hunt, and Uzgiris, in MS.; Uzgiris and Hunt, 1965).

Initial preferences were better controlled for the short-term variation in exposure by changing the familiarization pattern every other testing week, and by comparing the responsiveness to the particular pattern before and after the familiarization exposures. These exposures were given by attaching a duplicate of one of the test patterns (Pair 1) on the underside of the movable "stage" so that it was visible to the infant between each of the following test exposures until Pair 1 was again tested (usually following Pair 12). The results indicate decreasing relative fixation of the repeatedly-exposed pattern with increasing age (Fig. 20). The choice of the novel object was significant for both groups after 3 months of age; the suggested difference between groups, favoring the home sample, was not quite significant. Again it is apparent, from

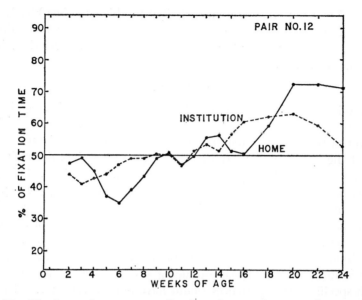

Fig. 17. Age-preference curves for the schematic face over the scrambled pattern.

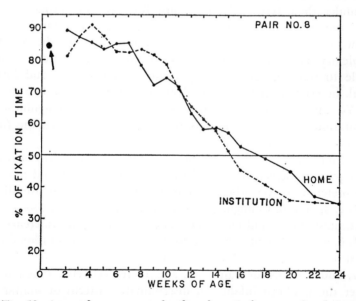

Fig. 18. Age-preference curves for the schematic face over the photographic reproduction of an actual face. Initial point (indicated by arrow) is for the unselected newborn infants.

the consistent pattern preferences elicited by this pair (see Fig. 13) that effects of previous experience on visual preferences are more difficult to bring out *by the present methods* than the effects of variations in the patterns themselves.

DISCUSSION

Several findings stand out forcibly from the mass of data obtained from young infants by the visual-preference method. First, the relative amount of time spent in looking at various targets is very largely a function of the stimulus properties of the target rather than determined by previous exposure history or similarity to familiar objects. This is, of course, limited to the experimental conditions—including the exposure of certain types of artificial or laboratory-specific stimuli in a reduced and unfamiliar stimulus situation for short periods of time, with no active contact or feedback from the stimuli—conditions which favor free visual exploration of the environment. It is likely that there are other conditions (e.g., a fear-producing situation or the home crib) in which specific past experiences would have more effect on visual preferences.

The determining stimulus variables are numerous and interrelated even under these restricted conditions. But certainly prominent—and more basic than color, reflectance, or size—are variations in *pattern*. And two important types of variation are the degree of the patterning (complexity) and the form of the patterning (configuration). It is not possible to state the relative importance of complexity and form in general, or even to make a clear distinction between the two in many cases. Yet many aspects of the results point to a special significance of configurational variations. This is the finding upon which the further interpretations will be based.

Configurational differences (form of contours, arrangement or orientation of pattern elements) elicited some of the strongest and most consistent preferences, even when the targets were quite similar overall (e.g., Figs. 1, 2, 3, and 9). Configurational differences brought out some of the earliest, most abrupt and most consistent age changes in preference (e.g., Figs. 1, 6, and 9). Infants can and do discriminate configurational differences at least by the second month of life (significant differentials shown at 5, 7, and 6 weeks for Pairs 3, 5, and 11 respectively). It is not clear whether the newborn infant can discriminate patterns of similar complexity or not; the age changes may represent the development of this ability (or this selectivity). The direction of the change is often towards circular or random configurations over linear or regular ones. Nevertheless, this generalization was reversed in one case (Fig. 13) and does not adequately describe the stimulus variation in other cases. Perhaps form is multidimensional for the infant as well as for the adult.

Configurational differences also brought out the most consistent differences in the age of preference-change between the two highly-selected samples of infants (e.g., Figs. 6, 9, and 13). This fact, with wide implications, must be interpreted carefully. That the two groups differed in rate of development of pattern preferences is quite clear from the data, but the meaning is less certain. We cannot differentiate among the various possible sources of difference, including genetic makeup, prenatal and postnatal care and nutrition, and early environment. Regarding the nature of the difference brought about by any or all of these factors, there is some basis for speculation.

The rough correlation between the pattern preference scores and the scores on a "mental development scale" (e.g., Figs. 8, 10, and 12) both supports the group difference and suggests that it involves basic aspects of psychological development, which are revealed earlier by pattern preference changes than by the appearance of various active, coordinated behaviors. The group difference was not related to sensory-motor development; the institution infants were actually a bit ahead in passing visual fixation and pursuit items. The preference changes most revealing of developmental differences involved selection and discrimination among similar forms or patterns—comparable to many items of intelligence tests given to children or adults (at least more so than the development of motor coordination or social responsiveness).

There is some basis for a tentative conclusion that the development of selective visual attention to configurational variables represents an early stage of basic perceptual-cognitive development—a stage which may be not only predictive of later stages in this development, but also may facilitate further development by making visual exploration of the environment a more effective learning process. At first glance, the latter possibility does not seem to be in accord with the various results failing to show an effect of experience on the attention value of stimuli, or even showing the opposite of the expected increased responsiveness to the familiar object or pattern (Figs. 19 and 20). But these results most likely indicate, not that learning through early visual explorations is absent, but that we are looking for the wrong effects of this learning. The primary effects of early visual experience are probably in the reception, organization, differentiation, and accumulation of information from the visual input, rather than in an increased or decreased tendency to fixate

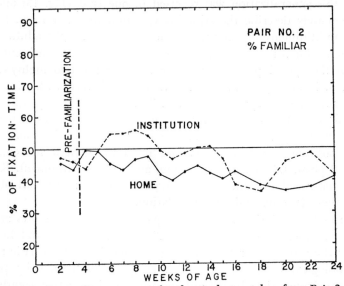

Fig. 19. Age-preference curves for the single toy taken from Pair 2, which was hung continually over the home crib of each infant from the third week to the end of the experiment.

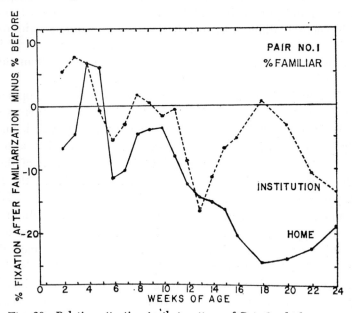

Fig. 20. Relative attention to that pattern of Pair 1 which was repeatedly exposed during the particular test session, compared with response to the same pattern at the beginning of each session.

a familiar target, or in any other change in response frequency or duration.

The latter kind of change may give little information about the former kind. Thus a change in duration of fixation of a target from one occasion to another in itself tells us nothing about what information was received and assimilated in the course of fixating the target on either occasion. But a change in the *relative* attention to several stimulus targets may do so. The development of a preference for one of several pattern arrangements, for example, indicates that certain configurational variations can now be discriminated and tend to be selected for attention. This has an effect comparable to putting the infant in a more enriched or variegated environment, and thus of giving increased and more selective opportunities for perceptual learning. For the development of such a pattern preference to occur earlier for a given infant may or may not have been the result of a prior stimulus-rich environment and more variegated experience. In either case the infant thereby has a head start in the opportunity to discriminate, become familiar with, and take in information from configurational parts of his surroundings. This analysis assumes a perceptual learning process such as that described by Gibson and Gibson (1955), progressing towards increasing stimulus differentiation. It also postulates an important role of selectivity, at both the peripheral and central level, in the learning process.

In other words, we are proposing that what goes on during the long hours the young infant spends in visual exploration and examination of his surroundings is not to be discovered in altered responsiveness to specific objects from reinforcement or repetition, since the primary changes are to be found in finer differentiations, better integrations, and more selective examinations of the total visual input. These cumulative, non-specific effects of experience are difficult to study directly. Some indirect information is given from changes in the stimulus variations which are selected and discriminated at successive points in development, and which can then affect what is subsequently learned through visual exploration.

Whether a difference of several weeks in the development of certain pattern preferences can be of any practical use in the prediction of future mental development or in the study of effects of varying early environmental circumstances remains to be determined. The possibilities might be summed up in this way: Could it be that the infant's future prospects, as well as his past experiences and present interests, are reflected in his eyes? With that bit of crystal-ball gazing, we rest our case.

REFERENCES

BAYLEY, NANCY. On the growth of intelligence. *Amer. Psychologist*, 1955, *10*, 805-818.

BERLYNE, D. E. The influence of albedo and complexity of stimuli on visual fixation in the human infant. *Brit. J. Psychol.*, 1958, *49*, 315-318.

BOWER, T. G. R. Stimulus variables determining space perception in infants. *Science*, 1965, *149*, 80-89.

BRENNAN, W. M., AMES, E. W., & MOORE, R. W. Age differences in infants' attention to patterns of different complexities. *Science*, 1966, *150*, 354-356.

FANTZ, R. L. A method for studying early visual development. *Percept. mot. Skills*, 1956, *6*, 13-15.

FANTZ, R. L. Visual discrimination in a neonate chimpanzee. *Percept. mot. Skills*, 1958, *8*, 59-66. (a)

FANTZ, R. L. Pattern vision in young infants. *Psychol. Rec.*, 1958, *8*, 43-47. (b)

FANTZ, R. L. The origin of form perception. *Scient. American*, 1961, *204*, 66-72.

FANTZ, R. L. Pattern vision in newborn infants. *Science*, 1963, *140*, 296-297.

FANTZ, R. L. Visual experience in infants: decreased attention to familiar patterns relative to novel ones. *Science*, 1964, *146*, 668-670.

FANTZ, R. L. Visual perception from birth as shown by pattern selectivity. In H. E. Whipple (Ed.), New issues in infant development. *Ann. N.Y. Acad. Sci.*, 1965, *118*, 793-814. (a)

FANTZ, R. L. Ontogeny of perception. In A. M. Schrier, H. F. Harlow, & F. Stollintz (Eds.), *Behavior of nonhuman primates. I.* New York: Academic Press, 1965. Pp. 365-403. (b)

FANTZ, R. L. Pattern discrimination and selective attention as determinants of perceptual development from birth. In Aline H. Kidd & J. L. Rivoire (Eds.), *Perceptual development in children.* New York: Internat. Univer. Press, 1966.

FANTZ, R. L. Visual perception and experience in early infancy: a look at the hidden side of behavior development. In H. W. Stevenson, E. H. Hess, & Harriet Rheingold (Eds.), *Early behavior: comparative and developmental approaches.* New York: Wiley, in press.

FANTZ, R. L. & NEVIS, SONIA. The predictive value of changes in visual preferences in early infancy. In J. Hellmuth (Ed.) *Exceptional Infant, Volume I.* Seattle: Special Child Publications, 1967, Pp. 351-415.

FANTZ, J. L., ORDY, J. M., & UDELF, M. S. Maturation of pattern vision in infants during the first six months. *J. comp. physiol. Psychol.*, 1962, *55*, 907-917.

GRAEFE, O. Versuche über visuelle Formwahrnehmung im Säugglingsalter. *Psychol. Forsch.*, 1963, *27*, 177-224.

GREENBERG, D. J., HUNT, J. McV., & UZGIRIS, I. C. Infants' preference for visual stimuli: the role of complexity and familiarity. Unpublished paper.

GRIFFITHS, R. *The abilities of babies.* New York: McGraw-Hill, 1964.

HAITH, M. M. The response of the human newborn to visual movement. *J. exp. Child Psychol.*, 1966, *3*, 235-243.

HAYEK, F. *The sensory order.* Chicago: Univer. Chicago Press, 1952.

GIBSON, J. J. & GIBSON, ELEANOR J. Perceptual learning: differentiation or enrichment? *Psychol Rev.*, 1955, *62*, 32.

HAYNES, H., WHITE, B. L., & HELD, R. Visual accommodation in human infants. *Science*, 1965, *148*, 528-530.

HERSHENSON, M. Visual discrimination in the human infant. *J. comp. physiol. Psychol.*, 1964, *58*, 270.

HERSHENSON, M., MUNSINGER, H., & KESSEN, W. Preference for shapes of intermediate variability in the newborn human. *Science*, 1965, *147*, 630-631.

HUBEL, D. H. & WIESEL, T. N. Receptive fields of cells in striate cortex of very young, visually inexperienced kittens. *J. Neurophysiol.*, 1963, *26*, 994-1002.

KAGAN, J. & LEWIS, M. Studies of attention in the human infant. *Merrill-Palmer Quart.*, 1965, *11*, 95-127.

LEWIS, M., MEYERS, W., KAGAN, J., & GROSSBERG, R. Attention to visual patterns in infants. *Amer. Psychologist*, 1963, *18*, 357.

SAAYMAN, G., AMES, E. W., & MOFFETT, A. Response to novelty as an indicator of visual discrimination in the human infant. *J. exp. Child Psychol.*, 1964, *1*, 189-198.

SACKETT, G. P. A neural mechanism underlying unlearned, critical period, and developmental aspects of visually controlled behavior. *Psychol. Rev.*, 1963, *70*, 40-50.

SPEARS, W. Assessment of visual preference and discrimination in the four-month-old infant. *J. comp. physiol. Psychol.*, 1964, *57*, 381-386.

STECHLER, G. The effect of medication during labor on newborn infants. *Science*, 1964, *144*, 315-317.

STECHLER, G., BRADFORD, S., & LEVY, H. Attention in the newborn: effect on motility and skin potential. *Science*, 1966, *151*, 1246-1248.

STIRNIMANN, F. Uber das Forbenempfinden Neugeborener. *Ann. Paedia.*, 1944, *163*, 1-25.

THOMAS, H. Visual fixation responses in infants to stimuli of varying complexity. *Child Develpm.*, 1965, *36*, 629-638.

UZGIRIS, I. C. & HUNT, J. McV. A longitudinal study of recognition learning. Paper presented at Soc. Res. Child Develpm., Minneapolis, March, 1965.

WOLFF, P. H. Observations on the early development of smiling. In B. M. Foss (Ed.), *Determinants of Infant behavior: II.* New York: Wiley, 1963. Pp. 113-114.

3

NONNUTRITIVE SUCKING AND RESPONSE THRESHOLDS IN YOUNG INFANTS

Peter H. Wolff, M.D.

Harvard Medical School and Children's Medical Center

and

Michael A. Simmons

Harvard Medical School

The motor response to tickling of 24 4-day-old healthy neonates was tested during ordinary restful sleep, when the infants were sucking on a pacifier in sleep, and during sleep when they had a pacifier in their mouth but were not sucking. The results indicate that sucking renders the sleeping infant unresponsive to an external stimulus. A similar but less marked rise in response thresholds was observed when a pacifier was in the baby's mouth but the baby was not sucking. In this condition, the infant usually responded to the stimulus with a new burst of sucking rather than a burst of diffuse motility, as in ordinary sleep. Various interpretations for these findings are considered.

The quieting effect of nonnutritive sucking on excited babies is so well known that mothers have exploited it in one or another form wherever the culture has not proscribed the use of pacifiers on medico-

Reprinted from CHILD DEVELOPMENT, Vol. 38, No. 3, September 1967, pp. 631-638. © 1967 by The Society for Research in Child Development, Inc. Work for this report was completed while the first author was supported by a Career Development Award, MH-K-3461, and a research grant, MH-06034, both of the U. S. Public Health Service, National Institute of Mental Health.

dental, aesthetic, or moral grounds (Peiper, 1963). Explanations offered for the inhibitory effect are as numerous as psychological theories of motivation, but no existing formulation is entirely satisfactory.

In home observations, one of us (P.H.W.) found that sleeping infants were less sensitive to external stimulation while sucking on the pacifier than without a pacifier in their mouth. Infants who, while sleeping, had a pacifier in their mouths, responded more vigorously to stimulation *between* bursts of rhythmical sucking than *while sucking,* but their primary response between bursts was usually a resumption of sucking rather than an increase of diffuse motility. The aim of the study was to test these observations systematically and to identify one possible mechanism for the inhibition of motility by nonnutritive sucking.

METHOD

The subjects for the study were 24 healthy full-term 4-day-old infants, born after uneventful pregnancies and uncomplicated deliveries. All infants were observed in an isolated nursery, in a standard hospital crib which was supported on metal runners, so that the baby's movements would shake the crib. Responsiveness was tested by gently tickling sensitive areas of the infant's face. Pretest trials had indicated that the nasal columna and the medial and lateral epicanthi were among the most sensitive areas of the face to tickling, and each infant was tested in these three areas under the following organismic conditions: during natural regular sleep (A), during regular sleep with the pacifier in the mouth but not sucking (B), and during regular sleep while sucking on the pacifier (C).

The stimulus was delivered by a camel's-hair brush from which all but five hairs had been removed. A single trial consisted of three slow strokes of the brush (back and forth at the lateral epicanthus, horizontally across the nasal columna, and up and down at the medial epicanthus). The method of stroking, which took about 2 seconds from the start to the end of a trial, had been practiced before the start of the experiment to achieve some uniformity of stimulus presentation. The duration of stimulation was also recorded on the polygraph record by a time marker, so that corrections for differences in length of stimulation could be made in the final tabulation, (i.e., dividing the obtained values of motor activity by a ratio of actual stimulation time over 2 seconds).

Infants were always tested during restful or "regular" sleep (for clinical criteria, see Wolff, 1966). Since the regular pattern of respiration was the major defining criterion for this state, respirations were monitored by a bellows pneumograph and pressure transducer to insure that the state remained clinically the same during the test. In Conditions B and C, the infant was tested while he had in his mouth an ordinary pacifier whose air space was connected to a pressure transducer (Sanborn pulse-wave attachment #374), from which sucking movements were monitored on a polygraph writer.

Earlier studies had shown that sleeping infants sucked in a pattern of bursts and rest periods that was sufficiently constant, so that one could predict within a second for how long after the start of a burst the infant would continue to suck, and how long the rest periods between bursts of sucking would last (Wolff, 1966).

In Condition C, the stimulus was presented while the infant was sucking and could, from his pretest performance, be expected to suck for another 3-6 seconds. In Condition B, the stimulus was presented at the start of a rest period when the infant was not sucking and would, under unstimulated conditions, *not* have sucked again for another 4-12 seconds even though the pacifier remained in his mouth.

The motor response to tickling was recorded from a phonograph pick-up crystal taped to the bottom of the crib, to which a wire coil was attached (see Crider, Shapiro, and Tursky, 1966). This coil translated the baby's movements into pendular movements and generated a small current that was recorded on the same Sanborn recorder as sucking movements, respirations, and duration of stimulation. The instrument was sufficiently sensitive to record the effects of the sucking movements on the crib when the infant was otherwise immobile.

By this method the infant's activity could not be measured in absolute values, since the wire coil oscillated for a few seconds after the movements had stopped. The oscillation also varied as a function of the baby's total body weight so that apparently equal displacements of the limbs in different infants did not always produce the same amount of oscillation. Comparisons were therefore only made for the same baby under different testing conditions, and each infant was taken as his own control. The results are reported in arbitrary units that have no direct bearing on the physical work performed.

A complete schedule for one infant called for nine separate trials (stimulation at each of three places under each of three organismic conditions), which were administered in a random sequence determined by a Latin square design. Since all cells of the square were not filled, the design was only used to generate a random order, and not as the basis for testing statistical significance.

To control for the arousal effects of removing the pacifier when testing for responsiveness in Condition A, all babies were allowed to go to sleep while sucking on the pacifier. As soon as the respirations had stabilized into a regular pattern, and the infant's clinical condition indicated that he was in regular sleep, 3 minutes of activity in the unstimulated condition were recorded while the infant was sucking. Then the infant was tickled at 1-minute intervals, at each of the three areas under each of the three organismic conditions.

Motor activity was measured in units of grid paper marked by the recording pen, and the responses were scored as total activity units in the 2 seconds after the start of the test stimulus, minus the activity units in the 2 seconds before stimulation. Because sucking without limb displacements was sufficient to activate the motility sensor, the 2 seconds before stimulation in which the infant was still sucking served as control values for Conditions B and C.

The immediate resumption of sucking after stimulation was a significant mode of response in Condition B that had to be distinguished from an increase in general motility. Therefore the response to each stimulation in Condition B was also scored as either a resumption of sucking before the expected time (inferred from his pretest performance) or as no shortening of the rest periods between bursts of sucking.

RESULTS

Table 1 summarizes the motor responses to tickling at the three sites under the three conditions, and for Condition B it indicates whether the infant responded by sucking before the expected time with or without diffuse motility $(+)$, or only by diffuse motility $(-)$. Infants who failed to suck altogether in regular sleep were rejected from the study during pretest trials. One of the infants in the sample was so sensitive to stimulation that he woke up whenever he was tickled. On three other infants the full schedule of nine tests could not be completed because they shifted to irregular or light sleep while being tested. The statistical evaluation was thus based on the findings of only twenty infants.

As a group, the infants were most responsive to tickling in Condition A, less responsive in Condition B, and least responsive in Condition C. Differences in motor responses from Condition A to B to C were statistically significant at each site of stimulation $(p = 0.001$, by Friedman Two-Way Analysis of Variance [Siegel, 1956]. In 16 of the 20 infants this relation between responsiveness and organismic state was consistent

TABLE 1

MOTOR RESPONSES TO TICKLING IN FIRST 2 SECONDS AFTER STIMULATION

	Site								
	Nasal Columna			Medial Epicanthus			Lateral Epicanthus		
Condition..........	A	B	C	A	B	C	A	B	C
Mean units of diffuse motor response........	137.1	95.7	37.8	139.2	87.1	40.5	123.2	76.0	39.4
$A > B > C$......		$p^a = .001$			$p = .001$			$p = .001$	
Type of motor response in B........		$\begin{cases} + = 16 \\ - = 3 \end{cases}$			$+ = 15$ $- = 4$			$+ = 14$ $- = 5$	
$+ > -$ (in B)........		$p^b < .002$			$p < .004$			$p < .05$	

NOTE.—A = no pacifier in mouth; B = pacifier in mouth, not sucking; C = sucking on pacifier; + = resumption of sucking before expected time; — = no resumption of sucking before expected time.
a By Friedman Two-Way Analysis of Variance.
b By one-tailed Sign Test.

at all three areas of the face, with a 25 per cent reduction of activity or more from A to C. The response patterns of the other four infants were variable, showing an increase of motility at one site, a decrease or no change at the others. For the 20 infants as a group, the differences in motor responses between Conditions A and B, B and C, or A and C, were also statistically significant ($p = .01$ by Wilcoxin Matched-Pairs Signed-Rank Test).

By comparing the mean duration of rest periods between bursts of sucking in the unstimulated condition and Condition B, it was possible to show that the test stimulus precipitated a burst of sucking before the expected time more often than not, and that this effect was statistically significant at two of the three sites ($p = .002$, nasal columna; $p < .004$, medial epicanthus; $p < .05$, lateral epicanthus; by one-tailed Sign Test). There were no significant differences in responsiveness of the three facial areas stimulated.

DISCUSSION

From these findings we concluded that sleeping infants are less responsive to tickling while they are sucking on a pacifier than in ordinary sleep. When infants are stimulated during sleep, while they are not sucking but the pacifier is in their mouth, they respond by a resumption of sucking rather than by diffuse motility alone.

A possible source of error in our findings was the lack of control over stimulus intensity. Since the face was tickled by hand rather than by instrument, there was no assurance that the intensity of stroking was the same in each condition, even though the physical features of the camel's-hair brush did not allow for great variations in pressure. We sacrificed control over stimulus intensity and did not use sound or other more easily controlled modalities of stimulation, in order to exploit the relatively slow rate of habituation to tickling (Benjamin, 1956). The instrumentation required to achieve satisfactory control over the intensity of tickling seemed too costly in time and money for this pilot study.

Another possible source of error was the absence of control over sensitivity of the receptor organs under the three organismic conditions. The skin of the nasal columna might have been under greater tension and the receptor organs consequently less (or more) sensitive when the pacifier was in the mouth (Conditions B and C) than during ordinary regular sleep (Condition A). It is unlikely, however, that the skin sensitivity of the lateral and medial epicanthi would have been affected by a pacifier in the same way.

The experiment was not critical in the sense that its results would admit one and only one interpretation. Certain explanations offered in the past for the quieting effect of pacifier sucking could, however, be ruled out in favor of others.

According to classic psychoanalytic theory, one might interpret the findings to mean that a specific quantity of painful internal excitations is discharged in non-nutritive sucking (Hug-Hellmuth, 1921) and that such instinctual drive discharge lowers the motivation for diffuse motor activity (Rapaport, 1951).

The familiar observation that sucking inhibits diffuse motility almost as soon as the infant starts to suck, while removal of a pacifier after a long period of sucking frequently reinstates the previous level of diffuse activity (Kessen and Leutzendorff, 1963; Peiper, 1963), argues against the assumption that sucking per se is an adequate channel for the discharge of instinctual drive tension. The fact that the inverse relation between pacifier sucking and responsiveness was present at the end, as well as at the beginning, of a prolonged period of sucking also argues against the assumption that a fixed quantity of psychological energy must be discharged before the infant becomes quiescent.

A second formulation is based on the observation that physical contact between a suitable sucking object and the lips inhibits diffuse motor activity. Some have suggested that lip stimulation is a specific inhibitor of diffuse motility (Wolff, 1959). Others have proposed that hunger satiation may reinforce the association between such inhibition of motor activity and mouth contact or that mouth contact "reminds" the infant of previous experiences of satisfaction (Peiper, 1963; Williams and Kessen, 1961). Since sustained mouth contact even without sucking inhibits the infant's motility in the first 24 hours after birth and therefore before he has been fed (Wolff, 1963), those formulations which explain the phenomenon in terms of reinforcement by drive reduction also do not seem satisfactory.

A third formulation, not incompatible with the concept that hand-mouth contact per se inhibits motility, is the one we believe to be most consonant with the reported findings. It assumes that the nervous system is organized at birth in a hierarchy of dominant and subordinate motor functions and that pacifier (or nipple) sucking inhibits diffuse motility in the same way that defecation inhibits other reflex activities (e.g., visual pursuit, sucking, crying), or sucking and swallowing modify the pattern of respiration (Peiper, 1963). When an infant with a pacifier in his mouth on which he is not sucking is tickled, he responds with an abortive episode of diffuse activity that includes the resumption of sucking (Balint, 1948; Peiper, 1963). According to our assumption, the onset of sucking immediately inhibits the generalized response so that one usually observes a burst of sucking with only a slight and transient increase of diffuse activity. Any latent tendency to respond diffusely therefore appears to be "channeled" into rhythmical mouthing, not because of some redistribution of excitations, but because sucking effectively blocks other responses.

Such an assumption might also account for the general quieting effect of pacifier sucking on an infant who has continued to cry and thrash long after the offending stimulus which precipitated the outburst ceased, but who quiets down almost as soon as he is offered the pacifier. As in temper tantrums of older children and hysterical attacks of adults, the aimless motility of the neonate seems to maintain itself once it is set into motion, even after the precipitating cause has been eliminated. Any intervention which blocks the self-stimulation of diffuse motility, whether it be pacifier sucking, swaddling, or other monotonous nonpainful stimulation, interrupts the self-activating cycle, reduces the infant's excitement, and eventually promotes sleep without necessarily removing the initial offending cause (Kessen & Mandler, 1961; Wolff, 1966).

REFERENCES

BALINT, M. Individual differences of behavior in early infancy and an objective method for recording them. *Journal of genetic Psychology,* 1948, *73,* 57-79, 81-117.

BENJAMIN, F. B. Effect of pain on simultaneous perception of non-painful sensory stimulation. *Journal of applied Physiology,* 1956, *8,* 630-634.

CRIDER, A., SHAPIRO, D., and TURSKY, B. Reinforcement of spontaneous electrodermal activity. *Journal of comparative and physiological Psychology,* 1966, *61,* 20-27.

HUG-HELLMUTH, H. *Aus dem Seelenleben des Kindes.* (2d German ed.) Leipzig: Deuticke, 1921.

KESSEN, W., and LEUTZENDORFF, A. M. The effects of non-nutritive sucking on movement in the human newborn. *Journal of comparative and physiological Psychology,* 1963, *56,* 69-72.

KESSEN, W., and MANDLER, G. Anxiety, pain, and the inhibition of distress. *Psychological Reviews,* 1961, *68,* 396-404.

PEIPER, A. *Cerebral function in infancy and childhood.* (Trans. of 3d German ed.) New York: Consultants Bureau, 1963.

RAPAPORT, D. The conceptual model of psychoanalysis. *Journal of Personality,* 1951, *20,* 56-81.

SIEGEL, S. *Nonparametric statistics for the behavioral sciences.* New York: McGraw-Hill, 1956.

WILLIAMS, J., and KESSEN, W. The effect of hand-mouth contacting on neonatal movement. *Child Development,* 1961, *32,* 243-248.

WOLFF, P. H. Observations on newborn infants. *Psychosomatic Medicine,* 1959, *21,* 110-118.

WOLFF, P. H. Observations of behavior in early infancy. Paper preesnted to the New Orleans Psychoanalytic Society, New Orleans, June, 1963.

WOLFF, P. H. The causes, controls, and organization of behavior in the neonate. *Psychological Issues,* 1966, Ser. No. 17.

4

COMPARATIVE DEVELOPMENT OF NEGRO AND WHITE INFANTS

C. Etta Walters

Institute of Human Development, Florida State University

A. INTRODUCTION

The paucity of recent investigations, conflicting results of other studies and their lack of statistical treatment and proper controls, and the age-old controversy of the superiority of the races make a comparative study of Negro and white development a vital area of research.

Williams and Scott[13] compared gross motor development, by means of the Gesell schedules, of a group of Negro infants from a low socio-economic background with those from a high socioeconomic background. They found the infants from the low socioeconomic group to be significantly accelerated in gross motor development over the higher group. They also found significant differences in the way the infants from the two groups were handled; the ones from the lower background came from homes where, comparatively, the atmosphere was more permissive and less exacting. From the results of their study they say, "the findings suggest that motor acceleration is not a 'racial characteristic' "[13] (p. 120).

Scott *et al.*[10] studied two groups of Negro infants from two contrasting socioeconomic backgrounds on 12 neuromuscular steps. They found the

Reprinted from The Journal of Genetic Psychology, 1967, *110*, pp. 243-251. Copyright, 1967, by The Journal Press. This investigation was supported by Research Grant No. MH8312-O1A1 from the National Institute of Mental Health of the National Institutes of Health, U.S. Public Health Service. Appreciation is extended to Mrs. Pat Rochester and to Miss Filiz Balkir for their testing of the subjects and for their dedication to the study.

Negro infant from the clinic to be accelerated over the Negro infants from private practice from the 8th to the 35th week of life; after that the development was similar. The babies in this group (lower socio-economic group) were accelerated in their development when compared with a group of white babies studied in a like manner by Aldrich,[1] except in the two patterns of "smiling" and "vocalization." When the Negro group from private practice was compared with Aldrich's white sample from private practice, they noted a marked similarity during the first 30 weeks of life in their development. They thus attributed the differences and similarities found in the three groups studied to environmental factors.

While McGraw[7] in her study found the development of Negro babies to be about 80 per cent as mature as that of white babies she tested, critics of her study have pointed out that the heights and weights of the Negro infants were considerably below those of the white babies, and, therefore, she did not have comparable groups.

Pasamanick[9] compared 53 Negro babies with 99 white infants and found Negro superiority in gross motor development, but no differences in the other categories measured by the Gesell test. In a follow-up on these infants, Knoblock and Pasamanick[5] found the Negro child to be equal in development to his white "coeval," but a definite acceleration was noted in the gross motor development of the Negro infant over the white child. In a later and more controlled study, Knoblock and Pasamanick[6] found no differences at 40 weeks of age between the two races. In an analysis of factors affecting development, they conclude that prenatal experience, birth weight, and later physical condition are the most important, "and, in essence, the only significant factors we have been able to discover at this point that result in group differences in developmental quotients"[6] (p. 214).

Solomons and Solomons[11] studied the factors affecting motor development of 4-month-old infants and found firstborns to have a significantly higher motor score than later-borns. They found no significant differences between the mean motor score of Negro and white infants, although the Negro score was slightly higher than the white score.

Meredith,[8] in summarizing weights and lengths of North American Negro infants, says that the Negro baby is, on the average, nearly 4 per cent lighter at birth than the average North American white infant and is .20 and .13 kilograms lighter at 6 months and 1 year, respectively. Although he found that the birth length of the American Negro was shorter by about 1.0 cm than that of the white infant, there was no difference in mean length between the two groups after six months of postnatal age. Crump et al.,[3] in discussing the factors influencing birth-weights in Negro infants, concludes that the Negro is smaller at birth than is the white baby. However, they point out that it has not been demonstrated that this is exclusively a racial characteristic. The factors they found to influence birthweight were age of mother at time of conception (younger mother has a lighter baby), prenatal supervision and care, and socioeconomic status of the Negro mother.

Bayley[2] gave the revised forms of the Bayley Scales of mental and motor development to a representative sample of 1409 infants, ages 1 to 15 months. The study was cross-sectional and included white, Negro, and a small sample of Puerto Rican babies. While she found no differences on either scale (mental or motor) for education of either parent, the number of babies tested at each month was small, varying in number from seven to 37 in each educational subgroup. While no differences were found between the Negroes and whites on the mental scale, the mean motor scores for the Negroes were higher at every age, except 15 months. These differences reached significance at the .01 level of con-fidence for the months of 3, 4, 5, and 9 months, and at the .05 level for 7 and 12 months. It is difficult to see the rationale for her statement in regard to the Negro-white differences for the motor scale when she says, "the lack of differences for educational subgroups in our sample tends to discredit the environmental explanation for the difference in score, at least for these U.S. children"[2] (p. 409). This is especially true in view of the small number of education subgroups which were used for comparison, and for the fact that 19.8 per cent of the Negro fathers and 5 per cent of the mothers did not report their education. The Negro and white groups were also not compared by educational background or socioeconomic status.

There is a fallacy in taking a representative sample when the problem is one of determining whether any differences found are of racial origin. It would appear to this investigator that a comparative study involving infant development should control for the variables affecting develop-ment. Many of the previous studies have controlled for one variable, but few have attempted to hold constant several factors affecting devel-opment.

B. PURPOSE

The purpose of this study was to compare the development of Negro and white infants by means of the Gesell developmental schedules at 12, 24, and 36 weeks.

The hypothesis was that, when influencing variables were controlled, there would be no differences between Negro and white infant development.

C. METHOD

The Negro and white samples came from Tallahassee, Florida, and environs and were chosen by the following criteria: full-term births, birthweight of at least 5½ pounds, a minimum of four months of maternal prenatal care, and delivery by an obstetrician and in a hospital. An effort was made in the selection of the sample to obtain comparable socioeconomic groups. All babies who had a difficult delivery or whose mothers had toxemia or any disease which might affect the developmental status of the baby were eliminated from the study. Of the 90 mothers of Negro babies and of the 116 white babies who fit the criteria, 51 Negro and 57 white subjects expressed willingness to participate in the study. Sixteen of the Negro parents had an education, occupation, and method of salary payment of the father which classified them, for this study, as being in the high socioeconomic group. Similarly 15 of the white sample could be so classified. The remaining sample was categorized, for descriptive purposes, as the low socioeconomic group. The term high and low will be used, hereafter, in reference to them. The total Negro and white samples were then equated on the basis of the combined education of the father and mother. From Table 1, it is apparent that the two groups were matched quite well as to socioeconomic background (see Method of Payment, Table 1) and for other factors affecting development: e.g., number of children in the family, age of mother, number of first births, and birthweight and length, as well as subsequent weight and length measurements (Tables 1 and 2), add validity to the fact that the groups were matched quite well as to background and factors influencing growth and development.[3, 6, 8] Since the majority of previous investigations have found no sex differences at these early months, the unequal number of males and females in the Negro group was not considered an influencing variable.

Babies were tested on the Gesell developmental schedules[4] within three days of their 12-week, 24-week, and 36-week birthday. Two trained Gesell testers were assigned at random to both Negro and white samples. For the majority of subjects testing was done in the laboratory, while some of the infants were examined in their homes. If, for any reason, the infant could not be tested at his regular time or within the three-day birthday limit, the test was postponed for four weeks. An infant from the opposite sample and from the same socioeconomic background was

TABLE 1

DESCRIPTION OF GROUPS

Variable	High Negro(a)	High White(b)	Low Negro(c)	Low White(d)
No. of children (M)	2	3	3	3
No. of first births	4	3	8	6
Brith weight (pounds)	7.13	7.26	7.26	7.58
Birth length (inches)	20.51	19.09	20.51	19.94
Mother works	12	5	25	9
Full	9	2	12	6
Part	3	3	13	3
Mother and father live together	All but 1	All	All but 6	All but 2
Mothers' age (M years)	27	29	25	26
Fathers' education (M years)	16	16	10	12
Mothers' education (M years)	15	14.5	10.5	11
Method of payment (% paid)				
Monthly	65	53	15	25
Bimonthly	12	27	32	33
Weekly	23	20	47	36
Hourly	0	0	6	6

(a) Males = 8, females = 9.
(b) Males = 6, females = 9.
(c) Males = 10, females = 24.
(d) Males = 22, females = 20.

TABLE 2

MEAN WEIGHT AND HEIGHT OF NEGRO AND WHITE INFANTS

Group	No. of cases	Test period	Weight (pounds)	Length (inches)
Negro	47	12 week	12.84	23.98
White	54		12.79	23.60
Negro	41	24 week	16.96	26.23
White	46		16.96	26.19
Negro	43	36 week	19.83	28.00
White	50		19.66	27.81

tested at this time, so that all tests were comparable. They were analyzed, however, with the closest regular test-period group. Data were scored as to the number of items passed in each behavioral area of the Gesell schedule and were totaled for the total Gesell developmental score.[12]

D. RESULTS AND DISCUSSION

The Mann-Whitney U test was used to determine the significance of the difference between the Negro and white groups. The level of significance was determined for a two-tailed test.

The only statistically significant difference between the two groups was in favor of the Negro infant in motor development at 12 weeks (.009 level of significance). However, the mean scores for the Negro group were higher than the white mean scores for all test areas of development at 12 weeks; after that, the means were comparable.

1. High Socioeconomic Negro and White Groups

(Sixteen Negro infants and 15 white babies comprised this sample.) From Table 1, it is evident that these two groups were fairly well matched on the factors affecting development. When the two groups were compared, significant differences were found, in favor of the Negro infant, in total development and in personal-social behavior at 12 weeks and in motor behavior at 24 weeks (.05 level of significance) .

2. Low Socioeconomic Negro and White Groups

Thirty-five Negroes and 42 white infants constituted this sample. From Table 1, it is apparent that these two groups also were equated quite well on factors affecting development. The only significant difference found between the two groups was in adaptive behavior at 24 weeks, in favor of the white infant (.05 level of significance).

3. Other Socioeconomic Group Racial Comparisons

Tests of significance were computed among all the other groups. Table 3 presents the results of these tests. While there are differences in sample size, such as in the comparisons of the high Negro and high white groups with the low groups, the results bear further scrutiny. The overwhelming superiority of the high Negro group over all other groups, especially the low Negroes, leads one to analyze the high Negro subject more closely. In the high Negro group, as in the white sample, both parents had a minimum of a high school education, with the exception of one Negro

TABLE 3

SIGNIFICANT INTERGROUP DIFFERENCES BY SOCIOECONOMIC CLASS

Class	High White	Low Negro	Low White
High Negro	12 weeks. Negroes better in total development & personal-social area. 24 weeks. Negroes better in motor area. 36 weeks. No differences.	12 weeks. High Negroes better in all areas but motor. 24 and 36 weeks. High Negroes better in total development, motor, and adaptive behavior.	12 weeks. Negroes better in all areas. 24 weeks. Negroes better in motor area. 36 weeks. No differences.
High White		12 weeks. No differences. 24 weeks. No differences. 36 weeks. No differences.	12 weeks. No differences. 24 weeks. No differences. 36 weeks. No differences.
Low Negro			12 weeks. No differences. 24 weeks. Whites higher on adaptive area. 36 weeks. No differences.

mother who had 11 years of education. The occupations of the Negro group included, among other occupations, three university professors, a high school teacher, and a professional football player. The Negro, in the South, who has had a minimum of a high school education, and who has attained the status of a college or high school teacher rates among the highest echelon in social status and in standard of living. The selective factors operating to enable this individual to reach and to strive for this attainment, no doubt, produce a quite superior individual. The white man and woman who have completed high school and who have gone into teaching and similar professions have had more opportunities to do so, and do not represent as highly selected a group. These factors may help to account for the superiority of the Negro group.

E. SUMMARY

Fifty-one Negro and 57 white babies were tested at 12, 24, and 36 weeks on the Gesell developmental schedules. They were equated for socioeconomic status and for other factors affecting development. When comparisons were made on the Gesell test and its component subdivisions (motor, adaptive, language, and personal-social) the only significant difference found at the three test periods was in motor behavior at 12 weeks, in favor of the Negro infant. This is in accord with other investigations which have found the Negro to have a higher motor quotient at the early months of growth. [2, 5, 9] The groups were divided into socioeconomic subgroups and compared for development at the three test periods. The high Negro group was superior to all other groups at various stages of development, and the greatest number of differences occurred between it and the low Negro group. This is at variance with other investigations which have found the low socioeconomic groups to be superior to the higher groups. When the two largest groups were compared—e.g., the low Negro and the low white—the only significant difference found was in favor of the white infant in adaptive behavior at 24 weeks. The results suggest that factors, other than racial, probably account for the few differences found between the two races. The overwhelming superiority of the small group of high Negroes leads one to speculate that the selective factors operating to produce their high educational and socioeconomic status may also be responsible for their superior development.

REFERENCES

1. ALDRICH, C. A., & NORVAL, M. A. A developmental graph for the first year of life. *J. Pediat.*, 1946, *29*, 304-308.

2. BAYLEY, N. Comparison of mental and motor test scores for ages 1-15 months by sex, birth, order, race, geographical location, and education of parents. *Child Devel.*, 1965, *36*, 379-411.
3. CRUMP, E. P., CARELL, H. P., MASUOKA, J., & RYAN, D. Growth and development. 1. Relation of birthweight in Negro infants to sex, maternal age, parity, prenatal care, and socio-economic status. *J. Pediat.*, 1957, *51*, 678-697.
4. GESELL, A., & AMATRUDA, C. S. Developmental Diagnosis (5th ed.). New York: Hoeber, 1952.
5. KNOBLOCK, H., & PASAMANICK, B. Further observations on the behavioral development of Negro children. *J. Genet Psychol.*, 1953, *83*, 137-157.
6. ————: Environmental factors affecting human development, before and after birth. *Pediatrics*, 1960, *26*, 210-218.
7. McGRAW, M. B. A comparative study of a group of Southern white and Negro infants. *Genet. Psychol. Monog.*, 1931, *10*, 1-105.
8. MEREDITH, H. V. North American Negro infants: Size at birth and growth during the first postnatal year. *Hum. Biol.*, 1952, *24*, 250-308.
9. PASAMANICK, B. A comparative study of the behavioral development of Negro infants. *J. Genet. Psychol.*, 1946, *69*, 3-44.
10. SCOTT, R. B., FERGUSON, A. D., JENKINS, M. E., & CULTER, F. F. Growth and development of Negro infants: V. Neuromuscular pattern of behavior during the first year of life. *Pediatrics*, 1955, *16*, 24-30.
11. SOLOMONS, G., & SOLOMONS, H. C. Factors affecting motor performance in four-month-old infants. *Child Devel.*, 1964, *35*, 1283-1295.
12. WALTERS, C. E. The prediction of postnatal development from fetal activity. *Child Devel.*, 1965, *36*, 801-808.
13. WILLIAMS, J. R., & SCOTT, R. B. Growth and development of Negro infants: IV. Motor development and its relationship to child rearing practices in two groups of Negro infants. *Child Devel.*, 1953, *24*, 103-121.

5

SEX, AGE, AND STATE AS DETERMINANTS OF MOTHER-INFANT INTERACTION

Howard A. Moss, Ph.D.

Child Research Branch, National Institute of Mental Health, Bethesda, Md.

A major reason for conducting research on human infants is derived from the popular assumption that adult behavior, to a considerable degree, is influenced by early experience. A corollary of this assumption is that if we can precisely conceptualize and measure significant aspects of infant experience and behavior we will be able to predict more sensitively and better understand adult functioning. The basis for this conviction concerning the enduring effects of early experience varies considerably according to the developmental model that is employed. Yet there remains considerable consensus as to the long term and pervasive influence of the infant's experience.

Bloom (1964) contends that characteristics become increasingly resistant to change as the mature status of the characteristic is achieved and that environmental effects are most influential during periods of most rapid growth. This is essentially a refinement of the critical period hypothesis which argues in favor of the enduring and irreversible effects of many infant experiences. Certainly the studies on imprinting and the

Reprinted from MERRILL-PALMER QUARTERLY OF BEHAVIOR AND DEVELOPMENT, Vol. 13, No. 1, 1967, pp. 19-36. Presented at The Merrill-Palmer Institute Conference on Research and Teaching of Infant Development, February 10-12, 1966, directed by Irving E. Sigel, chairman of research. The conference was financially supported in part by the National Institute of Child Health and Human Development. The author wishes to express his appreciation to Mrs. Helene McVey and Miss Betty Reinecke for their assistance in preparing and analyzing the data presented in this paper.

effects of controlled sensory input are impressive in this respect (Hess, 1959; White and Held, 1963). Learning theory also lends itself to support the potency of early experience. Since the occurrence of variable interval and variable ratio reinforcement schedules is highly probable in infancy (as in many other situations), the learnings associated with these schedules will be highly resistant to extinction. Also the preverbal learning that characterizes infancy should be more difficult to extinguish since these responses are less available to linguistic control which later serves to mediate and regulate many important stimulus-response and reinforcement relationships. Psychoanalytic theory and behavioristic psychology probably have been the most influential forces in emphasizing the long-range consequences of infant experience. These theories, as well as others, stress the importance of the mother-infant relationship. In light of the widespread acceptance of the importance of early development, it is paradoxical that there is such a dearth of direct observational data concerning the functioning of infants, in their natural environment, and in relation to their primary caretakers.

Observational studies of the infant are necessary in order to test existing theoretical propositions and to generate new propositions based on empirical evidence. In addition, the infant is an ideally suitable subject for investigating many aspects of behavior because of the relatively simple and inchoate status of the human organism at this early stage in life. Such phenomena as temperament, reactions to stimulation, efficacy of different learning contingencies, perceptual functioning, and social attachment can be investigated while they are still in rudimentary form and not yet entwined in the immensely complex behavioral configurations that progressively emerge.

The research to be reported in this paper involves descriptive-normative data of maternal and infant behaviors in the naturalistic setting of the home. These data are viewed in terms of how the infant's experience structures potential learning patterns. Although the learning process itself is of primary eventual importance, it is necessary initially to identify the organizational factors, in situ, that structure learning opportunities and shape response systems.

A sample of 30 first-born children and their mothers were studied by means of direct observations over the first 3 months of life. Two periods were studied during this 3-month interval. Period one included a cluster of three observations made at weekly intervals during the first month of life in order to evaluate the initial adaptation of mother and infant to one another. Period two consisted of another cluster of three observations, made around 3 months of age when relatively stable patterns of behavior were likely to have been established. Each cluster included two 3-hour observations and one 8-hour observation. The 3-hour observations were made with the use of a keyboard that operates in conjunction with a 20-channel Esterline-Angus Event Recorder. Each of 30 keys represents a maternal or infant behavior, and when a key is depressed it activates one or a combination of pens on the recorder, leaving a trace that shows the total duration of the observed behavior. This technique allows for a continuous record showing the total time and the sequence of behavior. For the 8-hour observation the same behaviors were studied but with the use of a modified time-sampling technique. The time-sampled units were one minute in length and the observer, using a stenciled form, placed a number opposite the appropriate behaviors to indicate their respective order of occurrence. Since each variable can be coded only once for each observational unit, a score of 480 is the maximum that can be received. The data to be presented in this paper are limited to the two 8-hour observations. The data obtained with the use of the keyboard will be dealt with elsewhere in terms of the sequencing of events.

The mothers who participated in these observations were told that this was a normative study of infant functioning under natural living conditions. It was stressed that they proceed with their normal routines and care of the infant as they would if the observer were not present. This structure was presented to the mothers during a brief introductory visit prior to the first observation. In addition, in order to reduce the mother's self-consciousness and facilitate her behaving in relatively typical fashion, the observer emphasized that it was the infant who was being studied and that her actions would be noted only in relation to what was happening to the infant. This approach seemed to be effective, since a number of mothers commented after the observations were completed that they were relieved that they were not the ones being studied. The extensiveness of the observations and the frequent use of informal conversation between the observer and mother seemed to contribute further to the naturalness of her behavior.

The observational variables, mean scores and sample sizes are presented in Table 1. These data are presented separately for the 3-week and the 3-month observations. The inter-rater reliabilities for these variables range from 7.4 to 1.00 with a median reliability of .97. Much of the data in this paper are presented for males and females separately, since by describing and comparing these two groups we are able to work from an established context that helps to clarify the theoretical meaning of the results. Also, the importance of sex differences is heavily emphasized in contemporary developmental theory and it is felt that infant data concerning these differences would provide a worthwhile addition to the literature that already exists on this matter for older subjects.

The variables selected for study are those which would seem to influence or reflect aspects of maternal contact. An additional, but related consideration in the selection of variables was that they have an apparent bearing on the organization of the infant's experience. Peter Wolff (1959), Janet Brown (1964), and Sibylle Escalona (1962) have described qualitative variations in infant state or activity level and others have shown that the response patterns of the infant are highly influenced by the state he is in (Bridger, 1965). Moreover, Levy (1958) has demonstrated that maternal behavior varies as a function of the state or activity level of the infant. Consequently, we have given particular attention to the variables concerning state (cry, fuss, awake active, awake passive, and sleep) because of the extent to which these behaviors seem to shape the infant's experience. Most of the variables listed in Table 1 are quite descriptive of what was observed. Those which might not be as clear are as follows: *attends infant*—denotes standing close or leaning over infant, usually while in the process of caretaking activities; *stimulates feeding*—stroking the infant's cheek and manipulating the nipple so as to induce sucking responses; *affectionate contact*—kissing and caressing infant; *stresses musculature*—holding the infant in either a sitting or standing position so that he is required to support his own weight; *stimulates/arouses infant*—mother provides tactile and visual stimulation for the infant or attempts to arouse him to a higher activity level; and *imitates infant*—mother repeats a behavior, usually a vocalization, immediately after it is observed in the infant.

The sex differences and shifts in behavior from 3 weeks to 3 months are in many instances pronounced. For example, at 3 weeks of age mothers held male infants about 27 minutes more per 8 hours than they held females, and at 3 months males were held 14 minutes longer. By the time they were 3 months of age there was a decrease of over 30% for both sexes in the total time they were held by their mothers. Sleep time also showed marked sex differences and changes over time. For the earlier observations females slept about an hour longer than males, and this difference tended to be maintained by 3 months with the female infants sleeping about 41 minutes longer. Again, there was a substantial reduction with age in this behavior for both sexes; a decrease of 67 and 86 minutes in sleep time for males and females, respectively. What is particularly striking is the variability for these infant and maternal variables. The range for sleep time is 137-391 minutes at 3 weeks and 120-344 minutes at 3 months, and the range for mother holding is 38-218 minutes

TABLE 1

Mean Frequency of Maternal and Infant Behavior
at 3 Weeks and 3 Months

Behavior	3-week observation		3-month observation [a]	
	Males [b] (N = 14)	Females (N = 15)	Males [b] (N = 13)	Females (N = 12)
Maternal variables				
Holds infant close	121.4	99.2	77.4	58.6
Holds infant distant	32.2	18.3	26.7	27.2
Total holds	131.3	105.5	86.9	73.4
Attends infant	61.7	44.2	93.0	81.8
Maternal contact				
(holds and attends)	171.1	134.5	158.8	133.8
Feeds infant	60.8	60.7	46.6	41.4
Stimulates feeding	10.1	14.0	1.6	3.6
Burps infant	39.0	25.9	20.9	15.3
Affectionate contact	19.9	15.9	32.8	22.7
Rocks infant	35.1	20.7	20.0	23.9
Stresses musculature	11.7	3.3	25.8	16.6
Stimulates/arouses infant	23.1	10.6	38.9	26.1
Imitates infant	1.9	2.9	5.3	7.6
Looks at infant	182.8	148.1	179.5	161.9
Talks to infant	104.1	82.2	117.5	116.1
Smiles at infant	23.2	18.6	45.9	46.4
Infant variables				
Cry	43.6	30.2	28.5	16.9
Fuss	65.7	44.0	59.0	36.0
Irritable (cry and fuss)	78.7	56.8	67.3	42.9
Awake active	79.6	55.1	115.8	85.6
Awake passive	190.0	138.6	257.8	241.1
Drowsy	74.3	74.7	27.8	11.1
Sleep	261.7	322.1	194.3	235.6
Supine	133.7	59.3	152.7	134.8
Eyes on mother	72.3	49.0	91.0	90.6
Vocalizes	152.3	179.3	207.2	207.4
Infant smiles	11.1	11.7	32.1	35.3
Mouths	36.8	30.6	61.2	116.2

[a] Four of the subjects were unable to participate in the 3-month observation. Two moved out of the area, one mother became seriously ill, and another mother chose not to participate in all the observations.

[b] One subject who had had an extremely difficult delivery was omitted from the descriptive data but is included in the findings concerning mother-infant interaction.

at 3 weeks and 26-168 minutes for the 3-month observation. The extent of the individual differences reflected by these ranges seems to have important implications. For instance, if an infant spends more time at a higher level of consciousness this should increase his experience and contact with the mother, and through greater learning opportunities, facilitate the perceptual discriminations he makes, and affect the quality of his cognitive organization. The finding that some of the infants in our sample slept a little over 2 hours, or about 25% of the observation time, and others around 6 hours, or 75% of the time, is a fact that has implications for important developmental processes. The sum crying and fussing, what we term irritability level of the infant, is another potentially important variable. The range of scores for this behavior was from 5-136 minutes at 3 weeks and 7-98 at 3 months. The fact that infants are capable through their behavior of shaping maternal treatment is a point that has gained increasing recognition. The cry is a signal for the mother to respond and variation among infants in this behavior could lead to differential experiences with the mother.

Table 2 presents t values showing changes in the maternal and infant behaviors from the 3-week to the 3-month observation. In this case, the data for the males and females are combined since the trends, in most instances, are the same for both sexes. It is not surprising that there are a number of marked shifts in behavior from 3 weeks to 3 months, since the early months of life are characterized by enormous growth and change. The maternal variables that show the greatest decrement are those involving feeding behaviors and close physical contact. It is of interest that the decrease in close contact is paralleled by an equally pronounced increase in attending behavior, so that the net amount of maternal contact remains similar for the 3-week and 3-month observations. The main difference was that the mothers, for the later observation, tended to hold their infants less but spent considerably more time near them, in what usually was a vis-à-vis posture, while interacting and ministering to their needs. Along with this shift, the mothers showed a marked increase in affectionate behavior toward the older infant, positioned him more so that he was required to make active use of his muscles, presented him with a greater amount of stimulation and finally, she exhibited more social behavior (imitated, smiled, and talked) toward the older child.

The changes in maternal behavior from 3 weeks to 3 months probably are largely a function of the maturation of various characteristics of the infant. However, the increased confidence of the mother, her greater familiarity with her infant, and her developing attachment toward him

TABLE 2

CHANGES IN BEHAVIOR BETWEEN 3 WEEKS AND 3 MONTHS $(N = 26)$

Maternal variables	t-values	Infant variables	t-values
Higher at 3 weeks:		*Higher at 3 weeks:*	
Holds infant close	4.43****	Cry	2.84***
Holds infant distant	.56	Fuss	1.33
Total holds	4.00****	Irritable (cry and fuss)	1.73*
Maternal contact		Drowsy	9.02****
(holds and attends)	.74	Sleep	4.51****
Feeds infant	3.49***		
Stimulates feeding	3.42***		
Burps infant	3.28***		
Rocks infant	1.08		
Higher at 3 months:		*Higher at 3 months:*	
Attends infant	5.15****	Awake active	2.47**
Affectionate contact	2.50**	Awake passive	5.22****
Stresses musculature	3.42***	Supine	1.75*
Stimulates/arouses infant	2.63**	Eyes on mother	3.21***
Imitates infant	4.26****	Vocalizes	3.56***
Looks at infant	.38	Infant smiles	6.84***
Talks to infant	2.67**	Mouths	3.69***
Smiles at infant	4.79****		

$* p < .10 \qquad ** p < .05 \qquad *** p < .01 \qquad **** p < .001$

will also account for some of the changes that occurred over this period of time.

By 3 months of age the infant is crying less and awake more. Moreover, he is becoming an interesting and responsive person. There are substantial increases in the total time spent by him in smiling, vocalizing, and looking at the mother's face, so that the greater amount of social-type behavior he manifested at three months parallels the increments shown in the mother's social responsiveness toward him over the same period. The increase with age in the time the infant is kept in a supine position also should facilitate his participation in vis-à-vis interactions with the mother as well as provide him with greater opportunity for varied visual experiences.

Table 3 presents the correlations between the 3-week and the 3-month observations for the maternal and infant behaviors we studied. These findings further reflect the relative instability of the mother-infant system over the first few months of life. Moderate correlation coefficients

TABLE 3

CORRELATIONS BETWEEN OBSERVATIONS AT 3 WEEKS AND AT 3 MONTHS
($N = 26$)

Maternal variables	$r =$	Infant variables	$r =$
Holds infant close	.23	Cry	.28
Holds infant distant	.04	Fuss	.42**
Total holds	.13	Irritable (cry and fuss)	.37*
Attends infant	.36*	Awake active	.25
Maternal contact		Awake passive	.26
(holds and attends)	.25	Drowsy	.44**
Feeds infant	.21	Sleep	.24
Stimulates feeding	.37*	Supine	.29
Burps infant	.20	Eyes on mother	—.12
Affectionate contact	.64****	Vocalizes	.41**
Rocks infant	.29	Infant smiles	.32
Stresses musculature	.06	Mouths	—.17
Stimulates/arouses infant	.23		
Imitates infant	.45**		
Looks at infant	.37*		
Talks to infant	.58***		
Smiles at infant	.66****		

$* p < .10$ $** p < .05$ $*** p < .01$ $**** p < .001$

were obtained only for the class of maternal variables concerning affectionate-social responses. It thus may be that these behaviors are more sensitive indicators of enduring maternal attitudes than the absolute amount of time the mother devoted to such activities as feeding and physical contact. The few infant variables that show some stability are, with the exception of vocalizing, those concerning the state of the organism. Even though some of the behaviors are moderately stable from three weeks to three months, the overall magnitude of the correlations reported in Table 3 seems quite low considering that they represent repeated measures of the same individual over a relatively short period.

Table 4 presents t-values based on comparisons between the sexes for the 3-week and 3-month observations. A number of statistically significant differences were obtained with, in most instances, the boys having higher mean scores than the girls. The sex differences are most pronounced at 3 weeks for both maternal and infant variables. By 3 months the boys and girls are no longer as clearly differentiated on the maternal variables although the trend persists for the males to tend to have higher mean scores. On the other hand, the findings for the infant variables

TABLE 4

Sex Differences in Frequency of Maternal and Infant Behaviors at 3 Weeks and 3 Months

Maternal variables	t-values 3 weeks	3 months	Infant variables	t-values 3 weeks	3 months
Male higher:			*Male higher*:		
Holds infant close	1.42	1.52	Cry	1.68	1.11
Holds infant distant	2.64**		Fuss	2.48**	3.47***
Total holds	1.65	1.12	Irritable (cry and fuss)	2.23**	2.68**
Attends infant	2.66**	1.10	Awake active	1.66	.57
Maternal contact			Awake passive	2.94***	1.77*
(holds and attends)	2.09**	1.57			
Feeds infant	.06	.27	Drowsy		.41
Burps infant	1.67	.69	Supine	2.30**	1.07
Affectionate contact	.90	1.00	Eyes on mother	1.99*	.75
Rocks infant	1.21		Mouths	.64	
Stresses musculature	2.48**	1.67			
Stimulates/arouses					
infant	2.20**	1.53			
Looks at infant	1.97*	1.36			
Talks to infant	1.02	.79			
Smiles at infant	.57				
Female higher:			*Female higher*:		
Holds infant distant		.05	Drowsy	.03	
Stimulates feeding	.62	1.47	Sleep	3.15***	2.87***
Rocks infant		.82	Vocalizes	1.34	.23
Imitates infant	.80	1.76*	Infant smiles	.02	.08
Smiles at infant		.44	Mouths		2.57**

* $p < .10$ \qquad ** $p < .05$ \qquad *** $p < .01$

concerning state remain relatively similar at 3 weeks and 3 months. Thus, the sex differences are relatively stable for the two observations even though the stability coefficients for the total sample are low (in terms of our variables).

In general, these results indicate that much more was happening with the male infants than with the female infants. Males slept less and cried more during both observations and these behaviors probably contributed to the more extensive and stimulating interaction the boys experienced with the mother, particularly for the 3-week observation. In order to determine the effect of state we selected the 15 variables, excluding those

TABLE 5

Sex Differences after Controlling for Irritability and Sleep Time through Analysis of Covariance[a]

Maternal or Infant Behaviors	Sleep time controlled for		Sex with higher mean score	Irritability controlled for		Sex with higher mean score
	3 weeks	3 months		3 weeks	3 months	
Variables	t	t		t	t	
Holds infant close	.30	1.22		.64	1.70	
Holds infant distant	.59	—.20		.92	—.20	
Total holds	.43	.88		.86	1.08	
Attends infant	1.12	1.36		1.91*	.94	Males
Maternal contact (holds and attends)	.62	1.04		1.20	1.12	
Stimulates feeding	.55	—1.12		—.09	—1.06	
Affectionate contact	—.46	.91		.56	1.27	
Rocks	.35	—.70		.44	—1.44	
Stresses musculature	1.84*	.71	Males	1.97*	1.40	
Stimulates/arouses infant	2.09**	1.82*	Males	2.43**	2.31**	Males
Imitates infant	—.91	—2.73**	Females	—.63	—2.14**	Females
Looks at infant	.58	1.35		1.17	1.02	
Talks to infant	—.48	.24		.70	.59	
Infant supine	.82	—.03		1.36	.69	
Eyes on mother	.37	.58		1.76*	—.37	Males

* p < .10   ** p < .05

a A positive t-value indicates that males had the higher mean score, and a negative t-value indicates a higher mean score for females.

dealing with state, where the sex differences were most marked and did an analysis of covariance with these variables, controlling for irritability and another analysis of covariance controlling for sleep. These results are presented in Table 5. When the state of the infant was controlled for, most of the sex differences were no longer statistically significant. The exceptions were that the t-values were greater, after controlling for state, for the variables "mother stimulates/arouses infant" and "mother imitates infant." The higher score for "stimulates/arouses" was obtained for the males and the higher score for "imitates" by the females. The variable "imitates" involves repeating vocalizations made by the child, and it is interesting that mothers exhibited more of this behavior with the girls. This response could be viewed as the reinforcement of verbal behavior, and the evidence presented here suggests that the mothers differentially reinforce this behavior on the basis of the sex of the child.

In order to further clarify the relation between infant state and maternal treatment, product-moment correlations were computed relating the infant irritability score with the degree of maternal contact. The maternal contact variable is based on the sum of the holding and attending scores with the time devoted to feeding behaviors subtracted out. These correlations were computed for the 3-week and 3-month observations for the male and female samples combined and separate. At 3 weeks a correlation of .52 ($p < .01$) was obtained between irritability and maternal contact for the total sample. However, for the female sub sample this correlation was .68 ($p < 0.2$) and for males only .20 (non. sig.). Furthermore, a somewhat similar pattern occurred for the correlations between maternal contact and infant irritability for the 3-month observation. At this age the correlation is .37 ($p < .10$ level) for the combined sample and .54 ($p < .05$ level) for females and —.47 ($p < .10$ level) for males. A statistically significant difference was obtained ($t =$ 2.40, $p < .05$ level) in a test comparing the difference between the female and male correlations for the 3-month observation. In other words maternal contact and irritability positively covaried for females at both ages; whereas for males, there was no relationship at 3 weeks, and by 3 months the mothers tended to spend less time with the more irritable male babies. It should be emphasized that these correlations reflect within group patterns, and that when we combine the female and male samples positive correlations still emerge for both ages. Since the males had substantially higher scores for irritability and maternal contact than the females, the correlation for the male subjects does not strongly attenuate the correlations derived for the total sample, even when the males within group covariation seems random or negative. That is, in terms of the total sample, the patterning of the males scores is still consistent with a positive relationship between irritability and maternal contact.

From these findings it is difficult to posit a causal relationship. However, it seems most plausible that it is the infant's cry that is determining the maternal behavior. Mothers describe the cry as a signal that the infant needs attention and they often report their nurturant actions in response to the cry. Furthermore, the cry is a noxious and often painful stimulus that probably has biological utility for the infant, propelling the mother into action for her own comfort as well as out of concern for the infant. Ethological reports confirm the proposition that the cry functions as a "releaser" of maternal behavior (Bowlby, 1958; Hinde, et al., 1964; Hoffman, et al., 1966). Bowlby (1958) states:

> It is my belief that both of them (crying and smiling), act as social releasers of instinctual responses in mothers. As regards crying, there

is plentiful evidence from the animal world that this is so: probably in all cases the mother responds promptly and unfailingly to her infant's bleat, call or cry. It seems to me clear that similar impulses are also evoked in the human mother. . . .

Thus, we are adopting the hypothesis that the correlations we have obtained reflect a causal sequence whereby the cry acts to instigate maternal intervention. Certainly there are other important determinants of maternal contact, and it is evident that mothers exhibit considerable variability concerning how responsive they are to the stimulus signal of the cry. Yet it seems that the effect of the cry is sufficient to account at least partially for the structure of the mother-infant relationship. We further maintain the thesis that the infant's cry shapes maternal behavior even for the instance where the negative correlation was noted at 3 months for the males. The effect is still present, but in this case the more irritable infants were responded to *less* by the mothers. Our speculation for explaining this relationship and the fact that, conversely, a positive correlation was obtained for the female infants is that the mothers probably were negatively reinforced for responding to a number of the boys but tended to be positively reinforced for their responses toward the girls. That is, mothers of the more irritable boys may have learned that they could not be successful in quieting boys whereas the girls were more uniformly responsive (quieted by) to maternal handling. There is not much present in our data to bear out this contention, with the exception that the males were significantly more irritable than the girls for both observations. However, evidence that suggests males are more subject to inconsolable states comes from studies (Serr and Ismajovich, 1963; McDonald, Gynther, and Christakos, 1963; Stechler, 1964) which indicate that males have less well organized physiological reactions and are more vulnerable to adverse conditions than females. The relatively more efficient functioning of the female organism should thus contribute to their responding more favorably to maternal intervention.

In summary, we propose that maternal behavior initially tends to be under the control of the stimulus and reinforcing conditions provided by the young infant. As the infant gets older, the mother, if she behaved contingently toward his signals, gradually acquires reinforcement value which in turn increases her efficacy in regulating infant behaviors. Concurrently, the earlier control asserted by the infant becomes less functional and diminishes. In a sense, the point where the infant's control over the mother declines and the mother's reinforcement value emerges could be regarded as the first manifestation of socialization, or at least represents the initial conditions favoring social learning. Thus, at first the mother is shaped by the infant and this later facilitates her shaping the behavior of the infant. We would therefore say that the infant, through his own temperament or signal system, contributes to establishing the stimulus and reinforcement value eventually associated with the mother. According to this reasoning, the more irritable infants (who can be soothed) whose mothers respond in a contingent manner to their signals should become most amenable to the effects of social reinforcement and manifest a higher degree of attachment behavior. The fact that the mothers responded more contingently toward the female infants should maximize the ease with which females learn social responses.

This statement is consistent with data on older children which indicate that girls learn social responses earlier and with greater facility than boys. (Becker, 1964). Previously we argued that the mothers learned to be more contingent toward the girls because they probably were more responsive to maternal intervention. An alternative explanation is that mothers respond contingently to the girls and not to the boys as a form of differential reinforcement, whereby, in keeping with cultural expectations, the mother is initiating a pattern that contributes to males being more aggressive or assertive, and less responsive to socialization. Indeed, these two explanations are not inconsistent with one another since the mother who is unable to soothe an upset male infant may eventually come to classify this intractable irritability as an expression of "maleness."

There are certain environmental settings where noncontingent caretaking is more likely and these situations should impede social learning and result in weaker attachment responses. Lennenberg (1965) found that deaf parents tended not to respond to the infant's cry. One would have to assume that it was more than the inability to hear the infant that influenced their behavior, since even when they observed their crying infants these parents tended not to make any effort to quiet them. The function of the cry as a noxious stimulus or "releaser" of maternal behavior did not pertain under these unusual circumstances. Infants in institutions also are more likely to be cared for in terms of some arbitrary schedule with little opportunity for them to shape caretakers in accordance with their own behavioral vicissitudes.

Although we have shown that there is a covariation between maternal contact and infant irritability and have attempted to develop some theoretical implications concerning this relationship, considerable variability remains as to how responsive different mothers are to their infants' crying behavior. This variability probably reflects differences in maternal attitudes. Women who express positive feelings about babies and who consider the well-being of the infant to be of essential importance should tend to be more responsive to signals of distress from the infant than women who exhibit negative maternal attitudes. In order to test this assumption, we first derived a score for measuring maternal responsiveness. This score was obtained through a regression analysis where we determined the amount of maternal contact that would be expected for each mother by controlling for her infant's irritability score. The expected maternal contact score was then subtracted from the mother's actual contact score and this difference was used as the measure of maternal responsivity. The maternal responsivity scores were obtained separately for the 3-week and the 3-month observations. The parents of 23 of the infants in our sample were interviewed for a project investigating marital careers, approximately 2 years prior to the birth of their child, and these interviews provided us with the unusual opportunity of having antecedent data relevant to prospective parental functioning. A number of variables from this material were rated and two of them, "acceptance of nurturant role," and the "degree that the baby is seen in a positive sense" were correlated with the scores of the maternal responsivity measure.* Annotated definitions of these interview variables are as follows:

> "Acceptance of nurturant role" concerns the degree to which the subject is interested in caring for others and in acquiring domestic and homemaking skills such as cooking, sewing, and cleaning house. Evidence for a high rating would be describing the care of infants and children with much pleasure and satisfaction even when this involves subordinating her own needs.
> The interview variable concerning the "degree that the baby is seen in a positive sense" assesses the extent to which the subject views a baby as gratifying, pleasant and non-burdensome. In discussing what she imagines infants to be like she stresses the warmer, more personal, and rewarding aspects of the baby and anticipates these qualities as primary.

Correlations of .40 ($p < .10$ level) and .48 ($p < .05$ level) were obtained between the ratings on "acceptance of nurturant role" and the maternal responsivity scores for the 3-week and 3-month observations, respectively. The "degree that the baby is seen in a positive sense" correlated .38 ($p < .10$ level) and .44 ($p < .05$ level) with maternal responsivity for the two ages. However, the two interview variables were so highly intercorrelated ($r = .93$) that they clearly involve the same

---

* Dr. Kenneth Robson collaborated in developing these variables, and made the ratings.

dimension. Thus, the psychological status of the mother, assessed substantially before the birth of her infant, as well as the infant's state, are
predictive of her maternal behavior. Schaffer and Emerson (1964) found
that maternal responsiveness to the cry was associated with the attachment behavior of infants. Extrapolating from our findings, we now
have some basis for assuming that the early attitudes of the mother
represent antecedent conditions for facilitating the attachment behavior
observed by Schaffer and Emerson.

The discussion to this point has focused on some of the conditions that
seemingly affect the structure of the mother-infant relationship and influence the reinforcement and stimulus values associated with the mother.
Next we would like to consider, in a more speculative vein, one particular
class of maternal behaviors that has important reinforcing properties for
the infant. This discussion will be more general and depart from a direct
consideration of the data. There has been mounting evidence in the
psychological literature that the organism has a "need for stimulation"
and that variations in the quantity and quality of stimulation received
can have a significant effect on many aspects of development (Moss, 1965;
Murphy, et al., 1962; White and Held, 1963). Additional reports indicate
that not only does the infant require stimulation, but excessive or
chaotic dosages of stimulation can be highly disruptive of normal functioning (Murphy, et al., 1962). Furthermore, there appear to be substantial individual differences in the stimulation that is needed or in the extremes that can be tolerated. As the infant gets older he becomes
somewhat capable of regulating the stimulation that is assimilated. However, the very young infant is completely dependent on the caretaking
environment to provide and modulate the stimulation he experiences. It
is in this regard that the mother has a vital role.

The main points emphasized in the literature are that stimulation
serves to modulate the state or arousal level of the infant, organize and
direct attentional progress, and facilitate normal growth and development. Bridger (1965) has shown that stimulation tends to have either an
arousing or quieting effect, depending on the existing state of the infant.
Infants who are quiet tend to be aroused, whereas aroused infants tend
to be quieted by moderate stimulation. Moreover, according to data collected by Birns (1965), these effects occur for several stimulus modalities
and with stable individual differences in responsivity. (We found that
mothers made greater use of techniques involving stimulation—"stresses
musculature" and "stimulates/arouses"—with the males who as a group
were more irritable than the females.)

The capacity for stimulus configurations to direct attention, once the infant is in an optimally receptive state, also has been demonstrated by a number of studies. Young infants have been observed to orient toward many stimuli (Razran, 1961; Fantz, 1963), and certain stimuli are so compelling that they tend to "capture" the infant in a fixed orientation (Stechler, 1965). Other studies have demonstrated that infants show clear preferences for gazing at more complex visual patterns (Fantz, 1963). Thus, stimulation can influence the set of the infant to respond by modifying the state of the organism as well as structure learning possibilities through directing the infant's attention. White (1959) has systematically described how stimulation contributes to the learning process in infants. He points out that the infant is provided with the opportunity to activate behavioral potentials in attempting to cope with control stimulation. Motor and perceptual skills eventually become refined and sharpened in the process of responding to stimulus configurations and it is this pattern of learning which White calls "effectance behavior."

Not all levels of stimulation are equally effective in producing a condition whereby the infant is optimally alert and attentive. Excessive stimulation has a disruptive effect and according to drive reduction theorists the organism behaves in ways aimed at reducing stimulation that exceeds certain limits. Leuba (1955), in an attempt to establish rapprochement between the drive reduction view and the research evidence that shows that there is a need for stimulation, states that there is an optimal level of stimulation that is required, and that the organism acts either to reduce or to increase stimulation so as to stay within this optimal range.

The mother is necessarily highly instrumental in mediating much of the stimulation that is experienced by the infant. Her very presence in moving about and caring for the infant provides a constant source of visual, auditory, tactile, kinesthetic and proprioceptive stimulation. In addition to the incidental stimulation she provides, the mother deliberately uses stimulation to regulate the arousal level or state of the infant and to evoke specific responses from him. However, once the infant learns, through conditioning, that the mother is a source of stimulation he can in turn employ existing responses that are instrumental in eliciting stimulation from her. Certain infant behaviors, such as the cry, are so compelling that they readily evoke many forms of stimulation from the mother. It is common knowledge that mothers in attempting to quiet upset infants, often resort to such tactics as using rocking motion, waving bright objects or rattles, or holding the infant close and thus provide warmth and physical contact. The specific function of stimulation in placating the crying infant can be somewhat obscured because of the possibility of confounding conditions. In our discussion so far we have indicated that stimulation inherently has a quieting effect irrespective of learning but that crying also can become a learned instrumental behavior which terminates once the reinforcement of stimulation is presented. However, it is often difficult to distinguish the unlearned from the learned patterns of functioning, since the infant behavior (crying) and the outcome (quieting) are highly similar in both instances. Perhaps the best means for determining whether learning has occurred would be if we could demonstrate that the infant makes anticipatory responses, such as the reduction in crying behavior to cues, prior to the actual occurrence of stimulation. In addition to the cry, the smile and the vocalization of the infant can become highly effective, and consequently well-learned conditioned responses for evoking stimulation from adult caretakers. Rheingold (1956) has shown that when institutional children are given more caretaking by an adult they show an increase in their smiling rate to that caretaker as well as to other adults. Moreover, for a few weeks after the intensive caretaking stopped there were further substantial increments in the smiling rate, which suggests that the infant after experiencing relative deprivation worked harder in attempting to restitute the stimulation level experienced earlier.

It seems plausible that much of the early social behavior seen in infants and children consists of attempts to elicit responses from others. We mentioned earlier that it has been stressed in recent psychological literature that individuals have a basic need for stimulation. Since the mother, and eventually others, are highly instrumental in providing and monitoring the stimulation that is experienced by the infant, it seems likely that the child acquires expectancies for having this need satisfied through social interactions and that stimulation comes to serve as a basis for relating to others. Indeed, Schaffer and Emerson (1964) have shown that the amount of stimulation provided by adults is one of the major determinants of infants' attachment behavior. Strange as well as familiar adults who have been temporarily separated from an infant often attempt to gain rapport with the infant through acts of stimulation. It is quite common for the father, upon returning home from work, to initiate actions aimed at stimulating the child, and these actions are usually responded to with clear pleasure. Because of the expectancies that are built up some of the provocative behaviors seen in children, particularly when confronted with a non-responsive adult, could be interpreted as attempts to elicit socially mediated stimulation.

The learning we have discussed is largely social since the infant is dependent on others, particularly the mother, for reinforcements. This dependency on others is what constitutes attachment behavior, and the specific makeup of the attachment is determined by the class of reinforcements that are involved. The strength of these learned attachment behaviors is maximized through stimulation, since the mother is often the embodiment of this reinforcement as well as the agent for delivering it. The social aspect of this learning is further enhanced because of the reciprocal dependence of the mother on the infant for reinforcement. That is, the mother learns certain conditioned responses, often involving acts of stimulation, that are aimed at evoking desired states or responses from the infant.

In conclusion, what we did was study and analyze some of the factors which structure the mother-infant relationship. A central point is that the state of the infant affects the quantity and quality of maternal behavior, and this in turn would seem to influence the course of future social learning. Furthermore, through controlling for the state of the infant, we were able to demonstrate the effects of pre-parental attitudes on one aspect of maternal behavior, namely, the mother's responsiveness toward her infant. Many investigators, in conducting controlled laboratory studies, have stressed that the state of the infant is crucial in determining the nature of his responses to different stimuli. This concern is certainly highly relevant to our data, collected under naturalistic conditions.

REFERENCES

BECKER, W. C.: Consequences of different kinds of parental discipline. In M. L. Hoffman & Lois W. Hoffman (Eds.), Review of child development research: I. New York: Russell Sage Found., 1964. Pp. 169-208.

BIRNS, B.: Individual differences in human neonates' responses to stimulation. Child Develpm., 1965, 36, 249-256.

BLOOM, B. S.: Stability and change in human characteristics. New York: Wiley, 1964.

BOWLBY, J.: The nature of a child's tie to his mother. Internat. J. Psychoanal., 1958, 39, 350-373.

BRIDGER, W. H.: Psychophysiological measurement of the roles of state in the human neonate. Paper presented at Soc. Res. Child Develpm., Minneapolis, April, 1965.

BROWN, JANET L.: States in newborn infants. Merrill-Palmer Quart., 1964, 10, 313-327.

ESCALONA, SIBYLLE K.: The study of individual differences and the problem of state. J. Child Psychiat., 1962, 1, 11-37.

FANTZ, R.: Pattern vision in newborn infants. Science, 1963, 140, 296-297.

HESS, E. H.: Imprinting. Science, 1959, 130, 133-141.

HINDE, R. A., ROWELL, T. E., & SPENCER-BOOTH, Y.: Behavior of living rhesus monkeys in their first six months. Proc. Zool. Soc., London, 1964, 143, 609-649.

HOFFMAN, H., et al.: Enhanced distress vocalization through selective reinforcement. Science, 1966, 151, 354-356.

LENNENBERG, E. H., REBELSKY, FREDA G., & NICHOLS, I. A.: The vocalizations of infants born to deaf and to hearing parents. Vita Humana, 1965, 8, 23-37.

LEUBBA, C.: Toward some integration of learning theories: The concept of optimal stimulation. Psychol. Rep., 1955, 1, 27-33.

LEVY, D. M.: Behavioral analysis. Springfield, Ill.: Charles C Thomas, 1958.

McDonald, R. L., Gynther, M. D., & Christakos, A. C.: Relations between maternal anxiety and obstetric complications. *Psychosom. Med.*, 1963, 25, 357-362.

Moss, H. A.: Coping behavior, the need for stimulation, and normal development. *Merrill-Palmer Quart.*, 1965, 11, 171-179.

Murphy, Lois B., et al. *The widening world of childhood.* New York: Basic Books, 1962.

Noirot, Elaine.: Changes in responsiveness to young in the adult mouse: the effect of external stimuli. *J. comp. physiol. Psychol.*, 1964, 57, 97-99.

Razran, G. The observable unconscious and the inferable conscious in current Soviet psychophysiology: Interoceptive conditioning, semantic conditioning, and the orienting reflex. *Psychol. Rev.*, 1961, 68, 81-146.

Rheingold, Harriet L.: The modification of social responsiveness in institutional babies. *Monogr. Soc. Res. Child Develpm.*, 1956, 21, No. 2 (Serial No. 23).

Schaffer, H. R. & Emerson, Peggy E.: The development of social attachments in infancy. *Monogr. Soc. Res. Child Develpm.*, 1964, 29, No. 3 (Serial No. 94).

Serr, D. M. & Ismajovich, B.: Determination of the primary sex ratio from human abortions. *Amer. J. Obstet. Gyncol.*, 1963, 87, 63-65.

Stechler, G.: A longitudinal follow-up of neonatal apnea. *Child Develpm.*, 1964, 35, 333-348.

Stechler, G.: Paper presented at Soc. Res. Child Develpm., Minneapolis, April, 1965.

White, B. L. & Held, R.: Plasticity in perceptual development during the first six months of life. Paper presented at Amer. Ass. Advncmnt. Sci., Cleveland, Ohio, December, 1963.

White, R. W.: Motivation reconsidered: the concept of competence. *Psychol. Rev.*, 1959, 66, 297-323.

Wolff, P. H.: Observations on newborn infants. *Psychosom. Med.*, 1959, 21, 110-118.

6

THE ROLE OF EYE-TO-EYE CONTACT IN MATERNAL-INFANT ATTACHMENT

Kenneth S. Robson, M.D.

Child Research Branch, National Institute of Mental Health, Bethesda, Maryland*

Among clinicians and researchers in child development there is general agreement that the character and quality of one's earliest relationships will contribute significantly to, and even predict the nature of, many later behaviours. Consequently, increasing attention is being focussed on the parameters of maternal-infant interaction in a search to define the more significant variables of this system. An eloquent attempt in this direction was made by Bowlby (1958) in a paper devoted to "The nature of the child's tie to his mother." After reviewing the relevant aspects of both psychoanalytic and learning theories, Bowlby takes an ethological position in describing the growth of the infant's first relationship. He cites five behaviours—crying, smiling, following, clinging, and sucking—as innate "releasers" of maternal caretaking responses.

The point of departure of the present report is to add another variable to Bowlby's list: eye-to-eye contact, an interchange that mediates a substantial part of the non-verbal transactions between human beings. This interaction (as will be noted later) is well known in the animal kingdom, and it is beginning to be studied by observers of adult behavior (Exline, 1963; Exline and Winters, 1965; Argyle and Dean, 1965) but has

* Present address: Department of Psychiatry, Tufts New England Medical Center, Boston, Massachusetts. Reprinted with permission from the *Journal of Child Psychology and Psychiatry*, Vol. 8, No. 1, May 1967, pp. 13-25, Pergamon Press.

received little consideration by child development researchers. In this report the vicissitudes of eye-to-eye contact will be followed through the first six months of life with an emphasis on attachment from the point of view of both mother and infant. The author's aim is to bring together a number of diverse but related observations in order to offer some ideas that can be subjected to experimental verification.

Some introductory comments on the visual mode

There are some unique peculiarities of the visual mode that favour its preeminence as a major vehicle of intra-psychic and inter-personal development. Greenman (1963) states that of all the neonatal reflexes visual fixation and following are the only ones that do not drop out over time, but, on the contrary, demonstrate increasing facility. Rheingold (1961) notes that this behavior ". . . is all the more remarkable . . . because of its maturity relative to . . . other patterns of behaviour . . . (so that by the end of the second month) . . . it is already in the form it will keep throughout life." Furthermore, following and fixation are among the first acts of the infant that are both intentional and subject to his control. Vision is the only modality which, by closure of the eyelids, gaze aversion, and pupillary constriction and dilation, is constructed as an "on-off" system that can easily modulate or eliminate external sensory input, sometimes at will, within the first months of life. And, finally, the appeal of the mother's eyes to the child (and of his eyes to her) is facilitated by their stimulus richness. In comparison with other areas of the body surface the eye has a remarkable array of interesting qualities such as the shininess of the globe, the fact that it is mobile while at the same time fixed in space, the contrasts between the pupil-iris-cornea configuration, the capacity of the pupil to vary in diameter, and the differing effects of variations in the width of the palpebral fissure.

Rheingold (1961) has suggested that ". . . not physical, but visual contact is at the basis of human sociability . . .", and she adds ". . . (that the) basic and primary activity is the infant's visual exploration of his environment . . .". In his observations of neonatal visual behaviour Greenman (1963) makes the point that the importance of vision ". . . exceeds the essential role it plays in perception of the outside world and in differentiating the self from the non-self . . . (in that) . . . one of the primary ways in which human beings communicate at a non-verbal level is by looking at one another . . . (and) . . . when visual communication does not exist between humans, something deviant or pathological often exists in the relationship."

The first comprehensive review of the functions of the distance receptors, vision and hearing, in the development of social responsiveness has been made by Walters and Parke (1965). As for vision, it is only recently that studies exclusively concerned with the role of this modality as an important avenue for accomplishing the tasks of early development have appeared in the literature. These have tended to fall into three categories, the first of which has been concerned with the evolution of perceptual and attentive capacities in the infant (Fantz, 1958; Greenman, 1963; Kagan, 1965; Kagan and Lewis, 1965; Lewis, Kagan and Kalafat, 1966; Kagan, Henker, Hen-Tov, Levine and Lewis, 1966; Stechler and Latz, 1966; White and Castle, 1964; White, Castle, and Held, 1964; Wolff and White, 1965; Wolff, 1965). Another group of papers has described, primarily from the psychoanalytic point of view, the effects of blindness on maturational processes (Burlingham, 1964; Fraiberg and Freedman, 1964; Nagera and Colonna, 1965; Sandler, 1953; Wills, 1955). Although these efforts have been useful, a reconstruction of the functions of vision built upon the effects of its absence is fraught with difficulties, not the least of which is maternal disturbance secondary to the birth of a severely defective child. A third series of reports approaches behaviour, broadly speaking, from the ethological position (Ambrose, 1961; Freedman, 1961 and 1964; Harlow, 1961; Szekely, 1954; Wolff, 1963). Of the latter type, three studies have particular relevance to eye-to-eye contact. Kaila (1935), Spitz and Wolff (1946) and Ahrens (1954) —all of whom were exploring the infant's social responses to faces— have established an important fact: that one of the earliest and most effective stimuli for eliciting social smiling is a visual gestalt ("key stimulus" in ethological terms) consisting of the two eyes and forehead configuration *en face,* i.e. such that the eyes of the infant and those of the observer meet fully in the same vertical plane of rotation. Indirect confirmation for this finding is implicit in Watson's (1965) work. Studying both smiling to, and fixation of, faces and face schemata, in infants from 7 to 26 weeks of age, he found that both behaviours were maximal in the *en face* position. Watson also noted that this facial orientation was not the most frequent in routine caretaking but that when mothers addressed their infants "socially," i.e. to the face, they used the *en face* orientation. But none of these authors, including Spitz (1965) in his recent text on the formation of early object relations, elaborate on the long-range significance of this eye-to-eye interaction in more than a passing way.

The beginnings of maternal attachment

The development of maternal attachments in most non-human mammals requires a comparatively short time span, and the ties that result are rather abruptly terminated by active discouragement of the infant's approach behaviour. Rosenblatt (1966) has recently summarized the course of these processes in a number of animal species. Even in those species where infancy is prolonged, these non-human mothers seem to need far less responsiveness from their offspring than would satisfy man. Eye-to-eye contact and precursors of the human smiling response (i.e. lip retraction in dogs and cats and the "grins" and "grimaces" of primates) play a minimal part in sub-human attachments. When these behaviours serve a social function it is mainly to indicate fear, "appeasement," or the intention to attack (Andrew, 1965; Lorenz, 1953). "Staring down" in man occurs in a similar context. Generally, however, the more usual pattern of intermittent gaze fixation between humans ". . . signifies a readiness to interact . . . (and) . . . little social interaction is possible without it" (Hutt and Ounsted, 1966).

The human mother is subject to an extended, exceedingly trying and often unrewarding period of caring for her infant. Her neonate has a remarkably limited repertoire with which to sustain her. Indeed, his total helplessness, crying, elimination behavior, and physical appearance frequently elicit aversive reactions. Thus, in dealing with the human species, nature has been wise in making both eye-to-eye contact, and the social smile that it often releases in these early months, behaviours that at this stage of development generally foster positive maternal feelings and a sense of payment for "services rendered." As others have suggested (Ahrens, 1954; Freedman, 1964; and Szekely, 1954), there is no reason to believe that smiling and eye contact in human babies differ in origin from the primarily defensive functions they play in the animal world. Lorenz (1966) views the human smile as a ritualized form of aggression comparable to the "greeting" ceremonies which inhibit intraspecific fighting in many lower animals. Hence, though a mother's response to these achievements may be an *illusion,* from an evolutionary point of view it is an illusion with survival value.

Both Greenman (1963) and Wolff (1963) note the pleasure that new mothers take when their infants begin to "see" them. The latter author notes that during the fourth week of life ". . . the baby now seems to focus on the observer's eyes as if there were true eye-to-eye contact . . . (and) . . . it appears to be specifically the contact between the eyes (of the infant and the observer) that is effective (in evoking a smile)." Three of his mothers, who spent little time playing with their infants before the fourth week, suddenly began doing so within 2 or 3 days of his first recording eye-to-eye contact, yet these mothers had no idea of why this was so. Unlike the smiling response, which follows soon after eye contact is established, the infant's fixing of his mother's gaze seems rarely available to her for conscious recall.

One aspect of a longitudinal study in which the author is participating involves rather extensive post-natal interviews with fifty-four primiparous mothers.* Most of these women describe some initial feelings of "strangeness," "distance" and unfamiliarity towards their offspring which persist for at least the first few weeks of life. When one inquires as to when the mother first felt love, when she ceased feeling "strange" with her child and when he "became a person" to her, the answer to these questions frequently involves the baby's "*looking*," as if recognizing objects in the environment. A small number specifically articulate that eye-to-eye contact releases strong positive feelings. These feelings have something to do with "being recognized" in a highly personal and intimate way.

The resolution of maternal anxiety

When one "sees eye-to-eye" with another person, exclusive communication, "resonance," and accord of a fundamental sort are implied. The often intense discomfort experienced in encounters with the blind or cross-eyed may indeed stem in part from a variety of unconscious fantasies. But the absence of eye-to-eye contact in these situations realistically leaves one feeling ill at ease, since it impedes the most usual form of mutual recognition, assessment and contact. Visual impairment interferes with the development of certain social responses that are derivatives of eye-to-eye contact. Freedman (1964) comments that although fleeting spontaneous smiles emerge at the usual time in blind infants ". . . prolonged social smiling seems to require visual regard as a maintaining stimulus." Selma Fraiberg (personal communication), in her observations of blind infants, has noted that she was unable to carry out a normal "dialogue" with her subjects, with one exception, a baby who was supposedly blind but demonstrated visual following. She also comments (Fraiberg and Freedman, 1964) that "When the mother sought contact through her eyes, the child's eyes did not meet hers, which feels curiously like a rebuff if you do not know the baby is blind. All those ways in which the eyes unite human partners (are) denied this mother and baby." In an attenuated form, the same situation—probably one of the sources of early maternal anxiety—obtains for a new mother before her infant establishes eye contact with her. In the course of several home observations, previously anxious and uncomfortable mothers have told the author that they feel somehow "more at ease" and "comfortable" with their infants. This shift coincides with the beginning of true eye-to-eye contact over a time span as brief as three days, but as in Wolff's (1963) study these mothers were unable to specify why they felt differently.

The eye gestalt as a perceptual organizer

Though up to 3 months eye contact has no true social relevance to the infant, it may fulfil another function. A baby of this age reacts to a wide variety of endogenous and exogenous stimuli. Yet in terms of orienting, attentive and discriminative capacities, his visual apparatus is manifestly advanced relative to other receptor systems. Eye-to-eye contact occurs either simultaneously with, or in close contiguity to, many non-visual stimuli. Furthermore, the eye gestalt is a highly discriminable stimulus configuration that can focus and hold the infant's attention more successfully than many competing internal and external perceptual events. One could then speculate that in the first months of life many forms of stimulation are experienced by the infant as "coming from" the eyes of his caretakers. If this speculation were even partially true, and relevant empirical data will be presented below, the vicissitudes of eye-to-eye contact would provide one starting point for examining the origins and persistence of perceptions in adults whereby internal experiences are attributed to external events.

Many mothers report that as soon as eye-to-eye contact is established it often dominates the feeding situation, so that their infants are totally distracted from sucking. Only much later does the sight of breast or bottle evoke excitement. It is perfectly possible that the oral and body contact sensations of feeding may, through contiguity, be attributed to the eyes of the caretaker. Spitz (1965) was the first to suggest that the Isakower phenomenon (1938) and Lewin's (1950) "blank dream screen" represent a fusion of the breast and the visually perceived face. Also, when an infant of this age is spoken to he ignores the mouth of the speaker and fixates the eyes. According to Ahrens (1954) the mouth is not involved in eliciting the smiling response until the fifth or sixth month, and even then eye fixation precedes the smile.

Though relatively little is known about the development of body

---

* The senior investigator in this research is Dr. Howard A. Moss, Chief of Maternal-Infant Interaction Section, Child Research Branch, National Institute of Mental Health.

image, if attention to eyes is dominant in early development it should be reflected in the emerging body concept of the young child. Thus, despite the fact that psychoanalytic theory has emphasized the mouth as an early focal point of body image (Spitz, 1955), in terms of their salience the eyes should have priority. Shapiro and Stine (1965) collected the figure drawings of 3- and 4-year-old children in order to test the primacy of mouth perceptions. In their younger sample, less than 46 months old, 89 per cent drew eyes while 22 per cent drew the mouth. Ninety-nine per cent of children older than 46 months drew eyes and 75 per cent the mouth. They also found that eyes were represented independently of the nose and mouth, both of which tended to appear simultaneously and usually later in time. Some children, when asked to draw a face, will represent the eyes alone. As to whether figure drawings in fact represent body image, a definitive answer must await further research. Nonetheless, Shapiro and Stine suggest that the earliest body representations are taken from visual experience while tactile experiences are only later "projected." These drawings, of course, bear a strong resemblance to the "two eyes" gestalt mentioned earlier, a fact that further supports the argument that this stimulus configuration is selectively attended to as the "locus vitae" of the infant's primary caretakers, and as such serves as an important organizer of his perceptual world.

FOUR TO SIX MONTHS

Reciprocal attachment

By the fourth month an infant shows differential reactions of anticipatory excitement to his mother's approaching step, her voice, and for the present purposes most important, her face, by his selective smiling response. Up to this time his smiles have been indiscriminate. Ahrens (1954) states that the ". . . absolute stimulus . . . which must stand at the root of social behaviour . . . (is) . . . the eye part (of a mask or an observer's face)." Rheingold (1961) has pointed out that the infant's capacity to initiate physical contact and clinging develops towards the end of the first year of life. For sub-human primates such "contact comfort" (Harlow, 1961) is essential in establishing their first relationships and can be sought out from birth. Schaffer and Emerson (1964b) found that "non-cuddly" infants displayed less intense social relationships in the first year of life when compared with a "cuddly" group; but by 18-months both populations were comparable in their attachment behaviours. Elsewhere (Schaffer and Emerson, 1964a) they observe that with increasing frequency during the first year of life, situations in which "visually maintained contact" is interrupted are the most provocative of separation protest.

Eye-to-eye contact is one of the most intense and binding visual interactions for an infant at this age. And though visual scanning of other facial characteristics becomes an associated behaviour, the maternal eye gestalt retains its salience. Kagan *et al.* (1966) found that 4-month-old infants smiled far more often to the presentation of a realistic face stimulus than to those where the features were either scrambled or lacking eye representations. Children for 4½ to 10½ years-of-age, given the task of identifying familiar peers from photographs showing isolated facial features, were far more successful when part or all of the two eyes and forehead configuration was displayed (Goldstein and Mackenberg, 1966).

Through repeated visual scrutiny of his mother's face, more particularly its eye area, the infant of 4-6 months comes to single out his primary caretaker. In a sense, one might say that this face—the most discrete and localizable human point of reference in the infant's world—is "mother." Only gradually, over many months, does the rest of her body become an integral part of his scheme of things.

A fundamental two-way process of communication—*looking at* and *being looked at* (Almansi, 1960)—is set in motion. In the normal course of events this process continues to operate in human relationships. The fulfilment of physical needs, and the experiencing of pleasurable stimulation through non-visual modes, are equally significant factors in the development of attachment. Eye-to-eye contact is one component in the matrix of maternal and infant behaviours that comprise reciprocal interaction. Yet the nature of the eye contact between a mother and her baby seems to cut across all interactional systems and conveys the intimacy or "distance" characteristic of their relationship as a whole.

The intensity of the first attachment

The strength of the infant's tie to his mother's face is affected both by his characteristics and those of the caretaking environment. In the course of close to four hundred hours of naturalistic observations of some thirty mother-infant pairs, the author has noted marked variations in the patterns of eye contact among infants. Certain visually alert infants engage in vigorous attempts to search out their mothers' eyes and when contact is achieved they appear totally engaged. Others may make contact but somehow never display the "fascination" that can occur during such an exchange. Still another class of infants seem to avoid their mothers' eyes and thus pre-empt reciprocal maternal eye contact. The factors that contribute to these differences seem to be accessible to systematic analysis.

Concepts such as attentiveness, arousal level, and orienting behaviour in the infant, are often based on visual functioning. The term *"alertness"* is frequently used to characterize the intensity of these behaviours. In the early months of life, when one describes an infant as alert or dull, that judgement is primarily based on his visual activities: how long his eyes remain open; how soon he seems to "see," i.e. follow and fixate; the duration of his fixations; and the intensity of his gaze.

Freedman (1965), in his twin studies, found that the age of onset and intensity of visual fixation of the mother's face was the same in monozygotic pairs. Wolff (1965) has established that the amount of time neonates spend in "alert inactivity," the state in which maximal visual attention occurs, varies enormously in individual infants but shows a steady increment over the first month of life. *Sex differences* in visual attentiveness are also evident. In a series of studies one group of investigators (Kagan, 1965; Kagan and Lewis, 1965; Lewis, Kagan and Kalafat, 1966, Kagan et al., 1966) has demonstrated that females exhibit greater attentiveness and more rapid habituation time to human faces. Girls are therefore likely to develop a differentiated percept of their mother's face earlier than boys. In general, one might suppose that a visually alert baby would attract early, frequent, and possibly more rewarding eye-to-eye contact from his mother, and that he would thereby develop a precociously differentiated and stronger bond with her face. Conversely, the tie of the blind infant to his mother, both in terms of specificity and intensity, should be significantly weaker than that of the sighted infant. According to workers in this area this is often the case (personal communications from Daniel Freedman, Selma Fraiberg and Dorothy Burlingham). Nagera and Colonna (1965) comment that these children ". . . sometimes give the impression that they readily and easily exchange objects, even for unfamiliar ones, as if object constancy had not been properly established."

Another infant characteristic that is likely to influence has to do with the differences that infants manifest in terms of *sensory modality preferences*. Benjamin (1959), for example, mentions that babies can be classified as visual, auditory, or tactile and kinesthetic, in the sense that they are predominantly soothed through and explore with one or another of these receptor systems. If such a categorization proves to be valid, then an infant who is a "visual responder" should be more likely to establish a stronger tie to his mother's face.

A fourth and final factor is the infant's *predisposition to gaze aversion*. The author has seen a number of babies during the first three months of life who persistently avoid maternal eye contact. One mother of such an infant, after vigorous but unsuccessful attempts to catch his eye, angrily exclaimed: "Look at me"—she obviously felt rebuffed. Stechler and Latz (1966) also observed gaze aversion to the human face in infants of less than 1 month of age. The determinants of infantile gaze aversion are far from clear but the most plausible explanation, in the author's opinion, rests with the ethological data on the potency of the "eye gestalt" as an evoker of gaze aversion or flight responses in animals. Szekely (1954) reviews the history of these avoidance reactions along the evolutionary ladder, and constructs an encompassing theory of infantile anxiety within this frame of reference. According to Lorenz (1953), in the overwhelming majority of animals ". . . empty gazing is the normal state of affairs . . . (and) . . . amongst themselves, animals only look at each other fixedly when they intend to take drastic measures or are afraid of each other . . . (hence) . . . they conceive a prolonged fixed gaze as being something hostile and threatening . . .".

Similarly, turning to caretaking behaviours that act as determinants of the infant's face-tie, the *maternal predisposition to gaze aversion* will obviously affect eye contact with the baby. After several episodes of her 3-week-old infant's attempting to capture her gaze, one mother commented, as if to explain and apologize for her looking away, "He looks daggers." Though total gaze aversion is relatively rare, a pattern of eye contact that permits only transient fleeting glances is not at all uncommon. And it seems reasonable to assume that the *quantity* of eye contact a mother provides her infant, both in terms of the frequency of this interchange and the degree to which it is sustained, should bear on the development of the face-tie. One would conjecture that only below a rather small magnitude of maternal eye contact would the quantity parameter be operative.

Support for this speculation is found in Schaffer and Emerson's (1964a) study of attachment behaviour. These authors conclude that maternal "availability" related neither to choice of most important object nor to intensity of attachment. They also found that the primary "need fulfiller" was not selected as the primary object of attachment in 39 per cent of their sample. These authors emphasize that ". . . (the) independence of the attachment system from the vicissitudes of physical needs is indicated." It would seem that, *per se,* the amount of time a mother spends in caring for her infant would not affect attachment intensity. Watson (1965) observed that most caretaking behaviours are administered with the mother's face at a 45° orientation relative to that of the infant, while social interaction accurs as a 0° orientation, i.e. *en face.* Hence, a mother who provides perfectly adequate bathing, changing, dressing, etc., but who initiates little or no simultaneous eye contact, may deprive her infant of the optimal conditions for developing the face-tie. The infant and maternal characteristics just discussed should influence the strength of that tie. But one must consider the qualitative aspects of the relationship.

The quality of the relationship—contingent maternal behaviour

In his formulation of early social and attachment behaviour, Gewirtz (1961) stresses that ". . . we must take account of the circumstances under which given stimuli are made available to (the baby) and in particular, whether these stimuli are functional, and with his behaviours enter into effective contingencies for learning." He notes, in discussing the deprivation of institutionalized infants, that what is lacking in such an environment is not contact *per se*, but caretaking behaviour that is contingent upon the baby's signals. It would seem worthwhile to differentiate at least three dimensions of such contingency.

First, a mother's responses should follow the infant's signals within a period of *time* that is sufficiently short for him to casually associate his behaviours with her actions. Schaffer and Emerson (1964a) found that "maternal responsiveness," the rapidity with which the mother responded to her infant's demands, yielded a positive and significant correlation with both choice of a favored caretaker and attachment intensity. A second parameter is the degree to which maternal responses accurately *meet the baby's immediate needs.* For example, one can often see mothers who are preoccupied with food intake interpret every fuss or cry as a sign of hunger and act accordingly. As a result, they may force feeding and prolong distress, or waken a drowsy, full but fretful infant from sleep. Although neither the time nor "need meeting" axes of contingent responses directly involve eye-to-eye contact, these two parameters apply to maternal behaviors which probably become associated through contiguity with the infant's "gestalt" of his mother's gaze.

The third aspect of contingent behaviour is less refined but no less important than the preceding two. It has to do with the affective accompaniment of maternal eye contact. Behaviorally speaking, this might be defined as the *degree of animation and modulation of facial expression,* particularly around the upper half of the face. During the first months of life mothers utilize the eye-to-eye interchange for a variety of purposes: it can be used as a means of establishing pleasant social contact with the infant in a contented state; on other occasions it is used to "figure out" what is going on with a fussy or distressed baby. Still another use of the eye-to-eye exchange is to activate a placid infant or calm a fussy one. In the latter case, it is interesting that a baby who is mildly upset can be quieted through eye contact and the concomitant caretaking behaviors, but an infant who is fussing or crying either averts his gaze or, if he makes contact, often becomes more upset.

In all of these examples an observer senses an emotional "climate" that is specifically apparent through the mother's facial expression. One sees a range of this behaviour: some mothers maintain a fixed and flat expression, others a fixed but unconvincing smile, and still others a highly animated facies that reflect joy, anger or anxiety. There is little data on the capacity of infants to perceive such differences, but both Benjamin (1963) and Meili (1957) note that from the fourth month onward, i.e. when the mother's face begins to be differentiated from others, infants are particularly sensitive to changes in the upper portion of her face. A sober maternal demeanor can produce a fearful reaction in the infant. Ahrens (1954) observed that around the fifth month responsiveness to eyes diminishes and the mouth becomes more effective in eliciting smiling and attention. But after the mouth, the baby's eyes invariably fixate the eyes of an observer or a stylized "dummy" face, and if the gaze of the former is averted or the eyes of the latter are missing, the smiling ceases.

One could easily rate the degree of animation of the maternal face. However, whether a mother modulates her expression to the particular circumstances of the infant so as to reassure rather than disrupt, or quiet rather than prolong distress, is also a critical dimension of the eye-to-eye exchange that should strongly influence the quality of the infant's face-tie. In optimal circumstances, all three dimensions of contingent maternal behaviour should function in parallel, but they can and often do operate quite independently of one another.

In passing, contingent behavior thus defined may be the basis for establishing trust and the subjective sense of "meaning" (both of which in a sense are derivatives of events being predictable). Their early contingency experience may also determine the extent to which older children and adults rely upon and utilize non-verbal forms of communication such as eye-to-eye contact. If this form of interchange is primarily non-contingent, one result may be inordinate attention to such cues—as in some psychotic states where the patient may invalidate verbal communications while depending exclusively on non-verbal behaviors in assessing, often incorrectly, the intentions of therapist or family member. Alternatively, the glance as a means of communication may be totally abandoned, as in people who exhibit persistent gaze aversion or in "infantile autism" (Kanner, 1949; Wolff and Chess, 1964).

For a particular infant one would like to dimensionalize the infant and maternal variables in predicting the intensity and quality of the face-tie. Yet, even then one is hard put to determine the direction of effects; that is, to what extent maternal behaviours are influenced by infant characteristics and vice-versa. Currently, the work of Kagan and his associates (Kagan, 1965; Kagan and Lewis, 1965; Lewis, Kagan, and Kalagat, 1966; and Kagan et al., 1966) offers a paradigm in which some of these dimensions can be assessed under laboratory conditions. Fixation time, frequency of smiling and vocalization, and cardiac deceleration to the presentation of face stimuli have already proven to be differentiating measures. Even more productive would be a combination of such studies with antecedent observations of the mother-infant pair from birth onwards.

In any event, if the face-tie is not established, or if its quality fosters disruption and distress, the infant will experience varying degrees of interference in forming his earliest—and probably future—human relationships. Enduring deviations in eye-to-eye contact should be concomitants of these attachment disturbances. As the concluding section of this report some of these deviations will be considered.

SOME RESIDUES OF THE FIRST 6 MONTHS

Because they are so obviously derived from the eye-to-eye interchange, and because they may emphasize some of the points just made, a number of phenomena that most likely represent "unfinished business" from the early months of life will be briefly discussed. In the examples to follow it is important to keep in mind that no reconstructions of past events can accurately determine the "causes" of behaviours observed or described in the present. An adult who reports disturbance in his parents may well be citing his own congenital characteristics, his parents' reactions to them, or both.

An affectively loaded phenomenon is that of "love at first sight." Singular facial characteristics, such as the quality and color of hair and the morphology of the eyes, probably operate to some degree in the choice of every human love object. For the most part, a unique face is not especially sought out, nor is it more than an initiator of the attraction. But there are a number of patients in the author's experience, all of whom have disturbed relationships, who are fascinated by and drawn to particular faces, wholly independent of any other qualities of the person. One schizoid patient was able to trace his attraction to such faces back to a "motherly" teacher and from there to that of his unpredictable, frankly paranoid mother. A male homosexual used the "look" of the eyes (he was unable to specify the qualities) in selecting his partners, with whom the sexual contact was unimportant compared to the sense of "communion" he felt in face-to-face interactions. These behaviors might be described as attempts to rectify a previously established but dysphoric face-tie.

Almansi (1960) describes eye-face hypnagogic phenomena in a series of patients preoccupied with feelings of ". . . oral deprivation and object loss." Of interest was the fact that most of these patients were also scoptophilic, a perversion that Shapiro and Stine (1965) allude to in interpreting their figure drawings: "Some voyeuristic perversions . . . could be related to events occurring in this developmental period. (i.e. infancy and early childhood)." In a sense, the scoptophilic does a great deal of "looking at" but in circumstances where he is not "looked at." One of Almansi's patients, whose mother was replaced by a "cruel wet nurse" at a young age, experienced resolution of his symptoms during an analytic hour in which he ". . . visualized with great clarity the dark, benevolent eyes of his mother, isolated and suspended in space, looking down upon him."

The most extreme examples of deviant eye contact are seen in "anaclitic depression" (Spitz, 1946b) and "infantile autism" (Kanner, 1949), in both of which total gaze aversion is the rule. Discussing their experience with the latter condition, Wolff and Chess (1964) state that "a diagnosis or at least a suspicion of autism is usually arrived at very quickly, and as if intuitively . . . one senses whether or not one is making contact (which seems largely based on) the experience of eye-to-eye contact with the other person and on the quality of this contact." Their patients displayed abnormalities of eye-to-eye contact, ranging from a blank stare to total gaze aversion, proportional to the level of disturbance. Like Wills' (1965) blind children, the autistic or anaclitically depressed infants may experience ". . . some critical period when they fail to cathect and organize their external world (and) subsequently withdraw from the attempt." This is not to imply that either of these clinical states is a simple manifestation of deviant eye contact, but rather that these visual avoidance behaviors are pathognomonic of as yet unidentified but probably gross disturbances in the mother-infant relationship.

SUMMARY

This paper considers the developmental significance of eye-to-eye contact, between mother and infant, in the first six months of life. In a variety of ways this interchange facilitates the attachment of mother and infant to one another. The biological roots of eye-to-eye behavior are discussed and infant and maternal characteristics that should predict to the quality and intensity of the infant's tie to his mother's face are described. The paper concludes with some psychopathological sequelae of deviant eye-to-eye contact.

Acknowledgements—The author is indebted to Dr. Stanley Palombo for his constructive suggestions when this paper was in its formative stages. He would also like to thank Drs. Richard Bell and Howard Moss for their critical comments on the manuscript.

REFERENCES

AHRENS, R. (1954): Beitrag zur entwichlung des physiognomie und mimikerkennens. *Z. exp. angew. Psychol. 2,* 412-454.

ALMANSI, R. J. (1960): The face-breast equation. *J. Am. psychoanal. Ass. 8,* 43-70.

AMBROSE, J. A. (1961): The development of the smiling response in early infancy. *Determinants of Infant Behavior Vol. II, 179-201.* (Edited by B. M. Foss). Wiley, New York.

ANDREW, R. J. (1965): The origins of facial expression. *Scient. Am. 213,* 88-94.

ARGYLE, M. and DEAN, J. (1965): Eye contact, distance and affiliation. *Sociometry, 28,* 289-304.

BENJAMIN, J. D. ((1959): Prediction and psychopathological theory. *The Psychopathology of Childhood.* (Edited by L. Jessner and E. Pavenstedt). Grune & Stratton, New York.

BENJAMIN, J. D. (1963): Further comments on some developmental aspects of anxiety. *Counterpoint,* (Edited by H. Gaskill). International Universities Press, New York.

BOWLBY, P. (1958): The nature of the child's tie to his mother. *Int. J. Psycho-Analysis. 39,* 350-373.

BURLINGHAM, D. (1964): Hearing and its role in the development of the blind. *Psychoanal. Study Child 19,* 95-112.

EXLINE, R. V. (1963): Explorations in the process of person perception: Visual interaction in relation to competition, sex, and need for affiliation. *J. Personality 31,* 1-20.

EXLINE, R. and WINTERS, L. (1965): The effects of cognitive difficulty and cognitive style upon eye-to-eye contact in interviews. Paper read at Eastern Psychological Association, Atlantic City.

FANTZ, R. L. (1958): Pattern vision in young infants. *Psychol. Rec. 8,* 43-57.

FRAIBERG, S. and FREEDMAN, D. A. (1964) Studies in the ego development of the congenitally blind child. *Psychoanal. Study Child 19,* 113-169.

FREEDMAN, D. G. (1964): Smiling in blind infants and the issue of innate vs. acquired. *J. Child Psychol. Psychiat. 5,* 171-184.

FREEDMAN, D. G. (1965): Hereditary control of early social behaviour. *Determinants of Infant Behavior Vol. III* (Edited by B. M. Foss). 149-159. Wiley, New York.

GEWIRTZ, J. L. (1961): A learning analysis of the effects of normal stimulation, privation and deprivation on the acquisition of social motivation and attachment. *Determinants of Infant Behaviour Vol. I* (Edited by B. M. Foss) 213-299. Wiley, New York.

GOLDSTEIN, A. G. and MACKENBERG, E. J. (1966): Recognition of human faces from isolated facial features: a developmental study. *Psychon. Sci. 6,* 149-150.

GREENMAN, G. W. (1963): Visual behaviour of newborn infants. In *Modern Perspectives in Child Development* (Edited by A. Solnit and S. Provence). International Universities Press, New York.

HARLOW, H. F. (1961): The development of affectional patterns in infant monkeys. In *Determinants of Infant Behaviour* Vol. I (Edited by B. M. Foss), 75-88. Wiley, New York.

HUTT, C. and OUNSTED, C. (1966): The biological significance of gaze aversion with perticular reference to the syndrome of infantile autism. *Behav. Sci. 11*, 346-356.

ISAKOWER, O. (1938): A contribution to the patho-psychology of phenomena associated with falling asleep. *Int. J. Psycho-Analysis 19*, 331-345.

KAGAN, J. (1965): The growth of the "face" schema: theoretical significance and methodological issues. Paper presented at the annual meeting of the American Psychological Association, Chicago.

KAGAN, J. and LEWIS, M. (1965): Studies of attention in the human infant. *Merrill-Palmer Q. 11*, 95-1227.

KAGAN, J., HENKER, B., HEN-TOV, A., LEVINE, J. and LEWIS, M. (1966): Infant's differential reactions to familiar and distorted faces. *Child Dev. 37*, 519-532.

KAILA, E. (1935) Die reaktionen des sauglings auf des menschliche gesicht. *Z. Psychol. 135*, 156-163.

KANNER, L. (1949): Early infantile autism. *Am. J. Orthopsychiat. 19*, 416.

LEWIN, B. (1950): *The Psychoanalysis of Elation.* Norton, New York.

LEWIS, M., KAGAN, J., and KALAFAT, J. (1966): Patterns of fixation in the young infant. *Child Dev. 37*, 331-341.

LORENZ, K. (1953): *Man Meets Dog* (Translated by M. Wilson). Penguin Books, Baltimore.

LORENZ, K. (1966): *On Aggression* (Translated by M. Wilson). Harcourt, Brace & World, New York.

MEILI, R. (1957): *Anfange der Charakterentwicklung.* Huber, Stuttgart.

NAGERA, H. and COLONNA, A. B. (1965): Aspects of the contribution of sight to ego and drive development. *Psychoanal. Study Child 20*, 267-287.

RHEINGOLD, H. L. (1961): The effect of environmental stimulation upon social and exploratory behaviour in the human infant. *Determinants of Infant Behaviour* Vol. I. (Edited by B. M. Foss). Wiley, New York, pp. 143-177.

ROSENBLATT, J. S. (1965): The basis of synchrony in the behavioural interaction between the mother and her offspring in the laboratory rat. *Determinants of Infant Behaviour* Vol. III (Edited by B. M. Foss), Wiley, New York, pp. 3-45.

SANDLER, A.-M. (1953): Aspects of passivity and ego development in a blind infant. *Psychoanal. Study Child 18*, 343-360.

SCHAFFER, H. R. and EMERSON, P. E. (1964a): *The Development of Social Attachments in Infancy.* Monog. No. 94, vol. 29, Society for Research in Child Development.

SCHAFFER, H. R. and EMERSON, P. E. (1964b): Patterns of response to physical contact in early human development. *J. Child Psychiat. 5*, 1-13.

SHAPIRO, T. and STINE, J. (1965): The figure drawings of 3-year-old children. *Psychoanal. Study Child 20*, 298-309.

SPITZ, R. A. (1946): Anaclitic depression: an enquiry into the genesis of psychiatric conditions in early childhood, II. *Psychoanal. Study Child 2*, 313-342.

SPITZ, R. A. (1950): Anxiety in infancy: a study of its manifestations in the first year of life. *Int. J. Psycho-Analysis 31*, 138-143.

SPITZ, R. A. (1955): The primal cavity: a contribution to the genesis of perception and its role for psychoanalytic theory. *Psychoanal. Study Child 10*, 215-240.

SPITZ, R. A. (1965): *The First Year of Life.* International Universities Press, New York.

SPITZ, R. A. and WOLF, K. M. (1946): The smiling response. *Genet. Psychol. Monogr.* no. 34.

STECHLER, G. and LATZ, E. (1966): Some observations on attention and arousal in the human infant. *J. Am. Acad. Child Psychiat. 5*, 517-525.

SZEKELY, L. (1954): Biological remarks on fears originating in early childhood. *Int. J. Psycho-Analysis 35*, 57-67.

WALTERS, R. H. and PARKE, R. D. (1965): The role of the distance receptors in the development of social responsiveness. *Advances in Child Development and Behaviour* (Vol. 2), (Edited by L. Lipsitt and C. Spiker). Academic Press, New York.

WATSON, J. S. (1965): Orientation-specific age changes in responsiveness to the face stimulus in young infants. Paper presented at the annual meeting of the American Psychological Association, Chicago.

WHITE, B. L. and CASTLE, P. W. (1964): Visual exploratory behaviour following postnatal handling of human infants. *Percept. Mot. Skills 18,* 497-502.

WHITE, B. L., CASTLE, P. W. and HELD, R. (1964): Observations on the development of visually-directed reaching. *Child Dev. 35,* 349-364.

WILLS, D. (1965): Some observations on blind nursery school children's understanding of their world. *Psychoanal. Study Child 20,* 344-364. International Universities Press, New York.

WOLFF, P. H. (1959): Observations on newborn infants. *Psychosom. Med. 21,* 110-118.

WOLFF, P. H. (1963): Observations on the early development of smiling. *Determinants of Infant Behaviour* Vol. II (Edited by B. M. Foss). Wiley, New York, pp. 113-138.

WOLFF, P. H. (1965): The development of attention in young infants. *Ann. N. Y. Acad. Sci. 118,* 815-830.

WOLFF, P. H. and WHITE, B. L. (1965): Visual pursuit and attention in young infants. *J. Am. Acad. Child Psychiat. 4,* 472-484.

WOLFF, S. and CHESS, S. (1964): A behavioural study of schizophrenic children. *Acta. psychiat scand. 40,* 438-466.

7

ON HUMAN SYMBIOSIS AND THE VICISSITUDES OF INDIVIDUATION

Margaret S. Mahler, M.D.

Clinical Professor of Psychiatry, Albert Einstein Medical College
Director of Research, Masters Children's Center, New York, N. Y.

The term symbiosis is borrowed from biology, where it is used to refer to a close functional association of two organisms to their mutual advantage.

In the weeks preceding the evolution to symbiosis, the newborn and very young infant's sleeplike states far outweigh in proportion the states of arousal. They are reminiscent of that primal state of libido distribution that prevailed in intrauterine life, which resembles the model of a closed monadic system, self-sufficient in its hallucinatory wish fulfillment.

Freud's[12] use of the bird's egg as a model of a closed psychological system comes to mind. He said: "A neat example of a psychical system

Reprinted from the *Journal of the American Psychoanalytic Association*, Vol. 15, 1967, pp 710-762. Presented at the Plenary Session of the Annual Meeting of The American Psychoanalytic Association, Detroit, Michigan, Sunday, May 7, 1967. This Paper represents an overview of and the title chapter of the forthcoming book: *On Human Symbiosis and the Vicissitudes of Individuation*, Vol. I: *Infantile Psychosis and Allied Conditions*. New York: International Universities Press.

This work is partly based on research supported by The National Institute of Mental Health, U.S.P.H.S., Bethesda, Maryland, Grant MH-08238, and previously by Grant M 3353; as well as by the Field Foundation, the Taconic Foundation, The National Association for Mental Health, Inc., and the Psychoanalytic Research and Development Fund, Inc.

I want to express my profound gratitude to my many co-workers, who have played such a significant role in my research on these questions. First of all to my associate, Dr. John McDevitt, and also to Emmogene Kamaiko, Anni Bergman, Laura Salchow, Dr. Ernest Abelin, and many others.

shut off from the stimuli of the external world, and able to satisfy even its nutritional requirements *autistically*. . . . , is afforded by a bird's egg with its food supply enclosed in its shell; for it, the care provided by its mother is limited to the provision of warmth" (p. 220 n.; my italics).

In a quasi-symbolic way along this same line, conceptualizing the state of the sensorium, I have applied to the first weeks of life the term *normal autism;* for in it, the infant seems to be in a state of primitive hallucinatory disorientation, in which need satisfaction belongs to his own omnipotent, *autistic* orbit.

The newborn's waking life centers around his continuous attempts to achieve homeostasis. The effect of his mother's ministrations in reducing the pangs of need-hunger cannot be isolated, nor can it be differentiated by the young infant from tension-reducing attempts of his own, such as urinating, defecating, coughing, sneezing, spitting, regurgitating, vomiting, all the ways by which the infant tries to rid himself of unpleasurable tension. The effect of these expulsive phenomena as well as the gratification gained by his mother's ministrations help the infant, in time, to differentiate between a "pleasurable" and "good" quality and a "painful" and "bad" quality of experiences.[33]

Through the inborn and autonomous perceptive faculty of the primitive ego[17] deposits of memory traces of the two primordial qualities of stimuli occur. We may further hypothesize that these are cathected with primordial undifferentiated drive energy.[33]

From the second month on, dim awareness of the need-satisfying object marks the beginning of the phase of normal symbiosis, in which the infant behaves and functions as though he and his mother were an omnipotent system—a dual unity within one common boundary.

My concept of the symbiotic phase of normal development dovetails, from the infant's standpoint, with the concept of the symbiotic phase of the mother-child dual unity, which Therese Benedek[3, 4, 5] has described in several classical papers from the standpoint of both partners of the primary unit.

It is obvious that, whereas, during the symbiotic phase, the infant is *absolutely* dependent on the symbiotic partner, symbiosis has a quite different meaning for the adult partner of the dual unity. The infant's need for the mother is absolute, while the mother's for the infant is relative.[4]

The term "symbiosis" in this context is a metaphor. It does not describe, as the biological concept of symbiosis does, what actually happens between two separate individuals.[2] It was chosen to describe that state of undifferentiation, of fusion with mother, in which the "I" is not yet differentiated from the "not-I," and in which inside and outside are only gradually coming to be sensed as different. Any unpleasurable perception, external or internal, is projected beyond the common boundary of the symbiotic *milieu intérieur* (cf. Freud's concept of the "purified pleasure ego"), which includes the mothering partner's Gestalt during ministrations. Only transiently—in the state of the sensorium that is termed alert inactivity—does the young infant take in stimuli from beyond the symbiotic milieu. The primordial energy reservoir that is vested in the undifferentiated "ego-id" still contains an undifferentiated mixture of libido and aggression. As several authors have pointed out, the libidinal cathexis vested in symbiosis, by reinforcing the inborn instinctual stimulus barrier, protects the rudimentary ego from premature phase-unspecific strain—from stress traumata.

The essential feature of symbiosis is hallucinatory or delusional, somatopsychic, omnipotent fusion with the representation of the mother and, in particular, delusion of common boundary of the two actually and physically separate individuals. This is the mechanism to which the ego regresses in cases of the most severe disturbance of individuation and psychotic disorganization, which I have described as "symbiotic child psychosis." [24, 33]

In the human species, the function of, and the equipment for, self-preservation is atrophied. The rudimentary ego in the newborn baby and the young infant has to be complemented by the emotional rapport of the mother's nursing care, a kind of social symbiosis. It is within this matrix of physiological and sociobiological dependency on the mother that there takes place the structural differentiation that leads to the individual's organization for adaptation: the ego.

Ribble[36] has pointed out that it is by way of mothering that the young infant is gradually brought out of an inborn tendency toward vegetative, splanchnic regression and into increased sensory awareness of, and contact with, the environment. In terms of energy or libidinal cathexis, this means that a progressive displacement of libido has to take place, from the inside of the body (particularly from the abdominal organs), toward the periphery of the body.[14, 24]

In this sense, I would propose to distinguish, within the phase of primary *narcissism*—a Freudian concept to which I find it most useful to adhere—two subphases: during the first few weeks of extrauterine life, a stage of *absolute* primary narcissism, which is marked by the infant's lack of awareness of a mothering agent. This stage I have termed "normal autism," as discussed above. In the other, the symbiotic stage proper (beginning around the third month)—while primary narcissism still prevails, it is not such an absolute primary narcissism, inasmuch as the infant begins dimly to perceive need satisfaction as coming from a need-satisfying part object—albeit still from within the orbit of his omnipotent symbiotic dual unity with a mothering agency, toward which he turns libidinally.[42]

Pari passu, and in accordance with the pleasure-pain sequences, demarcation of representations of the body ego within the symbiotic matrix takes place. These representations are deposited as the "body image."[41]

From now on, representations of the body that are contained in the rudimentary ego mediate between inner and outer perceptions. The ego is molded under the impact of reality, on the one hand, and of the instinctual drives, on the other. The body ego contains two kinds of self representations: there is an inner core of the body image, with a boundary that is turned toward the inside of the body and divides it from ego; and an outer layer of sensoriperceptive engrams, which contributes to the boundaries of the "body self."

From the standpoint of the "body image": the shift of predominantly proprioceptive-enteroceptive cathexis toward sensoriperceptive cathexis of the periphery is a major step in development. We did not realize its importance prior to psychoanalytic studies of early infantile psychosis. We know now that this major shift of cathexis is an essential prerequisite of body-ego formation. Another parallel step is the ejection, by projection, of destructive unneutralized aggressive energy beyond the body-self boundaries.

The infant's inner sensations form the *core* of the self. They seem to remain the central, the crystallization point of the "feeling of self," around which a "sense of identity" will become established. [15, 26, 38, 39] The sensoriperceptive organ—the "peripheral rind of the ego," as Freud called it—contributes mainly to the self's demarcation from the object world. The two kinds of intrapsychic structures *together* form the framework for self-orientation.[43]

The two partners of the symbiotic dyad, on the other hand, may be regarded as polarizing the organizational and structuring processes. The structures that derive from the double frame of reference of the symbiotic unit represent a framework to which all experiences have to be related, before there are clear and whole representations in the ego of the self and the object world! Spitz[44] calls the mother the auxiliary ego of the infant. In the same line, I believe the mothering partner's "holding behavior," her "primary maternal preoccupation," to be the symbiotic organizer.[47]

Hitherto, I have described, in a number of papers, extreme failures of these structuralization processes. In those papers I referred to and extrapolated from the most severe disturbances and disorganization of those structuralization principles in infantile psychosis. In this paper, I wish to draw heavily upon observations of normal development as well.

Greenacre[15] has remarked how "extremely difficult [it is] to say exactly at what time the human organism develops from a biological to a *psychobiological* organization." Schur[42] puts the time at the point when the "wish" replaces the purely "physiological need."

The implications of new sleep-physiological studies about REM activity in very young infants are most interesting and challenging indeed.[37, 9]

Experimental psychologists tell us that, in the first two months of life, learning takes place through conditioning. Toward the third month, however, the existence of memory traces can be demonstrated experimentally. This was referred to by Spitz[44] as the beginning of learning according to the human pattern. Learning by conditioning is then gradually replaced by learning through experience. Here is then the first beginning of symbiotic relationship as well. We may say that, whereas during the quasi-prehistoric phase of magic hallucinatory omnipotence, the breast of the bottle *belongs* to the self, toward the third month, the object begins to be perceived as an *unspecific, need-satisfying part object.*[11]

When the need is not so imperative, when some measure of development enables the infant to hold tension in abeyance, that is to say, *when he is able to wait for and confidently expect satisfaction*—only then is it possible to speak of the *beginning of an ego,* and of a symbiotic object as well. This is made possible by the fact that there seem to be memory traces of the *pleasures of gratification*—connected with the memory of the perceptual Gestalt of the mother's ministrations.

The specific smiling response at the peak of the symbiotic phase predicates that the infant is responding to the symbiotic partner in a manner different from that in which he responds to other human beings. In the second half of the first year, the symbiotic partner is no longer interchangeable; manifold behaviors of the five-month-old infant indicate that he has by now *achieved a specific symbiotic relationship with his mother.*[44]

In 1954, Anna Freud reminded us that we may think of pregenital patterning in terms of two people joined to achieve what, for brevity's sake, one might call "homeostatic equilibrium" (see Mahler, 25). The same thing may be referred to under the term "symbiotic relationship."

Beyond a certain, but not yet defined degree, the immature organism cannot achieve homeostasis on its own. Whenever during the autistic or symbiotic phase there occurs "organismic distress"—that forerunner of anxiety proper—the mothering partner is called upon, to contribute a particularly large portion of symbiotic help toward the maintenance of the infant's homeostasis. Otherwise, the neurobiological patterning processes are thrown out of kilter. Somatic memory traces are set at this time, which amalgamate with later experiences and may thereby increase later psychological pressures.[15]

Understanding of symbiotic phenomena, which I conceptualized initially through observation of mother-infant behavior in well-baby clinics, and also through reconstruction from systematic studies of severe symbiotic psychotic syndromes, I have since supplemented by way of our observational study of the average mothers with their normal infants during the first three years of life, during the process of separation-individuation.

We have supplemented the understanding of these processes by way of following them in an observational study of *average* mothers with their *normal* infants during the first three years of life. We follow them from symbiosis to the process of separation-individuation—and up to the period of the establishment of libidinal object constancy in Hartmann's sense.[18]

OUT OF SYMBIOSIS THE INTRAPSYCHIC PROCESS
OF SEPARATION-INDIVIDUATION EVOLVES

For more accurate conceptualization and formulation of these still (up to the third year) essentially preverbal processes, we have tried to determine characteristic behavioral concomitants of those intrapsychic events that seem to occur regularly during the course of separation-individuation. In previous papers, I have described the subphases of that process. The concept of subphases has been fruitful in that it has helped to determine the *nodal* points of those structuralization and developmental processes. We have found them to be characteristic at the crossroads of individuation. Their description has greatly facilitated the ordering of our data into the psychoanalytic frame of reference, in a meaningful way.

In the following, I wish to refer only to a few points that may illustrate and somewhat complement more recent metapsychological constructs. These have pointed to the significance of *optimal human symbiosis* for the vicissitudes of individuation and for the establishment of a *cathectically stable "sense of identity."*

I would like to mention a relevant physiological and experimental finding that bears upon the transition from the autistic to the symbiotic phase. These findings set the *beginning* of this transition at the *end* of the first month. There are corresponding findings—for example, by the late John Benjamin[6]—which show that around three to four weeks of age a maturational crisis occurs. This is borne out in electroencephalographic studies and by the observation that there is a marked increase in overall sensitivity to external stimulation. As Benjamin said, "Without intervention of a mother figure for help in tension reduction, the infant at that time tends to become overwhelmed by stimuli, with increased crying and other motor manifestations of undifferentiated negative affect."

Metapsychologically speaking, this seems to mean that, by the second month, the quasi-solid stimulus barrier (negative, because it is uncathected)—*this autistic shell,* which kept external stimuli out—begins to crack. Through the aforementioned cathectic shift toward the sensory-perceptive periphery, a protective, but also receptive and selective, positively cathected stimulus shield now begins to form and to envelop the symbiotic orbit of the mother-child dual unity.[31] This eventually highly selective boundary seems to contain not only the pre-ego self representations, but also the not yet differentiated, libidinally cathected symbiotic part objects, within the mother-infant symbiotic matrix.

At the height of symbiosis—at around four to five months— the facial expression of most infants becomes much more subtly differentiated, mobile, and expressive. During the infant's wakeful periods, he reflects many more nuances of *"states"*—by now "ego states"—than he did in the autistic phase.

By the "states" of the newborn—which Peter Wolff (49) has described —we gauge, in a very general way, the states of the sensorium. In the course of the symbiotic phase, we can follow by the "ego states" of the infant the oscillation of his attention investment between his *inner* sensations and the symbiotic, libidinal attractions. During this state of "alert inactivity" the infant's attention turns toward the outer world; this, however, as yet, comprises mainly percepts that are more or less *closely* related to the mother.

The indicator of outward-directed attention seems to be the prototypical biphasic visual pattern of turning to an outside stimulus and then checking back to the mother's Gestalt, particularly her face. From this kind of scanning, elements of strangeness reaction patterns will develop. Outward-directed perceptual activity gradually replaces the inward-directed attention cathexis that was, only recently, almost exclusively vested in symbiotically disoriented inner sensations. The process by which this occurs—and which might be appropriately termed *hatching*—can now begin.

The gratification-frustration sequences promote structuralization. It is important, however, as several writers have pointed out lately, that in the early months of life, tension should not remain on an inordinately high level for any length of time! If such stress traumata *do* occur during the first five months of life, the symbiotic partner—this *auxiliary ego*—is called upon to save the infant from the pressure of having to develop *his own resources prematurely.* As Martin James[19] put it: "Premature ego development would imply that the infant—during the phase of primary narcissism—took over functions from the mother *in actuality,* or started *as though to do* so." Winnicott[48] and other British analysts call such an occurrence development of a "false self,"—by which I believe they mean *the beginning of "as if" mechanisms!*

When pleasure in outer sensory perceptions as well as maturational pressure stimulate outward-directed attention cathexis—while inside there is an optimal level of pleasure and therefore *safe anchorage* within the symbiotic orbit—these two forms of attention cathexis can oscillate freely.[43, 38] The result is an optimal symbiotic state from which smooth differentiation—and *expansion beyond the symbiotic orbit*—can take place.

The hatching process is, I believe, a gradual ontogenetic evolution of the sensorium—of the perceptual-conscious system—which leads to the infant-toddler's having a *permanently alert sensorium,* whenever he is awake.

It has been fascinating to observe how the prototype of outward-directed attention cathexis evolves—how the normal infant's differentiation process is guided by the pattern of "checking back" to the mother, as a point of orientation.[38] This pattern of checking back, and also the behavior termed "custom inspection,"[7] which consists in the baby's careful, more or less deliberate examination (visually and tactilely) of all features of the "not-mother's" face and comparing it point by point with the preobject or part-object representation of the mother—both these comparing and checking patterns recur, in an expanded, more complex edition, in the period from about ten to sixteen months of age, during the practicing subphase of separation-individuation. It then is supplemented by what Furer has called "emotional refueling."

THE SECOND MASSIVE SHIFT OF CATHEXIS

The peak point of the hatching process seems to coincide with the maturational spurt of active locomotion, which brings with it increased maturational pressure "for action," to practice locomotion and to explore wider segments of reality. From the fourth quarter of the first year on, this activity motivates the infant to separate in space from his mother, and to practice active physical separation and return. This will have a greatly catalyzing influence on further development of the ego.

The more nearly optimal the symbiosis, the mother's "holding behavior," has been; the more the symbiotic partner has helped the infant to become ready to "hatch" from the symbiotic orbit smoothly and gradually—that is, without undue strain upon his own resources—the better equipped has the child become to separate out and to differentiate his self representations from the hitherto fused symbiotic self-plus-object representations. But even at the height of the second subphase of individuation—during the practicing period—neither the differentiated self representations nor the object representations seem to be integrated as yet into a whole self representation or a whole libidinal object representation.

Among the many elements of the mother-child relationship during early infancy, we are especially impressed with the mutual selection of cues. We observed that infants present a large variety of cues—to indicate needs, tension, and pleasure.[32] In a complex manner, the mother responds selectively to only *certain* of these cues. The infant gradually alters his behavior in relation to this selective response; he does so in a characteristic way—the resultant of his own innate endowment and the mother-child relationship. From this circular interaction emerge patterns of behavior that already show certain overall qualities of the child's personality. *What we seem to see here is the birth of the child as an individual.*[23]

It is the specific unconscious need of the mother that activates, out of the infant's infinite potentialities, those in particular that create for each mother "the child" who reflects her own *unique* and individual needs. This process takes place, of course, within the range of the child's innate endowments.

Mutual cuing during the symbiotic phase creates that indelibly imprinted configuration—that complex pattern—that becomes the *leitmotif for "the infant's becoming the child of his particular mother."*[22]

In other words, the mother conveys—in innumerable ways—a kind of "mirroring frame of reference," to which the primitive self of the infant automatically adjusts. If the mother's "primary preoccupation" with her infant—*her* mirroring function during earlier infancy—is unpredictable, unstable, anxiety-ridden, or hostile; if her confidence in herself as a mother is shaky, then the individuating child has to do without a reliable frame of reference for checking back, perceptually and emotionally, to the symbiotic partner.[43] The result will then be a disturbance in the primitive "self feeling," which would derive or originate from a pleasurable and safe state of symbiosis, from which he did not have to hatch prematurely and abruptly.

The primary method of identity formation consisted of mutual reflection during the symbiotic phase. This narcissistic, mutual libidinal mirroring reinforced the delineation of identity—through magnification and *reduplication*—a kind of echo phenomenon, which Paula Elkisch[8] and Lichtenstein[22] have so beautifully described.

In previous papers I have described, in some detail, the second massive shift of cathexis in ontogenetic development, which seems to take place when the practicing period begins.[30] At that point, a large proportion of the available cathexis shifts from within the symbiotic orbit to investing the autonomous apparatuses of the self and the functions of the ego—locomotion, perception, learning.

In our study, we observe the intrapsychic separation-individuation process: the child's achievement of separate functioning in the presence and emotional availability of the mother. Even in this situation, this process by its very nature continually confronts the toddler with minimal threats of object loss. Nevertheless, through the predominance of pleasure in separate functioning, it enables the child to overcome that measure of separation anxiety that *is* entailed by *each new* step of separate functioning.

As far as the mothering partner is concerned, the practicing period confronts her with the impact of the toddler's spurt in individual autonomy, which is buttressed by the rapidly approaching occurrence—important for intrapsychic separation and self-boundary formation—of the negativistic behavior of the anal phase.[10, 45]

The practicing period culminates around the middle of the second year in the freely walking toddler seeming to feel at the height of his mood of elation. He appears to be at the peak point of his belief in his own magic omnipotence, which is still to a considerable extent derived *from his sense of sharing in his mother's magic powers.*

CONCEPTUALIZATION OF THE INTRAPSYCHIC PROCESSES
OF THE SECOND YEAR OF LIFE

Many mothers, however, take the very first unaided step of their toddler, who is, intrapsychically, by no means yet hatched, as heralding: "He is grown up now!" These mothers may be the ones who interpret the infant's signals according to whether they feel the child to be a continuation of themselves or a separate individual. Some tend to fail their fledgling, by "abandoning" him at this point, more or less precipitately and prematurely, to his own devices. They react with a kind of relative ridding mechanism, to the traumatization of their own symbiotic needs. These needs have been highlighted by the fact that maturational pressure has both enabled and prompted the child, at the very beginning of the second year, to practice the new "state of self": physical separateness.

One example of this is the case of Jay, who, at ten and a half months, had already learned *precociously* to walk. At that time, his body schema and his spatial orientation were still at a stage of *symbiotic fusion* and *confusion*. One could see this by innumerable behavioral signs.

The infant of twelve to fourteen months, who is gradually separating and individuating, rises from his hitherto quadruped exercises, to take his first unaided steps—initially with great caution, even though exuberantly. He automatically reassures himself of some support within reach. He also relies on his own ability to slide safely down into the sitting position—when the going gets rough, so to say. Jay, however, even though he was most wobbly and unsure on his feet, did not do any of these.

Through maturation of the ego apparatuses—and facilitated by the flux of developmental energy[21]—a relatively rapid, yet orderly process of separation-individuation takes place in the second year of life. By the eighteenth month, the junior toddler seems to be at the height of the process of dealing with his continuously experienced physical separateness from the mother. This coincides with his cognitive and perceptual achievement of the permanence of objects, in Piaget's sense.[35] This is the time when his sensorimotor intelligence starts to develop into true representational intelligence, and when the important process of internalization, in Hartmann's sense[17]—very gradually, through ego identifications—begins.

Jay did not improve his skill in locomotion during his second year. He still impressed us with the impetuousness and repetitiveness of his locomotor activity, as well as with the frequency with which he got himself into dangerous situations and fell. He climbed onto high places and ran about, and peculiarly disregarded any obstacles in his way. All this time, his mother consistently and conspicuously made literally no move to protect him. Jay's behavior was—at least in the beginning—a tacit appeal to the mother. We assumed this because his falls definitely decreased when the mother was out of the room.

Jay's precocious locomotor maturation—with which the other, the developmental lines of his ego, did not keep pace—should have made it even more imperative for the mothering partner to continue functioning as the child's auxiliary ego, in order to bridge the obvious gap between his motor and perceptual cognitive development.

The mother's inner conflicts, however, resulted in her appearing transfixed, almost paralyzed, at the sight of her junior toddler son's dangerous motor feats.

As I said before, many mothers fail their fledgling, because they find it difficult to strike intuitively and naturally an optimal balance between giving support—and yet at the same time knowing when to just be available and to watch from a distance. In other words, for many mothers in our culture, it is by no means easy to give up smoothly their "symbiotic holding behavior"—and instead to give the toddler optimal support on a higher emotional and verbal level, while allowing him to try his new wings of autonomy—in the second year of life.

Jay's mother demonstrated this conflict to a bizarre degree; she continually watched from a distance like a hawk, but could not make a move to assist him. I believe that it was Jay's developmental lag—which the precocity of his locomotor maturation had created in him, combined with the mother's continued failure to protect Jay's body—that resulted in seemingly irreversible damage to each of the three essential structures of Jay's individuating personality.*

The sixteen- to eighteen-month level seems to be a *nodal* point of development. The toddler is then at the height of what Joffe and Sandler[20] have termed "the ideal state of self." This is, I believe, the complex affective representation of the symbiotic dual unity, with its inflated sense of omnipotence—now augmented by the toddler's feeling of his own magic power—as the result of his spurt in autonomous functions.

---

* Whether the obvious defect in his visual-motor coordination was on an organic or functional basis to begin with is a moot and at this point, I believe, indeterminable question, even though interesting.

THE SECOND EIGHTEEN MONTHS OF LIFE

In the next eighteen months, this "ideal state of self" must become divested of its delusional increments. The second eighteen months of life is *thus* a period of vulnerability. It is the time when the child's self-esteem may suffer abrupt deflation.

Under normal circumstances, the senior toddler's growing autonomy has already begun to correct some of his delusional overestimation of his own omnipotence. During the course of individuation, internalization has begun, by true ego identification with the parents.

Jay did not seem to be able to learn through experience. He continued to suffer his hard falls, and every so often, without appropriate affective reactions. He seemed to be peculiarly lacking in sensitivity to physical pain. This *denial of pain* appeared to be in compliance with his mother's reactive belief that her son was indeed impervious to pain. Jay thus earned, in addition to his mother's pride, the epitheton: "Jay, the Painless Wonder," from the mothers of other children in the group.

Even at twenty months, Jay was conspicuous for his poorly developed ability to "inhibit the immediate discharge of impulse, and the attack on materials." His behavior could be characterized as impulsive, repetitive, and disoriented in space; it seemed to lag in age-adequate reality testing. In pursuing a goal in space, he seemed to overlook obstacles that lay between his body and the point of destination he had set himself to reach—he bumped into them.

Examinations ruled out any neurological disturbance—a question which, of course, concerned us all along. Dr. Sally Provence, who examined and tested Jay, felt, as did *we*, that Jay was basically a well-endowed child whose intellectual development was being impaired by his psychological problems.

One of the crucial findings, if not *the main yield* of our study, concerns the *time lag that exists in normal intrapsychic development—between object permanency (in Piaget's sense) and the attainment of libidinal object constancy,* in Hartmann's sense.[34] Attainment of *libidinal object constancy* is much more gradual than the achievement of object permanency—and, at the beginning, at least, it is a faculty that is waxing and waning and rather "impermanent." Up to about thirty months, it is very much at the mercy of the toddler's own mood swings and "ego states" and dependent on the actual mother-toddler situation of the moment.

In Jay's case it seemed there was by far too little *neutralized* cathexis available by the end of the fourth subphase of individuation—the subphase of the gradual attainment of *libidinal object constancy*.

To repeat: during the second half of the second year of life, the infant has become more and more aware of his physical separateness. Along with this awareness, the relative obliviousness of his mother's presence, which prevailed during the practicing period, wanes.[28]

Instead, the toddler of sixteen to eighteen months may appear suddenly and quite conspicuously surprised by situations—for example, when he hurts himself—in which mother is not automatically at hand to prevent such an occurrence.

The previous relative obliviousness to mother's presence is gradually replaced by active approach behavior on a much higher level. As he realizes his power and ability to physically move away from his mother, the toddler now seems to have an increased need, and a wish, for his mother to share with him every new acquisition of skill and experience. We may call this subphase of separation-individuation, therefore, the period of *rapprochement*.[28, 29]

Jay's primary identity formation by thirty months of age showed, as if in a distorted mirror, the mother's unintegrated maternal attitudes, her schizoid personality traits.

The mother's perplexity seems to have been triggered by Jay's purely maturational spurt, in the physical sense, away from her. The mother was able to respond positively to Jay only when he went directly to her. But toddlers, especially in the period of rapprochement, do not run to their mothers to be hugged or picked up—they approach the mother on a higher emotional level by bringing things to her, making contact by gestures and words Jay usually played at some distance from his mother, but would occasionally glance in her direction. Proximal contact between the two was quite infrequent. When it did occur, it was either that the mother went to Jay with an offer to read to him; or Jay, in turn, approached his mother with a book in his hand, which she would then read to him.

Thus, we could see Jay picking up, for example, this one cue—echoing and magnifying the mother's wish which we knew from our ultimate knowledge of the mother that he be an "outstanding intellectual." One could almost predict one of the fateful variations of the *leitmotif*[22] that is so frequently conveyed to the children of our time, and which Helen Tartakoff has dealt with in her paper: "The Normal Personality in Our Culture and the Nobel Prize Complex."[46]

Already at the age of two, Jay had had great pleasure in the use of words. For a while, this acquisition of language had made for better communication between Jay and his mother. Yet, by the end of his third and *the beginning of his fourth year*, it became more and more apparent that there was a serious discrepancy in Jay's "lines of development" in Anna Freud's sense[11]—both as to their rate of growth and as to their quality. Thus there ensued a serious deficit in the integrative and synthetic functions of Jay's ego. By that time, the counterphobic mechanism (which we saw in Jay's second year)—the impulse-ridden discharge behavior—had given way to phobic avoidance mechanisms.

The point that I wish to make in this presentation calls for conceptualization of certain elements of Jay's faulty individuation. The crucial deficiency was, we felt, Jay's disturbed body image, which robbed him of the core of primary identity formation, and thus of a reliably cathected self feeling invested with neutralized energy. Furthermore, because the polarizing function of the symbiotic dual unity of this mother-child pair failed the individuating toddler, there was an obvious lack of a frame of reference for perceiving the extrasymbiotic external reality. In consequence, the intrapsychic representational world contained no clear boundaries between self and object—the boundaries between ego and id remained deficient and so did the boundaries and connections between the intersystemic parts of the ego. Thus, one might say, symbiotic confusion has been perpetuated. Two conspicuous behavioral signs were Jay's handling of his body in space and the disturbance he displayed, in words and actions, in projecting experiences in the dimension of time.

When Jay graduated from our study to nursery school, we predicted that he would attain a borderline adjustment with schizoid features—unless corrective emotional therapy in Alpert's[1] sense could be instituted. We felt that he had no valid footing in the formation of his core identity; nor were the boundaries—between id and ego, between self and object world—structured firmly enough and sufficiently cathected with neutralized energy. Furthermore, there was not enough neutralized energy available for ego development—thus the establishment of libidinal object constancy was also questionable. The possibility of secondary identity formation, by true ego identifications and internalization, was greatly reduced.

In a forthcoming paper I shall elaborate on the findings from our follow-ups, which were done several times—until Jay was seven years old—and which validated our predictions.

Our prediction *now* is that Jay will be compelled to develop as an adolescent and as an adult—as he has already started to do, at age seven—"as if" mechanisms, in order to be able to function with his "false self" in his social environment. Suffice it to say that Jay reminded me of several patients in analysis, whose central problem was their incessant search for their place in life—their search for an identity.[40]

He reminded me especially of one analytic patient, whom I had treated as a child abroad and in his adolescence in this country. Charlie's developmental history I could reconstruct with fair accuracy—through the material that his intermittent analyses have yielded, and with the aid of my intimate knowledge of his parents' personality.

I could reconstruct a very long symbiotic-parasitic phase with a narcissistic mother, who was highly seductive yet could accept Charlie only if she could regard him as a continuation of her own narcissistic self. She had no regard for the little boy as an individual in his own right. She constantly needed babies to cuddle and bore infants up to her climacterium.

After the symbiotic-parasitic relationship, the mother suddenly abandoned Charlie to his own devices, at the beginning of the third year. Subsequently, there was a strong mirroring identification—on Charlie's part—with his father. The latter, however, suffered from a paralyzing depression, and went into seclusion when Charlie was three years old. This coincided with the time when the mother gave birth to one of her many babies. Thus, *both* primary love objects were unavailable to Charlie for object cathexis and for true ego identification, in the fateful second eighteen months of life.

Charlie never achieved libidinal object constancy. Instead, his identification with his mother was a total one—so much so that, when his mother, while taking him by car to the kindergarten, accidentally hit a man, Charlie behaved as if *he* was the one who had *deliberately* hurt the man. He refused to go on to school: he was afraid that the police would arrest *him*. From then on, he insisted on wearing dark glasses—to hide behind. He became intolerably destructive, and attacked his mother by throwing objects at her—obviously aiming at her eyes. At the same time, he developed a phobia of fire and a fear of going blind.

His symptoms were understood, in child analysis, as an attempt to re-externalize—to eject—the dangerous maternal introject. In view of the unavailability of the father figure, however, this left Charley utterly depleted of object cathexis.

Between his child analysis and his early adolescence, I lost sight of Charlie for quite a while as he and his family continued to live abroad.

Charles was sixteen years old when his analysis was resumed, here in the States. During the interval he appeared to have undergone a profound personality change. The maturational and/or developmental process had changed—had transformed the exuberant, aggressive, and irrepressible Charlie of the prelatency and early latency period into a subdued, overcompliant, utterly passive, and submissive youngster with a well-hidden cruel streak, which he tried strenuously to conceal even from himself.

He had a lofty—and not internalized—ego ideal, and imitated his father, parroting his sayings. Even though he seemed to try ever so hard to extricate himself from the actual influence of his mother, his analytic material revealed that he was forever searching for the "good" need-satisfying mother of his symbiotic phase Yet, at the same time, he dreaded re-engulfment in symbiosis. As soon as he found an object, he arranged somehow to lose her, out of fear that she would engulf him and that he would thus *"lose himself."* This was the same mechanism, I believe, with which he had so strikingly fought, to eject the maternal introject, at the age of five and six.

For lack of secondary—that is to say, true identity formation—through ego identifications, Charles seemed to be compelled to search for his identity—to fill the painful void, the inner emptiness, about which he continually complained.

He set himself the goal—as several of these borderline cases do, either covertly or overtly—of becoming famous, or at least important. His quite good performance, however, measured up very unfavorably against his lofty ego ideal, with the result that Charles was left with an excruciatingly low self-esteem. For this discrepancy, Charles blamed his mother because she was the one who had made him believe—in his early childhod—that he was "a genius."

In adolescence, then, Charles displayed a peculiarly affectless state. He lacked the charm that Helene Deutsch and others have found to be one of the characteristics of true "as if" personalities.[40]

He repeatedly changed his allegiance to people and to groups, because he never did feel comfortable when he came close to them—*he could only long for them from a distance.* This intense longing was the strongest affect I have ever seen in Charles.

Like Greenson's patient,[16] Charles was continually seeeking the company of others; he was quite incapable of being alone. *But he was also incapable of being "à deux" for any length of time!* What Charles kept seeking was experiences that would reunite him with the lost symbiotic mother, whom he had never renounced—in the intrapsychic sense. His affectlessness seemed to be a deep defense against his anxiety—to ward off the feeling of emptiness at the loss of a part of himself, at a time when the loss of the symbiotic mother was still equivalent to losing part of the self!

I would like to close with a quotation from material during Charles's adolescent analysis. He complained: "I don't feel like anything—I start thinking a lot; and when I think, I am not very happy." At another time, he said: "I try to find out in how many ways we are alike with any person—anybody—but particularly with people I like and respect. First I did this with my parents, with their older friends, and now I do it usually with girls. I try to find out what kind of sports and songs they like."

Charles tried to compensate for the cathectic void by identification of the mirroring type. By literally mirroring others, and also himself, he tried to learn how to feel, how to have emotions. Here are some of the associations he made in analysis: "When I dance with a girl, she becomes just like all the other girls. I want to refresh myself that *she is the one who dances with me, and yet that she is still kind and sweet.* I put my head back to look at her face, and into her eyes." In another analytic hour Charles said: "I dance around by the mirror-glass door where I can look at my own face—see what I look like, *from the point of view of others;* and also I catch a glimpse of her face, to see whether she is enjoying the dance. One thing I notice—even if I enjoy dancing, I don't look too excited, so one cannot say whether I enjoy it. So perhaps this is not the way to find out about how the girl feels either."

This brief excerpt from Charles's analysis shows how he struggled with his lack of empathy and his lack of genuine affect. One can also see that he is searching incessantly for the girl who is still *kind* and *sweet*—the "good" symbiotic mother—whom he can reflect and whose eyes reflect love for him.

SUMMARY

I have brought these clinical sketches of Jay and Charles, because I felt that these patients illustrated—through their developmental failure—the significance of normal symbiosis, and the crucial necessity of gradual individuation—particularly in the vulnerable second and third years of life.

In Jay's case we observed this developmental failure in *statu nascendi.* His traumatization occurred in the second year, and, as a result, *both* his reality constancy[13] and his object constancy suffered.

In Charles's case, we could fairly accurately reconstruct—through analytic material—the severe traumata, at vulnerable, nodal points of his separation-individuation process, particularly toward the end of it, when libidinal object constancy becomes established.

The fact that this traumatization occurred later than Jay's—in Charles's third year—is perhaps the reason why Charles's reality constancy remained fairly intact.

Both cases had to fall back to the primary mode—the "mirroring" kind of maintenance of identity—because of the failure of true identificatory and internalization processes.

BIBLIOGRAPHY

1. ALPERT, A. Reversibility of pathological fixations associated with maternal deprivation in infancy. *The Psychoanalytic Study of the Child*, 14:169-185. New York: International Universities Press, 1959.
2. ANGEL, K. On symbiosis and pseudosymbiosis. *This Journal*, 15:294-316, 1967.
3. BENEDEK, T. The psychosomatic implications of the primary unit: mother-child. *Amer. J. Orthopsychiat.*, 19:642-654, 1949.
4. BENEDEK, T. Parenthood as a developmental phase. *This Journal*, 7:389-417, 1959.
5. BENEDEK, T. The organization of the reproductive drive. *Int. J. Psycho-Anal.*, 41:1-15, 1960.
6. BENJAMIN, J. The innate and the experiential. In: *Lectures on Experimental Psychology*, ed. H. W. Brosin. Pittsburgh: University of Pittsburgh Press, 1961.
7. BROBY, S. & AXELRAD, S. Anxiety, socialization and ego-formation in infancy. *Int. J. Psycho-Anal.*, 47:218-229, 1966.
8. ELKISCH, P. Psychological significance of the mirror. *This Journal*, 5:235-244, 1957.
9. FISHER, C. Psychoanalytic implications of recent research on sleep and dreaming. *This Journal*, 13:197-303, 1965.
10. FREUD, A. A connection between the states of negativism and of emotional surrender (*Hörigkeit*). Abstr. in *Int. J. Psycho-Anal.*, 33:265, 1952.
11. FREUD, A. *Normality and Pathology in Childhood: Assessments of Development.* New York: International Universities Press, 1965.
12. FREUD, S. Formulations on the two principles of mental functioning (1911). *Standard Edition*, 12:218-227. London: Hogarth Press, 1958.
13. FROSCH, J. A note on reality constancy. In: *Psychoanalysis—A General Psychology: Essays in Honor of Heinz Hartmann*, ed. R. M. Loewenstein, L. M. Newman, M. Schur, & A. J. Solnit. New York: International Universities Press, 1966, pp. 349-376.
14. GREENACRE, P. The biologic economy of birth. *The Psychoanalytic Study of the Child*, 1:31-51, 1945.
15. GREENACRE, P. Early physical determinants in the development of a sense of identity. *This Journal*, 6:612-627, 1958.
16. GREENSON, R. R. On screen defenses, screen hunger and screen identity. *This Journal*, 6:242-262, 1958.
17. HARTMANN, H. *Ego Psychology and the Problem of Adaptation* (1939). New York: International Universities Press, 1958.
18. HARTMANN, H. *Essays on Ego Psychology: Selected Problems in Psychoanalytic Theory.* New York: International Universities Press, 1964.
19. JAMES, M. Premature ego development: some observations on disturbances in the first three months of life. *Int. J. Psycho-Anal.*, 41:288-294, 1960.
20. JOFFE, W. G. & SANDLER, J. Notes on pain, depression, and individuation. *The Psychoanalytic Study of the Child*, 20:394-424. New York: International Universities Press, 1965.

21. KRIS, E. Neutralization and sublimation: observations on young children. *The Psychoanalytic Study of the Child*, 10:30-46. New York: International Universities Press, 1955.

22. LICHTENSTEIN, H. Identity and sexuality: a study of their interrelationship in man. *This Journal*, 9:179-260, 1961.

23. LICHTENSTEIN, H. The role of narcissism in the emergence and maintenance of a primary identity. *Int. J. Psycho-Anal.*, 45:49-56, 1964.

24. MAHLER, M. S. On child psychoses and schizophrenia. *The Psychoanalytic Study of the Child*, 7:286-305. New York: International Universities Press, 1952.

25. MAHLER, M. S. [In:] Problems of infantile neurosis: a discussion. *The Psychoanalytic Study of the Child*, 9:65-66, 1954.

26. MAHLER, M. S. On two crucial phases of integration of the sense of identity: separation-individuation and bisexual identity. In panel on: Problems of Identity, rep. D. L. Rubinfine. *This Journal*, 6:141-142, 1958.

27. MAHLER, M. S. Perceptual dedifferentiation and psychotic object-relationship. *Int. J. Psycho-Anal.*, 41:548-553, 1960.

28. MAHLER, M. S. Thoughts about development and individuation. *The Psychoanalytic Study of the Child*, 18:307-324. New York: International Universities Press, 1963.

29. MAHLER, M. S. On the significance of the normal separation-individuation phase. In: *Drives, Affects, Behavior*, ed. M. Schur. New York: International Universities Press, 1965, 2:161-169.

30. MAHLER, M. S. Notes on the development of basic moods: the depressive affect. In: *Psychoanalysis—A General Psychology: Essays in Honor of Heinz Hartmann*, ed. R. M. Loewenstein, L. M. Newman, M. Schur, & A. J. Solnit. New York: International Universities Press, 1966, pp. 152-168.

31. MAHLER, M. S. Development of defense from biological and symbiotic precursors: adaptive and maladaptive aspects. In panel on: Development and Metapsychology of the Defense Organization of the Ego, rep. R. S. Wallerstein. *This Journal*, 15:130-149, 1967.

32. MAHLER, M. S. & FURER, M. Certain aspects of the separation-individuation phase. *Psychoanal. Quart.*, 32:1-14, 1963.

33. MAHLER, M. S. & GOSLINER, B. J. On symbiotic child psychosis: genetic, dynamic, and restitutive aspects. *The Psychoanalytic Study of the Child*. 10:195-212. New York: International Universities Press, 1955.

34. MAHLER, M. S. & McDEVITT, J. Observations on adaptation and defense in *statu nascendi*: developmental precursors in the first two years of life. *Psychoanal. Quart.* (in press).

35. PIAGET, J. *The Origins of Intelligence in Children* (1936). New York: International Universities Press, 1952.

36. RIBBLE, M. A. *The Rights of Infants: Early Psychological Needs and Their Satisfaction*. New York: Columbia University Press, 1943.

37. ROFFWARG, H. P., MUZIO, J. N. & DEMENT, W. C. Ontogenetic development of the human sleep-dream cycle. *Science*, 152:604-619, 1966.

38. ROSE, G. J. Creative imagination in terms of ego "core" and boundaries. *Int. J. Psycho-Anal.*, 45:75-84, 1964.

39. ROSE, G. J. Body ego and reality. *Int. J. Psycho-Anal.*, 47:502-509, 1966.

40. ROSS, N. The "as if" concept. *This Journal*, 15:59-82, 1967.

41. SCHILDER, P. *The Image and Appearance of the Human Body* (1935). New York: International Universities Press, 1950.

42. SCHUR, M. *The Id and the Regulatory Principles of Mental Functioning*. New York: International Universities Press, 1966.

43. SPIEGEL, L. The self, the sense of self, and perception. *The Psychoanalytic Study of the Child*, 14:81-108, New York: International Universities Press, 1959.

44. SPITZ, R. A. *The First Year of Life*. New York: International Universities Press, 1965.
45. SPOCK, B. The striving for autonomy and regressive object relationships. *The Psychoanalytic Study of the Child*, 18:361-366. New York: International Universities Press, 1963.
46. TARTAKOFF, H. H. The normal personality in our culture and the Nobel Prize complex. In: *Psychoanalysis—A General Psychology: Essays in Honor of Heinz Hartmann*, ed. R. M. Loewenstein, L. M. Newman, M. Schur, & A. J. Solnit. New York: International Universities Press, 1966, pp. 222-252.
47. WINNICOTT, D. W. Primary maternal preoccupation (1956). *Collected Papers*. New York: Basic Books, 1958, pp. 300-305.
48. WINNICOTT, D. W. *The Maturational Processes and the Facilitating Environment*. New York: International Universities Press, 1965.
49. WOLFF, P. H. Observations on newborn infants. *Psychosom. Med.*, 21:110-118, 1959.
50. YAZMAJIAN, R. V. Biological aspects of infantile sexuality and the latency period. *Psychoanal. Quart.*, 36:203-229, 1967.

8

CHILD DEVELOPMENT: A BASIC SCIENCE FOR PEDIATRICS

Julius B. Richmond, M.D.

*Department of Pediatrics, State University of New York
Upstate Medical Center, Syracuse, New York*

Although I have considered presenting some of the work of our group on this occasion, I have elected, rather, to discuss an issue which I feel to be of importance not alone to those of us interested in child development, but to all pediatricians (and indeed to all interested in child welfare). I refer to the role of child development in pediatrics—most particularly academic pediatrics.

To the members of this section it is no surprise to observe that teaching and research in child development have not been integrated into the mainstream of academic pediatrics. It continues, with rare exceptions, to be treated as a minority group in the academic community, even though a knowledge of child development is a major concern of the practicing pediatrician. This relative neglect causes me to inquire as to whether we are to have two cultures or one in pediatrics. At the outset I wish to indicate that my bias is clearly in favor of a unitarian view. For, I believe we continue this dichotomy at our peril in pediatric teaching and research.

Perhaps we can deal with this problem better if we understand how we came to be this way. I will, therefore, attempt to develop my thesis from an historical perspective. These periods are arbitrarily defined;

Reprinted from PEDIATRICS, Vol. 39, No. 5, May 1967, pp. 649-658. Presented on acceptance of the C. Anderson Aldrich Award of 1966, Annual Meeting, Section on Child Development, American Academy of Pediatrics. Chicago, October 23, 1966.

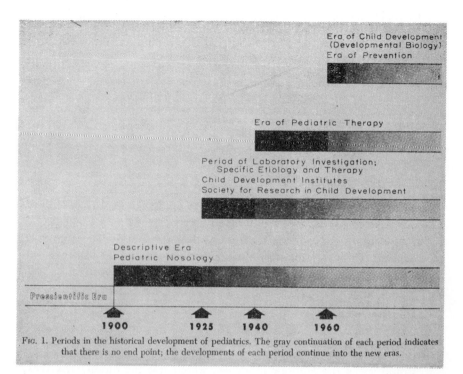

FIG. 1. Periods in the historical development of pediatrics. The gray continuation of each period indicates that there is no end point; the developments of each period continue into the new eras.

although starting dates are given, there are no end points, since each new period is telescoped into the rich history of its antecedents (Fig. 1).

The prescientific era in pediatrics (prior to 1900) was rich in contributions to our understanding of child development. Indeed, for those who consider our interest in child development as that of "Johnny-come-latelies," it is appropriate to observe that almost all of this early literature focused on the relationships of child rearing practices to child development. For example, let us recall the following observation:

> Infants who have just been weaned should be permitted to live at their ease and enjoy themselves: they should be habituated to repose of the mind and exercise in which little deceptions and gaiety play a part: . . . After the sixth or seventh year, little girls and boys should be confided to humane and gentle teachers. . . . It is not necessary either to torment children just beginning to learn by trying to teach them something through the whole length of the day: on the contrary, the greater part of the day should be devoted

to their games. In fact, even among the most robust people, who have already reached the age of complete development, deterioration of body is noticeable in those who have applied themselves too arduously and without interruption to the pursuit of learning. Children of twelve years should already frequent the grammarians and geometers and exercise their bodies; but it is necessary that they should have preceptors and supervisors who are reasonable and not entirely devoid of experience, so that they may know the amount and proper time for meals, exercise, bathing, sleeping and other details of personal hygiene. Most people will pay a high price for grooms for their horses, choosing for this purpose careful and experienced men, while they will select as teachers for their children individuals without experience. . . .

Remember, this is not from a recent issue of *Psychosomatic Medicine*, but was written by the Greek physician, Oribasius, in about 300 A. D.[1]

Or, in a more experimental manner, although not in keeping with modern day ethics concerning human experimentation, let us recall the following observations by Salimbene in the thirteenth century:[2]

. . . he wanted to find out what kind of speech and what manner of speech children would have when they grew up if they spoke to no one beforehand. So he bade foster mothers and nurses to suckle the children, to bathe and wash them, but in no way to prattle with them or to speak to them, for he wanted to learn whether they would speak the Hebrew language, which was the oldest, or Greek, or Latin, or Arabic, or perhaps the language of their parents, of whom they had been born. But he laboured in vain, because the children all died. For they could not live without the petting and joyful faces and loving words of their foster mothers. And so the songs are called "swaddling songs," which a woman sings while she is rocking the cradle, to put the child to sleep, and without them a child sleeps badly and has no rest.

And in our studies of swaddling we found a rich literature concerning this practice which raised many questions still unresolved.[3] Also we may observe that the origin of pediatrics as a discipline at the turn of the century was characterized by a concern about infant and child welfare— not exclusively health—in the developing infant welfare stations. The attention focused on feeding and other infant and child care practices, the living conditions of the family, and their consequences for the development of the child.

Although this concern with child development has remained a continuing, albeit somewhat submerged interest, it was historically inevitable that, with the coming of the scientific revolution, interests and priorities would be reordered. The rapid advances in microbiology and immunology, biochemistry, physiology, pathology, and pharmacology, among many other sciences, laid the basis for a reorganization of medical education and for the establishment of a research culture. The priorities very properly shifted toward the applications of our newer knowledge of biology to the saving of lives. That there have been great successes as a consequence of this approach is evident to anyone who cares to compare infant and child morbidity and mortality statistics on any basis between 1900 and today. To accomplish these changes, a sequence of historical development evolved as follows.

The period of descriptive pediatrics resulting in a pediatric nosology was from approximately 1900. As a prelude to more precise etiologic definitions of disease, clinical descriptions and classifications became necessary. During this period the unique aspects of disease in children became apparent to most and pediatrics was established as a discipline. (Let us recall there was considerable resistance to the acceptance of this concept and residua of resistance remain even to this day.) The textbooks of pediatrics of this era contain the most lucid descriptions of the natural history of disease in childhood.

Obviously this period was not confined exclusively to description. Many public health and therapeutic advances were taking place. The pasteurization of milk, the introduction of cod liver oil and orange juice for the prevention of rickets and scurvy on an empirical basis, and the introduction of parenteral fluid administration had much to do with lowering morbidity and mortality. For those who talk about research data in the social sciences today as "soft" data, I would recall that by modern standards the data of that era look rather "soft." But who would say that the Holts and Parks and many others of that era were "soft" in their approaches because they didn't anticipate the more precise quantification of the future.

The period of the rise of laboratory investigations into specific etiologies and therapies was from approximately 1925. During this period the elegant and elaborate studies of infant and child metabolism provided the basis for our better understanding of nutrition and the elaboration of our knowledge of specific food factors. These studies also provide the basis for modern parenteral therapy. The elucidation of specific infectious agents and the concomitant increase in our understanding of immunology led to the development of immunizing procedures which are still evolving. The basis for antibacterial therapy and its early successes developed during this period.

A parallel development was also occurring in this era. In the late 1920's the Laura Spelman Rockefeller Fund, largely at the urging of

Lawrence K. Frank, recognized the need for a better understanding of growth and development. Two very significant developments occurred as a consequence:

1. The establishment of a number of child research institutes. Although this took place in universities and largely outside the mainstream of medical centers, it is interesting to note that at least three or four child development research programs weer established under medical auspices. I refer of course, to the studies of Dr. Alfred Washburn at the Child Research Council in Denver, Dr. Harold Stuart at the Harvard School of Public Health, Dr. Lester Sontag at the Fels Research Institute at Yellow Springs, and Dr. Milton Senn, first at the Cornell Medical Center and then at the Yale Child Study Center. We should also note, although it is not widely heralded, that Dr. Arnold Gesell was also a pediatrician as he conducted his observations on the development of children.

2. The organization of the Society for Research in Child Development. Since there was no other scientific forum for communication among workers in the interdisciplinary field of child development, this development seemed logical. Over the years this organization has stimulated teaching and research in growth and development when the more clinically oriented disciplines were pursuing the control of pathology. This organization has facilitated the publication of work in this field, most notably the journal of *Child Development* and *Monographs of the Society for Research in Child Development*. I direct attention to this literature as one unfortunately largely neglected in pediatrics.

The golden era of pediatric therapy might also be called the period of the rise of molecular biology (from 1949).

Dr. Samuel Levine, in his presidential address before the American Pediatric Society,[4] summarized this period as follows: "From 1920 to 1950, many of us lived through and participated in what might be called the golden age of curative pediatrics—prophylactic immunization, the widespread use of vitamins, nutritional knowledge, water and electrolyte metabolism, discovery and availability of antibiotics, isolation and synthesis of hormones, tranquilizers and diuretics, plus an ever-growing body of scientific knowledge, led to radical changes in both the scope and direction of modern pediatrics."

But he also indicated the restlessness of some of the elder statesmen of pediatrics with the *status quo* by the following comment: "While a major revolution has taken place in community and individual child health needs during the past couple of decades, pediatric education would appear to be still plugging along in the pattern of the late 1920's or, at best, the early 1930's."

It was clear by the end of World War II that the dramatic declines in infant and childhood morbidity and mortality were coming to an end. I do not wish to minimize efforts to reduce morbidity and mortality as the continuing responsibility of pediatrics. But, as Dr. Levine indicates, there was a growing awareness that, if pediatrics was to continue to pursue its goal as defined by the American Academy of Pediatrics,* "to foster and stimulate interest in pediatrics and in all aspects of the work for the welfare of children," there would have to be an emphasis on all aspects of the life of the child and not exclusively his biological development. The conventional classifications of morbidity and mortality would no longer suffice. The new pediatric nosology would also need to be concerned with child ecology and child rearing practices and their consequences for the development of the child.

Certain sociological changes catalyzed the new concerns. The Selective Service statistics of World War II indicated a relatively high incidence of psychological and social ineffectiveness in our young adult population. It was reasonable that an expectation would develop that those of us in the child care professions might be in a position to minimize such developments. Also, with the increasing mobility of our population, parents came increasingly to look toward professional services for help with child rearing practices. Concomitantly, rapid urbanization came upon us with all of the complexities of rearing children in increasingly dense population areas. And, simultaneously, physicians and other health professionals were leaving the rural areas and the cities for the suburbs, leaving large numbers of children relatively unattended medically, particularly in the central cities. Dr. Christopherson has recently commented on this phenomenon as follows: "The practitioner has moved to the suburbs. I think a lot of men in practice don't see this thing occurring. They're taking care of a lot of people and doing a good job with those they see . . . but those they don't see . . . this bothers me."[5]

There were considerable efforts to deal with the pediatrician's potential concerns with the psychological and social development of children and their adaptations to a rapidly changing society during this period. But there were at least two factors which militated against more successful efforts. These were: (1) conceptual confusion concerning the defini-

---

* From the fellowship certificate of the American Academy of Pediatrics.

tion of the problem, and (2) resistance within the pediatric academic community to incorporating these efforts in a sophisticated way.

Conceptual confusion—As pediatricians came to realize the need for developing greater competence in guiding the psychosocial development of children in the period immediately following World War II, they turned predominantly to the field of child psychiatry for help. Within the Academy this was reflected in the establishment of a Section on Mental Health which had a checkered career for a variety of reasons.

I trust that my comments concerning this period will not be regarded as pejorative to individuals or disciplines (indeed, I lived through this period too). But, in retrospect, it seems clear to some of us that the stage of development of the field of child psychiatry ill-equipped it to provide the core conceptual and methodologic background and skills for pediatricians. Why was this so?

Child psychiatry grew out of a concern for the disturbed child and adult, although a few child psychiatrists who left their clinical settings contributed some original observations to normal development. As a consequence, child psychiatry was relatively rich in theory (drawn largely from retrospective reconstructions in the treatment of psychiatric patients) and relatively short on empirical observations of the development of children. Pediatricians have grown up in a culture based on empirical observation (and perhaps have been too atheoretical). Small wonder, therefore, that the teachings of child psychiatrists fell on relatively deaf ears of pediatric trainees, with the frustration level high on both sides—as it inevitably must be when there are inappropriate expectations by each.

I am not suggesting that the concerns of child psychiatry were and are inappropriate. The study of psychopathology and the management of disturbed children is a legitimate and socially necessary function. But pediatricians are concerned predominantly with the developmental process and prevention, which I submit is a quite different frame of reference which I would classify as child development. I refer to the dynamic development of individual differences in behavior patterns, the observation of child rearing practices and their consequences, the emergence of curiosity, learning patterns, coping behavior, and personality, and the capacities of children and families to master adversity. Such observations are available to pediatricians in their daily work; child psychiatrists must leave their settings to gain opportunities for such studies. In the face of these opportunities and challenges it is surprising, indeed, that pediatricians have with few exceptions so neglected research in child development.

Each clinical discipline, if it is to mature, must extend the knowledge in its field through investigation. And clinical investigation prospers most when it draws upon theory and method from a basic discipline. Thus, metabolic studies in pediatrics have drawn heavily on biochemistry and physiology; infectious disease studies have been based on epidemiology, microbiology, immunology, etc. By our dependence upon child psychiatry, we were looking to another clinical discipline (in this instance one which has not yet established a research tradition) for research orientation. This would be somewhat analogous to our metabolic investigators depending predominantly on workers in internal medicine for leadership; obviously there are lessons to be learned from other clinical disciplines, but they cannot be the primary source.

It may have been inevitable that it would take us two decades to become aware of the rapid developments in the social and biological sciences contributing to the growth of the field of child development. Perhaps this was due in part to their separation from clinical settings so that many of their studies seemed esoteric and without application. But would this be any more so than biochemical studies in the early decades of this century? It required a group of pioneering pediatricians—the Bambles and Darrows and many others—to effect the linkage. Certainly the application of the techniques of the social scientists and developmental biologists to clinical settings is destined to increase our knowledge of the development of children. For what richer opportunities are there for collaborative studies of varied patterns of child care occurring "spontaneously" than in our various clinical settings and in social agencies? I refer to foster care, adoptions, institutional care, the impact of physical illness, and handicapping conditions as challenging issues for study.

But there were other problems in our heavy dependence upon child psychiatry for the teaching of psychosocial deevlopment. In a review of the proceedings of the Conference on Training in Child Psychiatry[6] it is apparent that among child psychiatrists the concepts of development are largely limited to those stemming from psychiatry to the relative neglect of the very considerable literature in child development generally. Thus, our own neglect of this literature was reinforced. Also, since child psychiatrists know their own training programs best, they often cast the training of pediatricians in the same mold. Hence, such training often bore little relevance to the pediatrician's job. But, just as significantly, it often served to confuse the pediatrician concerning his basic professional identity.

This matter of identity merits further comment and has been discussed in more extensive terms by Erikson.[7] Since pediatricians were not conducting such training mainly (in contrast to training in metabolic, infectious diseases, and other areas), it undoubtedly was a source of confusion to the pediatrician as to whether this was a proper concern for him. Although I do not wish to oversimplify, this matter of identity-confusion was undoubtedly responsible for the fact that many pediatricians moved from pediatrics to child psychiatry (and in the process we hope that child psychiatry has been enriched). But I have looked—and thus far have not found—a single example of a child psychiatrist having moved into pediatrics What I am suggesting is that such teaching has not served to reinforce the pediatrician in terms of his professional identity.

But all of our problems do not stem from our dependence on another discipline. Some are of our own making, which I have referred to earlier as resistance to the incorporation of child development—especially its psychosocial aspects—within pediatrics, particularly by academic pediatrics. This has taken the following forms:

1. That psychosocial considerations are not a proper concern of pediatrics. Although by the Academy's definition this is untenable, it has been seriously held by some. In the face of increasing specialization and subspecialization (which I do *not* view with alarm) there is, among some, resistance to any new development. But progress is not achieved by burying our heads in the sand; rather, we must find ways of re-organizing our programs without sacrificing the basic, generic, clinical background of training which stamps each of us indelibly as pediatricians regardless of what we do later.

2. The rigid institutionalization (or bureaucratization) of our concepts and programs which inhibits new developments. It has been said that no institution is as resistant to change as one which has once attained excellence. But excellent institutions can deteriorate. It has been apparent that re-orientation of training programs has been difficult to achieve (as noted by Dr. Levine). Also, concepts can become rigid as well. Are we holding more tenaciously to disease oriented, rather than process oriented research? In other words, should not the concept of developmental biology become the pervasive orientation in pediatric education—and indeed in all of medical education? It is encouraging to note that Dr. Levine's successor, Dr. Wallace McCrory, reflects some growing interest in this direction among pediatric educators in his presidential address on "Psychometabolism" before the Society for Pediatric Research.[8]

Another comment on the institutionalization of pediatric education characterizes all successful institutions, that is the tendency to "play it safe." Bright trainees have a sure channel to success through the established laboratory fellowship programs. How many professors have encouraged their best trainees to pioneer in new ventures in child development? Yet this is what the pioneers in academic pediatrics did. The difference between their era and ours is that there were *no* sure channels to success then. There are many traditional ones now. Parenthetically I might add that those of us who have established such training programs in child development may not have promoted them sufficiently.

3. The "hard data" vs "soft data" concept. In many ways the most subtle resistance to research and training in child development has been the inference by many pediatric investigators that those who deal with biologic research have "hard data" while those interested in the social sciences have "soft data." I would be tempted to dismiss this as rubbish were it not for the considerable credence accorded this view by otherwise critical people.

At the risk of being pedantic, I would indicate that such positions have nothing in common with good science. For the scientific method demands excellence in experimental design, data collection, and data analysis. The question, therefore, is one of excellence—not of hardness or softness. As one who has been on the editorial board of several journals, I can vouch for the fact that there can be "soft data" in biological research as well as social science research. If we are unhappy about the state of development of a field, we have the obligation to help deepen and extend it—not to cast the first stone. Certainly, to go back to our early pediatric investigators, they had to make inferences from methods we would not be using today in many instances.

Another evidence of the view commonly held that there is no discipline or body of knowledge in child development was called to my attention by a colleague at another center. He pointed to the tendency for professors, as they taper off in their own investigative work, to take to lecturing on child development. This is reminiscent of a story the late Dr. Henry Sigerist, the eminent medical historian, was fond of telling. As he approached retirement, he received a letter from the professor emeritus of obstetrics at a western medical school explaining that he had retired and that he had always had an interest in medical history. He was, therefore, planning to teach a course to medical students and asked Dr. Sigerist to suggest a bibliography for him. Dr. Sigerist pondered over the letter, then replied that he, too, was retiring and that he had always had an interest in obstetrics. He was, therefore, planning to teach a course in obstetrics for medical students and wondered if the professor could suggest a bibliography.

But a critical analysis is not sufficient to meet our needs. A program of constructive action is necessary, in which the Section on Child Development can play a major role. For it came into being with our current era in pediatrics—what I would define as: the era of developmental biology and prevention.

As we developed greater conceptual and operational clarity concerning our needs in pediatrics, the Executive Board acted (for a variety of additional reasons, too) to terminate the Section on Mental Health. And, after much deliberation, it voted to establish the Section on Child Development, which defined its objectives as follows:

1. To stimulate interest, work, and research in the field of human development.

2. To advise the Executive Board of the American Academy of Pediatrics concerning developments in the field of human growth and development.

3. To establish a forum which will facilitate communication among professional workers in the field of growth and development.

4. To foster educational activities for pediatricians, other physicians and related professional groups to increase their understanding of and competence in the field of child development.

5. To stimulate programs for the education of non-professional citizens in the field of child development.

6. To engage in long-range evaluation of and planning for the Academy's varied interests in all matters concerning growth and development among appropriate agencies—governmental and non-governmental.[9]

But statements are not enough. If they were, the statement on training in growth and development published in 1951 by the American Board of Pediatrics[10] would have had a greater impact. It said, among other things:

> The Board does not believe that pediatricians should be less adequately trained in the care of the sick infant and child. It does believe, however, that a study of growth and developmental processes can be advantageously incorporated into such training. One of the outstanding defects of current candidates is the fact that on the basis of examination requirements they have didactically mastered a certain number of facts relating to growth and development without understanding the practical implications of these facts.
> It becomes obvious, therefore, that pediatric training centers must increasingly assume the responsibility for the day-to-day teach-

ing of growth and development in a clinical setting. This means a practical evaluation of the total development of each patient and its meaning to parents and physicians. It also means that some opportunity to observe presumably well infants and children become part of the training program where it is not at present. Intensive study of relatively few patients longitudinally provides an opportunity to teach not only growth and development but the importance of continuity of pediatric care which is an important element of pediatric practice.

It is to be emphasized that the Board recognizes that only pediatricians themselves adequately trained in growth and development can teach effectively. While other personnel (nutritionists, anthropologists, psychologists psychiatrists) may participate advantageously at various times, only the pediatrician is an a position to teach by example. At the resident level this is probably the most effective teaching technique.

This statement is presented, not with the idea of making something different of pediatricians or pediatric education. Rather it is intended to strengthen both, and to render both more adequate for their responsibility of caring for the total health of children.

What we need now is a strategy for incorporating teaching and research in child development into the mainstream of pediatrics. The strategy requires the development of a core of pediatric faculty members with a disciplined background of research and teaching analogous to our academic pediatricians in metabolism, infectious diseases, etc. This will necessitate the establishment of fellowships for pediatricians in child development (which includes a range of investigation from physical and physiological development—including developmental biochemistry, physiology, pharmacology—through psychophysiology and psychological and social development). The Section on Child Development of this Academy can become an advocate for the provision, by various granting agencies, of funds for this purpose. Training programs of this nature will require an investment of time and energy in the study of child development as a basic science for academic pediatricians.

Those of us interested in child development have an obligation to institutionalize such training for pediatricians, for as departments of pediatrics increasingly wish to add such faculty members, they find them relatively unavailable. This will mean, in addition to the few such fellowships now available in departments of pediatrics, periods of study by pediatricians in the social sciences—sociology, cultural anthropology, psychology, economics, and urban planning, among many others.

We also have a mission to bring developmental concepts into the mainstream of pediatric teaching if the goals of the American Board of Pediatrics are to be attained. And, perhaps even more significantly, the concept of human development must become a central theme of medical education if it is to meet the changing needs of society. I again come back to a shift in human biology—of which medicine is a division—from an emphasis on disease to one of process. And processes may be ordered around development as a unifying concept. And who will be the interpretors of these changes if not the members of this Section?

These developments have received some recognition through some disenchantment with the established categorical institutes of the National Institutes of Health organized as they have been around organ systems or diseases. The emergence of the new National Institute of Child Health and Human Development reflected this changing orientation. But new institutions do not emerge full blown and this one merits more support than we have given it. And its brief history reflects our weakness; there have been relatively few proposals for research in child development from pediatricians.

This emphasis on child development research by pediatricians does not reflect a proprietary interest on my part. It is not a matter of "if we don't do it, someone else will," for I have never considered such motivation to be wholesome. Rather, it reflects my conviction that the basic background of the pediatrician in biology—particularly his responsibility for enhancing the development of the nervous system—along with his opportunities through continuing health care to observe the unfolding of the child's psychological and social development, uniquely equips him to raise research questions concerning development which are rarely available to others. Indeed, this is the uniqueness of any pediatric investigator, for embryologists, biochemists, physiologists, pathologists, and many others can do research on development. The pediatrician's clinical orientation, however, marks his uniqueness.

Although we are relatively lacking in child development research in pediatrics, a word of caution is in order as we attempt to make up for deficits. There is no easy or quick road to competent scholarship. We have seen too many examples in recent years, because of the availability of money and of efforts to develop "instant" teachers and investigators—usually to the discredit of these programs. We must make haste slowly. As part of this caution, it is necessary to indicate that this area of pediatric interest cannot serve as a haven for people who are "fugitives from measurement" if it is to thrive. For to do research one must learn to measure something.

It would be inappropriate to discuss this era of preventive pediatrics without commenting on some of our social responsibilities. Our very considerable successes in reducing morbidity and mortality from many diseases have brought us face to face with new problems. And, precisely because of our past successes, society looks to us for new successes.

But many of our current problems are in large measure social problems. The leading cause of childhood mortality, accidents, will require the social applications of what we know in concert with other groups in society for its reduction. There is good reason to believe that further reductions in infant mortality will depend upon improvement of the living conditions of people in poverty and not alone on better medical care. The problems of delinquency and the addictions (to drugs, alcohol, and tobacco) will depend upon our better knowledge of the sociology of our communities.

As we continue to move rapidly toward an increasingly urban society, the needs of children must be considered in more dynamic terms. We have been slow, in all aspects of planning, to catch up with the rapid changes in our society. Pediatricians, while carrying on research to provide better data for planning, nonetheless can serve as advocates for the application of the knowledge we already have. I wish to emphasize that there are some who suggest that because we don't know everything that we propose nothing. This would be akin to our pediatric predecessors withholding cod liver oil as a preventive for rickets because biochemists had not yet learned that it contained Vitamin D.

For there are many things we do know. We know, for example, that environmental deprivation takes a heavy developmental toll among infants and young children. And we know that the consequence is a tremendous social loss in addition to the serious institutional problems presented to the schools. Although some of the new programs are endeavoring to deal with these problems, they represent only a start. More imagination, more planning, and more resources will be necessary. The greater cost to society will be to drift without such efforts.

It is clear that we must more explicity recognize that we are training pediatricians for a variety of functions which may be classified under the following divisions:

1. general clinical pediatrics,
2. subspecialties (including academic pediatrics),
3. institutional and public health pediatrics.

Each of these requires a generic training in clinical pediatrics. But, if we are to discharge our obligations to society, we cannot neglect any one of these functions in favor of the other.

We stand on the threshold of achieving the best health record for children the world has ever known. Whether we cross this threshold will depend upon the imagination, industry, and resourcefulness with which we expand and apply our knowledge of child development.

REFERENCES

1. RUHRAH, J.: Pediatrics of the Past. New York: Hoeber, p. 13, 1925.
2. ROSE, J. B., and McLAUGHLIN, M. M.: A Portable Medieval Reader. New York: Viking Press, 1949.
3. LIPTON, E. L., STEINSCHNEIDER, A., and RICHMOND, J. B.: Swaddling, a child care practice: Historical, cultural and experimental observations. *Pediatrics* (Suppl.), *35*:521, 1965.
4. LEVINE, S. Z.: Pediatric education at the crossroads: Presidential address, American Pediatric Society. Amer. J. Dis. Child., *100*:651, 1950.
5. CHRISTOPHERSON, E. H., M. D.: Modern Medicine, *34*:64, July 4, 1966.
6. Conference on Training in Child Psychiatry, Washington, D.C., January 10-15, 1963.
7. ERIKSON, E.: Identity and the life cycle. Psychological Issues, *1*:1, 1959.
8. McCRORY, W. W.: Psychometabolism. J. Pediat., *67*:894, 1965.
9. Section on Child Development, American Academy of Pediatrics. Statement of Objectives. Operations Manual, p. 137, April, 1960.
10. A statement by the American Board of Pediatrics on training requirements in growth and development. *Pediatrics*, 7:430, 1951.

9

THE RELATIONSHIP BETWEEN PSYCHIATRY AND PEDIATRICS: A DISPUTATIOUS VIEW

Leon Eisenberg, M.D.

Professor of Child Psychiatry, Harvard Medical School

The Aldrich Award Address by Dr. Julius Richmond[1] requires careful reading. Within its sober, low-keyed asesssment of the state of developmental research in pediatrics is a perceptive critique of the present and an exciting preview of a possible future. Writing as a pediatrician, Dr. Richmond chides, but only gently, my psychiatric colleagues and indicates, but only modestly, the potential contribution of pediatrics. As a child psychiatrist not under (or at least not admitting to) such restraints, I feel freer to comment on certain aspects of the relationship between the two specialties.

Child psychiatrists cite the importance of knowledge of child development for fully effective pediatric practice, bemoan the grossly inadequate training in medical psychology presently afforded pediatric house officers, and decry the unsympathetic reception they receive from pediatric faculties when they argue for more curriculum time. For each of these, they have ample justification. But, is the analysis complete when this much has been said? Not by a long shot!

Pediatricians have all too often gone to psychiatric rounds and come away none the wiser. In many centers, the pediatric house officer has been treated as though he were a sub-professional to whom the arcane art of psychotherapy and its theory of "depth" psychology were not to be entrusted. Pediatricians, with their grounding in laboriously acquired

Reprinted from PEDIATRICS, Vol. 39, No. 5, May 1967, pp. 645-647.

empirical data, controlled therapeutic trials, and action-oriented methods of intervention, find it difficult to swallow (having passed beyond the oral stage, to borrow Leo Kanner's pun) the untestable theories, the talmudical disputation based on appeal to authority, and the apparent indifference, at least until recently, to the public health aspects of psychiatric problems. They have been distressed by the commonly encountered ignorance of pediatrics, an area of training "recommended" to applicants for certification in child psychiatry, but clearly not considered necessary (since not obligatory) for the acquisition of competence. How absurd! Can disordered behavior be fully understood without regard to its neurophysiologic developmental underpinnings? If the physically ill child is inevitably troubled in his feeling and thinking, as psychiatrists properly remind pediatricians, is not the child with troubled emotions and faulty cognition equally characterized by physiologic malfunction? Or, does an illness, once its metabolic foundation has been identified, cease to be psychiatric? Quite to the contrary, what is specific to psychiatry as a medical discipline is its responsibility for the biologic as well as the psychologic aspects of behavior; what is specific to child psychiatry is its concern for an organism whose body, brain, and mind interact profoundly in the process of development.[2]

Let me pursue the heresy. In my experience with pediatric fellows who have elected a year of training in psychological pediatrics,[3] I repeatedly have been impressed that they start out ahead of the child psychiatry trainee and that they finish, surely not as knowledgeable as they would be after 2 or more years, but quite competent in the assessment and management of a wide range of developmental disorders. I must caution the reader that these fellows are, of course, not run-of-the-mine pediatric house officers; they are chosen from the self-selected few who enter this arena convinced of its importance and strongly interested in it. They have returned to pediatrics where they function, not as junior grade Dick Tracys, but as effective physicians sensitive to the body and soul and relatively expert in redressing disorders in each, at least insofar as expertness resides in today's methods.

Then, is original sin to be found only in child psychiatry? Not by a long shot! Psychiatrists do know some things which they can teach pediatricians, are not to be blamed for not knowing everything, and should be used charitably even if they sometimes affect to know more than they do, an affliction not unknown among physicians. But they are not often called upon to offer what they can. Moreover, pediatrics has long neglected its responsibility for the study of child development. The central nervous system, which quadruples its mass and undergoes an explosive proliferation in its interconnections as the infant progresses from birth to adolescence, is the most distinctive feature of the human species;[4] it is central to the understanding of the integrated function of the developing child, that with which the children's doctor is chiefly concerned. Academic pediatrics has, I believe, lagged in its interest in the clinical care of the non-hospitalized child. Its training has moved toward an ever more precious preoccupation with the exotic; it prepares its house officers exceedingly well for what they will rarely see and says hardly a word about what will confront them daily. Little wonder that so many are disaffected in the workaday world of practice.

Pediatrics is in ferment.[5] Should its training be lengthened? The answer should not be sought in status comparisons with other specialties but in the uses to which the additional time is to be put. If for more of the same, I say no; the exigencies of manpower cry out against it. If what is offered now be regarded as essential—and it may well be—then the extra year will be needed to provide a more profound experience in ambulatory care with major stress (1) on developmental problems—learning disorders, troubled behavior, mental retardation, CNS malfunction; (2) on the acquisition of skill in the delivery of medical care to those not now adequately served; and (3) on dynamic methods for disease prevention and health supervision.

All of this will require a solid base in research in child development, not simply borrowed from the behavioral sciences or from psychiatry but undertaken by pediatricians. For, the teachers of pediatricians must be pediatricians, with competence acquired precisely through investigation. With no intent to disparage the elegance of the DNA double helix, its further exploration is not more (neither less) of an intellectual challenge than the exploration of behavior. The dawning of a new era will be signaled when pediatric chairmen develop strategies to encourage their promising young people to acquire excellence in the disciplines pertinent to child development, for it will not happen of itself with manpower limited and with the lure of more established pathways to academic preferment. It will be heralded when senior pediatric faculty attend psychiatric conferences and when they discuss relevant psychosocial factors in evaluating patients (not merely their livers, enzymes or lungs) at pediatric grand rounds. It will have arrived when important faculty posts are awarded for contributions to the understanding of child development.

This is no call for the supplanting of the child psychiatrist by the pediatrician. The problems are too varied and the needs too great for any single specialty and, at the moment, for all.[6] It is an appeal, added to Dr. Richmond's, for the pediatrician to take his rightful and honored place. The justification for pediatrics as a medical specialty is precisely its concern with human development; in this sequence, the development of the brain and mind is at once the most truly human, the most important for the survival of the species, and the least understood.

REFERENCES

1. RICHMOND, J. B.: Child development: A basic science for pediatrics. *Pediatrics, 39*: 649, 1967.
2. EISENBERG, L.: A developmental approach to adolescence. *Children, 12*:131, 1965.
3. A fellowship program in the psychologic aspects of the medical care of children, supported originally by The W. T. Grant Foundation and currently by the Children's Bureau (Project Number 213).
4. EISENBERG, L.: A developmental approach to personality formation. *In* Freedman, A. M., and Kaplan, H., ed.: Comprehensive Textbook of Psychiatry. Baltimore: Williams and Wilkins, 1967.
5. WRIGHT, F. H., ed.: Pediatric residency training. Proceedings of an institute sponsored by the American Board of Pediatrics at Atlanta, Georgia, September 17-19, 1965. *Pediatrics, 38*:711, 1966.
6. LOURIE, R. S.: Problems of diagnosis and treatment: Communication between pediatrician and psychiatrist. *Pediatrics, 37*:1000, 1966.

10

WHAT IS THE OPTIMAL LEARNING ENVIRONMENT FOR THE YOUNG CHILD?

Bettye M. Caldwell, Ph.D.

Professor of Child Development and Education, Syracuse University, and Director, Children's Center, Department of Pediatrics, Upstate Medical Center, State University of New York, Syracuse, New York

This paper examines the validity of the premise that there is only one effective learning environment for the very young child—an intrafamily environment characterized by minimal disruption of primary social relationships. New evidence pointing to (1) the importance of the first three years for priming cognitive development and (2) the inability of many parents to provide the child with the priming ingredients suggests that alternative models involving home supplementation should be considered. If such supplementation is to have maximum effectiveness, careful thought should be given to the advisability of beginning it during the very earliest years of life during which time the child is maximally receptive.

A truism in the field of child development is that the milieu in which development occurs influences that development. As a means of validating the principle, considerable scientific effort has gone into the Linnaean task of describing and classifying milieus and examining de-

Reprinted from AMERICAN JOURNAL OF ORTHOPSYCHIATRY, January 1967, Volume XXXVII, Number 1, pp. 8-21. Copyright 1967, The American Orthopsychiatric Association, Inc., reproduced by permission. The author's work is supported by Grant Nos. MH-07649 and MH-08542, NIMH, U.S. Public Health Service, and by Grant No. D-156 (R), Children's Bureau, Social Security Administration, Department of Health, Education, and Welfare.

velopmental consequences associated with different types. Thus we know something about what it is like to come of age in New Guinea,[29] in a small Midwestern town,[4] in villages and cities in Mexico[25] in families of different social-class level in Chicago[12] or Boston,[27, 31] in a New York slum,[46] in Russian collectives,[9] in Israeli Kibbutzim,[23, 34, 41] in the eastern part of the United States,[33] and in a Republican community in Central New York.[10] Most of these milieu descriptions have placed great stress on the fact that they were just that and nothing more, i.e., they have expressed the customary scientific viewpoint that to describe is not to judge or criticize. However, in some of the more recent milieu descriptions which have contrasted middle- and lower-class family environments or highlighted conditions in extreme lower-class settings,[31, 46] often more than a slight suggestion has crept in that things could be better for the young child from the deprived segment of the culture. Even so, there remains a justifiable wariness about recommending or arranging any environment for the very young child other than the type regarded as its natural habitat, viz., within its own family.

Of course, optimizing environments are arranged all the time under one guise or another. For example, for disturbed children whose family environments seem effectively to reinforce rather than extinguish psychopathology, drastic alterations of milieu often are attempted. This may take the form of psychotherapy for one or both parents as well as the disturbed child, or it may involve total removal of the child from the offending environment with temporary or prolonged placement of the child in a milieu presumably more conducive to normal development. Then there is the massive milieu arrangement formalized and legalized as "education" which profoundly affects the lives of all children once they reach the age of five or six. This type of arrangement is not only tolerated but fervently endorsed by our culture as a whole. In fact, any subculture (such as the Amish) which resists the universalization of this pattern of milieu arrangement is regarded as unacceptably deviant and as justifying legal action to enforce conformity.

For very young children, however, there has been a great deal of timidity about conscious and planned arrangement of the developmental milieu, as though the implicit assumption has been made that any environment which sustains life is adequate during this period. This is analogous to suggesting that the intrauterine environment during the period of maximal cellular proliferation is less important than it is later, a suggestion that patently disregards evidence from epidemiology and experimental embryology. The rate of proliferation of new behavioral skills during the first three years of life and the increasing accumulation of data pointing to the relative permanence of deficit acquired when the environment is inadequate during this period make it mandatory that careful attention be given to the preparation of the developmental environment during the first three years of life.

CONCLUSIONS FROM INADEQUATE ENVIRONMENTS

It is, of course, an exaggeration to imply that no one has given attention to the type of environment which can nourish early and sustained growth and development. For a good three decades now infants who are developing in different milieus have been observed and examined, and data relating to their development have made it possible to identify certain strengths and deficiencies of the different types of environments. Of all types described, the one most consistently indicted by the data is the institution. A number of years ago Goldfarb[19] published an excellent series of studies contrasting patterns of intellectual functioning shown by a group of adopted adolescents who had been reared in institutions up to age three and then transferred to foster homes or else placed shortly after birth in foster homes. The development of the group that had spent time in the institution was deficient in many ways compared to the group that had gone directly into foster homes. Provence and Lipton[33] recently published a revealing description of the early social and intellectual development of infants in institutions, contrasting their development with that of home-reared children. On almost every measured variable the institutional infants were found wanting—less socially alert and outgoing, less curious, less responsive, less interested in objects, and generally less advanced. The findings of this study are almost prototypic of the literature in the field, as pointed out in excellent reviews by Yarrow[47] and Ainsworth.[1]

Although there are many attributes in combination that comprise the institutional environment, the two most obvious elements are (1) absence of a mother and (2) the presence of a group. These basic characteristics have thus been identified as the major carriers of the institutional influence and have been generalized into an explicit principle guiding our recommendations for optimal environments—learning or otherwise—for young children whenever any type of milieu arrangement is necessary. This principle may be stated simply as: the optimal environment for the young child is one in which the child is cared for in his own home in the context of a warm, continuous emotional relationship with his own mother under conditions of varied sensory input. Implicit in this principle is the conviction that the child's mother is the person best qualified to provide a stable and warm interpersonal relationship as well as the necessary pattern of sensory stimulation. Implicit also is the assumption that socio-emotional development has priority during the first three years and that if this occurs normally, cognitive development, which is of minor importance during this period anyway, will take care of itself. At a still deeper level lurks the assumption that attempts to foster cognitive development will interfere with socio-emotional development. Advocacy of the principle also implies endorsement of the idea that most homes are adequate during this early period and that no formal training (other than possibly some occasional supervisory support) for mothering is necessary. Such an operating principle places quite an onus on mothers and assumes that they will possess or quickly acquire all the talents necessary to create an optimal learning environment. And this author, at least, is convinced that a majority of mothers have such talents or proclivities and that they are willing to try to do all they can to create for their children the proper developmental milieu.

But there are always large numbers of children for whom family resources are not available and for whom some type of substitute milieu arrangement must be made. On the whole, such attempts have followed the entirely logical and perhaps evolutionary approach to milieu development—they have sought to create substitute families. The same is usually true when parents themselves seek to work out an alternate child-care arrangement because of less drastic conditions, such as maternal employment. The most typical maneuver is to try to obtain a motherly person who will "substitute" for her (not supplement her) during her hours away from her young child.

Our nation has become self-consciously concerned with social evolution, and in the past decade a serious attempt has been made to assimilate valid data from the behavioral and social sciences into planning for social action. In this context it would be meaningful to examine and question some of the hidden assumptions upon which our operating principle about the optimal environment for the young child rests.

EXAMINING THE HIDDEN ASSUMPTIONS

1. *Do intermittent, short-term separations of the child from the mother impair the mother-child relationship or the development of the child?* Once having become sensitized to the consequences of institutionalization, and suspicious that the chief missing ingredient was the continued presence of the mother, the scientific and professional community went

on the *qui vive* to the possibly deleterious consequences of any type of separation of an infant from its mother. Accordingly, a number of studies[10, 18, 21, 35, 39] investigated the consequences of short-term intermittent separation and were unable to demonstrate in the children the classical syndrome of the "institutional child." In reviewing the literature, Yarrow[47] stressed the point that available data do not support the tendency to assume that maternal deprivation, such as exists in the institutional environment, and maternal separation are the same thing. Apparently short cyclic interruptions culminated by reunions do not have the same effect as prolonged interruptions, even though quantitatively at the end of a designated period the amount of time spent in a mother-absent situation might be equal for the two experiences. Also in this context it is well to be reminded that in the institutional situation there is likely to be no stable mother-child relationship to interrupt. These are often never-mothered rather than ever-mothered children, a fact which must be kept in mind in generalizing from data on institutional groups. Thus until we have data to indicate that such intermittent separation-reunion cycles have similar effects on young children as prolonged separations, we are probably unjustified in assuming that an "uninterrupted" relationship is an essential ingredient of the optimal environment.

2. *Is group upbringing invariably damaging?* In studies done in West European and American settings, social and cognitive deficits associated with continuous group care during infancy have been frequently demonstrated. Enough exceptions have been reported, however, to warrant an intensification of the search for the "true" ingredient in the group situation associated with the observed deficits. For example, Freud and Dann[17] described the adjustment of a group of six children reared in a concentration camp orphanage for approximately three years, where they were cared for by overworked and impersonal inmates of the camp, and then transported to a residence for children in England. The children, who had never known their own mothers but who had been together as a group for approximately three years, were intensely attached to one another. Although their adjustment to their new environment was slow and differed from the pattern one would expect from home-reared children, it was significant that they eventually did make a reasonably good adjustment. That the children were able to learn a new language while making this emotional transition was offered as evidence that many of the basic cognitive and personality attributes remained unimpaired in spite of the pattern of group upbringing. The accumulation of data showing that Kibbutz-reared children[34] do not

have cognitive deficits also reinforces the premise that it is not necessarily group care *per se* that produces the frequently reported deficit and that it is possible to retain the advantages of group care while systematically eliminating its negative features. Grounds for reasonable optimism also have been found in retrospective studies by Maas[26] and Beres and Obers,[6] although in both cases the authors found evidence of pathology in some members of the follow-up sample. Similarly Dennis and Najarian[14] concluded from their data that the magnitude of the deficit varied as a function of the type of instrument used to measure deficit, and Dennis[13] showed that in institutions featuring better adult-child ratios and a conscious effort to meet the psychological needs of the infants the development of the children was much less retarded than was the case in a group of children residing in institutions with limited and unsophisticated staff. It is not appropriate to go into details of limitations of methodology in any of these studies; however, from the standpoint of an examination of the validity of a principle, it is important to take note of any exceptions to the generality of that principle.

In this context it is worth considering a point made by Gula.[20] He recently has suggested that some of the apparent consistency in studies comparing institutionalized infants with those cared for in their own homes and in foster homes might disappear if it were possible to equate the comparison groups on the variable of environmental adequacy. That is, one could classify all three types of environments as good, marginal, or inadequate on a number of dimensions. Most of the studies have compared children from palpably "inadequate" institutions with children from "good" foster and own homes. He suggests that, merely because most institutions studied have been inadequate in terms of such variables as adult-child ratio, staff turnover, and personal characteristics of some of the caretakers, etc., one is not justified in concluding *ipso facto* that group care is invariably inferior or damaging.

3. *Is healthy socio-emotional development the most important task of the first three years? Do attempts to foster cognitive growth interfere with social and emotional development?* These paired assumptions, which one finds stated in one variety or another in many pamphlets and books dealing with early child development, represent acceptance of a closed system model of human development. They seem to conceptualize development as compartmentalized and with a finite limit. If the child progresses too much in one area he automatically restricts the amount of development that can occur in another area. Thus one often encounters such expressions as "cognitive development at the *expense* of

socio-emotional development." It is perhaps of interest to reflect that, until our children reach somewhere around high school age, we seldom seem to worry that the reverse might occur. But, of course, life is an open system, and on the whole it is accurate to suggest that development feeds upon development. Cognitive and socio-emotional advances tend on the whole to be positively, not negatively correlated.

The definition of intelligence as *adaptivity* has not been adequately stressed by modern authors. It is, of course, the essence of Piaget's definition[32] as it was earlier of Binet.[7] Unfortunately, however, for the last generation or so in America we have been more concerned with how to measure intelligent behavior than how to interpret and understand it. Acceptance of the premise that intelligent behavior is adaptive behavior should help to break the set of many persons in the field of early child development that to encourage cognitive advance is to discourage healthy socio-emotional development. Ample data are available to suggest that quite the reverse is true either for intellectually advanced persons[42, 43] or an unselected sample. In a large sample of young adults from an urban area in Minnesota, Anderson[3] and associates found that the best single predictor of post-high school adjustment contained in a large assessment battery was a humble little group intelligence test. Prediction based on intelligence plus teacher's ratings did somewhat better, but nothing exceeded the intelligence test for single measure efficiency.

It is relevant here to mention White's[45] concept of competence or effectance as a major stabilizing force in personality development. The emotional reinforcement accompanying the old "I can do it myself" declaration should not be undervalued. In Murphy's report[30] of the coping behavior of preschool children one sees evidence of the adjustive supports gained through cognitive advances. In his excellent review of cognitive stimulation in infancy and early childhood, Fowler[16] raises the question of whether there is any justification for the modern anxiety (and, to be sure, it is a modern phenomenon) over whether cognitive stimulation may damage personality development. He suggests that in the past severe and harmful methods may have been the culprits whenever there was damage and that the generalizations have confused methods of stimulation with the process of stimulation *per se*.

4. *Do cognitive experiences of the first few months and years leave no significant residual?* Any assumption that the learnings of infancy are evanescent appears to be a fairly modern idea. In his *Emile*, first published in 1762, Rousseau[38] stressed the point that education should begin while the child is still in the cradle. Perhaps any generalization to the

contrary received its major modern impetus from a rather unlikely place—from longitudinal studies of development covering the span from infancy to adulthood. From findings of poor prediction of subsequent intellectual status[5] one can legitimately infer that the infant tests measure behavior that is somewhat irrelevant to later intellectual performance. Even though these behaviors predictive of later cognitive behavior elude most investigators, one cannot infer that the early months and years are unimportant for cognitive development.

Some support for this assumption has come from experimental studies in which an attempt has been made to produce a durable effect in human subjects by one or another type of intervention offered during infancy. One cogent example is the work of Rheingold,[36] in which she provided additional social and personal stimulation to a small group of approximately six-month-old, institutionalized infants for a total of eight weeks. At the end of the experimental period, differences in social responsiveness between her stimulated group and a control group composed of other babies in the institution could be observed. There were also slight but nonsignificant advances in postural and motor behavior on a test of infant development. However, when the babies were followed up approximately a year later, by which time all but one were in either adoptive or boarding homes or in their own natural homes, the increased social responsiveness formerly shown by the stimulated babies was no longer observed. Nor were the differences in level of intellectual functioning. Rheingold and Bayley[37] concluded that the extra mothering provided during the experimental period was enough to produce an effect at the time but not enough to sustain this effect after such a time as the two groups were no longer differentially stimulated. However, in spite of their conservative conclusion, it is worth noting that the experimentally stimulated babies were found to vocalize more during the follow-up assessments than the control babies. Thus there may have been enough of an effect to sustain a developmental advance in at least this one extremely important area.

Some very impressive recent unpublished data obtained by Skeels, offer a profound challenge to the assumption of the unimportance of the first three years of cognitive growth. This investigator has followed up after approximately 25 years most of the subjects described in a paper by Skeels and Dye.[40] Thirteen infants had been transferred from an orphanage because of evidence of mental retardation and placed in an institution for the retarded under the care of adolescent retardates who gave them a great deal of loving care and as much cognitive stimulation as they could. The 13 subjects showed a marked acceleration in development after this transfer. In contrast a group of reasonably well matched infants left on the wards of the orphanage continued to develop poorly. In a recent follow-up of these cases, Skeels discovered that the gains made by the transferred infants were sustained into their adult years, whereas all but one of the control subjects developed the classic syndrome of mental retardation.

The fact that development and experience are cumulative makes it difficult ever to isolate any one antecedent period and assert that its influence was or was not influential in a subsequent developmental period. Thus even though it might be difficult to demonstrate an effect of some experience in an adjacent time period, delayed effects may well be of even greater developmental consequence. In a recent review of data from a number of longitudinal studies, Bloom[8] has concluded that during the first three to four years (the noncognitive years, if you will) approximately 50 per cent of the development of intelligence that is ever to occur in the life cycle takes place. During this period a particular environment may be either abundant or deprived in terms of the ingredients essential for providing opportunities for the development of intelligence and problem solving. Bloom[8] states:

> The effects of the environments, appear to be greatest in the early (and more rapid) periods of intelligence development and least in the later (and less rapid) periods of development. Although there is relatively little evidence of the effects of changing the environment on the changes in intelligence, the evidence so far available suggests that marked changes in the environment in the early years can produce greater changes in intelligence than will equally marked changes in the environment at later periods of development. (pp. 88-89)

5. *Can one expect that, without formal planning, all the necessary learning experiences will occur?* There is an old legend that if you put six chimpanzees in front of six typewriters and leave them there long enough they eventually will produce all the works in the British Museum. One could paraphrase this for early childhood by suggesting that six children with good eyes and ears and hands and brains would, if left alone in nature, arrive at a number system, discover the laws of conservation of matter and energy, comprehend gravity and the motions of the planets, and perhaps arrive at the theory of relativity. All the "facts" necessary to discern these relationships are readily available. Perhaps a more realistic example would be to suggest that, if we surround a group of young children with a carefully selected set of play materials, they would eventually discover for themselves the laws of color mixture, of

form and contour, of perspective, of formal rhythm and tonal relationships, and biological growth. And, to be sure, all this *could* occur. But whether this will necessarily occur with any frequency is quite another matter. We also assume that at a still earlier period a child will learn body control, eye-hand coordination, the rudiments of language, and styles of problem solving in an entirely incidental and unplanned way. In an article in a recent issue of popular woman's magazine, an author[22] fervently urges parents to stop trying to teach their young children in order that the children may learn. And, to be sure, there is always something to be said for this caution; it is all too easy to have planned learning experiences become didactic and regimented rather than subtle and opportunistic.

As more people gain experience in operating nursery school programs for children with an early history deficient in many categories of experience, the conviction appears to be gaining momentum that such children often are not able to avail themselves of the educational opportunities and must be guided into meaningful learning encounters. In a recent paper dealing with the preschool behavior of a group of 21 children from multiproblem families, Malone[28] describes the inability of the children to carry out self-directed exploratory maneuvers with the toys and equipment as follows:

> When the children first came to nursery school they lacked interest in learning the names and properties of objects. Colors, numbers, sizes, shapes, locations, all seemed interchangeable. Nothing in the room seemed to have meaning for a child apart from the fact that another child had approached or handled it or that the teacher's attention was turned toward it. Even brief play depended on the teacher's involvement and support. (p. 5)

When one reflects on the number of carefully arranged reinforcement contingencies necessary to help a young child learn to decode the simple message, "No," it is difficult to support the position that in early learning, as in anything else, nature should just take its course.

6. *Is formal training for child-care during the first three years unnecessary?* This assumption is obviously quite ridiculous, and yet it is one logical derivative of the hypothesis that the only adequate place for a young child is with his mother or a permanent mother substitute. There is, perhaps unfortunately, no literacy test for motherhood. This again is one of our interesting scientific paradoxes. That is, proclaiming in one breath that mothering is essential for the healthy development of a child, we have in the very next breath implied that just any mother-

ing will do. It is interesting in this connection that from the elementary school level forward we have rigid certification statutes in most states that regulate the training requirements for persons who would qualify as teachers of our children. (The same degree of control over the qualifications and training of a nursery school teacher has not prevailed in the past, but we are moving into an era when it will.) So again, our pattern of social action appears to support the implicit belief in the lack of importance of the first three years of life.

In 1928, John B. Watson[44] wrote a controversial little trade book called *The Psychological Care of Infant and Child.* He included one chapter heretically entitled, "The Dangers of Too Much Mother Love." In this chapter he suggested that child training was too important to be left in the hands of mothers, apparently not because he felt them intellectually inadequate but because of their sentimentality. In his typical "nondirective" style Watson[44] wrote:

> Six months' training in the actual handling of children from two to six under the eye of competent instructors should make a fairly satisfactory child's nurse. To keep them we should let the position of nurse or governess in the home be a respected one. Where the mother herself must be the nurse—which is the case in the vast majority of American homes—she must look upon herself while performing the functions of a nurse as a professional woman and not as a sentimentalist masquerading under the name of "Mother." (p. 149)

At present in this country a number of training programs are currently being formulated which would attempt to give this kind of professional training called for by Watson and many others. It is perhaps not possible to advance on all fronts at the same time, and the pressing health needs of the young child demanded and received top priority in earlier decades. Perhaps it will now be possible to extend our efforts at social intervention to encompass a broader range of health, education, and welfare activities.

7. *Are most homes and most parents adequate for at least the first three years?* Enough has been presented in discussing other implicit assumptions to make it unnecessary to amplify this point at length. The clinical literature, and much of the research literature of the last decade dealing with social-class differences, has made abundantly clear that all parents are not qualified to provide even the basic essentials of physical and psychological care to their children. Such reports as those describing the incidence of battered children[15, 24] capture our attention, but reports concerned with subtler and yet perhaps more long-standing

patterns of parental deficit also fill the literature. In her description of the child-rearing environments provided by low lower-class families, Pavenstedt[31] has described them as impulse determined with very little evidence of clear planfulness for activities that would benefit either parent or child. Similarly, Wortis and associates[46] have described the extent to which the problems of the low-income mother so overwhelm her with reactions of depression and inadequacy that behavior toward the child is largely determined by the needs of the moment rather than by any clear plan about how to bring up children and how to train them to engage in the kind of behavior that the parents regard as acceptable or desirable. No social class and no cultural or ethnic group has exclusive rights to the domain of inadequate parentage; all conscientious parents must strive constantly for improvement on this score. However, relatively little attention has been paid to the possibly deleterious consequences of inadequacies during the first three years of life. Parents have been blamed for so many problems of their children in later age periods that a moderate reaction formation appears to have set in. But again, judging by the type of social action taken by the responsible professional community, parental inadequacy during the first three years is seldom considered as a major menace. Perhaps, when the various alternatives are weighed, it appears by comparison to be the least of multiple evils; but parental behavior of the first three years should not be regarded as any more sacrosanct or beyond the domain of social concern than that of the later years.

PLANNING ALTERNATIVES

At this point the exposition of this paper must come to an abrupt halt, for insufficient data about possible alternative models are available to warrant recommendation of any major pattern of change. At present there are no completed research projects that have developed and evaluated alternative approximations of optimal learning environments for young children in our culture. One apparent limitation on ideas for alternative models appears to be the tendency to think in terms of binary choices. That is, we speak of individual care *versus* group care, foster home *versus* institution, foster home *versus* own home, and so on. But environments for the very young child do not need to be any more mutually exclusive than they are for the older children. After all, what is our public education system but a coordination of the efforts of home plus an institution? Most of us probably would agree that the optimal learning environment for the older child is neither of these alone but rather a combination of both. Some of this same pattern of combined effort also may represent the optimal arrangement for the very young child.

A number of programs suggesting alternatives possibly worth considering are currently in the early field trial stage. One such program is the one described by Caldwell and Richmond.[11] This program offers educationally oriented day care for culturally deprived children between six months and three years of age. The children spend the better part of five days a week in a group care setting (with an adult-child ratio never lower than 1:4) but return home each evening and maintain primary emotional relationships with their own families. Well child care, social and psychological services, and parent education activities are available for participating families. The educational program is carefully planned to try to help the child develop the personal-social and cognitive attributes conducive to learning and to provide experiences which can partially compensate for inadequacies which may have existed in the home environment. The strategy involved in offering the enrichment experience to children in this very young age group is to maximize their potential and hopefully prevent the deceleration in rate of development which seems to occur in many deprived children around the age of two to three years. It is thus an exercise in circumvention rather than remediation. Effectiveness of the endeavor is being determined by a comparison of the participating children with a control group of children from similar backgrounds who are not enrolled in the enrichment program. Unfortunately at this juncture it is too early for such projects to do more than suggest alternatives. The degree of confidence plus replicated experience will have to wait a little longer.

Effective social action, however, can seldom await definitive data. And in the area of child care the most clamorous demand for innovative action appears to be coming from a rather unlikely source—not from any of the professional groups, not particularly from social planners who try to incorporate research data into plans for social action, but from *mothers*. From mothers themselves is coming the demand that professionals in the field look at some of the alternatives. We need not be reminded here that in America at the present time there are more than three million working mothers with children under six years of age.[2] And these mothers are looking for professional leadership to design and provide child-care facilities that help prepare their children for today's achievement-oriented culture. The challenge which has been offered is inevitable. After almost two decades of bombarding women with the importance of their mothering role, we might have predicted the weakening of their defenses and their waving the flag of truce as though to say, "I am not good enough to do all that you are saying I must do."

It is a characteristic of social evolution that an increased recognition of the importance of any role leads to the professionalization of that role, and there can be no doubt but that we are currently witnessing the early stages of professionalization of the mother-substitute role—or, as I would prefer to say, the mother-supplement. It is interesting to note that no one has as yet provided a satisfactory label for this role. The term "baby-sitter" is odious, reminding us of just about all some of the "less well trained" professionals do—sit with babies. If English were a masculine-feminine language, there is little doubt that the word would be used in the feminine gender, for we always speak of this person as a "she" (while emphasizing that young children need more contact with males). We cannot borrow any of the terms from already professionalized roles, such as "nurse" or "teacher," although such persons must be to a great extent both nurse and teacher. Awkward designations such as "child-care worker," or hybridized terms such as "nurse-teacher" do not quite seem to fill the bill; and there appears to be some reluctance to accept an untranslated foreign word like the Hebrew "metapelet" or the Russian "Nyanya." When such a word does appear, let us hope that it rhymes well and has a strong trochaic rhythm, for it will have to sustain a whole new era of poetry and song. (This author is convinced that the proper verb is *nurture*. It carries the desired connotations, but even to one who is not averse to neologisms such nominative forms as "nurturist," "nurturer," and "nurturizer" sound alien and inadequate.)*

Another basis for planning alternatives is becoming available from a less direct but potentially more persuasive source—from increasing knowledge about the process of development. The accumulation of data suggesting that the first few years of life are crucial for the priming of cognitive development call for vigorous and imaginative action programs for those early years. To say that it is premature to try to plan optimal environments because we do not fully understand how learning occurs is unacceptable. Perhaps only by the development of carefully arranged environments will we attain a complete understanding of the learning process. Already a great deal is known which enables us to specify some of the essential ingredients of a growth-fostering milieu. Such an environment must contain warm and responsive people who by

---

* In a letter to the author written shortly after the meeting at which this paper was presented, Miss Rena Corman of New York City suggested that the proper term should be "nurcher," a compound of the words, "nurse" and "teacher." To be sure, a "nurcher" sounds nurturant.

their own interests invest objects with value. It must be supportive and as free of disease and pathogenic agents as possibly can be arranged. It also must trace a clear path from where the child is to where he is to go developmentally; objects and events must be similar enough to what the child has experienced to be assimilated by the child and yet novel enough to stimulate and attract. Such an environment must be exquisitely responsive, as a more consistent pattern of response is required to foster the acquisition of new forms of behavior than is required to maintain such behavior once it appears in the child's repertoire. The timing of experiences also must be carefully programmed. The time table for the scheduling of early postnatal events may well be every bit as demanding as that which obtains during the embryological period. For children whose early experiences are known to be deficient and depriving, attempts to program such environments seem mandatory if subsequent learning difficulties are to be circumvented.

SUMMARY

Interpretations of research data and accumulated clinical experience have led over the years to a consensual approximation of an answer to the question: what is the optimal learning environment for the young child? As judged from our scientific and lay literature and from practices in health and welfare agencies, one might infer that the optimal learning environment for the young child is that which exists when (a) a young child is cared for in his own home (b) in the context of a warm and nurturant emotional relationship (c) with his mother (or a reasonable facsimile theerof) under conditions of (d) varied sensory and cognitive input. Undoubtedly until a better hypothesis comes along, this is the best one available. This paper has attempted to generate constructive thinking about whether we are justified in overly vigorous support of (a) when (b), (c) or (d), or any combination thereof, might not obtain. Support for the main hypothesis comes primarily from other hypotheses (implicit assumptions) rather than from research on experimental data. When these assumptions are carefully examined they are found to be difficult if not impossible to verify with existing data.

The conservatism inherent in our present avoidance of carefully designed social action programs for the very young child needs to be re-examined. Such a re-examination conducted in the light of research evidence available about the effects of different patterns of care forces consideration of whether formalized intervention programs should not receive more attention than they have in the past and whether attention should be given to a professional training sequence for child-care workers. The careful preparation of the learning environment calls for a degree of training and commitment and personal control not always to be found in natural caretakers and a degree of richness of experience by no means always available in natural environments.

REFERENCES

1. AINSWORTH, MARY. *1962*. Reversible and irreversible effects of maternal deprivation on intellectual development. Child Welfare League of America, 42-62.
2. AMERICAN WOMEN. *1963*. Report of the President's Commission on the Status of Women. (Order from Supt. of Documents, Washington, D.C.)
3. ANDERSON, J. E., ET AL. *1959*. A survey of children's adjustment over time. Minneapolis, Minn. University of Minnesota.
4. BARKER, R. G., and H. F. WRIGHT. *1955*. Midwest and its Children: The Psychological Ecology of an American Town. Row, Peterson, New York.
5. BAYLEY, NANCY. *1949*. Consistency and variability in the growth of intelligence from birth to eighteen years. J. Genet. Psychol. *75:* 165-196.
6. BERES, D., and S. OBERS. *1950*. The effects of extreme deprivation in infancy on psychic structure in adolescence. Psychoanal. Stud. of the Child. *5:* 121-140.
7. BINET, A., and T. SIMON, *1916*. The Development of Intelligence in Children. Elizabeth S. Kite, trans. Williams and Wilkins, Baltimore.
8. BLOOM, B. S. *1964*. Stability and Change in Human Characteristics. John Wiley and Sons, New York.
9. BRONFENBRENNER, URIE. *1962*. Soviet studies of personality development and socialization. *In* Some Views on Soviet Psychology. Amer. Psychol. Assoc., Inc. pp. 63-85.
10. CALDWELL, BETTYE M., ET AL. *1963*. Mother-infant interaction in monomatric and polymatric families. Amer. J. Orthopsychiat. *33:* 653-64.
11. CALDWELL, BETTYE M., and J. B. RICHMOND. *1964*. Programmed day care for the very young child—a preliminary report. J. Marriage and the Family. *26:* 481-488.
12. DAVIS, A., and R. J. HAVIGHURST. *1946*. Social class and color differences in child-rearing. Amer. Social. Rev. *11:* 698-710.
13. DENNIS, W. *1960*. Causes of retardation among institutional children. J. Genet. Psychol. *96:* 47-59.
14. DENNIS, W., and P. NAJARIAN. *1957*. Infant development under environmental handicap. Psychol. Monogr. *71:* (7 Whole No. 536).
15. ELMER, ELIZABETH. *1963*. Identification of abused children. Children. *10:* 180-184.
16. FOWLER, W. *1962*. Cognitive learning in infancy and early childhood. Psychol. Bull. *59:* 116-152.
17. FREUD, ANNA, and SOPHIE DANN. *1951*. An experiment in group upbringing. Psychoanal. Study of the Child. *6:* 127-168.
18. GARDNER, D. B., G. R. HAWKES, and L. G. BURCHINAL. *1961*. Noncontinuous mothering in infancy and development in later childhood. Child Develpm. *32:* 225-234.
19. GOLDFARB, W. *1949*. Rorschach test differences between family-reared, institution-reared and schizophrenic children. Amer. J. Orthopsychiat. *19:* 624-633.
20. GULA, H. *January, 1965*. Paper given at Conference on Group Care for Children. Children's Bureau.
21. HOFFMAN, LOIS WLADIS. *1961*. Effects of maternal employment on the child. Child Develpm. *32:* 187-197.

22. HOLT, J. *1965*. How to help babies learn—without teaching them. Redbook. *126* (1): 54-55, 134-137.

23. IRVINE, ELIZABETH E. *1952*. Observations on the aims and methods of child-rearing in communal settlements in Israel. Human Relations. *5:* 247-275.

24. KEMPE, C. H. ET AL. *1962*. The battered-child syndrome. J. Amer. Med. Asso. *181:* 17-24.

25. LEWIS, O. *1959*. Five families. New York: Basic Books.

26. MAAS, H. *1963*. Long-term effects of early childhood separation and group care. Vita Humana. *6:* 34-56.

27. MACCOBY, ELEANOR, and PATRICIA K. GIBBS. *1954* Methods of child-rearing in two social classes. *In* Readings in Child Developm. W. E. Martin and Celia B. Stendler, eds. Harcourt, Brace & Co., New York. Pp. 380-396.

28. MALONE, C. A. *1966*. Safety first: comments on the influence of external danger in the lives of children of disorganized families. Amer. J. Orthopsychiat. *36:* 3-12.

29. MEAD, MARGARET. *1953*. Growing up in New Guinea. The New American Library, New York.

30. MURPHY, LOIS B., ET AL. *1962*. The Widening World of Childhood. Basic Books, Inc., New York.

31. PAVENSTEDT, E. *1965*. A comparison of the child-rearing environment of upper-lower and very low-lower class families. Amer. J. Orthopsychiat. *35:* 89-98.

32. PIAGET, J. *1952*. The Origins of Intelligence in Children. Margaret Cook, trans. International Universities Press, New York.

33. PROVENCE, SALLY, and ROSE C. LIPTON. *1962*. Infants in institutions. International Universities Press, New York.

34. RABIN, A. I. *1957*. Personality maturity of Kibbutz and non-Kibbutz children as reflected in Rorschach findings. J. Proj. Tech. Pp. 148-153.

35. RADKE YARROW, MARIAN. *1961*. Maternal employment and child rearing. Children. *8:* 223-228.

36. RHEINGOLD, HARRIET. *1956*. The modification of social responsiveness in institutional babies. Monogr. Soc. Res. Child Develpm. *21:* (63).

37. RHEINGOLD, HARRIET L., and NANCY BAYLEY. *1959*. The later effects of an experimental modification of mothering. Child Develpm. *30:* 363-372.

38. ROUSSEAU, J. J. *1950*. Emile (1762). Barron's Educational Series, Great Neck, N. Y.

39. SIEGEL, ALBERTA E., and MIRIAM B. HASS. *1963*. The working mother: a review of research. Child Develpm. *34:* 513-42.

40. SKEELS, H. and H. DYE. *1939*. A study of the effects of differential stimulation on mentally retarded children. Proc. Amer. Assoc. on Ment. Def. *44:* 114-136.

41. SPIRO, M. *1958*. Children of the Kibbutz. Cambridge, Mass.: Harvard U. Press.

42. TERMAN, L. M., ET AL. *1925*. Genetic studies of genius: Vol. 1. Mental and physical traits of a thousand gifted children. Stanford University, Calif.: Stanford University Press.

43. TERMAN, L. M., and MELITA H. ODEN. *1947*. The gifted child grows up: twenty-five years' follow-up of a superior group. Stanford University, Calif.: Stanford University Press.

44. WATSON, J. B. *1928*. Psychological care of infant and child. Allen and Unwin, London.

45. WHITE, R. W. *1959*. Motivation reconsidered: the concept of competence. Psychol. Rev. *66:* 297-333.

46. WORTIS, H., ET AL. *1963*. Child-rearing practices in a low socio-economic group. Pediatrics. *32:* 298-307.

47. YARROW, L. J. *1961*. Maternal deprivation: toward an empirical and conceptual re-evaluation. Psychol. Bull. *58:* 459-490.

11

PARENTAL INFLUENCE ON COGNITIVE DEVELOPMENT IN EARLY CHILDHOOD: A REVIEW

Norman E. Freeberg

and

Donald T. Payne

Educational Testing Service

This review summarizes literature dealing with child-rearing practices that influence cognitive development. The 3 major aspects of the literature considered are: (1) studies that attempt to relate measures of the child's cognitive ability to particular parental rearing practices, (2) rearing practices characteristic of various social class levels as related to cognitive performance of children from those social classes, and (3) experimental attempts to enhance cognitive skills in the very young child by specialized training techniques. Despite increasing interest in this area, systematic research concerned with specific rearing practices as they affect particular cognitive skills is only beginning to become available.

Despite the extent of child development research on intellectual skills and learning, the answer to a parent who asks specifically "What can I do during my child's preschool years to improve his learning ability or intelligence?" would have to be couched in fairly broad and guarded generalizations. If the question were pressed further by our hypothetical

Reprinted from CHILD DEVELOPMENT, March 1967, Vol. 38, No. 1, pp. 65-87. This work was supported in part under a contract with the Institute for Educational Development, New York.

parent and an optimum sequence of training techniques was requested, the child specialist might feel that his recommendations were even further removed from a body of relevant literature. Perhaps little more than a generalization to provide "maximum environmental enrichment" could, at present, be supported with confidence. But it appears that evidence for an outline of more substantial proportions is beginning to emerge. The present review will attempt to deal with the extent and applicability of available literature to the question posed and those aspects of the research effort that remain to be undertaken if a more satisfactory answer is to be given.

SIGNIFICANCE OF EARLY LEARNING

It has been no small task to arrive at a point where one could speak with assurance of even as general a concept as the enhancing of human cognitive development through an early environment "rich in experience." To do so has required marshaling evidence for the effects of experience upon intellectual growth and against the two long-entrenched assumptions of fixed intelligence, and a maturational hypothesis that prescribes the unfolding of cognitive abilities in a predetermined relation to anatomic development. Hunt (1961) has dealt with the task incisively. With Hebb's (1949) work on the neurophysiological basis of intellectual growth as one theoretical cornerstone. Hunt builds his conception of learning and intelligence as a form of dynamic information processing dependent upon infantile experience.

In effect, Hebb (1949) concluded that experience is an essential mediator of neural connections and a requirement for the formation of so-called cell assemblies. These neural assemblies become relatively fixed functional units ("autonomous central processes") whose sequence and phasing in the associative cortex can only be formed by receptor inputs (i.e., sensory experience). Thus, it is the earliest experience or "primary" learning which forms much of the pattern for later information-processing capability in the system and serves as the "programmer of the human brain-computer" (Hunt, 1964, p. 242).

Evidence from animal studies of the effects of infantile experience on later learning lends substantial support to the above concepts and tends to negate consideration of a central nervous system that functions as a "passive switchboard" (Newell, Shaw, & Simon, 1958). Beach and Jaynes (1954) as well as Hunt (1961, chap. iv) review much of the work dealing with the enhancement of later learning by rich environmental stimulation in early life. Rats reared in darkness take longer to learn pattern discrimination than normals, and chimps reared in a darkened room for the first 16 months of life fail, initially, to show normal responses to moving objects in the visual field. Pets (cats and dogs) reared in the home perform better in learning situations than laboratory-reared animals. In addition, animals provided with the early experience of living with a variety of objects in their cages perform better in later learning situations and with less emotional interference than animals not exposed to such variations in the stimulus environment. The degree and permanence of this retardation depend largely upon the extent of deprivation. In the case of chimps reared in darkness, there is an eventual recovery of normal visual functioning if the deprivation does not go beyond an assumed critical point where physiological deterioration begins to occur (Riesen, 1958). Similarly, in human development, the ability to recover from the handicap of various forms of perceptual-motor deprivation (given sufficient time and opportunity to practice the requisite skills) indicates that, despite the importance of the early environment, maturational components cannot be ignored (Dennis & Najarian, 1957; Senden, 1932).

Although the behavioral evidence for the role of early learning has been impressive, the more recent works of Krech, Rosenzweig, and Bennett (1962) and Bennett, Diamond, Krech, and Rosenzweig (1964) have served to anchor this evidence in neural correlates. Behavioral measurement as well as chemical and neuroanatomical changes in the cortex of rats raised in enriched and impoverished environments (with and without designs and objects in the cage; variations in number of litter mates) have revealed significant differences in favor of the animals raised under conditions of greater environmental complexity. This improvement is evidenced by (a) superior learning ability on a variety of tasks, (b) neurochemical changes known to facilitate learning, and (c) increased quantity (weight) of cortical tissue in brain areas *specific* to those aspects of sensory stimulation provided by the environmental variables (e.g., greater development of the occipital cortex was related to greater environmental visual stimulation).

Evidence for early learning effects in children and "cumulative deficit" (decline in IQ scores) resulting from deprived environments have been reviewed extensively by Bloom (1964) and others (Anastasi, 1958; Bayley, 1955; Klineberg, 1963; Yarrow, 1964). Largely through studies of intellectual growth in twins reared apart, children separated from parents early in life by adoption, and effects of environmental deprivation in childhood, there has been mounting evidence for the potency of early environment in shaping later cognitive abilities. The extent to which such adverse environmental effects are reversible for retardation of higher-level cognitive skills in man remains poorly defined. But there appear to be extremes of social and cultural deprivation beyond which compensatory training provides only limited benefit (Zingg, 1940).

Bloom (1964) re-evaluates the data from longitudinal studies of the past four decades in an attempt to support a hypothesis of differential growth rate for human intellectual ability. He concludes that, in terms of intelligence measured at age 17, approximately 50 per cent of the variance can be accounted for by age 4 so that as much intellectual growth is achieved between birth and 4 years of age as is achieved for the remaining 13 years. (Assumptions of behavior overlap, absolute scaling, and a unidimensionality of measured intelligence, which are required for such a conclusion, remain open to contention.) Unfortunately, most of the evidence available has not dealt with specific mechanisms to explain conclusions regarding early environmental effects upon the child, and Bloom (1964) feels that it is now necessary to bridge the inferential gap with more detailed and meaningful measures of the environment in order to relate these to cognitive performance.

This brief discussion of an extensive and complex topic is intended only to serve as background for the assumption upon which the balance of this review is predicated, that is, that the formation of cognitive and intellectual skills can reasonably be conceived of as developmental in nature and modifiable by variation in the environment. If this is granted, then how might changes be effected in early intellectual development through the use of appropriate child-rearing and educational practices? Hunt touches upon the need for such knowledge when he states: "Various bits of the evidence reviewed hint that if the manner in which encounters with the environment foster the development of intellectual interest and capacity were more fully understood, it might be possible to increase the average level of intelligence within the population substantially" (Hunt, 1961, p. 346). Similarly, Bloom feels that we are at a level where one can "specify some of the major characteristics of an environment which will positively or negatively affect the development of general intelligence or school achievement" (Bloom, 1964, p. 196). If cultural effects on intellectual functioning are, in some measure, "from the outside in" (Bruner, 1964), then the techniques by which this process can be influenced through parental practices are certainly an area of legitimate concern.

Three major aspects of the literature can be utilized to deal with the problem. The first is of primary concern for this review and deals with those studies that attempt to relate parental influences directly to some aspect of the child's cognitive performance. Second are the studies of child-rearing behavior in various social classes as linked with the evidence of intellectual achievements of children from these classes, and third is the experimental and descriptive literature dealing with educational techniques that have been used for developing cognitive skills in the very young child.

DIRECT MEASURES OF PARENTAL INFLUENCE

Research concerned with direct relations between parental practices and child development has tended to focus upon dependent variables concerned with physical development, personality formation, and behavior adjustment. Attempts to incorporate measures of cognitive skill and intelligence are relatively recent by comparison. Where such studies have been undertaken, they generally deal with children of elementary school levels, and they rely heavily upon retrospective reports by the mother regarding parental practices in early childhood. If there is a willingness to accept a relative continuity of home environment for the period of years from early childhood to the later grades and/or some measure of accuracy for mothers' retrospective reporting, then a number of pertinent studies to be considered in this review can provide insight into the nature of those family influences that might affect intellectual achievement.

One such study by Bing (1963) used sixty mothers of fifth grade children. All of these children had similar total IQ scores and were divided by sex into "high" and "low" verbal groups. This grouping was based upon the contrast of verbal scores with spatial and numerical scores. For example, a "high verbal" subject was one whose verbal scores were high in relation to his numerical and spatial scores. Data were obtained from questionnaires and from interviews with the mother as well as from observation of an "interaction situation" during which the mother engaged in various problem-solving activities with the child. Responses on the retrospective questionnaire and interview indicated that mothers of "high verbal" children provided more verbal stimulation in early childhood (highly significant for boys but not for girls). These mothers also remembered more of the child's early accomplishments (significant for boys but not for girls), were more critical of poor academic achievement, provided the child with more storybooks, and let him take a greater part in mealtime conversations Time spent reading to the child by the father was associated with high verbal scores for girls only, although no comparable association was found for reading time spent by the mothers with the child of either sex. The various sex differences that characterized these results were often difficult to reconcile on the basis of any previously stated hypotheses. In the observational situation, mothers of children with high verbal ability generally provided more assistance voluntarily, provided it sooner when requested by the child, and pressured the child more for improvement.

This influence of the mother's pattern of interaction and communication with the child appears to play a pivotal role in cognitive skill level, as is also evident in the work by Hess (1965). Utilizing the observational situation, Hess is presently conducting a series of studies with preschool children that require mother-child interaction in a problem-solving situation. His focus is on the way in which the mother assists the child in solving problems and the nature of the "cognitive environment" which she provides. Results indicate that, when mothers provide "restrictive language codes" (i.e., language that provides a smaller number of alternatives for action, fewer choices to be made, and fewer possibilities for thought), the child's problem-solving ability is diminished.

Maternal behavior toward the preschool child, which includes emphasis on verbal skill acquisition along with other phases of achievement, has also been shown to be related to measured IQ scores. Data obtained from parents of middle-class children from the Fels Longitudinal Study (Moss & Kagan, 1958) were used to develop a "maternal acceleration" score derived from ratings of "pressure" for the child's achievement, as evidenced by the mother in interviews. A significant relation between the child's IQ and maternal acceleration was found only for boys at the 3-year level but not for either sex in the 6-year age group. The study was essentially repeated in a second phase using another sample of children. The child's IQ scores at the 3- and 6-year levels were positively correlated with the mother's IQ and educational level, but the maternal acceleration score was, again, found to be related only to the boys' IQ at the 3-year level. The authors note that one possible explanation lies in the fact that four of six items on the 2½-year scale of the Stanford-Binet test are of the type that mothers who had high maternal acceleration scores emphasized (i.e., identifying objects by use, naming objects and body parts, and picture vocabulary).

There is evidence that early childhood achievement behaviors, as well as parental practices, are age- and sex-dependent in their predictive ability for later adult achievement behavior (Sontag & Kagan, 1963). Indications of sex differences were not only apparent in the Moss and Kagan study (1958), but Bing (1963) also reported that variables derived from the retrospective interview, which distinguished between high and

low verbal groups, did so mainly for boys, while those from the con-
temporaneous observation situation indicated such differences primarily
for girls. This finding of sex differences, based upon parental recall of
earlier practices as contrasted with present behavior of the parent (observational data), represents a result that merits further verification. It is
hardly surprising that mothers would respond differently to broad classes
of behavior displayed by the male than they would for the female child
(Sears, Maccoby, & Levin, 1957). Such differences for intellectual and
achievement behaviors might also be culturally determined to some
extent and could stem from differences in parental expectation for
later intellectual and vocational achievement (Freeberg & Payne, 1955).

Age dependence has also become a variable of recent concern. Variations in the consequences of a parental practice, as a function of the
child's age level at the time the practice is introduced, have been termed
the "sleeper effect" by Kagan and Moss (1962). Evidence presented by
these authors indicates that there may be critical periods in the child's
development when a particular parental practice may be more effective
in shaping later development than if it is introduced at other than the
"optimum" age or developmental level. Obvious difficulties in evaluating
research and defining suitable criteria of cognitive development are
introduced by the need to identify such complex and incompletely understood effects of age and sex.

Another approach to uncovering pertinent aspects of parental influence is through the child's responses to questions about the home environment, an approach used by Milner (1951). First-grade children were
classed as "high" and "low" scorers on the Haggerty Reading Examination and the Language Factors subtest of the California Test of Mental
Maturity. The findings support the general pattern of subsequent studies,
with the "high scorers" showing significantly more responses for such
parental behavior-related items as: expressed appreciation for the time
the mother spent taking them places and reading to them, possession of
several or a great many storybooks, and the fact that the parents regularly read to them.

One of the most comprehensive, and apparently successful, attempts
to relate parental influence to intelligence test performance of the child
used data obtained from sixty fifth-grade students and from interviews
with their mothers (Wolf, 1964). Those aspects of the home which were
considered as most relevant to the development of general intelligence
were incorporated as items in an interview schedule of 63 questions. The
items were then used as a basis for ratings on 13 scales designated as
"Environmental Process Characteristics." The correlation of the total

score (which was a summation of the 13 scale scores) and the child's IQ score was a striking .69. Of particular interest for our purposes are the individual correlations of the 13 scales with the intelligence test score. The best relations were found for those scales dealing with the parents' intellectual expectations for the child, the amount of information that the mother had about the child's intellectual development, the opportunities provided for enlarging the child's vocabulary, the extent to which the parents created situations for learning in the home, and the extent of assistance given in learning situations related to school and nonschool activities. Dave (1963), using the same 63-item interview schedule as Wolf (1964) and apparently the same data, categorized the scales into five "Environmental Process Variables" that could be grouped to form an "Index of Educational Environment." The correlation of this overall "Index" with an "Educational Achievement Score" (composed of such areas as word knowledge, spelling, reading, and arithmetic computation) was found to be .80.

The findings from these two studies are indeed impressive as indications of parental influence on intellectual development. However, a number of the reported correlations between the intelligence measure and variables of social class are at odds with previous studies and require clarification. For example, the index of social class and parental education level were found to be unrelated to the child's intelligence test scores, whereas measures of this sort are customarily found to possess a moderate but significant degree of relation with intelligence. In any event, the general pattern of results from the several studies considered here is fairly consistent. Children of superior intellectual ability come from homes where parental interest in their intellectual development is evidenced by pressures to succeed and assistance in doing so, particularly in the development of the child's verbal skills.

Achievement

The concept of achievement has frequently been used as a criterion of performance for cognitive and intellectual development. As is the case for many of the criterion and predictor variables utilized in parent-child studies, the concept is not a unitary one. In this case it has been used to refer to "need," or motivation for achievement, measured proficiency, and opinions about achievement. Crandall lends some clarification to this widely used criterion variable. He distinguishes achievement variables from other behavior variables such as dependency, aggression, etc., on the basis of "positive reinforcement for demonstrated competence" and achievement situations from other social situations on the basis of the provision of "cues pertaining to some 'standard of excellence'" (Crandall, 1963, p. 418). Contrasted with these is the concept of achievement motivation or "need (n) achievement."

Several studies have attempted to relate specific parental child-rearing practices or attitudes to the development of either achievement behavior or achievement motives in the child. Ratings were obtained for: (a) achievement behavior in a nursery school free-play situation, (b) child-mother interaction in the home, and (c) mother reactions to child behavior (Crandall, Preston, & Rabson, 1960). The results depict a high-achieving child as one who is less dependent upon the mother for emotional support and whose mother frequently rewarded achievement efforts.

A series of studies conducted at the Fels Institute dealt with the relation of parents' attitudes concerning their own achievement to the achievement behaviors of their child (Crandall, Dewey, Katkovsky, & Preston, 1964; Katkovsy, Preston, & Crandall, 1964a; 1964b). The general findings of interest for this review include a similarity between intellectual achievement values that parents hold for themselves and those they expect for their child, as well as a relation between intellectual expectations and their participation with the child in intellectual activities. Academic achievement of children in the early grades and "general" parental behaviors (largely descriptive of "social climate") were found to be significantly related, but primarily with regard to mothers and daughters—such that mothers of academically competent girls were less affectionate and less nurturant toward their daughters than were mothers of less proficient girls. The essential distinction for fathers was a tendency for those who had academically proficient daughters to use praise more often and to criticize less. More "specific" variables, such as parents' expressed values for intellectual performance and satisfaction with the child's performance, were related to the child's achievement regardless of sex.

These findings of the Fels group are supported in general by the results of Callard's (1964) study with nursery school children and, in addition, by Rosen and D'Andrade (1959), who found that boys with high-need achievement scores had parents with higher aspirations for them and a higher regard for their competence and were fairly quick to disapprove if the child performed poorly. Biglin (1964), on the other hand, had little success in attempting to relate parents' attitudes (as measured by the Nebraska Parent Attitude Scale) to academic achievement when intellectual ability and socioeconomic status were controlled. The explanation for such differences would probably be found in the nature of the attitude scales utilized or in differences between interview results and those of attitude questionnaires. Moving from preschool and early elementary school to the high school level, some consistency of results can be demonstrated by reported relations of academic achievement with parental encouragement, approval, and sharing of activities (Mannino, 1962; Morrow & Wilson, 1961).

In the measurement of achievement, as for intellectual performance, the pattern of parental influence that emerges from these studies would appear to be sex-dependent as well as the result of overt parental pressures for achievement along with expressed attitudes indicating a high level of aspiration for the child.

Social Environment

One area of controversy that still requires clarification has centered about the social environment in the home and its effects upon the intellectual performance of the child. An early article by Baldwin, Kalhorn, and Breese (1945) reported that children reared in families characterized as Acceptant-Democratic-Indulgent showed higher IQ scores and more favorable changes in IQ, over several years, than children from authoritarian and rejecting homes. A controversy was sparked by Drews and Teahan (1957) who found that high achievers tend to have been reared in families where adult standards were not questioned and where mothers were more "authoritarian and restrictive." Hurley (1959) attempted to serve as mediator and re-evaluated the Drews and Teahan data (1957) to show that although mothers of high academic achievers tended to be more dominant and ignoring toward their children, mothers of "gifted" (high Binet IQ) children tended to be less so. Watson (1957) presented results that tend to favor the "permissive" home as one that stimulated intellectual activity of better quality. The controversy remains unresolved, and results have been difficult to reconcile simply on the basis of the techniques employed and the variables chosen.

To complicate the matter further, a similar and parallel controversy has arisen for what probably represents a related constellation of variables concerned with fostering dependence and independence in early childhood. It has been reported by Winterbottom (1958) that boys with high-need achievement had mothers who prompted earlier self-reliance and independence, while indulgent and overprotective mothers in Stewart's (1950) study had children who tended to be inferior in reading achievement. In support of this pattern, emotional dependence upon the mother by the preschool child was shown to be related to lower-need achievement and declining IQ scores, in a study by Sontag, Baker, and Nelson (1958). Shaw (1964) adds further positive evidence for early independence as a factor favoring academic achievement.

The trend toward agreement was upset, however, by Chance (1961) who found that first-grade children (particularly girls) whose mothers favored earlier demands for independence made less adequate school progress. Crandall et al. (1960) found that "neither maternal affection nor independence training was predictive of the children's achievement behavior." The results do indeed indicate, as Hurley (1959) has suggested, the "complex nature of relationships between maternal child rearing attitudes and children's behavior." Resolution of such a controversy can only be achieved by better understanding of the relations between those child-rearing variables that underlie the authoritarian-democratic, dependence-independence, and permissive-restrictive dimensions, along with greater precision of behavioral definitions for these concepts than has been shown in a number of the studies cited. Differences in criterion measures of achievement (i.e., academic performance, need achievement, measured intelligence) also require reconciliation in future attempts to deal with the controversy.

Cognitive Style

It has long been recognized that cognitive skill development and achievement are somehow related to personality characteristics. Linking of the causal sequence has been vague, however, until recent studies of cognitive style have attempted to deal with the relation of conceptual strategies in problem solving to personality correlates. Emotional dependence on parents, aggressiveness, self initiation, and competitiveness in the preschool years were found to be predictive of intellectual growth, from an analysis of the Fels Longitudinal Study data (Sontag et al., 1958). The problem remains one of defining consistent, specific differences in the individual's approach to the environment. Kagan, Moss, and Sigel (1963) have established measures of distinctive cognitive (conceptual) styles in grade-school children that indicate "analytic" and "relational" (nonanalytic) approaches which differentiate between males and females. These resemble the "field-dependent," "field-independent" dimension found by Witkin, Dyk, Faterson, Goodenough, and Karp (1962) who, in addition, attempted to relate the perceptual differences in cognitive styles to maternal influence in early childhood. "Field-independent" boys tended to be more resistant to social group pressure, showed greater consistency of behavior, used intellectualization as a defense mechanism rather than repression, and had mothers who encouraged greater autonomy and curiosity in early childhood. Hess and Shipman (1965) have argued that the child's style of response to problem-solving situations can be associated with the mother's ability to utilize verbal concepts in her interaction with him. Measures of cognitive style were obtained from a sorting task by Sigel (reported in Hess & Shipman, 1965) that defines the level and mode of abstraction displayed by the individual. One version of this instrument was used to obtain scores for the mothers' cognitive style and another was used for their children. Levels of conceptualization displayed by the mother were associated with the cognitive style and conceptual "maturity" of the child as well as with the child's performance on several problem-solving tasks. Cognitive style and levels of conceptual maturity were also found to be differentiated by the social status of the mothers and children.

Although the importance of maternal language style as a mediating factor may lead to stressing of environmental and situational variables in the shaping of cognitive patterns, the possibility of genetic influences has also been suggested, based upon two lines of evidence. First is the persistent finding of sex differences along the cognitive style dimensions reported by Kagan et al. (1963) and by Witkin et al. (1962). Second is a rather interesting discovery of unusual cognitive patterns among girls with Turner's syndrome, a genetic abnormality in the complement of x chromosomes (Witkin, Faterson, Goodenough, & Birnbaum, 1965). Intelligence test performance of twenty girls exhibiting Turner's syndrome was analyzed by these investigators using data from a study by Shafer (reported in Witkin et. al., 1965). Significant discrepancies were found between verbal intelligence and ability on "analytical" tasks (i.e., perceptual organization skills characterized by such Wechsler Adult Intelligence Scale subtests as Block Design, Picture Completion, and Object Assembly). Having previously found strong relations between such discrepancies and scores on the perceptual field-dependence, field-independence dimension, Witkin et al. (1965) hypothesize strong field dependency for girls with the Turner syndrome.

Accuracy of Parental Evaluation and Report

A number of the studies that have been cited depend heavily upon the parents' (most frequently the mother's) evaluation of the child. It is, therefore, pertinent to consider this source of data in terms of its error contribution to any study.

Crandall and Preston (1955) compared mothers' self-ratings of their behavior with psychologists' ratings of this same behavior based upon observations, and found that the simpler maternal self-rating scales were not correlated highly enough with the more time-consuming observational ratings to be considered as a substitute. Significant agreement between scales, where it existed, depended upon the particular area of maternal behavior evaluated. Similar use of the observational situation by Zunich (1962) resulted in negligible agreement when questionnaire results were compared with observational ratings.

Other studies have demonstrated either a selective accuracy or general distortion of mothers' reports on developmental data and child-rearing practices (Mednick & Shaffer, 1963; Pyles, Stolz, & MacFarlane, 1935). This has been found even in situations where parents participated in a longitudinal study and were virtually "practiced" respondents (Robbins, 1963). Among such respondents, it was found that mothers displayed greater accuracy in recall of the child's early behavior than fathers when their responses were compared with prior reports obtained during the course of the longitudinal study. Hefner (1963) found overall agreement to be poor between mothers' reports 2½ years apart, with wide variation for different aspects of child development. Somewhat superior reliability was found for mothers' reports on first-born children and for those mothers whose husbands were of higher occupational level.

Sources of bias and questionable validity were also reported for selected areas of parent-child behavior with the interview technique (McCord & McCord, 1961). Attitude scale biases based on social desirability effects have been shown to influence responses on a number of widely used scales (Taylor, 1961). Yarrow (1963) discusses some of these problems in parent-child research and reviews a number of studies that indicate low agreement between parent-child data contemporaneously obtained and retrospective interview reports. Only Walters (1960) defends the questionnaire as preferable to the more time-consuming interview method for measurement of family behavior, but this is based exclusively upon criteria of economy and reliability.

Since the questionnaire or interview are often the only practical sources of information for studies of parent-child relationships, knowledge of the extent of the deficiencies of these instruments is critical. A review by Bell (1958) lends some perspective to the methodological considerations and to the means of improving the research design for the retrospective parent-child study. It seems evident that there is a need to combine parental report with observational data or with other sources of verification where possible.

SOCIAL CLASS AND INTELLECTUAL GROWTH

One major area of the research literature that bears a largely circumstantial relation to parental practices and intellectual characteristics of the child is concerned with performance of children from families of different social classes. Considerable detail exists regarding the behavior of parents of different social classes during various stages of child rearing, but rarely has there been any effort to relate specific practices to specific cognitive skills. For example, only brief mention of intellectual concomitants of achievement behavior is given in the Sears et al. (1957) widely quoted study of child-rearing practices. Others have been concerned largely with measures of personality and behavior adjustment that derive from practices which might logically be related to such measures (Havighurst & Davis, 1955; Kohn, 1959; Minturn & Lambert, 1964; White, 1957). The middle-class values that stress consideration, self-control, and higher educational expectation have been contrasted with lower- or working-class values of neatness, cleanliness, and obedience. These differences have tended to hold up from study to study, although Havighurst and Davis' (1955) evidence leads them to caution against generalizing too broadly from samples taken in geographically restricted areas to an entire social class.

Differences in intellectual achievement among children of different social classes have long been known to exist (Anastasi, 1958; Eells, Davis, Havighurst, Herrick, & Tyler, 1951), but any inference that these differences stem from particular parental behaviors has been tenuous at best. Attempts to explain variations in intellectual skill among social strata (Eells et al., 1951) have been based on the argument that intelligence tests, in general, favor children from middle and upper social classes. Efforts to devise "culture-free" tests have been made in order to overcome this supposed unfair advantage. However, even if adequate tests of this sort could be devised, they do not solve the problems resulting from poor early learning environments, since children of lower social class are, in fact, less likely to succeed in an academic setting. Questions remain regarding specific parental practices requiring revision if changes are to be effected. Jensen (1964) addresses himself to the evidence that supports the relation of the child's social class membership to verbal learning and reviews the literature in the areas of early experience, perceptual development, environmental deprivation, and laboratory studies of verbal learning in an attempt to show that it is the verbal deficit to which much of the lower-class cognitive disadvantage can be attributed.

SOCIAL CLASS AND DEPRIVATION

Declines in IQ during early childhood have been shown to occur repeatedly under environmental conditions of extreme cultural deprivation (Stoddard, 1943; Wheeler, 1932). Similar trends in measured intellectual ability have been used to support a "cumulative deficit" hypothesis for children of the lower socioeconomic classes (Deutsch, 1965; Deutsch & Brown, 1964; Wiener, Rider, & Oppel, 1963) and a conception of their retarded intellectual development as being the result of "cultural deprivation." Support for the deprivation pattern comes from work by Milner (1951), in which differences in reading ability could be attributed to differences in verbal interaction with the child by parents of high and low social class, and from similar findings by Deutsch (1965) that associate poorer language functioning with lower-class groups. Bernstein (1960) explains these differences on the basis of verbal styles in the use of language by different classes, along a "convergent" ("restrictive")-"divergent" ("elaborative") dimension. His concepts have served as a framework for examination of maternal verbal styles in relation to the child's cognitive behavior by Olim, Hess, and Shipman (1965). Language scales have been developed by these investigators which served to differentiate among mothers on the basis of social class— primarily middle- from lower-class mothers—with the middle-class mother exhibiting a more elaborate language style that includes a greater degree of complexity and a higher level of abstraction. Their evidence points to the mother's language usage as the mediating factor in the child's conceptual development, rather than to the child's IQ or the verbal IQ of the mothers. Class differences in maternal verbal style are credited with the superior problem-solving performance for middle-class mothers working with their children than is found for mothers and children of lower social status. In the view of Hess and Shipman (1965, p. 885), "the meaning of deprivation is a deprivation of meaning."

Lower levels of achievement motivation and expectation for lower-class children can also be assumed to occur from long-term social deprivation and to be passed along to the child by the parents (Rosen, 1956; 1959). Such differences are intimately linked to variations in the way the child learns to perceive the environment and its rewards for achievement. For example, lower-class children were found to perform more effectively for a material incentive, whereas a nonmaterial incentive is just as effective as a material one for middle-class children (Terrell, Durkin, & Wiesley, 1959). Battle and Rooter (1963) showed that lower-class Negro children perceived themselves as having far less control over reinforcement in the environment than did middle-class white children. Such differences in perception of incentives could be a major factor in the focus and orientation of achievement behaviors.

A note of caution is in order for continued use of variables of parent-child interaction dependent upon social class distinctions. Bronfenbrenner (1961) has concluded, from an analysis of changes in parent-child relations over the past 25 years, that there are decreasing differences among classes with regard to such practices. More recently, Caldwell (1965) analyzed items that were used to rate the home environment and family interactions in homes classified as low or middle class on the basis of the customary criteria. Only a few of a large number of items differentiated lower- from middle-class homes, and these were entirely on the basis of physical environment. Hopefully, more specific and direct evidence relating parental practices to the child's intellectual growth is becoming available which will lessen dependence upon the grossly differentiating characteristics subsumed under the rubric of "social class."

TECHNIQUES FOR EARLY ENHANCEMENT OF COGNITIVE SKILLS

Systematically obtained evidence for parental use of specific instructional techniques to modify the young child's acquisition of cognitive skills is quite rare. A study by Irwin (reported in McCandless, 1961) indicated that working-class mothers who spent 10 minutes per day reading to the child, from 12 months to about 20 months of age, achieved improvement in "all phases of speech." Other available evidence of parental intervention is largely observational or anecdotal. Fowler (1962) summarizes a number of these "descriptive" surveys of gifted children who were early readers, including one with his own daughter. In such cases, children were generally exposed to instructional techniques developed by a parent, and the ability to read by age 3 was not uncommon. These same children often went on to outstanding intellectual achievement as adults.

One of the most extensive sources of potential didactic methods is the large number of studies by educators and psychologists who have evaluated techniques applied during the preschool years for modifying the child's intellectual development. The assumption is, essentially, that if such techniques have been effective they could constitute the framework for methods adaptable to parental use. The bulk of this evidence, to 1960, is covered in the comprehensive review by Fowler (1962) in which he summarizes the research which points to the possibility of modifying specific cognitive skills in children. His examination of the early studies, typified by those of Gesell (1954) and McGraw (1939), that attempted to support a maturational point of view, led him to conclude that the authors "often underplayed . . . the fact that specific training has invariably produced large gains regardless of whether training came early or late in development" (Fowler, 1962, p. 118). Studies cited on improvement of verbal memory and language, in that same review, point to the advantages of early verbal stimulation provided by oral, written, and pictorial material, as well as to the general experience gained in making observations and learning to discriminate between objects. Improvement in conceptual skills and increases in IQ score were also shown to be amenable to early training attempts which teach higher-order verbal abstractions and provide broad verbal stimulation in play situations of the sort found in a nursery school setting.

Some of the more recent work, during the present decade, delves into the problem in broader scope, dealing largely with culturally deprived children of preschool age and the attempts to improve intellectual performance through specialized training methods (Deutsch, 1963; 1964). One such program by Gray and Klaus (1965) resulted in significant increases in IQ scores for deprived Negro children of preschool age following training programs over two summers and periodic visits to the home during the other months of the year. A control group showed the customary "cumulative deficit" in IQ scores over this same period of time. Further evidence from the Project Headstart Program of the U.S. Office of Economic Opportunity (Dobbin, 1965) has shown that preschool "enrichment" programs might reasonably improve intellectual and social skills. Evaluations of specific methods utilized in this program are now being undertaken and should constitute a rich source of instructional techniques.

Results in teaching young children from a variety of backgrounds to read at earlier ages than usual have been reported for a technique known as the Initial Teaching Alphabet (Downing, 1964) under large-scale evaluation in England. Attempts to apply programed instructional techniques as a means of hastening the acquisition of reading skills by the preschool child include those of Staats, Minke, Finley, Wolf, & Brooks (1964) and of Moore (reported in Hunt, 1964), who adapted the typewriter to a method of teaching letter recognition by having the child press the keys and observe the appropriate letter displayed. Unfortunately, this initial success has been dampened by Rosenhan's (1965) failure to duplicate Moore's results when the possible Hawthorne effect, resulting from the "publicity spotlight," is absent.

Although the programs that attempt to overcome environmental deficit seem certain to continue and expand, questions remain of just how extensively conceptual processes in the young child can be modified. Bruner's (1960) position is that almost any subject matter, if properly organized, can be taught at the grade-school or preschool level. At somewhat the other extreme is the essentially maturational position of Inhelder and Piaget (1958) who argue for specific levels of cognitive development that must be achieved before certain conceptual strategies can be learned (e.g., those basic to inductive reasoning). Ausubel (1965) would also doubt any likelihood of teaching certain concepts at the "pre-operational" stage in Piaget's system (i.e., to about age 7). However, he looks upon these conceptual stages as "nothing more than approximations" that are "susceptible to environmental influences" (Ausubel, 1965, pp. 11-12).

While it is not our intention to explore this controversy through all of the developmental stages, some noteworthy attempts have been made to deal with the teachability of "processes" or "central concepts" in Piaget's formulation at earlier age levels than Piaget (Inhelder & Piaget, 1958) had observed them to occur. With some reservations, trainability of young children on concepts of "conservation" and "transitivity" have been demonstrated by Smedslund (1961a; 1961b; 1963), but there is some question about the permanence of the results and whether the child is able to generalize the principles learned. Anderson (1964) achieved some degree of success with first-grade children in teaching problem solving that required a level of inductive reasoning usually reserved for much older children under the Inhelder and Piaget (1958) scheme. The learning was also shown to be relatively permanent and transferable. But the author believes that the children achieved this result using different strategies than those employed by adolescents or adults.

The major focus of research, stimulated by Piaget's work, seems to have shifted from attempts to support his postulated sequence of conceptual development, which appears to have been demonstrated reasonably well (Braine, 1959; Peel, 1959), to the more fruitful one of analysis of the strategies involved at such stages and appropriate programing of the material to be learned (Gibson, 1965).

SUMMARY AND NEEDED RESEARCH

The direction of recent research suggests that attempts to define parental influences on the child's acquisition of cognitive skills have begun to expand beyond the rather vague concepts of "enriched experience" and "widening of interests" that have served too often as explanations for poorly understood learning mechanisms. It is largely over the past decade that various aspects of parent-child interaction have been investigated in an attempt to define their influence upon specific modes of cognitive responses, with the most compelling lines of evidence pointing to a critical role for verbal patterns established by the parent. Included in these verbal patterns are the manner or "style" of communicating information to the child and the opportunities for verbal stimulation provided in the home (e.g., in the sheer amount of verbal activity and in the provision of books or other devices that supply a wide range of opportunity for language usage). Many of the social class distinctions in intellectual achievement, which consistently have been found, are likely to center around parental stimuli to the development of language skills as the mediating variable. But much more remains to be delineated regarding the dimensions of parental linguistic styles: the way in which these affect particular forms of verbal development and the patterns of parent-child communication which have an impact on specific verbal and problem-solving abilities.

Still other phases of parental practice that indicate some promise for differentiating levels, as well as areas, of cognitive skill development have been dealt with in the framework of permissive-restrictive environments in the home and parental pressures for achievement. If these variables were to be more clearly defined operationally—so that present inconsistencies in research findings can be reconciled—the next steps would require determining their likely interaction with one another and their relation to the important role that seems to mark communication and language.

Any description of the processes by which parental behavior influences the development of cognition would be augmented considerably by knowledge of the parents' perception of their role in rearing practices and its influence on cognitive growth. One of the major research gaps has been the scarcity of information regarding parents' attitudes toward their own potential influence upon intellectual development—particularly for parents of different social classes. In a laboratory setting it has been found that inconsistencies in experimental results can occur if there is a failure to deal with data regarding the mother's feelings about interacting with the child in a problem-solving situation (Beller & Nash, 1965). Perhaps some appreciation of the child's views of the learning situation and of his mother's responses would also be in order.

The most pertinent and systematically obtained results dealing with relations between parental practices and the child's level of cognitive skill development have been (and are likely to continue to be) achieved by observation in the laboratory setting as opposed to questionnaire methods. However, there remains the more ultimate validation that can only be derived from the broad range of daily rearing practices in a home or "home-like" setting. Data obtained from this source will be essential for defining the more complex aspects of parental influences in the modification of the child's cognitive performance.

REFERENCES

ANASTASI, ANNE. Heredity, environment, and the question "How?" *Psychological Review*, 1958, *65*, 197-208.

ANDERSON, R. C. Shaping logical behavior in six- and seven-year-olds. Cooperative Research Project No. 1790A. Chicago: University of Illinois, 1964.

AUSUBEL, D. P. Stages of intellectual development and their implications for early childhood education. In P. B. Neubauer (Ed.), *Concepts of development in early childhood education*. Springfield, Ill.: Charles C Thomas, 1965. Pp. 8-51.

BALDWIN, A. L., KALHORN, JOAN, & BREESE, FAY H. Patterns of parent behavior. *Psychological Monographs: General and Applied*, 1945, *58*, No. 3 (Whole No. 268).

BATTLE, ESTHER S., & ROTTER, J. B. Children's feelings of personal control as related to social class and ethnic group. *Journal of Personality*, 1963, *31*, (4), 482-490.

BAYLEY, NANCY. On the growth of intelligence. *American Psychologist*, 1955, *10*, 805-818.

BEACH, F. A., & JAYNES, J. Effects of early experience upon the behavior of animals. *Psychological Bulletin*, 1954, *51*, 239-263.

BELL, R. Q. Retrospective attitude studies of parent-child relations. *Child Development*, 1958, *29*, 323-338.

BELLER, E. K., & NASH, A. Research with educationally disadvantaged preschool children. Paper presented at the annual meetings of the American Educational Research Association, Chicago, February 12, 1965.

BENNETT, E. L., DIAMOND, MARIAN C., KRECH, D., & ROSENZWEIG, M. R. Chemical and anatomical plasticity of brain. *Science*, 1964, *146*, No. 3644, 610-619.

BERNSTEIN, B. Language and social class. *British Journal of Sociology*, 1960, 11, 271-276.

BIGLIN, J. E. The relationship of parental attitudes to children's academic and social performance. Unpublished doctoral dissertation, University of Nebraska, 1964.

BING, ELIZABETH. Effect of childrearing practices on development of differential cognitive abilities. *Child Development*, 1963, *34*, (3), 631-648.

BLOOM, B. S. *Stability and change in human characteristics*. New York: Wiley, 1964.

BRAINE, M. D. S. The ontogeny of certain logical operations: Piaget's formulations examined by nonverbal methods. *Psychological Monographs: General and Applied*, 1959, *73*, No. 5 (Whole No. 475).

BRONFENBRENNER, U. The changing American child: a speculative analysis. *Journal of social Issues*, 1961, *17*, (1), 6-17.

BRUNER, J. S. *The process of education*. Cambridge, Mass.: Harvard University Press, 1960.

BRUNER, J. S. The course of cognitive growth. *American Psychologist*, 1964, *19*, 1-15.

CALDWELL, BETTYE. Infant and preschool socialization in different social classes. Paper presented at the meetings of the American Psychological Association, Chicago, September, 1965.

CALLARD, ESTHER D. Achievement motive in the four-year-old child and its relationship to achievement expectancies of the mother. Unpublished doctoral dissertation, University of Michigan, 1964.

CHANCE, JUNE E. Independence training and first graders' achievement. *Journal of consulting Psychology*, 1961, *25*, 149-154.

CRANDALL, V. J. Achievement. In H. W. Stevenson (Ed.), *Child psychology: the sixty-second yearbook of the National Society for the Study of Education*. Part I. Chicago: University of Chicago Press, 1963. Pp. 416-459.

CRANDALL, V. J., DEWEY, RACHEL, KATKOVSKY, W., & PRESTON, ANNE. Parents' attitudes and behaviors and grade-school children's academic achievements. *Journal of genetic Psychology*, 1964, *104*, 53-66.

CRANDALL, V. J. & PRESTON, ANNE. Patterns and levels of maternal behavior. *Child Development*, 1955, *26*, 267-277.

CRANDALL, V. J., PRESTON, ANNE, & RABSON, ALICE. Maternal relations and the development of independence and achievement behavior in young children. *Child Development*, 1960, *31*, 243-251.

DAVE, R. H. The identification and measurement of educational process variables that are related to educational achievement. Unpublished doctoral dissertation, University of Chicago, 1963.

DENNIS, W., & NAJARIAN, PERGROUHI. Infant development under environmental handicap. *Psychological Monographs: General and Applied*, 1957, *71*, No. 7 (Whole No. 436).

DEUTSCH, M. The disadvantaged child and the learning process: some social, psychological and developmental considerations. In A. H. Passow (Ed.), *Education in depressed areas*. Part II. New York: Bureau of Publications, Teachers College, Columbia University, 1963. Pp. 163-179.

DEUTSCH, M. Facilitating development in the preschool child: Social and psychological perspectives. *Merrill-Palmer Quarterly of Behavior and Development*, 1964, *10*, (3), 249-263.

DEUTSCH, M. The role of social class in language development and cognition. *American Journal of Orthopsychiatry*, 1965, *35*, (1), 78-88.

DEUTSCH, M., & BROWN, B. Social influences in Negro-white intelligence differences. *Journal of Social Issues*, 1964, *20*, (2), 24-35.

DOBBIN, J. E. Observations of Project Head Start: a report on 335 Project Head Start centers. Princeton, N. J.: Institute for Educational Development, October, 1965.

DOWNING, J. Teaching reading with i. t. a. in Britain. *Phi Delta Kappan*, 1964, *45*, 322-329.

DREWS, ELIZABETH M., & TEAHAN, J. E. Parental attitudes and academic achievement. *Journal of Clinical Psychology*, 1957, *13*, 328-332.

EELLS, K., DAVIS, A., HAVIGHURST, R. J., HERRICK, V. E., & TYLER, R. *Intelligence and cultural differences*. Chicago: University of Chicago Press, 1951.

FOWLER, W. Cognitive learning in infancy and early childhood. *Psychological Bulletin*, 1962, *59*, (2), 116-152.

FREEBERG, N. E., & PAYNE, D. T. A survey of parental practices related to cognitive development in young children. Princeton, N. J.: Institute for Educational Development, September, 1965.

GESELL, A. The ontogenesis of infant behavior. In L. Carmichael (Ed.), *Manual of child psychology*. New York: Wiley, 1954.

GIBSON, ELEANOR J. Learning to read. *Science*, 1965, *148*, 1066.

GRAY, SUSAN W., & KLAUS, R. A. An experimental preschool program for culturally deprived children. *Child Development*, 1965, *36*, (4), 887-898.

HAVIGHURST, R. J., & DAVIS, A. A comparison of the Chicago and Harvard studies of social class differences in child rearing. *American sociological Review*, 1955, *20*, 438-442.

HEBB, D. O. *The organization of behavior: a neuropsychological theory*. New York: Wiley, 1949.

HEFNER, LESLIE T. Reliability of mothers' reports on child development. Unpublished doctoral dissertation, University of Michigan, 1963.

HESS, R. D. Effects of maternal interaction on cognitions of pre-school children in several social strata. Paper presented at the meetings of the American Psychological Association, Chicago, September, 1965.

HESS, R. D., & SHIPMAN, VIRGINIA C. Early experience and the socialization of cognitive modes in children. *Child Development*, 1965, *36*, (4), 869-886.

HUNT, J. McV. *Intelligence and experience.* New York. Ronald Press, 1961.

HUNT, J. McV. The psychological basis for using pre-school enrichment as an antidote for cultural deprivation. *Merrill-Palmer Quarterly of Behavior and Development*, 1964, *10*, 209-248.

HURLEY, J. R. Maternal attitudes and children's intelligence. *Journal of clinical Psychology*, 1959, *15*, 291-292.

INHELDER, BARBEL, & PIAGET, J. *The growth of logical thinking.* New York: Basic Books, 1958.

JENSEN, A. R. Social class and verbal learning. Unpublished manuscript. Berkeley: University of California, 1964. (On file at Library, Educational Testing Service, Princeton, N. J.)

KAGAN, J., & MOSS, H. A. *Birth to maturity, a study in psychological development.* New York: Wiley, 1962.

KAGAN, J., MOSS, H. A., & SIGEL, I. E. Psychological significance of styles of conceptualization. *Monographs of the Society of Research in child Development*, 1963, *28*, No. 2 (Serial No. 86), 73-112.

KATKOVSKY, W., PRESTON, ANNE, & CRANDALL, V. J. Parents' attitudes toward their personal achievements and toward the achievement behaviors of their children. *Journal of genetic Psychology*, 1964, *104*, 67-82. (a)

KATKOVSKY, W., PRESTON, ANNE, & CRANDALL, V. J. Parents' achievement attitudes and their behavior with their children in achievement situations. *Journal of genetic Psychology*, 1964, *104*, 105-121. (b)

KLINEBERG, O. Negro-white differences in intelligence test performance: a new look at an old problem. *American Psychologist*, 1963, *18* (4), 198-203.

KOHN, M. L. Social class and parental values. *American Journal of Sociology*, 1959, *64*, 337-351.

KRECH, D., ROSENZWEIG, M. R., & BENNETT, E. L. Relations between brain chemistry and problem-solving among rats raised in enriched and impoverished environments. *Journal of comparative and physiological Psychology*, 1962, *55*, (5), 801-807.

McCANDLESS, B. *Children and adolescents: behavior and development.* New York: Holt, Rinehart & Winston, 1961.

McCORD, JOAN, & McCORD, W. Cultural stereotypes and the validity of interviews for research in child development. *Child Development*, 1961, *32*, 171-185.

McGRAW, MYRTLE B. Later development of children specially trained during infancy; Johnny and Jimmy at school age. *Child Development*, 1939, *10*, 1-19.

MANNINO, F. V. Family factors related to school persistence. *Journal of educational Sociology*, 1962, *35*, 193-202.

MEDNICK, S. A., & SHAFFER, J. B. P. Mothers' retrospective reports in child-rearing research. *American Journal of Orthopsychiatry*, 1963, *33*, 457-461.

MILNER, E. A. A study of the relationships between reading readiness in grade one school children and patterns of parent-child interactions. *Child Development*, 1951, *22*, 95-112.

MINTURN, L. & LAMBERT, W. *Mothers of six cultures: antecedents of child rearing.* New York: Wiley, 1964.

MORROW, W. R., & WILSON, R. R. Family relations of bright high-achieving and underachieving high school boys. *Child Development*, 1961, *32*, 501-510.

MOSS, H. A., & KAGAN, J. Maternal influences on early IQ scores. *Psychological Reports*, 1958, *4*, 655-661.

NEWELL, A., SHAW, J. C., & SIMON, H. A. Elements of a theory of human problem solving. *Psychological Review*, 1958, *65*, 151-166.

OLIM, E. G., HESS, R. D., & SHIPMAN, VIRGINIA. Maternal language styles and their implications for children's cognitive development. Paper presented at the meetings of the American Psychological Association, Chicago, September, 1965.

PEEL, E. A. Experimental examination of some of Piaget's schemata concerning children's perception and thinking and a discussion of their educational significance. *British Journal of educational Psychology*, 1959, *29*, 89-103.

PYLES, M. K., STOLZ, H. R., & MACFARLANE, J. W. The accuracy of mothers' reports on birth and developmental data. *Child Development*, 1935, *6*, 165-176.

RIESEN, A. H. Plasticity of behavior: psychological aspects. In H. F. Harlow and C. N. Woolsey (Eds.), *Biological and biochemical bases of behavior*. Madison: University of Wisconsin Press, 1958. Pp. 425-450.

ROBBINS, LILLIAN C. The accuracy of parental recall of aspects of child development and of child rearing practices. *Journal of abnormal and social Psychology*, 1963, *66*, 261-270.

ROSEN, B. C. The achievement syndrome: a psychocultural dimension of social stratification. *American sociological Review*, 1956, *21*, 203-211.

ROSEN, B. C. Race, ethnicity, and the achievement syndrome. *American sociological Review*, 1959, *24*, 47-60.

ROSEN, B. C., & D'ANDRADE, R. The psychosocial origins of achievement motivation. *Sociometry*, 1959, *22*, 185-218.

ROSENHAN, D. L. Cultural deprivation and learning: an examination of method and theory. Paper presented at the annual meetings of the American Educational Research Association, February, 1965.

SEARS, R. R., MACCOBY, ELEANOR E., & LEVIN, H. *Patterns of child rearing*. Evanston, Ill.: Row, Peterson, 1957.

SENDEN, M. VON., *Raum- und Gestaltauffassung bei operierten Blindgeborenen vor und nach der Operation*. Leipzig: Barth, 1932.

SHAW, M. C. Note on parent attitudes toward independence training and the academic achievement of their children. *Journal of educational Psychology*, 1964, *55*, (6), 371-374.

SMEDSLUND, J. The acquisition of conservation of substance and weight in children, II: External reinforcement of conservation of weight and of the operations of addition and subtraction. *Scandinavian Journal of Psychology*, 1961, *2*, 71-84. (a)

SMEDSLUND, J. The acquisition of conservation of substance and weight in children, II: Extinction of conservation of weight acquired "normally" and by means of empirical controls on a balance. *Scandinavian Journal of Psychology*, 1961, *2*, 85-87. (b)

SMEDSLUND, J. Patterns of experience and the acquisition of concrete transitivity of weight in eight-year-old children. *Scandinavian Journal of Psychology*, 1963, *4*, 251-256.

SONTAG, L. W., BAKER, C. T., & NELSON, VIRGINIA L. Mental growth and personality development: a longitudinal study. *Monographs of the Society for Research in child Development*, 1958, *23*, No. 2 (Serial No. 68).

SONTAG, L. W., & KAGAN, J. The emergence of intellectual achievement motives. *American Journal of Orthopsychiatry*, 1963, *33*, (3), 532-535.

STAATS, A. W., MINKE, K. A., FINLEY, J. R., WOLF, M., & BROOKS, L. O. A reinforcer system and experimental procedure for the laboratory study of reading acquisition. *Child Development*, 1964, *35*, 209-231.

STEWART, R. S. Personality maladjustment and reading achievement. *American Journal of Orthopsychiatry*, 1950, *20*, 410-417.

STODDARD, G. D. *The meaning of intelligence*. New York: Macmillan, 1943.

TAYLOR, J. B. What do attitude scales measure? the problem of social desirability. *Journal of abnormal and social Psychology*, 1961, *62*, 386-390.

TERRELL, G., JR., DURKIN, KATHRYN, & WIESLEY, M. Social class and the nature of the incentive in discrimination learning. *Journal of abnormal and social Psychology,* 1959, *59,* 270-272.

WALTERS, J. Relationship between reliability of responses in family life research and method of data collection. *Marriage and family Living,* 1960, *22,* 232-237.

WATSON, G. Some personality differences in children related to strict or permissive parental discipline. *Journal of Psychology,* 1957, *44,* 227-249.

WHEELER, L. R. The intelligence of East Tennessee mountain children. *Journal of educational Psychology,* 1932, *23,* 351-370.

WHITE, MARTHA S. Social class, child rearing practices, and child behavior. *American sociological Review,* 1957, *22,* 704-712.

WIENER, G. G., RIDER, R. V., & OPPEL, W. Some correlates of IQ changes in children. *Child Development,* 1963, *34,* (1), 61-67.

WINTERBOTTOM, MARIAN. The relation of need for achievement in learning experiences in independence and mastery. In J. Atkinson (Ed.), *Motives in fantasy, action and society.* Princeton, N. J.: Van Nostrand, 1958.

WITKIN, H. A., DYK, RUTH B., FATERSON, HANNA, GOODENOUGH, D. R., & KARP, S. A. *Psychological differentiation: studies of development.* New York: Wiley, 1962.

WITKIN, H. A., FATERSON, HANNA, GOODENOUGH, D., & BIRNBAUM, JUDITH. Cognitive patterning in high grade mentally retarded boys. Unpublished manuscript, Psychology Laboratory, Department of Psychiatry, State University of New York, Downstate Medical Center, 1965.

WOLF, R. M. The identification and measurement of environmental process variables related to intelligence. Unpublished doctoral dissertation, University of Chicago, 1964.

YARROW, L. J. Separation from parents during early childhood. In M. L. Hoffman and Lois Hoffman (Eds.), *Review of child development research.* New York: Russell Sage Foundation, 1964. Pp. 89-136.

YARROW, MARIAN R. Problems of methods in parent-child research. *Child Development,* 1963, *34,* 215-226.

ZINGG, R. M. Feral man and extreme cases of isolation. *American Journal of Psychology,* 1940, *53,* 487-517.

ZUNICH, M. Relationship between maternal behavior and attitudes toward children. *Journal of genetic Psychology,* 1962, *100,* 155-165.

12

CHILDREN'S BEHAVIORAL STYLE AND THE TEACHER'S APPRAISAL OF THEIR INTELLIGENCE

Edward M. Gordon, Ph.D.

School Psychologist, Leonia (N. J.) Public Schools

and

Alexander Thomas, M.D.

Professor of Psychiatry, New York University School of Medicine

The concept that psychological development is a function of an inter-action between organismic characteristics of the child and intra-and extrafamilial environmental influences has been receiving increasing emphasis in the child development literature, by such researchers as Korner (1964), Murphy (1962), and Thomas (1963). These authors have stressed that a child's response to a teacher or classroom situation will depend not only on the attitudes and behavior of the teacher but also on the child's own behavioral characteristics. A further implication is that children with dissimilar behavioral characteristics, or styles, may evoke different responses or behavior in the same teacher. The latter possibility has, however, received little attention in the literature, except for a few special considerations, such as the influence of the child's socio-cultural background on the teacher's attitudes toward him (Bloom, 1965).

The study reported here explored the influence of certain character-

Reprinted from JOURNAL OF SCHOOL PSYCHOLOGY, Summer 1967, Vol. V, No. 4, pp. 292-300. This investigation was supported in part by Grant MH-03614 from the National Institute of Mental Health.

istics of behavioral style of kindergarten pupils on their teachers' appraisal of their intelligence. The possibility that teachers' judgments of children's intelligence may be influenced by such nonintellective behavioral attributes is clearly of theoretical and practical importance. However, no references to this issue have been found in a search of the literature.

The specific hypothesis tested in the present study was that teachers would tend to overestimate the intelligence of children who react positively and quickly to new situations, and to underestimate the intelligence of children who react negatively to most new situations and who require a relatively long acclimatization period to change this initial response to one of full participation. This hypothesis was suggested by the finding in a New York longitudinal study (Chess & Birch, in press) that a number of teachers grossly underestimated the intelligence of several children who typically showed initial negative reactions to the new, followed by a slowly developed positive adaptation.

PROCEDURE

The subjects were all the children (N=93) enrolled in the four kindergarten classes of the Anna C. Scott School, Leonia, N. J., in May 1964 and their two teachers,[1] each of whom taught a morning and an afternoon class of approximately 23 children. Leonia is a very small middle-class residential community whose families are of relatively high socioeconomic status and well above the average in educational background. The two teachers, each with at least 30 years of kindergarten teaching experience, were considered unusually competent by their peers and administrators.

The particular aspect of children's behavior studied is called *Quality of Participation*. This category refers to the child's characteristic style of reaction to new activities and situations in the classroom. Four types of children were defined:

1. The kind of child who plunges into new activities and situations quickly, positively and unhesitatingly (*plungers*).

2. The kind of child who goes along in a positive manner but clearly does not plunge right in (*go-alongers*).

[1] The sensitive and wholehearted participation of Miss Emily Baxter and Miss Dorothy Whitney, who retired from teaching at the end of the 1964-65 year, is gratefully acknowledged. This study could not have been completed without the additional generous cooperation of Mr. Irving S. Ziegler, Principal of the Anna C. Scott School, and Mr. Stephen B. Sims, Superintendent of Schools.

3. The kind of child who stands on the sidelines waiting, then slowly and gradually gets involved in the new activity (*sideliners*).

4. The kind of child who remains negative and a non-participator in a new situation either for weeks and months on end, or even indefinitely (*non-participator*).

Quality of Participation can be considered to be a combination of the child's initial response to a new situation, (i.e. a positive approaching one, or a negative withdrawal response), and of the ease with which an initial negative response will change to a positive one with repeated contact with the situation. These two characteristics have been identified in a current ongoing longitudinal study (Thomas, et. al. 1963), as present in the behavioral functioning of children from early infancy onward. They have been categorized as Approach-Withdrawal and Adaptability. The latter also includes the ease with which a socially desirable modification in the child's behavior is obtainable when a situation to which he is already adapted is altered. It should be pointed out that these categories do not carry with them any assumption as to the existence or absence of "anxiety" or "insecurity." It is considered that non-participation of a child may be the result of "anxiety" or may reflect a child's customary behavioral response to newness.

Near the end of the school year, in May, the teachers were asked to characterize all of their children as to their *Quality of Participation,* using the four categories of participation listed above.[2] Two training sessions were first held with the teachers one and two weeks prior to making their categorizations, in which they were instructed in the definitions and criteria for the variable by the senior author. They were told to take into consideration all of their observations of the experiences with each child since the beginning of the school year and to focus their thinking on the child's actual behavior rather than on any interpretations as to its meaning or causation. The teachers subsequently reported that they did not in fact find this categorizing procedure difficult. Whether less experienced teachers would do as well we cannot say.

Following their categorizing of the children on *Quality of Participation,* the teachers were asked to make a judgment as to each child's intelligence, in the form of an answer to the following question: What do you estimate this child's general mental ability or native intelligence

---

[2] It is important to distinguish between the children's actual behavior and *Quality of Participation* as perceived and categorized by the teachers. It is the latter with which this particular study is concerned. Independent classroom observations of the children's behavior as a study of the validity of the teachers' categorizations of *Quality of Participation* would be of interest and value, but is not essential to the interpretation of the data reported here.

to be? A 7-point scale was provided, which included very inferior, inferior, below average, average, above average, superior, and very superior. The children had not been given psychometric tests in school, so that neither the teachers nor the authors had any knowledge of their measured intellectual ability.

The Anna C. Scott School regularly administers the Kuhlmann-Anderson Tests of Academic Potential (Book A, 7th Ed.) to all first grade children in the late fall. The IQ's of the children in this study were determined in November, several months after the kindergarten teachers had categorized them on *Quality of Participation* and estimated their intelligence. The test was administered to the children in groups by their regular classroom teachers under the supervision of the senior author.

RESULTS

The distributions of the teachers' categorizations of *Quality of Participation* and estimates of intelligence are shown in Tables 1 and 2. Each teacher used only four out of the seven given points of the intelligence scale. The distributions of the two teachers' ratings are similar and when pooled together form a distribution which is skewed toward the "above average" side, as would be expected in such a sample of children where the median IQ customarily hovers in the neighborhood of 114.

Kuhlmann-Anderson IQ's were grouped conventionally into a 5-step scale; the distribution of scores is shown in Table 3. The IQ distribution is shaped differently from the teacher estimates, but agrees in that the central tendency is above the conventional "average" range.

The successive categories of each of the three variables were assigned weights on a linear scale and product-moment correlations calculated among them. The relationships are shown in Tables 4, 5, and 6 and the correlation coefficients in Table 7. As might be expected, the overall relationship between the teachers' estimates of intelligence and Kuhlmann-Anderson IQ's is positive and significant. The teachers differed in the accuracy of their intelligence estimates, the r for one being .53 ($p < .01$) and for the other .26 (N.S.).

The correlation between the teachers' categorizations of *Quality of Participation* and Kuhlmann-Anderson IQ's is similarly positive and significant. (As with the correlation between teachers' estimates of intelligence and Kuhlmann-Anderson IQ's the r's for the teachers separately are different, the one being .37 ($p < .01$) and the other .19 (N.S.)). One interpretation of this positive correlation is that the Kuhlmann-Anderson Test actually measures the children's quality of participation, as per-

TABLE 1

TEACHER CATEGORIZATIONS OF QUALITY OF PARTICIPATION[a]

Category	N
Plungers	25
Go-alongers	47
Sideliners	20
Non-participators	1
	—
Total	93

[a] One teacher categorized almost twice as many of her children *plungers* as *sideliners,* while the other had one and a half times as many *sideliners* as *plungers.* When their categorizations are pooled, however, they are approximately symmetrically distributed over the first three "points" of the participation scale.

TABLE 2

TEACHER ESTIMATES OF INTELLIGENCE

Estimates	N
Superior	3
Above Average	26
Average	55
Below Average	8
	—
Total	92[a]

[a] One teacher failed to estimate the intelligence of one of her children.

TABLE 3

KUHLMANN-ANDERSON IQ's

Score	N
Very Superior (130+)	9
Superior (120-129)	25
High Average (110-119)	23
Average (90-119)	28
Low Average (80-89)	4
	—
Total	89[a]

[a] Four children moved from the school district during the summer between kindergarten and 1st grade.

ceived by the teacher, as well as their academic potential. Or stated differently, it may be that the quality of a child's participation in new and altered situations and his academic potential are dynamically related. Another possibility is that *Quality of Participation* as a behavioral characteristic influences immediately and directly the child's level of performance in a new test situation. These are not mutually exclusive interpretations. The data of the present study, however, are not adequate for dealing with this question.

The correlation between the teachers' categorizations of *Quality of Participation* and their estimates of the children's intelligence was similarly positive and significant (*r*'s of .53 and .58). The interpretation of this finding was possible only after the influence of the children's actual measured intelligence on the teachers' ratings was first estimated. For this reason, a partial coefficient of correlation was calculated, taking out the effects of Kuhlmann-Anderson IQ's. The obtained partial r was .49, which is still significant at better than the .01 level of confidence.[3] This indicates that the teachers were influenced in their judgments of the children's intelligence by their perception of the non-intellective behavior characteristics of the children, namely the tendency to approach or withdraw from new experiences and the quickness of adaptability to such school situations.

The next question concerns the direction of the influence of the child's characteristics on the teachers' appraisals (i.e. which children were underestimated and which children overestimated in intelligence). The intelligence of six children in the study was overestimated by the teachers. Five of these six children were categorized as *plungers,* the sixth a *sideliner.* The five *plungers* had Kuhlmann-Anderson IQ's in the average range but they were rated by their teachers as above average. The *sideliner* had an IQ which was below average, but he was judged average by his teacher. The intelligence of 50 children was underestimated by the teachers. This group comprised 11 *plungers,* 28 *go-alongers,* and 11 *sideliners.*[4] An examination of the size of the teachers' underestimations of the 30 children in this group who were of superior measured intelligence plainly reveals the direction of influence of the children's *Quality of Participation* on the teachers' judgments. Of the seven children in this superior group who were *plungers,* six were rated as above average in intelligence and only one average. Of the four children who were *side-*

---

[3] Although normality assumptions are not met, the N is so large that the statistical test is nevertheless valid.

[4] The child who had been categorized a *non-participator* was one of those who moved out of the school district before the Kuhlmann-Anderson Test was administered.

TABLE 4

RELATIONSHIP BETWEEN TEACHERS' ESTIMATES OF INTELLIGENCE AND KUHLMANN-ANDERSON IQ'S

IQ's	Below Average	Estimates of Intelligence Average	Above Average	Superior	N
Very Superior		3	5	1	9
Superior		14	8	2	24
High Average	1	15	7		23
Average	4	19	5		28
Low Average	3	1			4
Total	8	52	25	3	88

TABLE 5

RELATIONSHIP BETWEEN TEACHERS' CATEGORIZATIONS OF QUALITY OF PARTICIPATION AND KUHLMANN-ANDERSON IQ'S

IQ's	Non-participator	Quality of Participation Sideliner	Go-alonger	Plunger	N
Very Superior		1	3	5	9
Superior		3	18	4	25
High Average		4	12	7	23
Average		7	13	8	28
Low Average		4			4
Total		19	46	24	89

TABLE 6

RELATIONSHIP BETWEEN TEACHERS' ESTIMATES OF INTELLIGENCE AND CATEGORIZATIONS OF QUALITY OF PARTICIPATION

Quality of Participation	Below Average	Estimates of Intelligence Average	Above Average	Superior	N
Plunger		8	15	2	25
Go-alonger	2	32	11	1	46
Sideliner	6	14			20
Non-participator		1			1
Total	8	55	26	3	92

TABLE 7

CORRELATIONS AMONG TEACHERS' ESTIMATES OF INTELLIGENCE, KUHLMANN-ANDERSON IQ'S, AND TEACHERS' CATEGORIZATIONS OF QUALITY OF PARTICIPATION

	Estimated Intelligence	Measured Intelligence
Quality of Participation	.54**	.24*
Estimated Intelligence		.49**

* p < .05
**p < .01

liners, however, all were judged to be of only average intelligence. The underestimate was therefore larger for those children whom the teachers perceived as *sideliners* than for those perceived as *plungers.* The degree of underestimation was intermediate for the 19 superior children with the intermediate categorization in *Quality of Participation* (i.e. the *go-alongers*: seven were rated as above average and 12 as average).

In summary, then, the nature of the influence of *Quality of Participation* on the teachers' estimates of the children's intelligence was as predicted. If a child is a *plunger* and unhesitatingly jumps into new situations and accommodates himself easily and quickly, he is likely to be judged more intelligent by his teacher than the child who is a *sideliner* and tends to withdraw from new situations and adapts only after some warm-up period, even though the two types of children are of the same measured intelligence. This conclusion emerges irrespective of any assumptions that might be made as to the teachers' own personal rating scheme of different levels of intelligence. In other words, the correlations emerge simply from the teachers' ratings of the children on the two variables.

DISCUSSION

The findings reported above indicate that teachers' judgments of their children's intelligence are significantly distorted by their perceptions of specific aspects of the children's behavioral style or temperament. Theoretically the results of this study tend to support an interactional view of child development, in which characteristics of the child himself, as experienced by an adult, evoke responses in the adult that are likely, in turn, to influence significantly the future course of the child's development. The characteristics in question—the quality of a child's adaptation to newness—are considered to be within the range of "normal" behavioral variation. The two very experienced teachers who participated in the study recognized this, for none of the children in their classes was referred to the school psychologist because he was thought to be pathologically non-adaptable, not even the one child who had been categorized a *non-participator.* The teachers also remarked, when they were being trained to make categorizations and ratings, that they considered all their children quite well adapted by that time of the year to classroom and school routines. Yet, as the distribution of categorizations on *Quality of Participation* in Table 1 reveals, they had no difficulty in discriminating among the children as to the nature of their response to the new.

The findings also have practical implications for education and child development. Children develop images of themselves from the judgments significant adults in their lives make of them. If their teachers under- or overestimate their intelligence, children may come to under- or overestimate themselves. This study indicates that a child's customary responses to newness are capable of producing such distortions in the teacher's judgment which in turn may distort the child's self-image and self-esteem. In addition, the teacher's estimate can influence the demands she makes on the child. A child whose intelligence is overestimated may be thought to be performing below his capacity and be exposed to excessive expectations and pressures in school. On the other hand, a child whose intelligence is underestimated by his teachers may be exposed to insufficient expectations and stimulation.

It can be suggested that teachers will have fewer distorted judgments of their pupils if they can be taught to recognize and understand temperamental characteristics such as *Quality of Participation* for what they are and to accommodate themselves to the requirements of differing behavioral styles. Thus, for example, if a child who is a *sideliner* can be accepted simply as someone who requires additional time and patience to overcome his typical negative and slowly adaptive response to newness, there will undoubtedly be greater ability on the teacher's part to estimate his intellectual capacities accurately. Similarly, the teacher will also be able to make a more realistic appraisal of the intelligence of the child who adapts quickly and easily and never seems overwhelmed by new situations.

REFERENCES

BLOOM, B. S., DAVIS, A., & HESS, R. *Compensatory education for cultural deprivation.* New York: Holt, Rinehart & Winston, 1965.
CHESS, STELLA, THOMAS, A., & BIRCH, H. G. Behavior problems revisited: findings of an anterospective study. *J. Amer. Acad. Child Psychiat.,* in press.

KORNER, A. F. Some hypotheses regarding the significance of individual differences at birth for later development. In Ruth S. Eissler, et. al. (Eds.) *Psychoanalytic study of the child.* New York: International Universities Press, 1964, *19,* 58-72.

MURPHY, LOIS B. & ASSOCIATES. *The widening world of childhood.* New York: Basic Books, 1962.

THOMAS, A., CHESS, STELLA, BIRCH, H. G., HERTZIG, MARGARET E., & KORN, S. *Behavioral individuality in early childhood.* New York: New York University Press, 1963.

13

READING DISABILITY: TEACHING THROUGH STIMULATION OF DEFICIT PERCEPTUAL AREAS

Archie A. Silver, M.D., Rosa A. Hagin, Ph.D., and Marilyn F. Hersh, M.A.

Department of Psychiatry and Neurology
New York University Medical Center

A crossover experiment, using the method of stimulation of deficit perceptual areas, is designed to determine whether perception can be modified by training and whether increased accuracy of perception is reflected in improved reading achieveemnt. The method itself is discussed in terms of historical and experimental antecedents. Experimental design, training procedures, and case materials are described.

Basing our work on the hypothesis that increased accuracy of perception will be reflected in improved reading achievement, we are engaged in a four-year study to devise methods for the stimulation of deficit perceptual areas in children with reading disability and to subject these methods to controlled evaluation. This paper will outline methods of perceptual stimulation, describe our experimental procedure, and present preliminary findings in the clinical application of these methods. Quan-

Reprinted from AMERICAN JOURNAL OF ORTHOPSYCHIATRY, July 1967, Volume XXXVII, Number 4, pp. 744-752. Copyright the American Orthopsychiatric Association, Inc. Reproduced by permission. This study was made possible in part by funds granted by the Carnegie Corporation of New York. The statements made and views expressed are solely the responsibility of the authors.

titative evaluation will be presented upon completion of our study in January 1968.

DEVELOPMENT OF METHODS

Previous studies made in our clinic[25-28] offered a method for constructing a perceptual profile of the child with a reading disability and demonstrated the tenacity with which perceptual defects persist even ten to twelve years after such a child received what was considered effective remedial teaching. These follow-up studies suggested a need for departure from established procedure.

We chose to make a direct attack upon the perceptual problems which clinical studies of retarded readers had revealed. We postulated that a total remedial program would include teaching at three levels: (1) *An accuracy level* to develop accuracy of perception within a given modality. (2) *An intermodal level* to relate two or more perceptual modalities. (3) *A verbal level* to insure the transfer of perceptual abilities to language skills.

The experiment reported here, however, has been confined to the accuracy level, and has been designed to answer only the following questions: What is the effect of perceptual training on perception? What is the effect of perceptual stimulation on reading and spelling achievement? What is the effect of perceptual stimulation on cerebral dominance for language?

REVIEW OF THE LITERATURE

Itard may be regarded as an innovator in the educational application of theories of perceptual stimulation. In his attempts to educate the wild boy found in the woods near Aveyron,[12] he showed that various modalities differ in response to training and that perception is basic to learning. The painstaking detail with which Itard recorded the use of his "comparative method" of teaching pointed a way which Seguin was then to follow in his physiological approach.[24] Seguin emphasized the importance of isolating and stimulating single modalities, in a manner in keeping with the present information-processing theory.[18] Montessori demonstrated the applicability of these methods, not only to handicapped learners but to the education of all young children.[17]

Recent studies have shown that at least the beginning aspects of reading are closely related to perceptual abilities. This relationship has been shown in a variety of ways: predictive studies of reading progress—Barrett[2] and de Hirsch, Jansky, and Langford[8]; comparisons of the perceptual functioning of good and poor readers, such as differentials in visual and aural learning—Budoff and Quinlan[5]; difficulties in auditory-visual integration—Birch and Belmont[4]; systematic reversal in right-left discrimination—Benton[3]; "peculiarities in acoustic perception"—Levina.[16]

Although there seems to be theoretical and experimental support for recognition of a relationship between perceptual abilities and reading, the problem of enhancing perceptual abilities in retarded readers is touched very lightly in the literature. Some investigators have designed experiments in which a specific aspect of perception is investigated—Levin and Watson[15]; Staats and Schultz[29]—but these are classical experimental designs and provide neither the opportunity for application in the total process of learning to read nor evaluation of effects of training beyond the brief duration of the study. Informal "pilot studies" with limited N's or lack of controls have also been published.[1, 19]

A few objective reports are available. Chansky,[6, 7] for example, has continued to replicate his findings with different diagnostic groups as a means of evaluating the nature and permanence of changes following perceptual training. Robbins'[22] study has raised questions about the replicability of results claimed for Delcato's theory of neurological organization. Rutherford,[23] on the other hand, has shown that a group program of perceptual-motor skills training, as described by Kephart,[13-14] could have a significant effect upon reading but not upon number readiness test scores earned by kindergarteners, while Roach[21] found that although group work was not effective with older elementary school children, individual training utilizing Kephart's approach accelerated reading achievement in retarded readers. These studies show the value of such research not only to replicate findings but to ensure more specific application of these innovations.

PROCEDURE

Our project has been designed to encompass 80 boys, all referred to Bellevue Hospital Mental Hygiene Clinic because of school learning and behavior problems. The boys range in age from seven to eleven years, earn full scale scores not lower than 85 on the Wechsler Intelligence Scale for Children, and demonstrate at least one year's retardation in reading when achievement and expectancy are compared.

Two groups of 40 boys each are identified (arbitrarily labeled E_1 and E_2), with boys paired on the basis of age, IQ, and neurological and psychiatric diagnosis. Assignment to the groups is random.

Each child receives a clinical examination, including psychiatric,

TABLE 1

Perceptual Stimulation Techniques Accuracy Level

I. VISUAL MODALITY
  A. Forms
    1. Simple
    2. Asymmetric
    3. Matrix-like
    4. Complex
    5. Letters
    6. Review Games:
        Form Dominoes
        Concentration
  B. Spatial Orientation
    1. Orientation Lockplate
    2. Square Puzzles
    3. Pythagoras Puzzle
  C. Visual Figure-Background
    1. Patterns
    2. Single Letters
    3. Letter Sequences

II. AUDITORY MODALITY
  A. Code Patterns
  B. Sequencing
    1. Alphabet
    2. Telephone Game
    3. Xylophone Game
    4. Pictures
    5. Song Chains
  C. Sound Discrimination
    1. Initial Sounds

    2. Final Sounds
  D. Word Discrimination
  E. Rhyming
    1. Discriminating Rhymes
    2. Picture Strips
    3. Supplying Rhymes
    4. Review Game:
        Rhyming Dominoes

III. TACTILE MODALITY
  A. Discrimination of Textures
  B. Discrimination of Sizes
  C. Discrimination of Forms
    1. Tactile Templates
    2. Sandpaper and Smooth Forms
    3. Sandpaper Letters
  D. Tactile Dot Forms

IV. KINESTHETIC MODALITY
  A. Directionality Board
  B. Tracing Movements
  C. Tracing Forms
  D. Rhythmic Writing

V. BODY IMAGE
  A. Finger Number Game
  B. Hand Puzzle
  C. Rope Trick
  D. States
  E. Mirror Portraits

neurological, psychological, and educational functioning, to provide data for a profile of perceptual assets and deficits. The tests used in this assessment are those we have previously described.[25-28] This perceptual profile becomes the heart of the teaching program, with teaching focused on the deficit areas revealed by it. The teacher selects, from a pool of accuracy-level techniques (Table 1), those techniques appropriate to each child's perceptual deficits.

The experiment is designed so that each child has two teaching sessions a week for a period of one year, a total of approximately 100 sessions. These sessions are individual ones with the same teacher throughout the year, each lasting for 45 minutes. For the remainder of the school day the child continues his schooling in regular classes of public or parochial schools.

For the first six months of their part of the experiment, the children designated as E_1 receive perceptual stimulation; for the second six months they receive "contact appointments." The contact appointments are individual sessions held twice weekly between the same teacher and child who worked together on perceptual stimulation activities. During these "contact" sessions, the teacher tutors the child in the appropriate level of a basal reader using conventional teaching procedures. These procedures follow the teachers' guidebook of a reading series through developmental lessons which include: building experiential background, guided reading, phonetic analysis, comprehension, and word recognition practice in a drill pad. The purpose of the contact appointments is to minimize the effect of individual attention on reading achievement.

The children designated as E_2 receive contact appointments for the first six months of the experiment, perceptual stimulation during the second six months. E_1 and E_2 differ then only in the order of presentation of the treatments. The purposes of this crossover design are (1) to minimize the effect of spontaneous maturation independent of treatment, (2) to determine the extent to which gains achieved during stimulation are maintained after the termination of training, and (3) to determine whether there is a practical advantage, in terms of reading achievement, to offering perceptual training *before* verbal material is introduced.

All children are given the test battery, cited above, again at the end of 50 sessions and at the end of 100 sessions. In this manner, each child serves as his own control and, in addition, group contrasts are made possible.

TRAINING TECHNIQUES

The training techniques used in this experiment are directed only toward improvement of the accuracy of perception of visual, auditory, tactile, and kinesthetic stimuli and the awareness of body orientation in space through single channel input. Since this experiment merely attempts to determine whether perception is modifiable and whether such modification contributes to improved reading achievement, the training techniques do not offer the practice at the intermodal level or the provision for relating perception to written and oral language that we feel is essential to any well rounded remedial program. These techniques, numbering 41 at the accuracy level, have been defined in terms of purpose, materials, content, procedure, and mastery criteria and are collated in an instruction manual. Techniques within each modality are listed in order of increasing complexity and clinical difficulty.

In the visual modality, for example, our first task was to teach the perception of form. These forms start with the relatively simple circle, square, rectangle, triangle, and diamond, then proceed to asymmetric forms, to matrix-like forms, and, finally, to complex forms adjacent and overlapping. Accuracy is taught through the process of visual recognition, copying, and, finally, recall. Each step in the sequence must be mastered at three correct performances during three consecutive weeks before the next step is taken. If there is difficulty at any stage, cues are used, still within the same modality. For example, the child begins by visually matching simple cut-out forms. If this is failed, then color cues are used. At the copying stage, point-to-point cues on incomplete forms are given with gradual reduction of cues to the point of mastery. This process also provides immediate feedback. Just how difficult this sequence can be for these children is seen from our records which show that one child required 36 sessions, another 21, one 16, and four 13 to master the recognition, copying, and recall of complex overlapping forms. One child required 11 sessions to master the perception of simple forms.

In the visual modality, spatial orientation and visual figure-background perception is stressed through the use of Pythagoras puzzles. The materials for this technique are plastic or wooden pieces distributed commercially, consisting of seven geometric forms that include four triangles of various sizes, a parallelogram, and a square. These are to be put together to make various geometric forms which have been prepared. Two drawings are made for each form, one showing the elements of the design, the other showing the figure in outline only. Here again the sequence of recognition, copying, and recall is repeated.

In the auditory modality, the recognition and recall of patterns is taught through the use of a Morse Code signal set. The teacher begins by demonstrating the long and short tones until the child is able to differentiate them accurately.

It is important that she screen her hand from view so that the response is to auditory cues only and not to the visual perception of her hand movements. The sequences consist of various combinations of long and short tones. For the recognition stage, the teacher taps out the sequences in pairs so that the child can learn to discriminate between similar and different patterns. For the recall stage, the teacher taps out the pattern and the child reproduces it on the signal set.

These particular descriptions of techniques are examples drawn from Table 1. The perceptual stimulation approach uses a variety of techniques chosen on the basis of the child's profile of deficits.

RESULTS

The effect of the training on a matched pair of cases, one from Group E_1 and one from Group E_2, is presented here. Quantitative analysis will be available at the completion of this study in 1968.

J. (Group E_1)

J. is a 7½-year-old second-grader who was referred by his mother. She wrote: "He has a tendency to reverse letters, words, and often starts reading at the right-hand side of the page. He simply cannot learn how to do manuscript. He has difficulty expressing his ideas, sometimes blocking on words he knows well. He cannot tie a shoestring or button his shirt."

On initial testing he earned an oral reading score of 1.5, a reading comprehension score of 2.7, and a spelling score (if one could decipher his handwriting) of 2.0. His functioning on the Wechsler Intelligence Scale for Children was at the high end of the average range, with a full scale IQ of 110. There was a significant differential between performance and verbal IQs (VIQ—116: PIQ—101) and a high degree of variability among subtests, with scaled scores ranging from 18 on Comprehension and 14 on Similarities and Picture Arrangement to 4 on Coding.

Initial physical examination revealed a disheveled child with shoelaces untied, shirttail out, and fingers of his left hand in his mouth. He was in constant restless motion, with showers of jerky muscle movements easily seen in shoulders and trunk. His extended arms showed marked choreoform movements and tended to converge, with the left hand held distinctly higher than the right. His muscle tone was increased. Synkinetic activity was apparent on both sides, but especially marked on the left side. Finger-to-finger and finger-to-nose tests were poorly performed. Marked praxic difficulties were apparent. His deep reflexes were brisk but equal. No pathological reflexes were found. His speech was mildly dysarthric. There was a mild perioral pallor. These findings are greater than those described for children with developmental language defects and suggest superimposed, mild, structural central nervous system defect.

Perceptual study showed defects in every modality. His productions of the Bender Gestalt Test were disorganized. He could not draw straight horizontal or vertical lines, much less diagonals; his reproduction of the sinusoidal curves were scallops. Visual figure-background problems were seen on the Marbleboard Test in his difficulty with diagonals and his inability to build interlocking figures. Even the use of brightly colored marbles did not enable him to detach figure and background. J's drawings also illustrated this problem. For example, in his figure drawings he was impelled to draw not only the figure but the furnishing of the room—desk, chairs, even the objects on the desk. Figure-background interference was seen in the tactile modality also. In the auditory area, he had difficulty in discriminating differences and similarities of words presented orally, making 11 errors in 40 presentations. His trouble in auditory sequencing was illustrated by his pronunciation of his cat's name as "Amonymous." He managed to identify right and left on himself by using a ring as a cue. Handwriting, in which he used his right hand in the "crooked arm" fashion of some left-handers, was illegible. He sometimes "forgot" the directions for forming letters. It was noted that he used both right and left hands for a number of the tasks.

J. became a member of the E_1 group, which received perceptual stimulation for the first six months of the experiment. In the visual modality, emphasis was placed upon accurate perception of form and orientation of figures in space. In the auditory modality, activities dealt with the problem of sequencing and the discrimination and matching of initial and final sounds in words. Tactile activities included discrimination of textures, sizes, and forms. Kinesthetic activities, most important to J. because of his severe praxic deficits, included the use of the directionality board, the tracing of movements in media such as clay, and rhythmic writing on the chalkboard.

At the end of six months his oral reading score was found to have accelerated 2.5 grade points, to a score of 4.0; his spelling score increased .9, to 2.9; his reading comprehension increased 1.2 grade points, to 3.9. Perceptual re-examination at that time showed improvement in organization of visual stimuli, maturation of visual motor control and directionality, reduction in auditory discrimination errors, and improvement in body image as seen in the figure drawing and in the awareness of the finger schema. Although there was some improvement in tactile figure-background perception, visual figure-background problems persisted.

During the control phase of the experiment, J. worked in the third-grade-level basal reader. At the end of this period, approximately one year after the start of the experiment, his educational test scores were as follows: oral reading, grade 5.2; spelling, grade 2.6; reading comprehension, grade 4.4. Perceptual-motor gains were maintained. Further improvement was seen in the perception of visual stimuli and in body image. On extension of his arms, the right hand tended to be elevated. Auditory discrimination showed a slight improvement.

The above findings suggest that perceptual maturation can be effected by specific stimulation and that it is accompanied by improved educational achievement. One could wonder whether these changes might have occurred as a result of maturation alone, without training directed to perceptual defects, and whether a careful reteaching with conventional materials might have resulted in the same kind of educational gains. These questions may be answered by examining the other member of the experimental pair, C.

C. (Group E₂)

C. was 7 years 4 months of age when we first saw him. Except for a bilateral ptosis, he resembled J. in his disheveled appearance, his hyperkinetic, impulsive, and aggressive behavior, his excellent verbal abilities, his warm affective relationship, and his level of intellectual functioning on the WISC. His initial comprehension level was lower than J.'s, at grade 1.7.

Physical examination revealed, in addition to bilateral congenital ptosis, a diffuse hyperkinesis, an increase in muscle tone particularly on the left side, and fine showers of myoclonic activity bilaterally. Synkinetic activity was particularly marked, fine motor tasks poorly performed, and the ability to imitate fine movements impaired. Pupils were eccentric, and there was sustained nystagmus on lateral gaze. There was autonomic lability with perioral pallor and cyanotic nailbeds. Deep reflexes were brisk but equal bilaterally.

Perceptual defects were marked in all modalities. Severe body image confusion was found, not only in errors in right-left orientation but also in finger gnosis. On the extension test the left hand was elevated although C. preferred his right hand.

Retesting, after six months of contact appointments showed an increase in oral reading score to grade 2.3, an improvement of .8 of a grade. Spelling, however, improved only .3 of a grade, while reading comprehension score fell .2 of a grade. Perceptual testing showed no significant improvement. The Bender Gestalt figures, Marbleboard Test, auditory discrimination and sequencing, finger gnosis, Goodenough drawing, and the extension test showed no change. There was a decrease in the number of errors on tactile figure-background tests.

When the perceptual stimulation phase of the experiment was started, activities were directed toward C.'s problems in perception of form, difficulties in left-to-right sequencing, and errors in orientation of asymmetric stimuli. Auditory techniques included sound discrimination, matching initial sounds, and recognizing and supplying rhymes. Tactile activities directed toward the orientation of figures in space were used. When C. first began to work at the chalkboard, he was highly distractible, with scribbling and rapid, jerky movements seen. He commented himself, "My arm wants to go fast." A decrease in this hyperactivity as well as an improvement in his ability to deal with sequences was noted and he continued to work.

At the end of the six-month perceptual stimulation phase of the experiment, C. earned an oral reading score of 3.0. His spelling score had shown a very slight gain from 1.8 to 2.1, and his reading comprehension score rose from 1.5 to 2.5. There were perceptual changes as well. Growth in the visual modality was seen in the more accurate production of the figures of the Bender Gestalt Test, in a rise in score on the Marble-board Test. Some decrease in auditory discrimination errors was seen. Evidence of improvement in body image concepts was seen in improved right-left discrimination, in the correct orientation of the figure drawing, in the rise in score on the Finger Schema Test. The tendency for the right hand to elevate on the extension test (when before training, the left had done so) suggested that C. had established more clear-cut laterality for language. None of these perceptual changes had been seen during the control phase of the experiment.

In short, in both J. and C. the stimulation of the deficit perceptual areas in the manner described resulted in generally improved perception in those areas. It is as though a function left behind in successive waves of maturation may be stimulated to a level more appropriate to the child's total development.

The results so far suggest that where perceptual defects are first trained out, reading instruction at intermodal and verbal levels will have a better chance of success. This is particularly true of the more severe language disabilities, those with defects in multiple modalities and those in whom "soft" neurological signs may be found.

This principle of enhancing neurophysiological maturation before intermodal and verbal methods are introduced has direct implication in the prevention of reading and language disability. Perceptual training at that critical age when the function normally develops may indeed enable the child to grasp language material which would otherwise escape him. The variety of perceptual and neurological defects which we have found in the course of this study suggests the need for careful individual diagnosis and treatment appropriate to the pattern of defects thus revealed.

REFERENCES

1. ALLEN, R. M., and I. DICKMAN. *1966.* A pilot study of the immediate effectiveness of the Frostig-Horne training program with educable retardates. Exceptional Children. *33:* 41-42.
2. BARRETT, T. C. *1965.* Visual discrimination tasks as predictors of first grade reading achievement. Reading Teacher. *18:* 276-282.
3. BENTON, A. L. *1958.* Significance of systematic reversal in right-left discrimination. Acta Psychiatrica et Neurologica. *33:* 129-137.
4. BIRCH, H., and L. BELMONT. *1964.* Auditory-visual integration in normal and retarded readers. Amer. J. Orthopsychiat. *34:* 852-862.
5. BUDOFF, M., and D. QUINLAN. *1964.* Reading progress as related to efficiency of visual and aural learning in the primary grades. J. Educ. Psychol. *55:* 247-252.
6. CHANSKY, N., and M. TAYLOR. *1964.* Perceptual training with young retardates. Amer. J. Mental Deficiency. *68:* 460-468.
7. CHANSKY, N. *1965.* Effect of perceptual training on intelligence and achievement Coop. Res. Proj. #5-060. Mimeo.
8. DE HIRSCH, K., J. JANSKY, and W. S. LANGFORD. *1966.* Early prediction of reading failure. Bulletin of Orton Soc. *16:* 1-13.
9. GIBSON, E. J. *1965.* Learning to read. Science. *148:* 3673-3679.
10. HAGIN, R. A. *1961.* Some practical applications of diagnostic studies of children with specific reading disability. Bulletin of Orton Soc. *11:* 13-18.
11. HELD, R. *1965.* Plasticity in sensory motor systems. Scient. Amer. *213:* 84-94.
12. ITARD, J. The Wild Boy of Aveyron. Appleton, Century, Crofts, New York. 1962 reprint.
13. KEPHART, N. C. *1960.* The Slow Learner in the Classroom. C. E. Merrill, Columbus, Ohio.
14. KEPHART, N. C. *1965.* Perceptual-motor aspects of learning disabilities. Excep. Chil. *31:* 201-206.
15. LEVIN, H., and J. S. WATSON. *1964.* Writing as pretraining for association learning. J. Educ. Psychol. *55:* 181-184.
16. LEVINA, R. E. *1966.* Peculiarities of acoustic perception in children with speech defects. *In* Symposium 33, Mental Development and Sensory Defects, Internat. Cong. of Psychol., Moscow, USSR: 309-321.
17. MONTESSORI, M. The Montessori Method. Schocken, New York. 1964 reprint.
18. MOWBRAY, G. H. *1964.* Perception and retention of verbal information presented during auditory shadowing. J. Acoust. Soc. of Amer. *36* (8): 1459-1464.
19. PAINTER, A. *1966.* The effect of rhythmic and sensory motor activity progress on perceptual motor spatial abilities of kindergarten children. Excep. Chil. *33:* 113-116.
20. ROACH, E. G. *1966.* Evaluation of an experimental program of perceptual motor training with slow readers. Paper presented at the annual convention of the Internat. Reading Assn. Mimeo.
21. ROACH, E. G., and N. C. KEPHART. *1966.* The Purdue Perceptual-Motor Survey. C. E. Merrill, Columbus, Ohio.
22. ROBBINS, M. P. *1966.* The Delcato interpretation of neurological organization. Reading Res. Quart. *1:* 57-78.
23. RUTHERFORD, W. L. *1965.* Perceptual-motor training and readiness. *In* Reading and Inquiry, proceedings of the annual convention of the Internat. Reading Assn: 294-296.
24. SEGUIN, E. *1866.* Idiocy and Its Treatment by the Physiological Method. William Wood and Co., New York.
25. SILVER, A. A. *1950.* Neurological and perceptual survey of children with reading disability. Presented at Section of Neurology Psychiatry, N. Y. Acad. of Med.

26. SILVER, A. A., and R. A. HAGIN. *1960*. Specific reading disability: Delineation of the syndrome and relationship to cerebral dominance. Comprehen. Psychiat. *1* (2): 126-134.

27. SILVER, A. A. *1961*. Diagnostic considerations on children with reading disability. Bulletin of Orton Soc. *11:* 5-12.

28. SILVER, A. A., and R. A. HAGIN. *1964*. Specific reading disability: follow-up studies. Amer. J. Orthopsychiat. *34* (1): 95-102.

29. STAATS, C. K., A. W. STAATS, and R. E. SCHULTZ. *1962*. The effects of discrimination pretraining on textual behavior. J. Educ. Psychol. *53:* 32-37.

14

STIMULUS COMPETITION AND CONCEPT UTILIZATION IN BRAIN DAMAGED CHILDREN

Herbert Birch, M.D.

Research Professor, Dept. of Pediatrics
Albert Einstein College of Medicine

and

Morton Bortner, Ph.D.

Kennedy Foundation Scholar, Dept. of Special Education
Ferkauf Graduate School of Humanities and Social Sciences
Yeshiva University

INTRODUCTION

Brain injured children perform particularly poorly on a variety of tasks designed to test conceptual abiilty (Cotton 1941, Dolphin and Cruickshank 1951, Birch 1964, Jordan 1956, Strauss and Werner 1942, 1943, Werner and Strauss, 1941). The deficiencies observed include a tendency to be attracted by details or an excessive fluidity of association (Werner and Strauss 1943), difficulty in changing set (McMurray 1954), and in making insufficient use of function in definitions (Bijou and Werner 1945). A few reports have appeared (Stephenson 1956, Osborn 1960, Halpin and Patterson 1954) in which no consistent pattern of difficulty in conceptual behaviour was found in brain-damaged children. These failures to find difficulty seem to derive from the examination methods used. Deficits are most marked when the task situation is free

---

Reprinted from DEVELOPMENTAL MEDICINE AND CHILD NEUROLOGY, Vol. 9. No. 4. August, 1967. pp. 402-410.

and relatively undefined, and least noticeable when it is highly structured (Gallagher 1956).

Little is yet known about specific causes for such difficulties in brain injured children. An analysis of the demands made by tests of conceptual functioning may clarify the problem. In many tests the subject matches or groups objects or other stimuli with one another. In terms of Pavlov's hypothesis of two signal systems (Pavlov 1928) the responses are capable of being based on at least two levels of organization of afferent input. In the first, integration of the properties takes place, and in the second, a level of generalization and abstraction which goes beyond the immediately perceived properties of the stimuli and relates the objects to one another in terms of functional attributes or class membership takes place. Thus, in some of the more frequently used object matching tasks (e.g. Klapper and Werner 1950, Vigotsky 1934, Goldstein and Scheerer 1941), responses can be made by reacting to (a) common stimulus properties in the objects to be matched, (b) common functions which the objects might be used to perform, or (c) to features of common class membership. Such tasks therefore need not necessarily test the possession of, or the ability to have performed concepts.

They may be viewed as tests of the tendency to use functional or class attributes in preference over immediately given stimulus properties as the basis for responding. Failure to respond 'conceptually' and the tendency to be 'stimulus bound' on such tests need not reflect the absence of or the inability to use concepts of class and function but rather their hierarchical subordination under conditions in which they compete with immediately present stimuli as bases for the organization of a response.

The value of such a competition hypothesis has been illustrated in a recent study on object matching behavior in young normal children (Birch and Bortner 1965). In that study the hypothesis tested was that preferential responsiveness to stimulus factors and not the lack of possession of concepts of class and function underlies the failure of young children to use class and function in making categorical choices. In order to test this hypothesis the object matching behavior of normal children was studied under two conditions. In both conditions the identical index object was presented together with 3 objects from among which a matching choice had to be made. In one situation the objects from which matches with the index object were to be made had properties which could be related to it through stimulus similarity, function, or class membership. In the second task situation the set of three objects from which a matching choice to an index object had to be made included one with common functional or class attributes, and two other objects which were 'neutral' with respect to such attributes as common stimulus properties, class membership, and function. When object choices permitted the child to use stimulus similarity as well as class membership and function, younger children preferentially matched for stimulus properties rather than for functional relations or common class membership. When, in the second task, stimulus competition was eliminated, many of these younger children exhibited the capacity to use previously unexpressed concepts of class and functional relatedness in matching. It appeared, therefore, that one characteristic of early development was the domination of response by the first signal system with a consequent inhibition of the later developed second signal system. The elimination of first signal system competition then permitted the response within the second signal system.

The repeated finding of stimulus domination in brain damaged children could be the result of continued first signal system domination and not due to the lack of higher order concepts of function or class membership. The brain damaged children might, therefore, use concepts of function and class with increased frequency under circumstances in which stimulus competition was reduced. In the present study, this hypothesis is tested by analyzing the effects of stimulus competition and its systematic elimination on the object matching behavior of cerebral palsied children.

SUBJECTS AND PROCEDURES

The age and intellectual status of the cerebral palsied children and the normal children studied are given in Table 1. The cerebral palsied children ranged in age from 5 to 21 years and were all pupils in a special school. As there are no known differences between the different clinical categories of cerebral palsy with respect to the functions studied all clinical classes were grouped together. Estimates of intellect were obtained from the school records, and were based on the Stanford-Binet, Form L and the Wechsler Intelligence Scale for Children. They ranged from 30 to 118 and clustered in the mild to moderate subnormal range. There were significant differences in mean IQ between the ataxic and athetoid children at the .01 level of confidence; and between the ataxic and spastic children at the .05 level of confidence.

The normal children ranged in age from 3 to 10 years and were all pupils in nursery or elementary school. No mentally subnormal children were present in the group, and IQ's clustered in the bright normal

TABLE 1

AGE AND INTELLECTUAL STATUS OF THE CHILDREN STUDIED
Cerebral Palsied Children

Type	N	C.A.		M.A.		I.Q.	
		Mean	S.D.	Mean	S.D.	Mean	S.D.
Spastic	46	13.62	4.30	9.64	3.21	77.15	20.09
Athetoid	34	13.63	4.40	10.87	3.66	81.35	18.31
Ataxic	20	12.40	3.69	8.11	2.08	68.40	12.60
Mixed	4	13.27	3.87	8.41	2.21	67.25	5.97
TOTAL	104						

Normal Children

Grade	N	C.A.		M.A.		I.Q.	
		Mean	S.D.	Mean	S.D.	Mean	S.D.
Nursery 1	18	3.63	0.17	4.28	0.65	108.61	9.78
Nursery II	30	4.50	0.26	5.63	1.01	109.83	10.77
Kindergarten	24	5.42	0.26	6.25	0.64	115.67	12.58
First	28	6.20	0.31	7.66	0.87	123.75	13.51
Second	35	7.32	0.29	9.16	0.88	125.17	12.34
Third	32	8.28	0.32	9.93	0.90	120.25	12.29
Fourth	21	9.39	0.30	10.56	0.95	112.48	9.83
TOTAL	188						

category. They were obtained by means of the Peabody Picture Vocabulary Test in the nursery school and kindergarten children and with the Otis Quick-Scoring Mental Abilities Test in the remaining children. We did not attempt to use controls with similar IQ's to the cerebral palsied group as this would have meant using mentally subnormal children who are themselves suspect of having brain damage.

Each child was tested individually and given two sets of tasks—Tests A and B (Table 2). On every Task in both tests the child was required to match an index object with one of a group of three choice objects. As may be seen in the table, each pair of tasks used an identical index object as well as an identical choice object related to it by class or function. In test A the remaining two choice objects resembled the index object in either color or form whereas in Test B the remaining choice objects did not share any obvious stimulus property with the index object. Thus, in Test A, the child when he made a functional or class categorical choice, did so in the presence of stimulus competition, whereas in Test B such competition had been systematically eliminated. Each test contained ten items and the positions of the categorical choice

TABLE 2

MATCHING TESTS A AND B

Test A and B Index Objects	Test A Stimulus Competition Choices	Test B Stimulus Non-Competition Choices
1. Metal bottle top	a. metal spring b. *cork** c. red disc	a. clothespin b. *cork* c. card
2. Ink bottle with red and white label	a. *white bottle* b. sunglass lens c. red and white matchbox cover	a. *white bottle* b. candle c. brush
3. Metal bell	a. thimble b. *toy church* c. silver button	a. cigar b. *toy church* c. pliers
4. Red tea pot	a. pipe bowl with half stem b. red pill c. *saucer*	a. bow tie b. key c. *saucer*
5. Black rubber wheel	a. stick b. *wagon wheel* c. black round box top	a. fish b. *wagon wheel* c. small box
6. Red button	a. blue poker chip b. *thread* c. red lipstick case	a. blue nut b. *thread* c. cup
7. White plastic hat	a. *red glove* b. white box c. red dome	a. *red glove* b. ABC block c. eraser
8. Hour glass	a. *wrist watch* b. whiskey glass c. diaper pin	a. *wrist watch* b. pipe c. lock
9. Yellow lady	a. *white man* b. yellow ape c. blue clothespin	a. *white man* b. car c. bulb
10. Cow	a. lion b. tiger c. *hen*	a. scissor b. checker c. *hen*

* Italicized objects were scored as categorical choices.

objects were varied systematically. Positional placements are indicated in Table 2 where *a, b,* and *c* refer respectively to positions from left to right.

The index object and the choice objects were placed before the child with the index object nearest to him. The child was permitted to inspect the objects and their names were given him by the examiner. The child was then asked to choose the object that 'goes best' with the index object.

After he made a choice he was asked, 'Why do these go together?' Both the choice and the verbal responses were recorded.

All subjects were given Test A first and then Test B. This was necessary since Test A contained all competitive distractor items. Thus, if test A were given second, the 'pull' of the competitive stimulus properties might have been vitiated by the prior experience with Test B. Since it was possible that better performance on Test B could derive from prior experience with Test A, two additional groups not in the study population, each containing 15 normal children, were studied. These children were in the 5-6 years of age range and were matched for age and IQ. One of the groups received Test A only and the other Test B only. The superiority of the group taking Test B only was of the same magnitude as that found when comparable children in the study population had taken both tests. Therefore, the improvement found on Test B in the main study did not reflect an experience effect due to having Test A.

The reliability of the tests was established on the entire sample of 188 normal children. Using the Kuder-Richardson formula, the reliabilities of both Test A and Test B were 0.86.

RESULTS

Since the capacity (Birch and Bortner 1965) to match according to class and function in a context containing stimulus competition is an age related phenomenon, it was necessary to compare the category usage of cerebral palsied children with that of normal children comparable in chronological and mental age. Tables 3 and 4 show that when the factors of chronological and mental age respectively are held constant, normal children tend to match on the basis of class and function more frequently than do the cerebral palsied children. This difference is shown at all chronological age ranges studied and in the mental age range of 6 to 11.9 years. In the mental age range below six years no differences are found, since both the normal and cerebral palsied children of this age were matching on a chance basis.

As may be seen from Table 5 all the cerebral palsied children, regardless of category of disability, performed significantly better on Test B than on Test A. That is, with the elimination of the stimulus competition of form and color (present only in Test A), these children showed an increased tendency to make matching choices according to class and functional characteristics rather than on the basis of stimulus similarities.

TABLE 3

COMPARISON OF NORMAL AND CEREBRAL PALSIED CHILDREN ON TEST A ACCORDING TO CHRONOLOGICAL AGE

C.A.	N	Normal Mean	S.D.	N	Cerebral Palsied Mean	S.D.	p value*
6.0–6.9	23	8.43	1.93	5	5.00	1.90	$< .003$
7.0–7.9	40	9.18	1.02	8	5.00	2.83	$< .001$
8.0-8.9	29	9.28	1.36	8	6.00	2.18	$< .001$
9.0–9.9	17	9.41	0.69	8	4.50	2.18	$< .001$

* Level of confidence according to Mann-Whitney U Test.

TABLE 4

COMPARISON OF NORMAL AND CEREBRAL PALSIED CHILDREN ON TEST A ACCORDING TO MENTAL AGE

Mental Age	N*	Normal Mean	S.D.	N	Cerebral Palsied Mean	S.D.	p value
3.0– 5.9	49	3.6	1.87	11	3.6	1.65	N.S.
6.0– 8.9	70	7.2	2.71	39	5.7	2.48	.01
9.0–11.9	66	9.3	1.28	26	8.8	1.34	.05

* Total N does not equal 188 because one child was slightly below M.A. of 3, and two children obtained M.A. scores slightly higher than 11.9.

TABLE 5

CONCEPT SCORES OF CEREBRAL PALSIED CHILDREN

Type	Test A Mean	S.D.	Test B* Mean	S.D.
Spastic	7.22	2.74	8.26	2.18
Athetoid	7.62	2.84	8.71	2.32
Ataxic	6.65	2.50	8.15	1.93
Mixed	7.25	1.92	8.00	1.87

* For all groups Test B scores are significantly higher than Test A scores at $p < .005$ level of confidence according to Wilcoxon matched pairs signed ranks test.

If stimulus competition did interfere with the use of function and class as bases for matching in brain damaged children to a greater extent than in normal children, then brain damaged children, when such competition is eliminated, should perform like normal children of comparable mental age who are tested under conditions of stimulus competition. Such a comparison was carried out by contrasting scores of normal children on Test A with scores of cerebral palsied children on Test B. Table 6 shows that under the conditions of Test B where stimulus competition was reduced, the cerebral palsied children matched objects according to class and functional categories equally as frequently as did normal children on Test A. Thus, it can be concluded that the *ability* to match for class and functional characteristics is present in brain damaged children. However, its expression is facilitated by the systematic elimination of stimulus competition.

Since both chronological and mental ages varied widely, it was essential to note the influence of chronological and mental age on the degree of benefit deriving from the altered conditions of Test B as contrasted with Test A. It will be noted in Table 7 where cerebral palsied children are classified according to chronological age that performance on Test B is consistently different from that on Test A at all age ranges considered except in children aged between 14.0 and 16.9 years. That is, regardless of age (with the exception noted) the children showed an increased capacity to match by class category and function in the absence of stimulus competition.

In Table 8 the cerebral palsied children are classified according to mental age. The children continued to perform significantly differently on Test B at all except the highest levels of mental age.

When mental age is controlled there is, of course, a wide chronological age dispersion. Some children within a given mental age category are therefore 'brighter' than others in the sense that their IQ's are higher. It was, therefore, necessary to inquire whether IQ as such directly influenced the concept scores of either Test A or Test B when mental age was held constant. This question was dealt with by calculating the median IQ's of cerebral palsied children within successive mental age ranges of three years, *i.e.* 3.0 to 5.9, 6.0 to 8.9, etc. Within a given mental age range the concept scores of children above and below the median IQ were compared. This was done for Test A and Test B separately. There were no significant differences in performance on either test within any three year mental age range between groups of children dichotomized in this way.

TABLE 6

COMPARISONS OF NORMALS ON TEST A AND CEREBRAL PALSIED ON TEST B WITH MENTAL AGE CONTROLLED

Mental Age	Normals Test A			Cerebral Palsied Test B			p value
	N*	Mean	S.D.	N	Mean	S.D.	
3.0– 5.9	49	3.6	1.87	11	5.0	2.00	.05
6.0– 8.9	70	7.2	2.71	39	7.6	2.12	N.S.
9.0–11.9	66	9.3	1.28	26	9.4	1.22	N.S.

* Total N. does not equal 188 because one child was slightly below M.A. of 3, and two children got M.A. scores of slightly higher than 11.9.

TABLE 7

CONCEPT SCORES OF CEREBRAL PALSIED CHILDREN ACCORDING TO CHRONOLOGICAL AGE ON TESTS A AND B

N	C.A.	Test A		Test B		p value
		Mean	S.D.	Mean	S.D.	
14	5.0– 7.9	4.86	2.47	6.93	2.55	.01
18	8.0–10.9	5.55	2.36	7.39	2.52	.01
25	11.0–13.9	6.68	2.72	7.64	2.28	.01
20	14.0–16.9	9.65	0.57	9.80	0.51	N.S.
27	17.0–20.9	8.33	2.03	9.41	0.99	.01
104						

TABLE 8

CONCEPT SCORES OF CEREBRAL PALSIED CHILDREN ACCORDING TO MENTAL AGE ON TESTS A AND B

N	M.A.	Test A		Test B		p value
		Mean	S.D.	Mean	S.D.	
11	3.0– 5.9	3.63	1.66	5.00	2.0	.01
39	6.0– 8.9	5.71	2.47	7.58	2.11	.01
26	9.0–11.9	8.84	1.34	9.38	1.17	.01
21	12.0–14.9	9.23	1.14	9.85	0.34	.025
7	15.0–17.9	9.42	1.04	9.85	0.34	N.S.
104						

DISCUSSION

The findings of this study accord with the hypothesis that brain damaged children possess higher order concepts of functional relations and class membership, but that their expression in behavior is inhibited by the activation of the dominant first signal system. The presence of an objective basis for matching to immediately present stimulus properties results in the child using these rather than concepts of function and class as a basis for matching. In the usual test of category usage where the stimulus properties—form and color—compete with more abstract attributes, the cerebral palsied children were dominated in their matching choices by the prepotency of the immediately present stimulus features. This was true when either the factors of chronological or mental age were held constant.

A clue as to the mechanism underlying this type of matching behavior is found in the observation that the tendency to use class membership and functional characteristics as bases for matching was facilitated in brain damaged children when the competition of immediately present stimulus properties was systematically reduced. Moreover, the brain damaged subjects matched in terms of function and class as frequently and correctly in the context of Test B as did normals in Test A. This result demonstrates that these children possessed and were able in the context of Test B to use higher order abstractions less readily expressed in the context of stimulus competition.

In normal children increases in age are accompanied by hierarchical changes in the organization of responsiveness in matching tasks. In the main the shift involves an increased inhibition of response to stimulus attributes and an increased domination of behavior by concepts of function and class. In brain damaged children a significant lag in this progression was noted. Despite their possession of class and functional concepts they continued in their matching behavior to be dominated by stimulus features. The possession of concepts was ineffectual in directing behavior. Thus despite second signal system organization, hierarchical domination by the first signal system resulted in lower level response on the matching tasks. Only when the task had been so structured as to reduce stimulus competition did the brain damaged children function at a more advanced level.

A major educational implication of this finding may be that the systematic elimination of competing, immediately present stimuli can facilitate the utilization of higher order concepts of class membership and function. Educators who are concerned with the development of special procedures for brain damaged children may, therefore, find the competition hypothesis relevant to the problem of structuring more optimal learning situations.

Acknowledgements—The research reported stems from the work of a Program on Normal and Aberrant Behavioral Development in Children, supported in part by the National Institutes of Health, National Institute of Child Health and Human Development (HD 00719); by the Association for the Aid of Crippled Children; and by the National Association for Retarded Children. We would like to thank Mrs. Juliet Bortner and Mrs. Linda Levy for their help in the conduct of the study; the educational authorities of the West Hempstead School District, Nassau County, New York; and Dr. Leon Charash, Medical Director and Mr. Emil Lombardi, Principal, Roosevelt Center, for their co-operation and helpfulness in making this study possible.

SUMMARY

The hypothesis that defective conceptual functioning in brain damaged children is due to the domination of behavior by immediately present stimulus properties and not by the child's failure to possess concepts of a higher order was tested. Object matching behavior in 104 cerebral palsied (aged 5-21 years) and of 188 normal children (aged 3-10 years) was studied under two conditions. In the first condition the key object could be matched on the basis of stimulus similarity, common function, or common class membership. In the second condition the competitive presence of stimulus similarities was markedly reduced. Cerebral palsied children who could not express concepts of function and class membership under conditions of stimulus competition did so when such competition was systematically eliminated. The findings were discussed in the context of Pavlov's conception of first and second signalling systems.

REFERENCES

BIJOU, S. W., WERNER, H. (1945) 'Language analysis in brain injured and non-brain injured mentally deficient children.' *J. genet. Psychol., 66,* 239.

BIRCH, H. G. (1964) (ed.) Brain Damage in Children: Biological and Social Aspects. Baltimore: Williams and Wilkins.

———— BORTNER, M. (1966) 'Stimulus competition and category usage in normal children.' *J. genet. Psychol., 109,* 195.

COTTON, C. B. (1941) 'A study of the reactions of spastic children to certain test situations.' *J. genet. Psychol., 58,* 27.

DOLPHIN, J., CRUICKSHANK, M. (1951) 'Pathology of concept formation in children with cerebral palsy.' *Amer. J. ment. Def., 56,* 386.

GOLDSTEIN, K., Scheerer, M. (1941) 'Abstract and concrete behavior: An experimental study with special tests.' *Psychol. Monogr., 53;* no. 2, no. 239.

GALLAGHER, J. J. (1956) 'A comparison of brain injured and non-brain injured mentally retarded children on several psychological variables.' *Monogr. Soc. Res. Child Develop., 19,* 101.

HALPIN, V. G., PATTERSON, R. M. (1954) 'The performance of brain injured children on the Goldstein-Scheerer Tests.' *Amer. J. ment. Def., 59,* 91.

JORDAN, J. E. (1956) 'An investigation of the nature of concept formation in cerebral palsied children.' Unpublished doctoral dissertation. New York University.

KLAPPER, Z., WERNER, H. (1950) 'Developmental deviations in brain-injured (c.p.) members of identical twins.' *Quart. J. Child Behav., 2,* 288.

McMURRAY, J. G. (1954) 'Rigidity in conceptual thinking in exogenous and endogenous mentally retarded children.' *J. cons. Psychol., 18,* 366.

OSBORN, W. J. (1960) 'Associative clustering in organic and familial retardates.' *Amer. J. ment. Def., 65,* 351.

PAVLOV, I. P. (1928) Lecture on Conditional Reflexes. Liveright.

STEPHENSON, G. R. (1956) 'Form perception, abstract thinking and intelligence test validity in Cerebral Palsy.' Unpublished doctoral thesis. Columbia University.

STRAUSS, A. A. (1944) 'Ways of thinking in brain-crippled deficient children.' *Amer. J. Psychiat., 100,* 639.

—— WERNER, H. (1942) 'Disorders of conceptual thinking in the brain injured child.' *J. nerv. ment. Dis., 96,* 153.

—— —— (1943) 'Comparative psychopathology of the brain injured and traumatic brain injured adult.' *Amer. J. Psychiat., 99,* 835.

VIGOTSKY, L. S. (1934) 'Thought in schizophrenia.' *Arch. Neurol. Psychiat. (Chic.), 31,* 1063.

WERNER, H., STRAUSS, A. A. (1941) 'Experimental analysis of conceptual thinking in brain injured children. *Psychol. Bull. 38,* 538.

—— —— (1943) 'Impairment in thought processes of brain injured children.' *Amer. J. ment. Def., 47,* 291.

15

LEARNING PATTERNS IN THE DISADVANTAGED

Susan S. Stodolsky, Ph.D.

Department of Education, University of Chicago

and

Gerald Lesser, Ph.D.

Harvard University

GENERAL REVIEW OF RESEARCH

In a review of learning patterns in the disadvantaged, it is necessary to delimit certain key concepts: (1) Which population groups shall be included in the "disadvantaged"? (2) Which constructs or variables shall we consider as relevant indicators of learning?

We shall return at several points in this paper to the problem of definition of the term "disadvantaged." Since each new issue raised forces revision and refinement of this definition, we shall offer successive approximations to a useful definition as we proceed. For the review of research with which we begin this paper, we will follow the usual conventions regarding delimitation of the disadvantaged or deprived popu-

Reprinted from HARVARD EDUCATIONAL REVIEW, 37, Fall, 1967, pp. 546-593. Copyright © 1967 by President and Fellows of Harvard College. The preparation of this paper was supported in part by the Harvard Research and Development Center and the Conference on "Bio-Social Factors in the Development and Learning of Disadvantaged Children." Dr. Stodolsky has primary responsibility for the sections on General Review of Research and New Directions for Research. Dr. Lesser supplied the Specific Case of Research. The sections on Implications for Educational Policy were a joint effort. However, each author will blame the other for errors of fact or interpretation which appear anywhere throughout the paper.

lation. Typically included under this rubric are children who come from families of low socio-economic status (as measured by occupation of the breadwinner, educational attainment of the parents, income, place of residence, etc.) and children from minority groups (as determined by recent immigration of families from countries outside the United States or notable lack of acculturation of groups that may have been residents for generations) and minority racial status (in particular, Negroes and Indians who have been in a caste-like status in this country for generations). Also included in this population are children from rural areas which have been isolated from the mainstream of American culture (see Havighurst, 1964). These definitions usually have in common the element of poverty or low income in relation to the median income of Americans.

We have chosen to examine five classes of learning indicators: general intelligence, specific mental abilities, school achievement, laboratory learning, and expressions of cognitive development deriving from stage theory. Although these constructs vary in their clear-cut relevance to educational procedures and outcomes, we believe they all contribute some important insights in the learning patterns of the disadvantaged. We shall judge the approaches to research using each of these constructs in light of the power of the findings for improvement of the educational experiences of diasdvantaged learners.

General Intelligence

The performance of children from low socio-economic status and minority groups on intelligence tests has been quite well documented. Studies of intelligence test performance and social-class status have provided the broad outlines of a picture which generally fits a *deficit* or less-than model. Mean differences between children of high SES and low SES have been found consistently when measures of intelligence are administered. These differences are unequivocally present at age four and have occasionally been demonstrated at younger ages (Bereiter, 1965; Pasamanick & Knobloch, 1955; Bloom, 1964).

With increases in children's age, such intelligence test differences tend to increase. Thus, there are larger mean differences in intelligence between low and high SES children in adolescence than in the early years of school. This fanning-out effect and the evidence to support it has been carefully reviewed by a number of workers (Bloom, 1964; Hunt, 1961; Silverman, 1965; Gordon, 1965; Davis, 1948; Karp & Sigel, 1965; Coleman et al., 1966).

The nature of the tests and conditions of administration have been an object of considerable study. The hallmark work of Eells and Davis (1951) on cultural biases in intelligence tests spurred a multitude of studies which demonstrated inadequacies in the tests themselves as good samples of general intelligence in diverse populations. Factors which might influence test performance such as rapport, speed, motivation, and reward conditions were also studied (e.g., see Haggard, 1954). It appears clear now that Davis and his colleagues in their attempt to develop a culture-free measure of intelligence were accepting the idea that it was in fact possible to measure innate ability independent of cultural and experiential factors. They were assuming that it would be possible to tap the genotype of intelligence, and that intelligence would in fact be a stable quantity, randomly distributed by social class. (See Charters, 1963.)

Partly through the failure of the *Davis-Eells Games* and through increasing evidence from other quarters, both the belief in fixed intelligence and the notion of ridding intelligence measurement of cultural contamination have been abandoned. Now, rather than rejecting cultural effects as contaminants, researchers study them and take them into account in test construction and prediction. However, the notion of "culture-fair" testing has been widely accepted in the interest of making comparative statements about groups. Thus, as exemplified in one study of mental abilities (Lesser, Fifer, & Clark, 1965), items are based on a pool of experiences common to the subject population to be studied. Conditions of administration are arranged to minimize differences in rapport, motivation, and prior experiences with testing when intergroup comparisons are being made. Further, validity and reliability must be established for the relevant population. An excellent review of factors to be considered in testing minority groups is available (Deutsch et al., 1964).

The most important outgrowth of the work in the 1950's is the changed conception of intelligence. Only a few hardy souls will now maintain that intelligence tests measure something innate, fixed, and pre-determined. (Hunt, 1961, reviews these ideas.) The validity of intelligence tests for predicting school achievement cannot be doubted, but the ability (aptitude) *versus* achievement distinction has been attenuated. Intelligence tests must now be thought of as samples of learning based on general experiences. A child's score may be thought of as an indication of the richness of the milieu in which he functions and the extent to which he has been able to profit from that mileu. In contradistinction, school achievement tests assume deliberate instruction oriented to the outcomes measured in the tests.

We have indicated that consistent differences on general intelligence tests are found when groups of children from varying SES backgrounds are compared. Some of the determinants of such differences have been explored and a new understanding of the construct of intelligence has been presented. Nevertheless, it is important to keep in mind that the procedures for test construction and administration now recognized as essential were not consistently followed in much past research on group comparisons.

Differences in intelligence-test performance have been found when Negroes and whites are compared. In general, Negroes have been found to have lower tested intelligence than whites even when social class is controlled (Dreger & Miller, 1960; Deutsch & Brown, 1964), although the difficulties of measuring social status within the Negro population for comparisons with the white population have not been adequately overcome. Studies of other minority groups, though not nearly as plentiful as Negro-white comparisons, generally indicate similar mean differences. (See Anastasi, 1958, Ch. 15, for a review.)

It should be remembered that the studies we have reviewed deal only with group differences using social class, ethnicity, or both as classificatory variables. Although mean differences favor majority group and high SES children, the overlap in distributions is great. It is by now a truism that *all* disadvantaged children do not fall below their more advantaged peers on tested intelligence and mental abilities. The deficit model applies to groups only. Individual differences within groups must also be examined.

A number of recent studies (e.g., Karnes et al., 1965; Mackler et al., 1966; McCabe, 1964) attempt to locate and study disadvantaged children who in fact are superior to the normative status of the disadvantaged. These researchers are attempting to characterize successful children and to study environmental factors which may account for success in disadvantaged children. The ability of these workers to locate children who test above average on intelligence tests and who perform above grade level on achievement tests is witness to the overlap in populations of advantaged and disadvantaged children. It should be noted, however, that the criteria on intelligence tests for "gifted" are typically lower than those employed with a middle-class population.

Diverse Mental Abilities

Early research in subcultural differences attempted to demonstrate that minority-majority group differences were attributable to the verbal nature of most general intelligence tests. The results of investigations which utilized tests of a less verbal character are equivocal (Higgins & Sivers, 1958; Fowler, 1957; Stablein et al., 1961; MacCarthur & Elley, 1963). The most adequate conclusion for the moment seems to be that although group differences may be reduced somewhat by eliminating verbal components from the tests, other factors (such as experimental differences, attitudes toward test-taking, and speed) still affect test performance. And for certain groups such as Negroes, eliminating verbal items results in lower performance levels.

Coleman et. al. (1966), as a part of a massive survey on equality of educational opportunity in the United States, administered a verbal and nonverbal (reasoning) measure to first graders of various backgrounds at the beginning of the school year. He found that children of low social status and children from minority groups (Negroes, Mexican-Americans, Puerto Ricans, and American Indians) start school at grade one with mean scores on verbal and nonverbal tests of general ability that are below the national white average. The only exception to this general finding is that Oriental children score at the national average on the verbal measure at grade one and above the average on the nonverbal measure. In addition, the American Indian group that was sampled scored at the national average on the nonverbal measure at grade one.

Aside from comparisons of verbal and nonverbal abilities, little in the way of study of other mental abilities has been systematically undertaken. Especially limited is such information with young subject populations. One exception is the work of Lesser, Fifer, and Clark (1965) who have studied four mental abilities (Verbal ability, Reasoning, Number facility, and Space Conceptualization) in first-grade children. They compared performance of four subcultural groups (Chinese, Jews, Negroes, and Puerto Ricans) of high and low social status, studying the organization (patterns) of these abilities as well as level of performance. The study will be described in greater detail later in this paper.

The organization of mental abilities in disadvantaged groups as studied through factor analysis has received relatively little attention. Recent work by Lovinger et al. (1966) with junior-high-school students and Semler and Iscoe (1966) with elementary-school children makes an important contribution. Lovinger found that a factor analysis of the WISC responses of Negro lower-class seventh graders produced a factor structure which was congruent with that found for the normative group (Cohen, 1959), although level of performance on the WISC was considerably lower for his population and subtest scores were also variable. Semler and Iscoe (1966) administered the WISC and Progressive Matrices to white and Negro children who were seven to nine years of age. They found sufficient incongruity in the intercorrelations of the WISC subtests by race to warrant separate factor analyses. Intercorrelations among the Progressive Matrices subtests, however, were highly similar for both groups.

In summary, many data are available for purposes of comparing social-class groups on tests of general intelligence. When one wants to make more detailed analyses, however, either by minority-group membership or on particular mental abilities, the data become sparse. In addition, data on the organization of mental abilities within sub-groups are just becoming available. Testing of the same samples on a number of mental abilities (such as the PMA) has been done only occasionally (Havighurst & Breese, 1947; Havighurst & Janke, 1944; Lesser, Fifer & Clark, 1965).

School Achievement

Massive amounts of data are now available on a national sample of children at grades one, three, six, nine, and twelve in regard to school achievement (Coleman et al., 1966). The Coleman study employed verbal and nonverbal measures and tests of reading and mathematics achievement. As indicated in the previous section, most groups of minority children and those of low SES scored below the national average on verbal and nonverbal tests at the beginning of their school careers. The findings from this study are consistent with earlier ones dealing with the school achievement of disadvantaged children. Indications of social-class and racial differences, in favor of majority and high SES groups, had been found earlier when reading and arithmetic readiness tests[1] were administered to children at the kindergarten level (Brazziel & Terrel, 1962; Montague, 1964).

As minority-group children (with the exception of Orientals at grade three) proceed through school, they continue to perform below the national average at all grade levels on all measures: the relative standing of these groups in relation to the white population remains essentially constant in terms of standard deviations, but the absolute differences in terms of grade-level discrepancies increase (Coleman et al., 1966). This increase in the number of grade levels behind the normative population is what is commonly referred to as the "cumulative deficit" (Deutsch, 1960).

---

[1] The readiness tests, as opposed to the general ability tests, are more specifically oriented to learning necessary for successful achievement of a school subject. In fact predictive validities of the two types of tests do not differ appreciably.

The Coleman survey is cross-sectional. The few longitudinal studies of achievement in the literature reflect essentially the same pattern: as disadvantaged children move through the current school system, their achievement in grade levels as compared to the normative population becomes increasingly discrepant and low (Osborne, 1960).

The picture of educational disadvantage which emerges with examination of achievement data is a clear indication of the failure of the school systems. When intelligence test data and early achievement data are combined, we have a predictor's paradise, but an abysmal prognosis for most children who enter the school system from disadvantaged backgrounds. At the very least, this ability to predict school failure should be better exploited by the schools in an effort to remedy the situation. Payne (1964) has demonstrated that by the end of grade one, over one-half of the children who will be failing in arithmetic in grade six can be identified on the basis of socio-economic data, intelligence test scores, and an arithmetic achievement test. By the end of grade two, two-thirds of the failing children can be identified. This provides the school not with group tendencies but with individual tagging of children for whom the usual curriculum will surely fail. It also provides five years of lead time to remedy the situation.

Taken together, the data on general intelligence, mental abilities, and school achievement all give indications that general learning, first in the home and community and later within the school as well, is clearly associated with socio-economic status: the level of such learning is generally lower for children of most minority groups and children in low socio-economic status. Important variations in patterning of such learnings have yet to be studied systematically, with a few notable exceptions. Even in the school achievement area, data regarding progress in school subjects other than reading and mathematics are not readily available. It can perhaps be safely assumed that achievement in social studies, science, and other academic areas will be highly correlated with achievement in reading and arithmetic. Nevertheless, studies of performance of disadvantaged children in these areas should be carried out.

Laboratory Learning

There are only a few studies which have used laboratory learning paradigms to compare performance of children from different social and cultural backgrounds. As Jensen (1967a) has pointed out, it is somewhat inconsistent with the traditions of the learning laboratory to introduce examinations of individual difference variables. Thus, Subjects x Independent Variables interactions are usually considered to contribute to error variance (Jensen, 1967a, p. 117).

Semler and Iscoe (1963) compared the performance of Negro and white children on four conditions of paired-associate learning tasks; they also obtained WISC data on the children who ranged from five to nine years. Although significant racial differences were present on the WISC, they were not found in the paired-associate learning. Correlations between IQ and learning-task scores were low for both groups (.09 for whites, .19 for Negroes).

Zigler and DeLabry (1962) compared groups of middle-class, lower-class, and retarded subjects on a concept switching task, using different reward conditions. They found that when each group performed under the reward condition considered optimal, there were no group differences in performance. The intangible reward condition was considered optimal for the middle class; tangible reinforcement was optimal for the lower-class group and the retardates. A similar study using a discrimination task was carried out by Terrell, Durkin, and Wiesley (1959). They also found material reward produced better performance in lower-class children and nonmaterial reward proved more effective with middle-class children.

Rohwer (1966), Jensen (1961), and Rapier (1966) have found that performance of lower- and middle-class Negroes, Mexican-Americans and Anglo-Americans, and lower- and middle-class Caucasians, respectively, does not differ markedly in laboratory-learning tasks such as selective trial-and-error learning and paired-associate learning. These workers find that the relation between tested intelligence and performance on the learning tasks is high for the upper-status groups but negligible for the lower-status groups. Jensen (1967b) suggests that the equivalence of performance of the lower-status children with middle-class children on these tasks which do not require transfer from previous learning suggests the learning ability of children from lower-status backgrounds is not adequately reflected in general intelligence tests. Taken together with the findings of high correlations on these learning tasks and intelligence tests for upper-status groups and low correlations for low-status groups, he argues that research is needed to clarify the reasons for these unique relationships which probably reflect that intelligence tests are "truer" estimates of ability for the middle-class groups than for the lower-class groups.

Whether or not one wishes to join Jensen in his search for more accurate measurements of ability in low-status populations—it is admittedly reminiscent of the quest for culture-free measurement—his findings and those of his colleagues suggest the relevance of combining differential psychology with the tools of the learning laboratory in studying the learning patterns of the disadvantaged.

Along these lines, some recent factor analytic studies have been carried out with measures of various abilities and measures of learning on laboratory tasks. Illustrative of this work is a study by Duncanson (1966) who administered concept-formation, paired-associates, and rote-memory tasks to sixth-grade students, along with a number of tests from the Reference Tests for Cognitive Factors, the Kuhlman-Anderson Test, and some parts of the Stanford Achievement Battery. The socio-economic level of the students sampled is not specified in this study. However, the factor analysis carried out on these data did show common variance between certain ability tests and the laboratory tasks, with the exception of the concept-formation tasks. In addition, there were unique learning-task factors. Such factor analytic studies should help clarify the nature of learning-task performance and ability measurements on populations of different ages and backgrounds.

Other Studies of Cognitive Development

A number of other studies have been undertaken which deal with cognitive functioning but come from traditions other than the psychometric or learning laboratory. One such dimension of cognitive functioning is classificatory behavior. Classificatory behavior has often been considered a language function and has been studied along with other linguistic behaviors. Although we have not reviewed language studies of the disadvantaged, classificatory behavior can be seen as representative of linguistic or cognitive functioning. John (1963) asked children to sort pictures of common objects and to label the piles they created; she studied first- and fifth-grade Negro children of varying social class. With the fifth-graders, she found that lower-class children made more piles and gave fewer verbalizations about their sorting than did middle-class children. Hess and Shipman (1965), in presenting the Sigel Sorting Task to four-year-old Negro children of varying social class, also found that level of abstraction was related to social class, although the number of unscorable responses was extremely high for all children of this age.

Although child psychologists are showing increasing interest in the work of Piaget, few studies from a stage theoretic point of view have been undertaken with children from disadvantaged backgrounds. In one study, a sorting task and a class-inclusion task were administered to part of the Hess and Shipman (1963) sample when they reached age five. The tasks had been developed by Kohlberg (1965). In a middle-class sample of children, patterns of responses had been found to form a Guttman scale reflecting a Piaget-based developmental sequence. The developmental sequence was found to exist within this Negro population of mixed social class; that is, the Guttman scale was reproduced. There were differences by social class in the developmental level attained, the upper-middle-class group being more advanced developmentally (Stodolsky, 1965).

Other work from the stage theoretic point of view is reported by Wallach (1963). He reports studies by Hyde and Slater dealing with conservation of number in samples of children of differing social background. According to Wallach, these researchers have found variations in age norms in differing social groups but no indication of discrepancies in developmental sequences.

From the limited evidence to date, it appears reasonable to expect that the stage theory of Piaget is generally applicable to all children regardless of social-class background. Nevertheless, longitudinal studies and studies of older children are needed. The studies which have found developmental sequence to apply to diverse samples of children have been with young children. It is still not known how much of the developmental sequence is general. Thus, we might find a truncated developmental sequence if we tested children of disadvantaged background in adolescence. In other words, such children might display the sequence to a point, but the stage of development reached might be lower than that achieved by their more advantaged peers. Such studies should be considerably aided by the availability of standard testing techniques (Laurendeau & Pinard, 1962).

A Note on Testing

The types of achievement and intelligence tests which are most often used can have only limited value in describing the cognitive functioning of children. In almost all instances, we are concerned with scratchings on an answer sheet, not with the ways in which a student arrived at a conclusion. No matter how much we may think we know by looking at scores on such psychometric procedures, unless tests are constructed deliberately to reveal reasoning processes, these processes will not be identified. Zigler (1966), in discussing mental retardation, points out this content-versus-process distinction, making a plea for testing procedures which give us information about the "cognitive structures and processes that give rise to content" (p. 113).

Historically, there has been some incompatibility between test constructors working within the measurement tradition and those psychologists interested in cognitive processes. There does not seem to be any necessary reason for this split. The testing procedures developed by Smedslund (1963), Laurendeau and Pinard (1962), and by the Educational Testing Service (in the new series "Let's Look at First Graders") are procedures which allow statements about individual differences and also provide information about cognitive processes of children. These tests are outgrowth of Piaget's theories of cognitive development.

NEW DIRECTIONS FOR RESEARCH

Although the above review of recent studies relating to learning in the disadvantaged does not pretend to be totally comprehensive, it does give representation to the various emphases in prior research. There are at least two major orientations which research on the learning of disadvantaged students can take. Both seem important, but have different pay-offs in terms of relevance to educational procedure and outcomes.

Developmental Origins

The explanatory, developmental direction of research would be oriented to tracing the origins of the characteristics which have been observed in the disadvantaged, as well as to charting the etiology of characteristics not studied to date.

Beginning with a broad description of the relation between a characteristic such as general intelligence and social-class status, one might ask: How can we account for the observed differences in performance among groups? What does it mean in psychological-process terms to be a member of a given social class? In order to answer these questions one moves quickly to variables which are more detailed and which should explain within-class variations as well as between-class variations.

A start in this research direction has been made in a number of quarters. Milner (1951) assessed parent-child relations and certain attributes of the home environment in relation to reading readiness. She used interview procedures in her study of first-grade children and their parents. More recently, Davé (1963) and Wolf (1965) related indices of home environment to school achievement and intelligence test scores respectively, in a fifth-grade white population of varying social class. These workers began by conceptualizing the home in terms of environmental process variables believed to be salient for the development of the outcome measures in which they were interested. They also used interviews to assess these environmental characteristics. They rated such characteristics as press for achievement, language models in the home, academic guidance provided by the home, and provisions for general learning. The ratings which they derived on the environmental process variables were then correlated with children's performance. Davé found a multiple correlation of .80 between his environmental indices and over-all achievement on a standard test battery. Wolf achieved a multiple correlation of .69 between his ratings and intelligence-test performance.

From the point of view of prediction, these correlations represented a considerable advance over the usual relation found between social class and achievement or intelligence-test performance. More important, however, is the direction in which they orient future research. It is clearly demonstrated that one can move beyond gross classificatory variables, such as social class, to much more detailed assessment of environments. Although these studies are correlational, they move us conceptually in the direction of experimental studies of development by viewing environmental variables in dynamic, process-oriented terms.

A study reported by Peterson and DeBord (1966) investigated various home factors and their relation to achievement in eleven-year-old Negro and white lower-class boys in a southern city. Using interview procedures, they assessed family composition, economic and social stability of the family, social participation, cultural level of the home, educational press, and certain aspects of the parents' orientation to the world. Peterson and DeBord performed separate multiple regressions on their data by race. For both groups, they achieved high multiple correlations between certain home variables and achievement: multiple correlation for Negroes was .82 using eleven variables regressed on achievement scores; the comparable correlation for whites was .75 using fourteen home variables. Although there were certain variables which were significantly correlated for both the Negroes and whites, others were unique for each group. The fact that such multiple correlations were obtained *within* a lower-class sample indicates the extent to which home conditions vary within social-class groups.[2]

Another important step in this direction is the research of Hess and Shipman (1965). In an extensive project studying Negro pre-school children, they have assessed numerous maternal characteristics including language (Olim, Hess, and Shipman, 1965) and teaching style (Jackson, Hess, and Shipman, 1965). Maternal teaching style is assessed in an experimental interaction session in the laboratory in which the mother is

---

[2] These multiple correlations have not been cross-validated.

instructed in a simple task and then instructs her child. All interactions, both verbal and physical, are recorded and later analyzed into a number of dimensions. Olim, Hess, and Shipman report that maternal language is a better predictor of child's abstraction score on a sorting task than either the mother's IQ or the child's IQ. Jackson, Hess, and Shipman found that certain teaching variables were highly related to the learning outcome of the child in the experimental teaching situation. In addition, Stodolsky (1965) has extended these findings to predict a child's vocabulary at age five using a combination of maternal language and teaching variables assessed when the child was four. The multiple correlation of these process variables and the child's language score was .63, very close to the theoretical limits imposed by the reliability of the vocabulary test. She found that the quality of the mother's own language, the mother's use of reinforcement in a teaching situation, and the extent to which the mother made task-relevant discriminations in teaching a task were highly related to the child's vocabulary level.

The Hess and Shipman work posits that the mother's behavior, especially her linguistic and teaching behavior, is a key to the child's learning in the home. By drawing on learning theory and theories of language learning, they are able to point to relations between developments in the child and the mother's behavior which are both theoretically reasonable and have great heuristic power. The Hess and Shipman study is clearly an advance in the direction of explaining the origins of cognitive abilities in young children. Their work is more embedded in natural observation than the interview studies previously cited, but still does not go the whole way in assessment of what actually takes place in the home.

It should be clear that it will eventually be necessary to execute detailed observational studies of children in home environments if one wants to arrive at valid hypotheses about the dynamics of development in interaction with environment. The dearth of naturalistic data about children's behavior and concomitant environmental circumstances is most regrettable. Some atttempts are now being made to remedy this situation in Harvard University's Pre-School Project under the general direction of Burton White. This project is planned as a long-term study of pre-school children in home and school environments to trace the development of various abilities which promote educability. Beginning with first-hand observations of children and environments, this project will generate ideas about developmental regularities which will be tested through longitudinal studies of children from birth through six years of age. In addition, the project will generate hypotheses regarding environmental factors which interact in important ways with the developmental phenomena which are isolated. In the long run, these hypotheses will be subject to experimental test through manipulations of environmental conditions.

In order to extend knowledge of the development of intellectual abilities and learning in children, more investment in longitudinal studies which chart the course of growth within individuals will be needed. Such studies should be accompanied by investigations of relevant environmental circumstances. The longitudinal work of Thomas and his colleagues on the development of personality and temperamental characteristics in infants and young children is illustrative of the power of this approach (Thomas, Chess, Birch, Hertzig, & Korn, 1964).

The types of studies we were suggesting here clearly need not be restricted to disadvantaged populations. It is to be hoped that such research would include children of diverse backgrounds. From a methodological point of view, variations in environmental circumstances and variation in child characteristics would be less restricted by studying a wide range of children. On the other hand, it is altogether possible that circumstances which are relevant in one subcultural context would not generalize across subcultures.

Is such developmental research of highest priority for school people? In many ways, we think not. We think we should assume for the moment that the job of the schools is a limited one (however arduous and complex). Children are sent to schools for a limited part of their daily lives to acquire certain knowledge and skills and ways of thinking which are considered essential for functioning in the society—in the world of work, leisure, and citizenship.

Some compensatory programs have operated on the assumption that school programs should be oriented toward changing home conditions relevant to educability. If school people want to take on the job of changing home conditions, for example, changing parent-child interactions in the home, then the study of developmental origins becomes more relevant. But we should also like to suggest that such home-based interventions will probably not be sufficient. Let us remember that life styles are usually quite adaptive to life circumstances (Lewis, 1961). We are not suggesting that it is impossible to achieve some modification of parental behaviors to facilitate the educational progress of students, but we would probably be a lot more successful if we were to modify the conditions which probably lead to many of these behaviors: namely, lack of money and of access to jobs.

Now perhaps we are talking about politically-based action research!

But while we are keeping psychologists and anthropologists busy studying the characteristics of people who are poor, might it not also be advisable to assess the degree to which these characteristics are situation-dependent? We are suggesting here a rather simple experiment which seems very important. Would poor people, given jobs and money, change in their behaviors relevant to the child's educability? Would parental behaviors such as cognitive level, teaching style, values, and attitudes change with a change in economic conditions? We do not know; but we think the matter bears empirical investigation.

We are suggesting that heavy investment in investigations of children in conditions (low income, poor housing, etc.) which are modifiable through political and economic actions should be accompanied by knowledge of the outcomes of changing these conditions. We must know to what extent poor children's characteristics are simply a function of their economic circumstances. Further, we suggest that the type of research which is both legitimate and important for developmental psychologists is not the most direct route to solving the educational problems which the schools have to tackle right now. It is our opinion that a more ostrich-like approach to the learning of disadvantaged students might have salutary effects.

School-Based Research

The schools have a job to do. Ask any teacher; he knows what he is to "cover" in a term. How can researchers assist teachers in doing this job better?

First, one assumption must be made explicit. Most, if not all, teachers want to teach effectively and to see their students learn. We do not believe the cumulative deficit in achievement of disadvantaged students reflects any willful or determined attempts on the part of teachers to "keep these students down." Nor do we think it reflects laziness. The most parsimonious assumption would seem to be that teachers are not effective and students are not learning at an adequate rate because techniques have not been devised which produce desired learning outcomes in many children whom we label disadvantaged.

What can researchers do to help change this situation? One strategy would be to start where the teacher has to start; that is, with a curriculum to be taught and a group of students who are to learn it. Two broad questions can be asked: What is required in the way of student behaviors and attributes to begin the prescribed learning task? How does the student's current state match these requirements?

We are suggesting here that we formalize that process which typically goes on in a teacher's mind. The teacher attempts at some level to analyze the objective he wants his student to achieve into a logical sequence of learnings. He concomitantly assesses the state of readiness of the student in terms of prior learnings and behaviors which seem relevant to the learning task at hand. He then devises an instructional strategy which takes both curricular and student facts into account. We are talking here about the old-fashioned process of diagnostically-based instruction.

It seems that we could dramatically affect the educational progress of all students if a large investment were made along these lines. The idea, though simple to state, would be extremely laborious to execute. What would be needed first would be detailed analyses of tasks or objectives expressed in behavioral terms. We know of two groups who have attempted such work to date. Gagné (1966) describes a number of such analyses of cumulative learning in mathematics. For example, he attempts to analyze the task of learning to "add integers" into a hierarchical sequence of learnings which begins with the least complex learnings (associations) and proceeds in hierarchical fashion to the learning of simple and complex rules and principles. The task analysis which begins as a logical one can then be verified in part in the actual performance of students. Gagné has found that learning to add integers does in fact follow the hierarchical sequence he proposed; that is, students who learn higher-level tasks have achieved the lower levels; children who have not mastered the lower-level tasks in the hierarchy do not learn the higher-level tasks.

This type of task analysis provides sequencing for the instructional program and diagnostic power. Such analyses, since they are made in behavioral terms, could be readily translated into quick testing procedures to assess a student's readiness for learning a given task. Such testing would immediately orient the teacher to the appropriate part of the instructional sequence to begin with a particular student.

Another example of this type of work is provided by Smilansky (1964). Her interest was in the development of a kindergarten curriculum which would provide disadvantaged Israeli children with the necessary skills and behaviors to enter the first-grade curriculum. The approach she used was to begin with first-hand observations of successful first-grade children in classrooms. She analyzed the behaviors required of the students in these classrooms, compiling a long list and then constructed assessment techniques which would give evidence about these behaviors in five-year-old children. Simultaneously, she and her colleagues started to develop curricular approaches which would develop these behaviors in children who had not achieved them. The final success of their intervention program will be judged in terms of the achievement of these objectives in disadvantaged children.

Both the Gagné and Smilansky approaches result in very detailed statements of behavioral requirements for a learning task. They do not specify how the teacher would proceed in the instructional program, but they do pinpoint where to begin. In addition, the effort invested in the logical analysis of the task requirements, or the actual observation of children achieving tasks, is highly suggestive of instructional strategies. A heavy investment in such analyses of curriculum, and the development of diagnostic techniques which are curriculum-specific could make high-value information readily available to the teacher.

The task-analysis approaches described should serve as first steps in an iterative matching strategy. One begins with a set of behavioral characteristics which fit a learning task. Students are assessed to see which behaviors and prerequisite skills they display. Then an instructional procedure is adapted for the student. The process is iterative in that we can anticipate continuous refinements of both the assessments of students and the instructional procedures in the context of a given task. In addition, the process should be a continuous one, applying to each new task as it is reached.

The matching of instructional procedures to student characteristics could take at least two forms. One would be essentially remedial; that is, an instructional method considered suitable for all students would be settled on in advance. Therefore, only one set of prerequisite skills would have to be achieved by all students. After assessment of students, the teacher's first job would be to bring all students to this one configuration of necessary minimal skills before proceeding with the preselected regimen. Although this remedial strategy would clearly improve much current practice, as there often is only one instructional method sanctioned by a school system, it is not the most desirable approach.

The second approach would make use of multiple instructional methods. Certain initial patterns of skills and learnings would be associated with certain instructional procedures. Optimal matching of students to curricular approaches could then be executed on the basis of initial assessments. Such matching would be far more diagnostic and precise than the usual sort of tracking which goes on in the schools. Presently, tracking, at least in the early grades, is usually based entirely on *level* of student ability. Under such a procedure, student characteristics are not meaningfully articulated with curricular content or requirements.

The real power of the matching procedure we are suggesting would be in the extent to which alternative instructional strategies could be generated which would be based on a complex analysis of student characteristics and curricular contents.

The research program we are suggesting would be tedious. First, a large-scale investment in curricular analyses would be necessary. Once such analyses were completed, an enormous effort would have to be expended in the development of diagnostic methods which could be used effectively by teachers. Some of these methods might be widely useful whereas others might be very specific to a given school or classroom.

Once this approach is begun, it would feed into a deeper understanding of the conditions of learning which are appropriate for children with various characteristics. It is to be hoped that it would lead to much more pointed learning experiments in which children could be selected on the basis of a wide variety of characteristics.

Extension of test construction from the point of view of the psychologist (as in Lesser, Fifer, & Clark, 1965) should also contribute to this approach. Although it appears most efficient to start building diagnostic tools on the basis of curricular approaches, theories of intellect should also lead to profitable constructs. Once the matching procedure gets started, it has built-in corrective features. Analysis of curricular approaches leading to diagnostic tools will lead in turn to new insights into student performance and curriculum. The beginning point is not crucial as long as the process gets under way.

We have proposed a program of school-based research which we believe would enormously assist the work of teachers on a day-to-day basis. Most important it should have great value in creating more successful students because it recognizes the background they bring with them.

A SPECIFIC CASE OF RESEARCH

The Original Study

Aims. Our goal was to examine the patterns among various mental abilities in six- and seven-year-old children from different social-class and ethnic backgrounds. We accepted the definition of intelligence which postulates diverse mental abilities and proposes that intelligent behavior can be manifested in a wide variety of forms, with each individual displaying certain areas of intellectual strength and other forms of intellectual weakness. A basic premise of this study is that social-class and ethnic influences differ not only in degree but in kind, with the consequence that different kinds of intellectual skills are fostered or hindered in different environments.

Designs. Hypotheses were tested regarding the effects of social-class and ethnic-group affiliation (and their interactions) upon both the level of each mental ability considered singly and the pattern among mental abilities considered in combination. Four mental abilities (Verbal ability, Reasoning, Number facility, and Space Conceptualization) were studied in first-grade children from four ethnic groups (Chinese, Jewish, Negro, and Puerto Rican). Each ethnic group was divided into two

Ethnic Group

		CHINESE	JEWS	NEGROES	PUERTO RICAN
	BOYS				
MIDDLE					
Social	GIRLS				
Class					
LOWER					

Total │ N = 320

social-class components (middle and lower), each in turn being divided into equal numbers of boys and girls.

Thus, a 4 x 2 x 2 analysis-of-covariance design included a total of sixteen subgroups, each composed of twenty children. A total sample of 320 first-grade children was drawn from forty-five different elementary schools in New York City and its environs. Three test influences were controlled statistically: effort, responsiveness to the tester, and age of the subject.

The selection of four mental abilities (Verbal ability, Reasoning, Number facility, and Space Conceptualization) is described in detail elsewhere (Lesser, Fifer, & Clark, 1965, pp. 32-43). To obtain a first approximation to the assessment of intra-individual profiles of scores for the various mental abilities of children, these skills were assessed:

Verbal—The skill is defined as memory for verbal labels in which reasoning elements, such as those required by verbal analogies, are reduced to a minimum. Verbal ability has long been regarded as the best single predictor of success in academic courses, especially in the language and social-science fields. It is involved to a marked degree in the work of all professions and in most semiprofessional areas.

Reasoning—Reasoning involves the ability to formulate concepts, to weave together ideas and concepts, and to draw conclusions and inferences from them. It is, almost by definition, the central element of aptitude for intellectual activities and, therefore, is of primary importance in all academic fields and in most vocations.

Number—The ability is defined as skill in enumeration and in memory and use of the fundamental combinations in addition, subtraction, multiplication, and division. It is of great importance in arithmetic in elementary schools and in mathematics in secondary schools.

Space Conceptualization—The ability refers to a cluster of skills related to spatial relations and sizes of objects and to visualizing their movements in space. It is involved in geometry, trigonometry, mechanics, and drafting; in elementary-school activities, such as practical arts and drawing; and in occupations such as mechanics, engineering, and architecture.

Procedural Issues. In this brief report, it is impossible to describe all the details of the procedures employed. Yet since research on the intellectual performance of "disadvantaged" children does impose some unique demands upon the investigator, at least the following procedural issues should be outlined.

a. Gaining access to the schools: Perhaps the most formidable problem was that of gaining the cooperation of school boards and school authorities for research on such a supposedly controversial issue. An honest approach by the researcher to the school authorities must contain the words "ethnic," "Negro," "Jewish," and "lower-class," and yet it is precisely these loaded words which arouse immediate anxiety and resistance in those who are authorized to permit or reject research in the schools. We believed that our objective of supplying information and understanding about the intellectual strengths and weaknesses of the children being taught in school would be a strong inducement to participation. Not so. Only enormous persistence and lengthy negotiation—during which the researcher must agree to a succession of incapacitating constraints—permits such research at all.

Surely there are serious problems of ethics in educational research. Researchers should be (and most often are) as scrupulous as school authorities in maintaining the conditions of consent and confidentiality which protect subjects from unwarranted intrusions of privacy. But the legitimate ethical issues of privacy and free inquiry are not those that block access to the schools—the fear of controversy over racial issues seems to immobilize school authorities.

Beyond our own experiences in gaining access to the schools, numerous examples exist of how research on the disadvantaged is prevented or distorted by the decisions of school authorities. For example, in Coleman's (Coleman et al., 1966) study of *Equality of Educational Opportunity,* requested by the President and Congress of the United States, many major cities refused to participate, often because comparisons among racial groups were being made (although reasons for refusal were rarely stated).

Later in this paper, we shall discuss several new directions for future research comparing "disadvantaged" and "non-disadvantaged" children. These suggestions will remain the mental exercises of the academics unless some reasonable policies can be developed by researchers and school authorities to provide honest access to the school children, their parents, and their teachers.

b. Locating social-class and ethnic-group samples: An associated problem was to achieve an unambiguous definition and assessment of social-class and ethnic-group placement. (The detailed procedures used for sample selection are described in Lesser, Fifer, & Clark, 1965, pp. 21-32.) Both variables are clearly multidimensional in character, and to define and measure the necessary components in each is a formidable task. Since members of each ethnic group were to be located in both lower- and middle-class categories, additional problems arose in attempting to maintain an equal degree of separation between the two social-class categories for each ethnic group.

In addition, obtaining the data necessary to identify the social-class and ethnic-group placement of each child presented many practical problems. There are strong legal restrictions in New York State upon collecting the data necessary for social-class and ethnic identification— and these restrictions are perhaps quite justified—but since we were not allowed to ask parents or school authorities directly about education, or religion, or even occupation, we were forced to use information gathered indirectly through twenty-three different community agencies and four sources of Census and housing statistics. Among sources such as the New York City Regional Planning Association, the Commonwealth of Puerto Rico, the China Institute in America, the Demographic Study Committee of the Federation of Jewish Philanthropies, and the *New York Daily News* Advertising Department, our best single source of information was one of the largest advertising agencies in New York City, which has within its "Component Advertising Division" (which develops special marketing appeals for different ethnic groups) enormous deposits of information on the locations of the many cultural groups in New York City. There was little willingness, of course, to allow us to use these data. But after endless sitting-in and sheer pestering, we were given access to this information. We could not possibly have completed this study without it.

c. Developing "culture-fair" test materials: Perhaps the major technical problem was to insure the fact that observed differences among social-class and ethnic groups are in the children and not in the test materials themselves (or in the definitions upon which the tests are based). Therefore, tests were constructed which presuppose only experiences that are common and familiar within all of the different social-class and ethnic groups in an urban area. We had no intention to "free" the test materials from cultural influence, but rather to utilize elements which appear commonly in all cultural groups in New York City. If, for example, other Picture Vocabulary tests use pictures of xylophones or giraffes (which a middle-class child is more likely than a lower-class child to encounter in a picture book or in a zoo), we used pictures of buses, fire hydrants, lamp posts, garbage trucks, and police cars—objects to which all urban children are exposed.

d. Controlling "examiner bias": Each child was tested by an examiner who shared the child's ethnic identity in order to maintain chances of establishing good rapport and to permit test administration in the child's primary language, or in English, or, more often, in the most effective combination of languages for the particular child. Thus, we had a Negro tester, a Spanish-speaking Puerto Rican tester, a Yiddish-speaking Jewish tester, and three Chinese-speaking Chinese testers to accommodate the eight different Chinese dialects encountered among our Chinese children. Each tester had been trained beyond the Master's degree level, and each had extensive experience administering psychological tests; but the tendency of the testers to empathize with the children from their own cultural groups demanded careful control of the testing procedures to insure uniform test administration. This standardization was accomplished through extensive video-tape training in which each examiner observed other testers and himself administer the test materials.

Some Findings. Hypotheses were tested regarding the influence of social class and ethnicity (and their interactions) upon the levels of the four mental-ability scores and upon the patterns among them. The results are summarized in Table 1.

a. Distinctive ethnic-group differences: Ethnic groups are markedly

TABLE 1

Summary of Results

Source of Influence	Level	Effect upon Mental Abilities Pattern
Ethnicity	Highly Significant*	Highly Significant*
Social Class	Highly Significant*	Nonsignificant
Social Class x Ethnicity	Significant**	Nonsignificant

* p < .001
** p < .05

different (p<.001) *both* in the absolute *level* of each mental ability and in the *pattern* among these abilities. For example, with regard to the effects of ethnicity upon the *level* of each ability, Figure 1 shows that

(1) on Verbal ability, Jewish children ranked first (being significantly better than all other ethnic groups), Negroes second, Chinese third (both being significantly better than Puerto Ricans), and Puerto Rican fourth.

(2) on Space Conceptualization, Chinese ranked first (being significantly better than Puerto Ricans and Negroes), Jews second, Puerto Ricans third, and Negroes fourth.

But the most striking results of this study concern the effects of ethnicity upon the patterns among the mental abilities. Figure 1 (and the associated analyses-of-variance for group patterns) shows that these *patterns* are different for each ethnic group. More important is the finding depicted in Figures 2-5. Ethnicity does affect the pattern of mental abilities *and, once the pattern specific to the ethnic group emerges, social-class variations within the ethnic group do not alter this basic organization.* For example, Figure 2 shows the mental-ability pattern peculiar to the Chinese children—with the pattern displayed by the middle-class Chinese children duplicated at a lower level of performance by the lower-class Chinese children. Figure 3 shows the mental-ability pattern specific to the Jewish children—with the pattern displayed by the middle-class Jewish children duplicated at a lowel level of performance by the lower-class Jewish children. Parallel statements can be made for each ethnic group.

The failure of social-class conditions to transcend patterns of mental ability associated with ethnic influences was unexpected. Social-class influences have been described as superceding ethnic-group effects for such diverse phenomena as child-rearing practices, educational and occupational aspirations, achievement motivation, and anomie. The greater

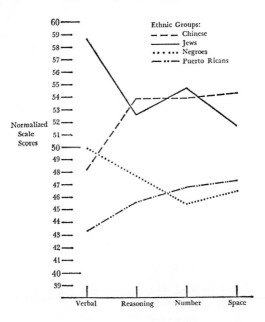

Fig. 1. *Pattern of Normalized Mental-Ability Scores for Each Ethnic Group*

salience of social class over ethnic membership is reversed in the present findings on patterns of mental ability. Ethnicity has the primary effect upon the organization of mental abilities, and the organization is not modified further by social-class influences.

Many other findings are described in our full report of this original study (Lesser, Fifer, & Clark, 1965). Only a few additional findings will be mentioned here, either because they are prominent in our recent replication study or in our plans for future research.

b. Interactions between social-class and ethnicity: Table 1, summarizing our earlier findings, indicates significant interactions (p<.05) between social class and ethnicity on the level of each mental ability. Table 2 shows the mean level of each mental ability for Chinese and Negro children from each social-class group; the same interaction effects appear when Jewish and Puerto Rican children are included, but the present table has been reduced to the Chinese and Negro children to simplify the present discussion. Two effects combine to produce the interaction effect between social class and ethnicity:

(1) On each mental-ability scale, social-class position produces more of a difference in the mental abilities of the Negro children than for the

TABLE 2

MEAN MENTAL-ABILITY SCORES FOR CHINESE AND NEGRO CHILDREN
FOR EACH SOCIAL-CLASS GROUP

| | Verbal | | | | Reasoning | | |
	Chinese	Negro			Chinese	Negro	
Middle	76.8	85.7	81.3	Middle	27.7	26.0	26.9
Lower	65.3	62.9	64.1	Lower	24.2	14.8	19.5
	71.1	74.3	72.7		25.9	20.4	23.2

Class x ethnicity, $F = 7.69, p < .01$ (Verbal)
Class x ethnicity, $F = 11.32, p < .01$ (Reasoning)

| | Number | | | | Space | | |
	Chinese	Negro			Chinese	Negro	
Middle	30.0	24.7	27.4	Middle	44.9	41.8	43.4
Lower	26.2	12.1	19.2	Lower	40.4	27.1	33.8
	28.1	18.4	23.3		42.7	34.4	38.6

Class x ethnicity, $F = 8.91, p < .01$ (Number)
Class x ethnicity, $F = 10.83, p < .01$ (Space)

other groups. That is, the middle-class Negro children are more different in level of mental abilities from the lower-class Negroes than, for example, the middle-class Chinese are from the lower-class Chinese.

(2) On each mental-ability scale, the scores of the middle-class children from the various ethnic groups resemble each other to a greater extent than do the scores of the lower-class children from the various ethnic groups. That is, the middle-class Chinese, Jewish, Negro, and Puerto Rican children are more alike in their mental ability scores than are the lower-class Chinese, Jewish, Negro, and Puerto Rican children.

Some earlier research (see Anastasi, 1958, Chapter 15) suggested that social-class influences upon intelligence are greater in white than in Negro groups. No distinct contrast with white children was available in our study, but the evidence indicates that social-class influences upon the mental abilities of Negro children are very great compared with the other ethnic groups represented. One explanation for the apparent contrast between the earlier and present findings is that the earlier research, perhaps, did not include middle-and lower-class Negro groups that were distinctively different. In any event, our findings show that the influence of social class on the level of abilities is more powerful for the Negro group than for the other ethnic groups.

c. Group data vs. individual data: The data analyses described to this point refer to differences in the performance of groups and not to the

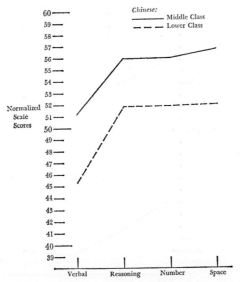

Fig. 2. *Patterns of Normalized Mental-Ability Scores for Middle- and Lower-Class Chinese Children.*

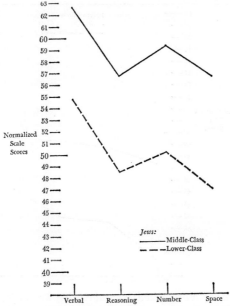

Fig. 3. *Patterns of Normalized Mental-Ability Scores for Middle- and Lower-Class Jewish Children.*

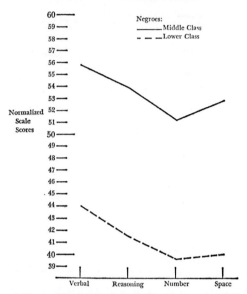

Fig. 4. *Patterns of Normalized Mental-Ability Scores for Middle- and Lower-Class Negro Children*

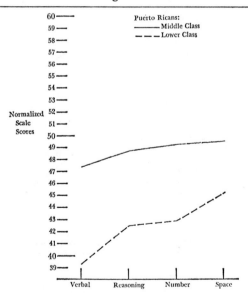

Fig. 5. *Patterns of Normalized Mental-Ability Scores for Middle- and Lower-Class Puerto Rican Children.*

TABLE 3

CLASSIFICATION ANALYSIS

Group N = 40, each Group	M Ch	L Ch	Group patterns M J	L J	M N	L N	M PR	L PR
Middle Chinese	13*	10	6	1	5	1	2	2
Lower Chinese	6	14	2	4	3	1	1	9
Middle Jewish	4	0	32	4	0	0	0	0
Lower Jewish	0	1	9	18	7	4	0	1
Middle Negro	5	1	11	10	11	0	0	2
Lower Negro	1	3	0	3	0	28	0	5
Middle Puerto Rican	6	6	3	6	4	0	3	12
Lower Puerto Rican	0	7	1	1	0	8	3	20

* Figures to read across as follows: The scores of 13 middle-class Chinese subjects fit the middle-class Chinese pattern and level on the four mental ability scales; 10 middle-class Chinese look like lower-class Chinese; 6 look more like middle-class Jews, 1 more like a lower-class Jew, etc.

performance of individuals. These analyses do not indicate how an individual will perform, but they suggest how he is likely to perform if he belongs to one of these eight groups. One technique we have used to proceed from group analyses to identifying particular patterns for individuals is called a "classification analysis" (see Table 3). This analysis allows the researcher to compare the pattern of mental-ability scores for each individual subject with the pattern profiles of his group and other groups. It yields data on the degree to which a subject's profile resembles the profile of his or the other groups (Tatsuoka, 1957). If mental-ability scores were not associated significantly with social class and ethnicity and hence a chance frequency of correct placement of individuals occurred, random cell assignment in Table 3 would be approximately five cases per cell. Thus, if the forty middle-class Chinese children showed no distinctive pattern of their own, they would be expected to be distributed equally among all eight group patterns. The deviation of the actual frequencies in the underlined diagonal cells from the chance frequency of five indicates the degree of correct classification beyond chance obtained through knowledge of the individual's mental-ability scores. Thus, thirty-two middle-class Jewish children and twenty-eight lower-class Negro children fit their group patterns. In contrast, only three middle-class Puerto Rican children (two less than chance) were classified correctly. It is clear that the middle-class Puerto Rican children were the most heterogeneous of the eight groups. Overall, the number of cases classified correctly through knowledge of the mental-ability pattern surpassed chance classification at a probability value associated with thirty-six zeroes; i.e., the probability value for correct classifications was less than one in ten to the thirty-fifth exponent. In short, knowledge of the child's pattern of mental abilities allows the correct identification of his social-class and ethnic-group membership to a degree far exceeding chance expectations.

We note this analysis for two reasons. Methodologically, it provides a useful device for moving from group data to the analysis of the individual case. Substantively, it has allowed us to identify the children who fit closely the profile of their group and those who are exceptions in their group but resemble the profile of some other group. This capability allows us to pinpoint cases in exploring questions about the origins of patterns of mental ability and about the fitting of school practices to these patterns.

Some Conclusions. The study demonstrated that several mental abilities are organized in ways that are determined culturally. Referring to social-class and ethnic groups, Anastasi (1958) proposed that "groups differ in their relative standing on different functions. Each . . . fosters the development of a different pattern of abilities." Our data lend selective support to this position. Both social-class and ethnic groups do "differ in their relative standing on different functions"; i.e., both social class and ethnicity affect the *level* of intellectual performance. However, only ethnicity "fosters the development of a different *pattern* of abilities," while social-class differences within the ethnic groups do not modify these basic patterns associated with ethnicity.

To return to our continuing discussion of defining and delimiting the term "disadvantaged": Defining the "disadvantaged" as belonging to a particular ethnic group has one set of consequences for the development of intellectual skills—ethnic groups differ in both level and pattern of mental abilities. Defining the term using the social-class criteria of occupation, education, and neighborhood leads to quite different consequences—social-class affects level of ability, with middle class being uniformly superior, but does not alter the basic patterns of mental ability associated with ethnicity. Still other definitions—for example, unavailability of English language models, presence of a threatening and chaotic environment, matriarchal family structure, high family mobility, parental absence or apathy, poor nutrition—probably generate still other consequences, although we really know very little empirically about these relationships.

A Replication Study[3]

Since our early results were both surprising and striking in magnitude, our next step was to conduct a replication and extension with first-graders in Boston. The replication was conducted with middle-class and lower-class Chinese and Negro children (the samples of Jewish and Puerto Rican children who fit our social-class criteria were not available); the extension included an additional ethnic group—children from middle- and lower-class Irish-Catholic families.

Once again, the results were both striking and surprising. The replication data on Chinese and Negro children in Boston duplicated almost exactly our earlier data on similar samples in New York City. The striking, almost identical test performances in the original and replication study are shown in Figures 6-10. The raw mean scores of the Chinese children in Boston and in New York were different by an average of one-third of one standard deviation (Figure 6), and the Negro children in Boston and in New York were one-fifth of one standard deviation different from each other (Figure 7). Only one mean difference (numerical scores of Boston and New York Chinese) slightly exceeded one-half of one standard deviation.

The resemblance of the original and replication samples in patterns of mental ability is shown in Figure 8 (which contrasts the ethnic groups in the two cities with middle- and lower-class samples combined), Figure 9 (which displays the Chinese patterns in Boston and New York for each social-class group), and Figure 10 (which displays the Negro patterns in Boston and New York for each social-class group). With very few exceptions (number skills, especially multiplication and division, of the middle-class Chinese in Boston are slightly superior to the middle-class Chinese in New York), both the levels and patterns of mental ability in the Boston data almost duplicate the New York City data for Chinese and Negro children.

This replication study also included an ethnic group not previously studied in New York City: middle- and lower-class Irish-Catholic children. These first-grade Irish-Catholic children, in contrast to all the other ethnic groups tested, displayed neither a distinctive ethnic-group pattern nor similarity of patterns for middle- and lower-class segments of

---

[3] This replication study was conducted under the direction of Dr. Jane Fort, Laboratory of Human Development, Harvard University.

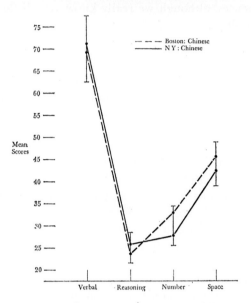

Fig. 6. *Mean Mental Ability Scores for* Chinese *Children in Boston (N = 20)
and New York (N = 80).*

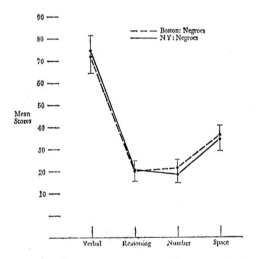

Fig. 7. *Mean Mental Ability Scores for* Negro *Children in Boston (N = 20)
and New York (N = 80).*

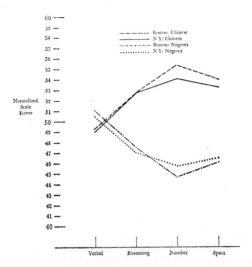

Fig. 8. *Patterns of Mental Ability for Chinese and Negro Children: NY vs. Boston.*

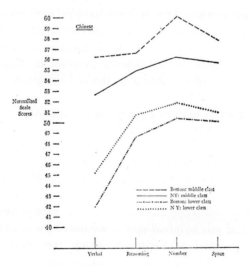

Fig. 9. *Patterns of Mental Ability for Chinese Children; Middle- and Lower-Class, NY vs. Boston.*

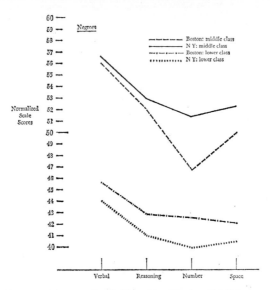

Fig. 10. *Patterns of Mental Ability for Negro Children; Middle- and Lower-Class, NY vs. Boston.*

the Irish-Catholic sample. Although we have no definitive explanation of this finding as yet, the absence of a distinctive ethnic-group pattern may be related to our failure to locate homogeneous concentrations of middle- and lower-class Irish Catholic families in Boston. The Irish-Catholic families are less confined to limited geographic areas than the other ethnic groups. We could not locate either middle- or lower-class Irish-Catholic families who fit clearly the occupational, educational, and neighborhood criteria for social-class placement. In short, there are at least two plausible explanations for the failure to replicate our results on other ethnic groups with the Irish-Catholic children: poor sampling of middle-class and lower-class Irish-Catholic families (due to their un-expected unavailability in Boston) or a real difference between Irish-Catholic children and those from other ethnic groups tested.

In the report of our original study, we noted an interaction effect be-tween social class and ethnicity in which the social-class difference produces more of a difference in the mental abilities of the Negro chil-dren than for the other ethnic groups. In the replication study, this finding reappeared: the middle-class Negro children are more different in level of mental abilities from the lower-class Negro children than the middle-class Chinese or Irish-Catholic children are from the lower-class

TABLE 4

PERCENTAGE OF VARIANCE CONTRIBUTED BY EACH ETHNIC GROUP
TO THE GROUP x TESTS INTERACTION TERM

Ethnic Group	% of Variance
Chinese	39
Irish-Catholic	1
Jewish	38
Negro	13
Puerto Rican	9

Chinese or Irish-Catholic children. It was also true in the replication, as in the original data, that the scores of the middle-class children from the various ethnic groups resembled each other more than the scores of the lower-class children from these ethnic groups. That is, the middle-class Chinese, Irish-Catholic, and Negro children are more alike in their mental ability scores (with the one exception of the middle-class Chinese in numerical ability) than are the lower-class Chinese, Irish-Catholic, and Negro children.

One further specific analysis should be noted before proceeding to a discussion of future research and the implications for educational policy. We have assessed the relative contributions of the five ethnic groups tested to the distinctiveness of ethnic-group patterning. The percentage of total ethnicity variance contributed by each ethnic group appears in Table 4. While the groups differ markedly in their relative contributions to the distinctiveness of ethnic-group patterns, all except the Irish-Catholic contribute to a statistically significant degree.

Some results of Coleman's recent study, *Equality of Educational Opportunity,* are compatible with these findings. The study included children from Oriental-American, Negro, Puerto Rican, Mexican, Indian-American, and white groups. This study does not include all our mental-ability variables nor does it provide a good assessment of social-class for the younger children, but Coleman's data for Chinese, Negro, and Puerto Rican children on Verbal and Reasoning tests show patterns very similar to ours.

We have some confidence, then, in our earlier findings on the effects of social-class and ethnic-group influence on the development of patterns of mental abilities in young children: at least several mental abilities are organized in ways that are determined culturally, social-class producing differences in the *level* of mental abilities (the middle-class being higher) and ethnic groups producing differences in both *level* and *pattern* of mental abilities.

Future Research

To pursue the educational relevance of these findings, we are now studying the following questions:

(1) What actual school behaviors are predicted by the patterns of mental ability?

(2) Are the differential patterns related to ethnic-group differences stable over time or do intervening experiences modify them?

(3) What are the specific origins or antecedents of differential patterns of mental ability?

(4) How can our knowledge about patterns of mental ability be fitted to the content and timing of instruction?

Mental-Ability Patterns as Predictors of School Achievement. We have stressed the importance of examining a variety of criteria related to school achievement in research on the "disadvantaged." We are assessing the predictive value of our mental-ability data for forecasting various patterns of school achievement, asking these questions: Is there an optimal pattern of mental abilities that results in superior school performance; or are different optimal patterns associated with superior school performance in different subject-matter areas? If optimal patterns are identified, can the child's abilities be reinforced differentially so that these optimal patterns are produced; or should the educational program adjust itself to the relative strengths and weaknesses of the child?

Convincing laboratory demonstrations (e.g., Duncanson, 1966) exist of the interrelations between measures of abilities and performance on several learning tasks. Using our mental-ability measures as predictors, we are attempting to extend these analyses to classroom learning performance.

In the research effort on matching instructional strategies and patterns of abilities, which we describe below, we go more deeply into the relations between types of intelligence and school performance. The achievement test measures used in our predictive validity study are static criteria of school performance; what really interests us is the predictive value of the mental-ability measures in forecasting learning in response to variations in instructional strategies. The relationships between mental-ability patterns and achievement test measures do, however, provide some assessment of the predictive validity of the mental-ability patterns.

Stability over Time of Mental-Ability Patterns. Will the major finding of this study, that differential patterns of ability are related to ethnic-group differences, remain stable across age groups? That is, does ethnic-group membership continue to determine the pattern of abilities for children with increasing maturity? Do the relative strengths and weaknesses of the subjects represent different rates of learning that eventually level off to a more or less common mean for all groups, or do they indeed represent stable cognitive organizations? What is the role of school experience in modifying distinctive ethnic-group patterns? That is, do the different patterns of mental ability persist in spite of the possible homogenizing effects of schooling through the heavy emphasis on verbal forms of instruction and the de-emphasis on the use of other intellectual skills?

To answer these questions, we have recently completed the construction of an upward extension of the tests of mental ability, providing appropriate measuring instruments for fifth- through eighth-grade children. Since our original New York City sample will be entering sixth-grade and we have located about 85 per cent of them, we will attempt to assess the size and magnitude of changes in mental-ability patterns over a five-year period.

There are few empirical precedents here. Studies of the differentiation of mental ability have not traced the course of social-class and ethnic influences through the use of samples followed longitudinally. Evidence on ethnic-group variations on samples of older subjects is conflicting: Stewart, Dole, and Harris (1967) do not find variations in the factorial structures of different ethnic groups, but Guthrie (1963) does. Cross-sectional findings (e.g., Meyers, Dingman, & Orpet, 1964) show stability in factorial structure across three age groups (two-, four-, and six-year-olds). But no direct evidence tells us whether there are ethnically distinctive patterns of mental ability which persist, dissolve, or change with age.

Developmental Origins: Antecedents of Diverse Mental Abilities. What early experiences produce the particular patterns of mental ability in different ethnic groups?[4] Many different environmental influences may be operating: the reinforcements the parents offer for different types of intellectual performance, opportunities inside and outside the home for learning different skills, the value placed on different forms of intel-

---

[4] We assume that our ability tests reflect student development produced by the interaction of environmental and genetic conditions. We are exploring the modifiability of these abilities and the degree to which they can be used in maximizing instruction.

lectual performance, the parents' intellectual aspirations for the child, work habits developed in the home, and so forth. Some suggestions exist in the literature (e.g., Bing, 1963) that less direct child-rearing influences —for example, the fostering of dependence or independence or the presence of a tense parent-child relationship—affect the development of mental abilities differentially.

We are now setting out to investigate the variations among ethnic groups in the history of differential experience in learning different mental skills. We assume that different emphases exist among ethnic groups in the specific intellectual functions that are stimulated and encouraged and that these different emphases are reflected in their different organizations of mental abilities. This research demands a longitudinal analysis which begins very early in the child's life as well as naturalistic observation in and out of the home. Since the little empirical research on the history of differential mental abilities is essentially retrospective in design, extensive methodological development is demanded by this research.

School-Based Research: Matching Instructional Strategies to Patterns of Mental-Ability. How can knowledge of a child's pattern of mental abilities be fitted to the content and timing of his instruction? How can instruction be adjusted to the child's particular strengths and weaknesses, or the child's abilities modified to meet the demands of instruction? In the context of individualizing instruction, we are attempting to fit instruction to particular forms of ability and *vice versa.* In the context of research design, we are searching for the interactions between instructional treatments and the abilities of the learner in order to determine how selected mental-ability variables are differentially related to learner performance under different treatments or conditions of instruction.

Answering these questions requires continuous, successive approximations to an analysis of the child's special combination of intellectual resources and the demands for intellectual resources placed upon him by the curriculum. We have begun two preliminary studies, one in the teaching of beginning reading, another in learning the concept of mathematical functions at the sixth-grade level. One approach we have used begins with an assessment of the child's particular pattern of mental ability and seeks to build an instructional strategy to capitalize on the child's intellectual strengths and minimize his weaknesses. For example, in teaching mathematical functions to children strong in Space Conceptualization but weak in Numerical facility, we use graphical presentation; in teaching the same concept to a child strong in Number facility but weak in Space Conceptualization, we rely on the manipulation of numbers in a tabular form. Using this approach, a correct matching of child and curriculum (e.g., a spatial child given a spatially-oriented curriculum) results in some learning for most children; however, there is wide variation in amounts of gain within the correctly-matched group. Incorrect matching (e.g., a numerical child given a spatially-oriented curriculum) results uniformly in insignificant gain. That is, at this point we seem to be able to create destructive mismatches more successfully than constructive matches. Practically, this is not much of a gain. Conceptually, however, we are discovering the forms that the matching and mismatching of intelligence and curriculum can take. We consider this research a useful first approximation to the iterative process of matching curriculum and individual differences. We now have identified one set of necessary conditions for fitting instruction and individual differences: to learn a space-oriented curriculum, the child must possess (or be taught first) a specifiable minimum skill in space conceptualization. How far and how rapidly he progresses in responding further to the space-oriented curriculum is not explained by his initial status. It is therefore necessary to extend our assessment to other relevant attributes of the child and thereby extend the iterative process of matching curriculum and individual differences in intelligence.

Another approach to intelligence-curriculum matching starts with a task analysis of the intellectual demands imposed by a curriculum and proceeds to an analysis of the intellectual skills available to the child, with the purpose of modifying or developing these skills to the requisite levels necessary to the task. Our only attack on this approach to date is some preliminary analysis of the modifiability of mental-ability variables. Some earlier work by Thelma Thurstone (1948) and more recent work at Educational Testing Service (Bussis, 1965) for first-graders in New York City and by Julian Stanley at Wisconsin hold promise that mental abilities can be modified to match the demands of the curriculum.

It is clear that knowledge of four mental abilities is insufficient to the task of matching individual differences in intelligence to the demands of complex curricula. It is also clear that we have few tools available for the adequate task analysis of different instructional strategies. Additional preliminary research is attempting to expand our conceptualization based on mental abilities by categorizing both the intellectual skills and the curriculum demands by means of three-dimensional models of intelligence, such as Guilford's (1959) scheme which includes not only mental operations (related to mental abilities) but contents and products as well, or Jensen's (1967a) model which includes not only modality variables (related to mental abilities) but types of learning and procedures for presenting learning materials.

Thus, we are applying our analysis of patterns of mental ability to an issue which we believe has promise for classroom learning and teaching —how to match instructional strategies and individual differences in intelligence to produce effective learning performance.

Implications for Educational Policy

Coleman's Argument in "Equality of Educational Opportunity:" Equal Opportunity for Equal Development. We mentioned earlier the recent study on *Equality of Educational Opportunity* directed by James S. Coleman. The results and particularly the interpretation of this study provide a useful point of departure for analyzing the implications for educational policy of the data described here on ethnic-group and social-class differences in mental-ability patterns.

Coleman failed to find what he expected to find, direct evidence of large inequalities in educational facilities in schools attended by children from different majority or minority groups. The study set out to document the fact that for children of minority groups school facilities are sharply unequal and that this inequality is related to student achievement. The data did not support either conclusion. What small differences in school facilities did exist had little or no discernible relationship to the level of student achievement.

Starting with these facts, Coleman develops an argument which we shall contrast with the implications of our mental-ability study. Inequality of educational opportunity still prevails, he says, because white and Negro (and other minority-group) students do not display equal levels of educational achievement when they complete high school. *Ipso facto,* the schools are unequal, despite the absence of direct evidence of such inequality.

Coleman's argument starts with the premise that the proper function of the schools in a democracy is to produce equal achievement levels among different groups in our society. Arguing from this premise, the demonstrated fact that Negroes and whites are unequal in level of educational attainment testifies to the inequality of educational opportunities provided by the schools. That is, by definition, schools are designed to make groups equal. They do not do so. Therefore, schools are unequal in the educational opportunities they provide. Indeed following this argument, the single decisive criterion for judging equal educational opportunity is that mean school performance of all groups be equal.

Coleman makes his position clear by saying that the role of the schools is to "make achievement independent of background" and to "overcome the differences in starting point of children from different social groups" (Coleman, 1966, p. 72). This position is shared by much research on the "disadvantaged," where the objective is to seek means to reduce the discrepancy in achievement levels between "deprived" and "nondeprived" children.[5]

The "Equal-Footing" Basis of Coleman's Argument. At one level—the "equal-footing" level—Coleman's line of reasoning seems to epitomize logic, common sense, and compassion. It seems to ask only that we give children from "disadvantaged" backgrounds a fair shake—that through the educational system, we educate all children to a point of equality in school achievement so that all groups can compete on equal terms for jobs or future educational opportunities.

However, it is our contention that Coleman's analysis does not go far enough, does not tell the whole story or consider all the evidence, and therefore is misleading and perhaps destructive. It fails to consider either the role of diversity and pluralism in our society or several alternative definitions of the function of schooling. Should schools provide equal opportunities to promote the *equal* development of all groups and individuals or equal opportunities for the *maximum* development of each group or individual? Can schools aim to do both?

An Alternative Argument: Equal Opportunity for Maximum Development. We believe that our data on patterns of mental ability clarify these two alternative and perhaps complementary assumptions regarding the function of education: (1) to provide equal opportunity for *equal* development, or (2) to provide equal opportunity for *maximum* development of each group or individual, whether or not group differences remain, enlarge, or disappear as a consequence. These positions are apparently incompatible but need closer examination in the light of empirical evidence.

---

[5] The counterpart to Coleman's reasoning about equal educational opportunity exists in the history of "culture-free" test construction, another topic of great relevance to the education of the disadvantaged. Early developers of "culture-free" tests (e.g., Eells et al., 1951) argued that only tests which eliminated items distinguishing among groups were free of "bias." The parallel to Coleman's argument is apparent: (1) the proper function of a "culture-free" test is to produce equal test scores for different social-class and ethnic groups; (2) if equal scores are not obtained, the fault is that the test (or some kinds of test items) produce the difference. Difference in test scores, *ergo,* bias in test items. The logical fallacy of this argument is now well-documented (e.g., Anastasi, 1958; Lorge, 1952), but the simple and surface persuasiveness of the argument stalled progress for many years in the study of cultural influences upon intelligence.

a. Data on social class: From our mental-ability data, what would we predict would happen if we modified the social-class characteristics of all our lower-class families—elevating the jobs, educations, and housing of the lower-class families in all ethnic groups? Within each ethnic group, we would expect to elevate the mental abilities of the lower-class children to resemble those of the middle-class children in that ethnic group, making them more similar to their middle-class counterparts in that ethnic group in level of ability. In this sense, we would be making groups of children more similar, removing the differences in mental ability associated with differences in social-class position.[6]

If we elevated the social-class position of lower-class families, we might produce still another effect which increases the similarity among groups. The interaction effect between social class and ethnicity showed that the mental-ability scores of middle-class children from various ethnic groups resembled each other more than the scores of the lower-class children from these ethnic groups. This interaction can be described as a convergence effect: the scores of the middle-class children across ethnic groups converge to a greater extent than the scores of lower-class children.

Thus, by elevating the occupations, educations, and neighborhoods of our lower-class families, our data would lead us to expect an increased resemblance of mental-ability levels for children within each ethnic group and, in addition, a convergence of scores of children across ethnic groups. To the extent that level of performance on mental abilities predicts school achievement, these convergences would narrow the range of differences in school achievement among social-class and ethnic groups.

b. Data on ethnic groups: To this juncture, our analysis supports the argument for equal educational opportunities for *equal* development: our data on level of mental ability suggest that elevating social-class characteristics of lower-class families would contribute to a greater degree of equality of development in level of intellectual functioning. Now, what of the alternative conception that the proper function of education is to provide equal opportunity for *maximum* development no matter what the consequences for the absolute magnitude of group differences? Since the data on patterns of intellectual functioning indicates that

---

[6] We noted earlier that social-class position produces more of a difference in the mental abilities of Negro children than for the other groups. From this finding, it is possible to speculate that elevating the social-class characteristics of lower-class Negro families would produce a more dramatic increase in the level of the Negro children's abilities than would a comparable change in social-class position affect the children from other ethnic groups.

once the mental-ability pattern specific to the ethnic group emerges, social-class variations within the ethnic group do not alter the basic organization associated with ethnicity, this finding suggests that lower-class children whose social-class position is elevated would still retain the distinctive mental-ability pattern associated with their ethnic group. The implication is that no matter what manipulations are undertaken to modify the social-class positions of children within an ethnic group, the distinctive ethnic group pattern of abilities will remain.

From this set of observations, the question then arises: how can we make *maximum* educational use of the distinctive patterns of ability the child possesses? We do not have definite answers to this question, which forces us to consider the line of future research discussed earlier on matching instructional strategies to the patterns of mental ability. In our discussion of school-based research, we called for a program to identify and explore mental attributes of children and the instructional methods which could be matched most effectively to these attributes to produce successful learning. In the simplest case, we can conceive of successful matching producing equal levels of achievement for children; such an outcome would be consistent with Coleman's argument. We think that at least for basic skills (e.g., literacy) the achievement of equal levels by all children is desirable.

Two possible contradictions to Coleman's argument remain, however. Beyond deploying all necessary resources to achieve minimal equality in essential goals, further development of students may well be diverse. A continuous utilization of student strengths and weaknesses may well lead to diverse development beyond a minimal set of achievements. To the extent that past experience, interests, and achievements of students are regularly related to subcultural membership, educational outcomes may differ. Second, we do not know what effects the matching procedure will have over time. We start, let us say, by using suitable alternative routes to identical educational objectives. Assuming we successfully achieve these outcomes, what else have we done? Have we, perhaps, reinforced and strengthened abilities, interests, or personality characteristics which are in fact associated with subcultural membership? In the long run, will we develop more diverse students than we started with?

Let us take a specific, if partially hypothetical, case. Our evidence indicates (see Figure 1) that young Chinese children have their strongest skill in Space Conceptualization and their weakest in Verbal ability. Conversely, young Jewish children are strongest in Verbal ability and weakest in Space Conceptualization. Following our principle of matching instruction and ability, we incidentally may enhance the initial strengths which each group possesses. For example, through the incidental enhancement of the space-conceptualization skills of the Chinese children, we may produce proportionally more Chinese than Jewish architects and engineers. Conversely, through incidental enhancement of verbal skills of the Jewish children, we may produce proportionally more Jewish than Chinese authors and lawyers. We will not have put members of these two ethnic groups on an "equal footing" for entering a particular occupation. But can we say that we have produced a socially-destructive outcome by starting with the knowledge of differences in ability patterns and adapting our instructional strategies to this knowledge to produce a maximum match for each child, even if this process results in inequality of certain educational and professional attainments? We are willing to accept, then, one possible consequence of arranging instruction to capitalize maximally on distinctive patterns of ability: that, in certain areas of intellectual accomplishment, rather than reducing or bringing toward equality the differences among various groups, we may actually magnify those differences.[7]

A Summary. We challenged Coleman's "equal-footing" argument on the grounds that it did not tell the whole story or use all known data. Some of these data, mainly the effects of social class upon level of mental ability, testify in favor of the argument for equal educational opportunity for *equal* development. Other data, namely the effects of ethnicity upon patterns of mental ability, testify to the importance of providing equal educational opportunities for the *maximum* development of groups and individuals, even if inequality of groups occurs as a consequence.

Are equalization and diversification necessarily incompatible goals? We do not believe so. If accelerating the feasible gains in jobs, education, and housing of lower-class families accelerates the gains in intellectual development of their children and reduces the difference in intellectual performance between social-class groups, we can all agree on the desirability of this outcome. On the other hand, if recognizing the particular patterns of intellectual strengths and weaknesses of various ethnic groups and maximizing the potential power of these patterns by matching

---

[7] At this point in the argument, the counterpart topic is that of the difference between "compensatory" and "supportive" educational programs for "disadvantaged." "Compensatory" programs aim to compensate, to make amends, to eradicate symptoms and causes—to give "disadvantaged" children what they need to make them like everyone else. In contrast, the aim of what might be termed "supportive" education is to give disadvantaged children what they need and can use maximally in order to learn to cope with and change their particular environments, even if they are made more different from everyone else in the process.

instructional conditions to them makes the intellectual accomplishments of different ethnic groups more diverse, we can all accept this gain in pluralism within our society. Thus, if lower-class children now perform intellectually more poorly than middle-class children—and it is clear that they do—and lower-class status can be diluted or removed by a society truly dedicated to doing so, this gain in equalization seems to be one legitimate aim of education. If the maximum educational promotion of particular patterns of ability accentuates the diverse contributions of different ethnic groups, this gain in pluralism seems another legitimate aim of education.

Our main point is that the study of mental abilities suggests that there may be patterns of attributes (cognitive, personality, motivational, and so forth) which are related in some regular way to ethnic-group membership. School-based research has not as yet identified the particular patterns of attributes which are educationally important and which (when matched with the appropriate instructional strategies) will maximize school achievement. Thus, we do not yet know if attribute patterns associated with ethnic-group membership will, in fact, be identified as educationally important. We believe, however, that data such as those derived from the current mental-abilities study must be considered since their implications may in fact require revisions of Coleman's position. We raise the issue because we are committed to our program of school-based research; whether ethnic- group differences are in fact minimized, held constant, or inflated by the programs which match individual differences to instructional strategies, we believe it important to pursue these programs nonetheless.

Perhaps this position asks no more than to change what is bad and changeable in education and society (resulting perhaps in greater equalization) and to use maximally what is good in education and society (resulting perhaps in increased diversity). Logic—and the empirical evidence—endorses both conclusions.

TOWARD A NEW DEFINITION OF THE DISADVANTAGED

Let us start with the simplest possible definition of "disadvantaged," i.e., the "not advantaged." Given this definition, one might argue that the "advantaged" have something (or many things) that the "disadvantaged" do not have, that these "have not's" should be given what the "have's" already possess, and then we shall all be equal. Certainly, matters are not that simple.

Defining the "disadvantaged" in terms of differences in social-class position adds some precision to the definition of "not advantaged." It identifies more clearly some of the characteristics on which the "have's" and the "have not's" differ: jobs, education, housing. A social-class definition thus specifies three dimensions of the limited social boundaries within which the lower-class child may move. The empirical implications of the social-class definition are not very different in substance, however, from the definition of "not advantaged." We have argued from our data that providing a lower-class family with what a middle-class family has— better jobs, education, and housing—will produce levels of mental ability resembling those of middle-class children. We thus provide equal education and social opportunities for equal development.

What happens, however, when we introduce ethnicity into our definition of "disadvantaged"? The consequences now change. It is no longer possible to follow the strategy of giving the "have not's" what "have's" possess; changing ethnic membership cannot be accomplished through the social decree of federal action programs. We know ethnic groups differ in patterns of ability no matter what the social-class level within the ethnic group, and our educational problem now becomes that of providing equal educational opportunity to all ethnic groups to maximize their development, even at the expense of magnifying differences among the groups.

The point for defining the term "disadvantaged" is clear. The many different meanings assigned to this label may have accumulated arbitrarily according to the idiosyncratic choices of the various users of the term. But it is not merely a matter of whose definition sounds most convincing, or elegant, or compassionate. Each definition brings different empirical results and suggests different implications for educational policy and social action. We cannot afford this confusion; we are forced to be clearer about our definitions and their educational and social consequences.

We began this paper by accepting the common definition of disadvantaged status based on gross environmental characteristics: social class and ethnicity. This definition of disadvantaged is strictly environmental and pre-assigned; it ignores the child's characteristics completely. It is a gross classification of children according to group membership only, and what we can learn about children by using this definition is usually expressed in terms of group tendencies (although we have suggested some techniques for moving from group data to individual analysis). Our suggestions for future research, both of developmental origins and school-based studies, direct us to some necessary refinements and extensions of these gross classifications.

Our recommendations for studies of developmental origins or environmental process analyses move us strongly in the direction of more precision and detail about environmental circumstances. Developmental research demands that a new definition of disadvantaged status be based on a much more refined assessment of environmental circumstances. Such an assessment would proceed far beyond the group characteristics we have dealt with in the past, specifying environmental circumstances which are closely articulated with developmental processes and which vary considerably within and across social-class and ethnic lines. Particular clusterings of environmental circumstances known to be related to developmental processes would lead to identification of disadvantaged status in more complex but precise terms.

Our discussions of school-based research suggest that disadvantaged status be expanded to include characteristics of the child. We refer now to assessments of children which are intimately connected with instructional objectives and procedures. From this point of view, a multiplicity of child attributes would have to be used to assess readiness for learning a variety of school tasks. Such measurements of readiness would give much power and operational substance to the concept of disadvantage.

We are therefore suggesting that an important advance in definition could be made by joining more precise descriptions of environments with instructionally-based assessments of child characteristics. Beginning with environmental characteristics and then assessing children's learning patterns would lead to one grouping of those we would class as disadvantaged; the other direction of attack, starting with child characteristics and then assessing environments, would lead to another grouping. The usefulness and desirability of each direction of approach must await both empirical and practical assessment. In either case, the lesson is clear: a new definition of "disadvantaged" should include psychologically-meaningful statements about the environment and the child. The complexity of such statements will reflect a plethora of constructs and if-then statements about child-environment interactions but will be a realistic reflection of the diversity and individuality of children and the lives they lead.

REFERENCES

ANASTASI, ANNE. *Differential psychology*. New York: Macmillan, 1958.

BEREITER, C.. et al. An academically-oriented preschool for culturally deprived children. Paper presented at AERA meeting, Chicago, Illinois, February, 1965.

BING, ELIZABETH. Effect of child-rearing practices on development of differential cognitive abilities. *Child Develpm.*, 1963, *34*, 631-648.

BLOOM, B. S. *Stability and change in human characteristics*. New York: Wiley, 1964.

BRAZZIEL, W. F. & TERRELL, MARY. An experiment in the development of readiness in a culturally disadvantaged group of first-grade children. *J. Negro Educ.*, 1962, *31*, 4-7.

BUSSAS, ANNE M. *From theory to the classroom.* Princeton, N. J.: Educational Testing Service, 1965.

CHARTERS, W. W. Social class and intelligence tests. In Charters, W. W. & Gage, N. L. (Eds.), *Readings in the social psychology of education.* Boston: Allyn & Bacon, 1963, 12-21.

COHEN, J. The factorial structure of the WISC at ages 7-6, 10-6, and 13-6. *J. consult. Psychol.*, 1959, *23*, 285-299.

COLEMAN, J. S. Equal schools or equal students? *The Public Interest*, 1966, *4*, 70-75.

COLEMAN, J. S. et al. *Equality of educational opportunity.* Washington, D. C.: U. S. Government Printing Office, 1966.

DAVE, R. H. The identification and measurement of environmental process variables that are related to educational achievement. Unpublished doctoral dissertation, Univer. of Chicago, 1963.

DAVIS, A. *Social class influences on learning.* Cambridge, Mass.: Harvard Univer. Press, 1948.

DEUTSCH, M. Minority group and class status as related to social and personality factors in scholastic achievement. *Applied Anthropology Monograph*, No. 2, Ithaca, N. Y., 1960.

DEUTSCH, M. & BROWN, B. Social influences in Negro-white intelligence differences. *J. soc. Issues*, 1964, *20*, 24-35.

DEUTSCH, M., FISHMAN, J., KOGAN, L., NORTH, R., & WHITMAN, M. Guidelines for testing minority group children. *J. soc. Issues*, 1964, *20*, 129-145.

DREGER, R. M. & MILLER, K. S. Comparative psychological studies of Negroes and whites in the United States. *Psychol. Bull.*, 1960, *57*, 361-402.

DUNCANSON, J. P. Learning and measured abilities. *J. educ. Psychol.*, 1966, *57*, 220-229.

EELLS, K. W., et al. *Intelligence and cultural differences.* Chicago: Univer. of Chicago Press, 1951.

FOWLER, W. L. A comparative analysis of pupil performance on conventional and culture-controlled mental tests. *Fourteenth Yearb. Nat. Council on Measmts. in Educ.* Princeton, N. J.: 1957, 8-20.

GAGNE, R. M. Contributions of learning to human development. Address of the Vice-President, Section I—Psychology, Amer. Assoc. for the Advancemt. Sci., Washington, D. C., December, 1966.

GORDON, E. W. Characteristics of socially disadvantaged children. *Rev. educ. Res.*, 1965, *35*, 377-388.

GRAY, SUSAN W. & KLAUS, R. A. An experimental preschool program for culturally deprived children. *Child Develpm.*, 1965, *36*, 887-898.

GUILFORD, J. P. Three faces of intellect. *Amer. Psychologist*, 1959, *14*, 469-479.

GUTHRIE, M. Structure of abilities in a non-Western culture. *J. educ. Psychol.*, 1963, *54*, 94-103.

HAGGARD, E. A. Social status and intelligence: an experimental study of certain cultural determinants of measured intelligence. *Genet. Psychol. Monogr.*, 1954, *49*, 141-186.

HAVIGHURST, R. J. Who are the socially disadvantaged? *J. Negro Educ.*, 1964, *33*, 210-217.

HAVIGHURST, R. J. & BREESE, F. H. Relation between ability and social status in a mid-western community: III. Primary mental abilities. *J. educ. Psychol.*, 1947, *38*, 241-247.

HAVIGHURST, R. J. & JANKE, L. L. Relation between ability and social status in a mid-western community: I. Ten-year-old children. *J. educ. Psychol.*, 1944, *35*, 357-368.

HESS, R. D. & SHIPMAN, VIRGINIA. Cognitive environment of urban pre-school children. *Progress report.* Urban Child Center, Univer. of Chicago, 1963.

HESS, R. D. & SHIPMAN, VIRGINIA. Early experience and the socialization of cognitive modes in children. *Child Develpm.*, 1965, *36*, 869-886.

HIGGINS, C. & SIVERS, CATHRYNE M. A comparison of the Stanford-Binet and the Colored Raven Progressive Matrices IQ's for children with low socio-economic status. *J. consult. Psychol.*, 1958, *22*, 465-468.

HUNT, J. McV. *Intelligence and experience.* New York: Ronald Press, 1961.

JACKSON, J. D., HESS, R. D., & SHIPMAN, VIRGINIA. Communication styles in teachers: an experiment. Paper presented at AERA meeting, Chicago, February, 1965.

JENSEN, A. R. Learning abilities in Mexican-American and Anglo-American children. *Calif. J. educ. Res.*, 1961, *12*, 147-159.

JENSEN, A. R. Varieties of individual differences in learning. In Gagné, R. M. (Ed.), *Learning and individual differences.* Columbus, Ohio: Charles E. Merrill, 1967 (a).

JENSEN, A. R. Social class, race, genes and educational potential. Paper presented at AERA meetings, New York, February, 1967 (b).

JOHN, VERA P. The intellectual development of slum children: some preliminary findings. *Amer. J. Orthopsychiat.*, 1963, *33*, 813-822.

KARNES, MERLE B., ZEHRBACH, R. R., STUDLEY, W. M., & WRIGHT, W. R. Culturally disadvantaged children of higher potential: intellectual functioning and educational implications. Champaign, Ill.: Community Unit and Schools, September, 1965.

KARP, JOAN M. & SIGEL, I. Psychoeducational appraisal of disadvantaged children. *Rev. educ. Res.*, 1965, *35*, 401-412.

KOHLBERG, L. Stages in children's conceptions of physical and social objects in the years four to eight. Unpublished monograph, Univer. of Chicago, 1965.

LAURENDEAU, MONIQUE & PINARD, A. *Causal thinking in the child.* New York: International Univer. Press, 1962.

LESSER, G. S., FIFER, G., & CLARK, D. H. Mental abilities of children from different social-class and cultural groups. *Monogrs. Soc. for Res. in Child Develpm.*, 1965, *30*, (4).

LEWIS, HYLAN. Child rearing practices among low-income families in the District of Columbia. Paper presented at Nat. Conf. soc. Welfare, Minneapolis, May, 1961.

LORGE, I. Difference or bias in tests of intelligence. In Anne Anastasi (Ed.), *Testing problems in perspective.* Washington, D. C.: Amer. Council on Educ., 1966.

LOVINGER, R. J., HARRIS, A. J. & COHEN, J. Factor analysis of intellectual performance in disadvantaged Negro adolescents. Paper presented at AERA meeting, Chicago, February, 1966.

McCABE, ALICE R. The intellectually superior child in a deprived social area. *Progress Report,* Harlem Demonstration Center, Community Serv. Soc. of New York, 1964.

MacCARTHUR, R. S. & ELLEY, W. B. The reduction of socio-economic bias in intelligence testing. *Brit. J. educ. Psychol.*, 1963, *33*, 107-119.

MACKLER, B., CATALANA, THELMA P., & HOLMANN, W. D. The successful urban slum child: a psychological study of personality and academic success in deprived children. Unpublished Progress Report and prospectus, Columbia Univer., 1965.

MEYERS, C. E., DINGMAN, H. F., & ORPET, R. E. Four ability-factor hypotheses at three preliterate levels in normal and retarded children. *Monogrs. Soc. for Res. in Child Develpm.*, 1964, *29*, (5).

MILNER, ESTHER. A study of the relationship between reading readiness in grade-one schoolchildren and patterns of parent-child interactions. *Child Develpm.*, 1951, *22*, 95-122.

MONTAGUE, D. O. Arithmetic concepts of kindergarten children in contrasting socio-economic areas. *Elem. School J.*, 1964, *64*, 393-397.

OLIM, E. G., HESS, R. D. & SHIPMAN, VIRGINIA. Relationship between mothers' abstract language style and abstraction styles of urban pre-school children. Paper presented at the Midwest Psychological Association Meetings, Chicago, April, 1965.

OSBORNE, R. T. Racial differences in mental growth and school achievement: a longitudinal study. *Psychol. Rep.*, 1960, *7*, 233-239.

PASAMANICK, B. & KNOBLOCH, HILDA. Early language behavior in Negro children and the testing of intelligence. *J. abnorm. soc. Psychol.*, *50*, 401-402.

PAYNE, ARLENE. Early prediction of achievement. *Administrator's notebook*, 1964, *13*, (1).

PETERSON, R. A. & DEBORD, L. Educational supportiveness of the home and academic performance of disadvantaged boys. *IMRID Behavioral Sci. Monogr.*, George Peabody Coll., 1966, No. 3.

RAPIER, JACQUELINE. The learning abilities of normal and retarded children as a function of social class. Unpublished doctoral dissertation, Univer. of California, Berkeley, 1966.

ROHWER, W. D. Verbal and visual elaboration in paired-associate learning. *Project Literacy Rep.*, 1966, No. 7, 18-28.

SEMLER, I. J. & ISCOE, I. Comparative and developmental study of the learning abilities of Negro and white children under four conditions. *J. educ. Psychol.*, 1963, *54*, 38-44.

SEMLER, I. J. & ISCOE, I. Structure of intelligence in Negro and white children. *J. educ. Psychol.*, 1966, *57*, 326-336.

SILVERMAN, SUSAN. An annotated bibliography on education and cultural deprivation. In Bloom, B. S., Davis, A. & Hess, R. D., (Eds.) *Compensatory education for cultural deprivation*. New York: Holt, Rinehart, & Winston, 1965, 65-179.

SMEDSLUND, J. Concrete reasoning: a study of intellectual development. *Monogrs. Soc. for Res. in Child Develpm.*, 1964, *29*, No. 2.

SMILANSKY, SARAH. Progress report on a program to demonstrate ways of using a year of kindergarten to promote cognitive abilities, impart basic information, and modify attitudes which are essential for scholastic success of culturally deprived children in their first two years of school. Jerusalem, Israel: Henrietta Szold Institute, 1964.

STABLEIN, J. E., WILLEY, D. S., & THOMSON, C. W. An evaluation of the Davis-Eells Test using Spanish and Anglo-American children. *J. educ. Sociol.*, 1961, *35*, 73-79.

STEWART, L. H., DOLE, A. A., & HARRIS, Y. Y. Cultural differences in abilities during high school. *Amer. educ. Res. J.*, 1967, *4*, 19-30.

STODOLSKY, SUSAN S. Maternal behavior and language and concept formation in Negro pre-school children: an inquiry into process. Unpublished doctoral dissertation, Univer. of Chicago, 1965.

TATSUOKA, M. M. *Joint probability of membership and success in a group*. Cambridge, Mass.: Harvard Grad. School of Educ. Rep., 1957.

TERRELL, G., DURKIN, KATHRYN, & WIESLEY, M. Social class and the nature of incentive in discrimination learning. *J. abnorm. soc. Psychol.*, 1959, *59*, 270-272.

THOMAS, A., CHESS, STELLA, BIRCH, H. G., HERTZIG, MARGARET E., & KORN, S. *Behavioral individuality in early childhood*. New York: New York Univer. Press, 1964.

THURSTONE, THELMA G. *Learning to think series. Teacher's manual for play and learn. The red book*. Chicago: Science Research Associates, 1948.

WALLACH, M. A. Research on children's thinking. *NSSE Yearb.*, *62*, Part I. Chicago: Univer. of Chicago Press, 1963, 236-276.

WOLF, R. M. The measurement of environments. *Proceedings of 1964 Invitational Conf. on Testing Problems*. Princeton, N. J.: Educational Testing Service, 1965.

ZIGLER, E. Mental retardation: current issues and approaches. In Hoffman, M. L. & Hoffman, Lois W., (Eds.) *Review of child development research*, Vol. 2. New York: Russell Sage Foundation, 1966, 107-168.

ZIGLER, E. & DELABRY, J. Concept switching in middle-class, lower-class and retarded children. *J. abnorm. soc. Psychol.*, 1962, *65*, 267-273.

16

VIOLENCE IN GHETTO CHILDREN

Robert Coles, M.D.

Harvard University Health Services

When I worked as a child psychiatrist in a children's hospital, I spent most of my time with middle class children whose parents very often seemed earnest and sensitive; certainly they were worried about their children, at times excessively so. The boys and girls, for their part, were usually quiet and controlled. They were suffering from "school phobias" or the various fears and anxieties that have been described by a generation of psychiatrists. If they were disobedient and loud, usually it was a specific form of disobedience I saw, a very particular noisiness I heard, all connected to something they dreaded or dared not to look at. In a sense, then, the unruliness I noticed only confirmed my impression of a general restraint (emotional tidiness, I suppose it could be called) that middle class children by the time they are 2 or 3 years old are likely to have acquired, never to lose.

Yes, there are the usual signs of aggressive tendencies in the "latency years" (the years preceding puberty when sexual urges are quiescent)— the bold and even nasty games, the play that seems involuntarily brutish —until a long look reveals how curiously formal, even restrained, the unruliness of these children actually is. Despite all the "drives" one hears psychologists and psychiatrists talk about—the surges of desire, spite, and hate that continuously press upon the child's mind and in dreams or daytime fantasies gain control of it—the fact remains that by the time middle class American children first reach school, at age 5 or 6, they are remarkably in control of themselves. As a result, when the violence in such children erupts in a psychiatrist's office during a

Reprinted from CHILDREN, May-June 1967, Vol. 14, No. 3, pp. 101-104.

session of drawing or in the midst of a game played by the psychiatrist and the child, it is almost a caricature of violence—violence so safe, so exaggerated, so camouflaged, and so quarantined that the very word seems inappropriate.

We in psychiatry are often accused of seeing only the drab and morbid side of human nature. If it would be any comfort to people, I suppose we could easily make partial amends for that morbid bias by letting it be known how overwhelmingly law-abiding man is: if he is vindictive, he is likely to be so toward himself. Psychiatrists spend most of their time helping people take a look at violence removed enough from their own recognition to be, in effect, somebody else's property. If in time the patient, whether child or adult, owns up to what he secretly or temporarily senses, he will be in greater, not less, control of himself. Thus, I remember treating a 10-year-old boy who drew wild and vicious scenes, filled with fire and death or at least an injury or two. When I wanted to know about what was going on, he let me know the score rather quickly by pointing to the people in his pictures and saying, "I don't know, you'd have to ask them."

A DIFFERENT "BALL GAME"

Not everyone in America is brought up to disown violence so consistently that its very presence in his own drawings can be adroitly (that is, innocently) denied. In the past few years, as I have worked with children in both southern rural slums and northern "ghettos," I have come to appreciate how useless it is to think of, or judge, the growth and development of the children of the depressed poor in the same way I ordinarily view the development of middle class children. It is, as one boy in a Boston ghetto recently reminded me, "a different ball game when you're out in left field, instead of in there pitching."

If we consider what a child of the slums goes through, from birth on, and if we keep a special eye on what in his experience may make him "violent" even at the age of 7 or 8, we may well gain, rather than lose, respect for the upbringing he receives. In fact, I have seen how much childbearing means to poor women: it is the one thing *they* can do, and do creatively. It is the the one chance they have to show both themselves and others that there is hope in this world, as well as the next.

By pointing this out, I am not arguing against keeping families to a sensible size, nor overlooking the impulsive, dreary background that is also commonly associated with pregnancies among the poor, whether in or out of wedlock. I am simply saying to others what a mother once felt she had to let me know:

> They all tell us to cut down on the kids, cut down on the kids, because you can't keep up with them as it is, and even a few is too much if you're on welfare for life, the way we has to be, like it or not. I tries to cut down, and I want to, but it's not so easy. You have to watch your step all the time, and we can't afford the pills they have for others.
>
> Anyway, it's the one time in my life I really feel like I'm *somebody*, like I'm doing something. People come around and expect me to feel ashamed of myself, like I've done something wrong, and I'm adding to crime on the streets—that's all you hear these days, *our* crime, not anyone else's—but instead, I feel proud of myself, like I can at least make a baby, and maybe he'll have it better than us, who knows, though I doubt it.

If we want to help this woman keep her family small, I hope we also want to give her what she needs to feel like the somebody she still desires to be.

I know this woman's children, and already I have seen them readying themselves for what their mother herself calls "the goddam street." Each one of those children has been held and breast fed in ways I think some middle class mothers might have cause to envy. The flat is cold and rat infested, but there is real and continuing warmth between that mother and her babies. "Symbiotic" some of my colleagues—who have a name for everything—might call the relationship of that mother and her children; it is also a bond that unites the fearful and hungry against the inevitable day when the home has to yield to the outside.

PREPARATION FOR THE STREET

Slum children do not go unprepared when that time comes, contrary to the assumptions of some social critics who can only see the life of the poor as aimless, neglected, and always "deprived." Chances are these children receive specific and brutal instruction about the "realities" of life at the age of 2, 3, or 4 so that when they emerge from the home the police, the hoods, the addicts, the drunks are already familiar, and what happens in the schools or on playgrounds is not disappointing but expected. The mother I have already quoted has also testified to the morality and lawfulness she tries to inspire in her children:

> I don't know how to do it. I don't know how to keep my kids from geting stained and ruined by everything outside. I keep them

close to me, and sometimes I feel like everything will be O.K., because they know how much I want for it to be, and they'll go make it be, the way I thought I could. But after a while they want to go out. You know how a kid is when he's 3 or 4, he wants to *move*, no matter where, so long as he keeps going. And where can he move in here? So I let them go, and I stop and say a prayer every morning, and ask for them to be saved, but I have to say it, I'm not expecting my prayers to be answered, not around here, I know.

And when the kids come back upstairs, I give them a look, if I have the time, to see what's on their face, and what they've learned that'll make a mess of everything I try to teach. And I can tell—I can tell from day to day what's getting into them. You know what it is? It's the Devil and he tells them to give up, because there's no other choice, not around here there isn't.

She is a churchgoing woman, as are many of her neighbors. I have found that she knows her Bible better than I or my neighbors, and in fact she doubtless puts more store in prophetic, messianic Christianity than most Americans do. When her children start walking and talking, she starts teaching them rules and fears—enough of both to satisfy anyone who is worried about the decline of "morality" in America. At least in that home, and others like it I have visited, children are not allowed free reign. Instead they are told to obey, and they are swiftly slapped or punched if they falter.

Over the years I have learned how loyal slum families can be to America's ethic of "rugged individualism." Children are taught through the ubiquitous television to seek after all the products of our proud technology: the cars that can speed faster than any law allows; the records and clothes whose worth can only be seasonal; the bright and shiny places to frequent; the showy, gadget-filled places that not only shelter people but also make statements about their power, influence, and bank accounts. At 5 and 6 years old, ghetto children in today's America share through television a world quite similar to the one known by their wealthy age-mates. I find it almost unnerving when I see drawings from a child not yet old enough to attend school that show the appetites and yearnings our advertisers are able to arouse. Precisely what do such children do with such wishes and fantasies, besides spell them out on paper for someone like me?

IN SCHOOL

When a child of 6 or 7 from the ghetto meets up with the politics of the street or the schoolyard, he brings along both the sensual and the fearfully moral experience he has had at home. Slum children live at close quarters to their parents and their brothers or sisters. They are often allowed to be very much on their own, very free and active, yet they are also punished with a vengeance when distracted or forlorn parents suddenly find an issue forced, a confrontation inevitable. They face an ironic mixture of indulgence and fierce curtailment.

Such children come to school prepared to be active, vigorous, perhaps much more outgoing on an average than middle class children. But they are quick to lose patience, sulk, feel wrong and wronged and cheated by a world they have already learned to be impossible, uncertain, and contradictory. Here are the words of an elementary-school teacher who has worked in a northern ghetto for 3 years and still feels able to talk about the experience with hope as well as bitter irony:

> They're hard to take these kids, because they're not what you think when you first come, but they're not what you'd like for them to be either. (I don't mean what I *used* to like for them to be, but what I want for them now.) They're fast and clever, and full of life. That was the hardest thing for me to realize—that a boy or girl in the ghetto isn't a hopeless case, or someone who is already a delinquent when he comes into the first grade. The misconceptions we have in the suburbs are fantastic, really, as I think back—and remember what I used to think myself.

> I expected to find children who had given up, and were on the way to fail, or to take dope, or something like that. Instead it was in a lot of ways a breath of fresh air, talking with them and teaching them. They were friendlier, and they got along better with one another. I didn't have to spend half the year trying to encourage the children to be less competitive with one another. We don't call middle class children "culturally deprived," but sometimes I wonder. They're so nervous and worried about everything they say—what it will mean, or what it will cost them, or how it will be interpreted. That's what they've learned at home, and that's why a lot of them are tense kids, and, even worse, stale kids, with frowns on their faces at ages 6 or 7.

> Not a lot of the kids I teach now. They're lively and active, so active I don't know how to keep up with them. They're not active learners, at least learners of the knowledge I'm trying to sell them, but they're active and they learn a lot about the world, about one another. In fact, one of the big adjustments I've had to make is realizing that these kids learn a lot from one another. They are smart about things my kids will never understand. They just don't think school is worth a damn. To them it's part of a big outside world that has a grip on them, and won't let them get any place, no matter how hard they try. So what's the use, they ask themselves;

and the answer is that there isn't any use—so they go right on marking time in class until they can get out.

We teachers then figure they're stupid, or they're hopelessly tough and "delinquent," or their homes are so bad they'll always be "antisocial" or "incorrigible." I've found that when they're playing and don't know I'm looking they are different kids—spontaneous, shrewd, very smart, and perceptive. Then we go back into the classroom, and it's as though a dense fog has settled in on all of us. They give me a dazed look, or a stubborn, uncooperative one, and they just don't do anything, unless forced to—by being pushed and shoved and made to fear the authority they know I have.

We have compared notes many times, this teacher and I. One child we both know is a boy of 8 who does very poor work in school. He is a belligerent child, a troublemaker. I see him in his home because his brother is going to a predominantly white suburban school, one of the very few children in the neighborhood who does. Their mother, living on public assistance with six children and no husband, has her hands full. She finds her "difficult child" smarter than her "model" one, the boy I watch riding a bus that takes him away from the ghetto.

The teacher and I agree, the "difficult boy" is a smart boy, but an impatient, agile, and provocative boy. He is headed for trouble, but as I talk with him I find *myself* in trouble. I have asked him to draw pictures—of himself, of his school, of his home, of anything he wishes. I get from him devastating portrayals: schools that look like jails; teachers whose faces show scorn or drowsiness; streets and homes that are as awful to see on paper as they are in real life; "outsiders" whose power and mercenary hostility are all too obvious; and, everywhere, the police, looking for trouble, creating trouble, checking up, hauling people to court, calling them names, getting ready to hurt them, assault them, jail them, and beat them up—even if they are children.

Once I asked the boy whether he *really* thought the police would hurt someone of his age. He said: "To the cops, everyone around here is a little bad boy, no matter how old he is or how many grandchildren he has around."

At moments like that my psychiatric, categorical mind finds itself stunned and for a change ready to grant that boy and others like him freedom from the various diagnostic, explanatory, or predictive schemes people like me learn so well and find to be (in our world) so useful.

AN IMPOSSIBLE SITUATION

I often find welfare workers as well as the police present in the pictures ghetto children draw. They stand near the police like dogs, caricatures of themselves, with huge piercing eyes, ears that seem as twisted as they are oversize, and mouths either noticeably absent or present as thin lines enclosing prominent and decidedly pointed and ragged teeth. To ghetto children, as to their parents, the welfare worker is the policeman's handmaiden, and together they come, as one child put it, "to keep us in line, or send us away."

I have listened to public welfare workers and their "clients" talk, and I recognize the impossible situation they both face, the worker often as insulted as the family he visits by the rules and regualtions they must contend with—and find a way around. I often compare the relationship between the workers and their clients with one that develops in psychotherapy as for a while powerful forces pull both doctor and patient backward in time toward those early years when parents check up on children, trying to keep them on the right side of a "line" that constantly puzzles the child and perhaps also the parent more than she or he realizes.

One welfare worker recently summarized the situation for me:

> They behave like evasive kids, always trying to avoid getting caught, for this or that. And me, I'm like a child myself, only an older one—always trying to take care of my poor brothers and sisters, but also trying to get them in trouble or find them in trouble, so I can squeal on them.

No wonder I encounter anger, frustration, and violence in ghetto children. Everywhere things go wrong: the lights don't work; the stairs are treacherous; rats constantly appear, and they are not timid; uniformed men patrol the streets, certain that trouble will appear; teachers work in schools they are ashamed to call their own, at work they judge hopeless, under a bureaucratic system that stifles them, that is, if they are still alive; jobs are few, and "welfare" is the essence of the economy.

Yet—and I am writing this article chiefly to say so—the ghetto does not kill its young children. That perhaps comes later, at age 12 or 14, when idleness becomes a way of life, when jobs are nowhere to be had. For a while, during the first decade of their existence, ghetto children huddle together, learn about the world they have inherited, and go on to explore it, master its facts, accept its fate, and burn from day to day their inner energy and life, able for a while to ignore the alien outside world.

I find in these children a vitality, an exuberance, that reminds me often of the fatally ill I once treated on hospital wards: for a long time they appear flushed with life, even beautiful, only to die. I remember hearing from a distinguished physician who supervised a few of us who were interns: "They're fighting the battle of tuberculosis, and they're going to lose, but not without a brilliant flash of energy. It's a shame we can't intervene, right at the critical moment, and help them win."

He, of course, had the faith that some day medicine would intervene —with one or another saving treatment. Ghetto people have no such confidence, and I am afraid that I, at least today, share their outlook.

17

FAMILIAL MENTAL RETARDATION:
A Continuing Dilemma

Edward Zigler

*Associate Professor in the Department of Psychology and the
Child Study Center, Yale University, New Haven, Connecticut.*

The past decade has witnessed renewed interest in the problem of
mental retardation. The interest has resulted in vigorous research activity and the construction of a number of theories which attempt an
explanation of attenuated intellectual functioning. However, much of
the research and many of the theoretical efforts in the area appear to
be hampered by a variety of conceptual ambiguities. Much of this
ambiguity is due to the very heterogeneity of phenomena included
within the rubric of intellectual retardation. A portion of this ambiguity
also appears to be the product of many workers' general conceptual
orientation to the area of mental retardation.

The typical textbook pictures the distribution of intelligence as
normal or Gaussian in nature, with approximately the lowest 3 percent
of the distribution encompassing the mentally retarded (see Fig. 1a).
A homogeneous class of persons is thus constructed, a class defined by
intelligence-test performance which results in a score between 0 and 70.
This schema has misled many laymen and students, and has subtly influenced the approach of experienced workers in the area. For if one
fails to appreciate the arbitrary nature of the 70-I.Q. cutoff point, it is
but a short step to the formulation that all persons falling below this
point compose a homogeneous class of "subnormals," qualitatively dif-

Reprinted from SCIENCE, Vol. 155, pp. 292-298, Jan. 20, 1967. Copyright 1967 by the
American Association for the Advancement of Science.

ferent from persons having a higher I.Q. The view that mental retardates comprise a homogeneous group is seen in numerous research
studies in which comparisons are made between retardates and normal
individuals with the two groups defined solely on the basis of an I.Q.
classification.

This practice gives rise to a "difference," or "defect," orientation to
mental retardation. Such an approach historically included the notion
of moral defect and had many origins, ranging from the belief that
retardates were possessed by a variety of devils to the empirical evidence
of the higher incidence among them of socially unacceptable behaviors,
such as crime and illegitimacy. More recently, the notion of defect has
referred to defects in either physical or cognitive structures. This defect
approach has one unquestionably valid component. There is a sizable
group of retardates who suffer from any of a variety of known physical
defects. For example, mental retardation may be due to a dominant gene,
as in epiloia; to a single recessive gene, as in gargoylism, phenylketonuria, and amaurotic idiocy; to infections, such as congenital syphilis, encephalitis, or rubella in the mother; to chromosomal defects, as in
mongolism: to toxic agents, as in retardation caused by radiation in
utero, lead poisoning, or Rh incompatibility; and to cerebral trauma.

The diverse etiologies noted above have one factor in common; in
every instance, examination reveals an abnormal physiological process.
Persons who are retarded as a result of an abnormal physiological process
are abnormal in the orthodox sense, since they suffer from a known
physiological defect. However, in addition to this group, which forms a
minority of all retardates, there is the group labeled "familial"—or,
more recently, "cultural-familial"—which compromises approximately
75 percent of all retardates. This group presents the greatest mystery
and has been the object of the most heated disputes in the area of mental
retardation. The diagnosis of familial retardation is made when an
examination reveals none of the physiological manifestations noted
above, and when retardation of this same type exists among parents,
siblings, or other relatives. Several writers have extended the defect
notion to this type of retardate as well, although they differ as to what
they propose as the specific nature of the defect. On the basis of differences in performance between retardates and normals on some experimental task, rather than on the basis of physiological evidence, they
have advanced the view that all retardates suffer from some specifiable
defect over and above their general intellectual retardation.

Some order can be brought to the area of mental retardation if a distinction is maintained between physiologically defective retardates, with

retardation of known etiology, and familial retardates, with retardation of unknown etiology. For the most part, work with physiologically defective retardates involves investigation into the exact nature of the underlying physiological processes, with prevention or amelioration of the physical and intellectual symptoms as the goal. Jervis[1] has suggested that such "pathological" mental deficiency is primarily in the domain of the medical sciences, whereas familial retardation represents a problem to be solved by behavioral scientists, including educators and behavioral geneticists. Diagnostic and incidence studies of these two types of retardates have disclosed certain striking differences. The retardate having an extremely low I.Q. (below 40) is almost invariably of the physiologically defective type. Familial retardates, on the other hand, are almost invariably mildly retarded, usually with I.Q.'s above 50. This difference in the general intellectual level of the two groups of retardates is an important empirical phenomenon that supports the two-group approach to mental retardation, the approach supported in this article.

A TWO-GROUP APPROACH

Hirsch[2] has asserted that we will not make much headway in understanding individual differences in intelligence, and in many other traits, unless we recognize that, to a large degree, such differences reflect the inherent biological properties of man. We can all agree that no genotype spells itself out in a vacuum, and that the phenotypic expression is finally the result of environment interacting with the genotype. However, an appreciation of the importance of genetic differences allows us to bring considerable order to the area of mental retardation.

We need simply to accept the generally recognized fact that the gene pool of any population is such that there will always be variations in the behavioral or phenotypic expression of virtually every measurable trait or characteristic of man. From the polygenic model advanced by geneticists, we deduce that the distribution of intelligence is characterized by a bisymmetrical bell-shaped curve, which is characteristic of such a large number of distributions that we have come to refer to it as the normal curve. With the qualification noted below, this theoretical distribution is a fairly good approximation of the observed distribution of intelligence. In the polygenic model of intelligence,[2-4] the genetic foundation of intelligence is not viewed as dependent upon a single gene. Rather, intelligence is viewed as the result of a number of discrete genetic units. (This is not to assert, however, that single gene effects are never encountered in mental retardation. As noted above, certain relatively rare types of mental retardation are the product of such simple genetic effects.)

Various specific polygenic models have been advanced which generate theoretical distributions of intelligence that are in keeping with observed distributions.[3, 5, 6] An aspect of polygenic models of special importance for the two-group approach is the fact that they generate I.Q. distributions of approximately 50 to 150. Since an I.Q. of approximately 50 appears to be the lower limit for familial retardates, it has been concluded[4, 5, 7] that the etiology of this form of retardation reflects the same factors that determine "normal" intelligence. With this approach, the familial retardate may be viewed as normal, where "normal" is defined as meaning an integral part of the distribution of intelligence that we would expect from the normal manifestations of the genetic pool in our population. Within such a framework it is possible to refer to the familial retardate as less intelligent than other normal manifestations of the genetic pool, but he is just as integral a part of the normal distribution as are the 3 percent of the population whom we view as superior, or the more numerous group of individuals whom we consider to be average.[8]

The two-group approach to mental retardation calls attention to the fact that the second group of retardates, those who have known physiological defects, represents a distribution of intelligence with a mean which is considerably lower than that of the familial retardates. Such children, for the most part, fall outside the range of normal intelligence— that is, below I.Q. of 50—although there are certain exceptions. Considerable clarity could be brought to the area of mental retardation through doing away with the practice of conceptualizing the intelligence distribution as a single, continuous, normal curve. Perhaps a more appropriate representation of the empirical distribution of intelligence would involve two curves, as Fig. 1b illustrates. The intelligence of the bulk of the population, including the familial retardate, would be depicted as a normal distribution having a mean of 100, with lower and upper limits of approximately 50 and 150, respectively. Superimposed on this curve would be a second, somewhat normal distribution having a mean of approximately 35 and a range from 0 to 70. (That the population encompassed by the second curve in Fig. 1b extends beyond the 70-I.Q. cutoff point is due to the fact that a very small number of individuals with known defects—for example, brain damage—may be found throughout the I.Q. continuum.) The first curve would represent the polygenic distribution of intelligence; the second would represent all those individuals whose intellectual functioning

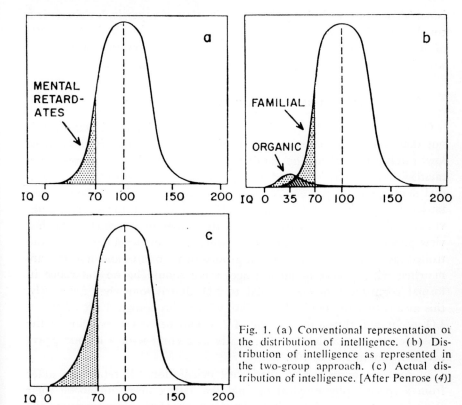

Fig. 1. (a) Conventional representation of the distribution of intelligence. (b) Distribution of intelligence as represented in the two-group approach. (c) Actual distribution of intelligence. [After Penrose (4)]

reflects factors other than the normal polygenic expression—that is, those retardates having an identifiable physiological defect. This two-group approach to the problem of mental retardation has been supported by Penrose,[4] Roberts,[9] and Lewis.[10] The very nature of the observed distribution of I.Q.'s below the mean, especially in the range of 0 to 50 (see Fig. 1c), seems to demand such an approach. This distribution, in which we find an overabundance of individuals at the very low I.Q. levels, is exactly what we would expect if we combined the two distributions discussed above, as is the general practice.

Limitations of space prevent consideration here of the controversy concerning the role of environmental factors in the etiology of familial retardation. Although such factors cannot be ignored by the serious student of mental retardation, the general dispute, discussed below, between adherents of the defect theory and of the general developmental theory can be examined somewhat independently of the environmental issue. That there will always be a distribution of a particular shape is a conclusion inherent in the polygenic argument, but the absolute amounts of intelligence represented by the various points on the distribution would still depend in large part on environmental factors.

DEVELOPMENTAL VERSUS DEFECT ORIENTATION

Once one adopts the position that the familial mental retardate is not defective or pathological but is essentially a normal individual of low intelligence, then the familial retardate no longer represents a mystery but, rather, is viewed as a particular manifestation of the general developmental process. According to this approach, the familial retardate's cognitive development differs from that of the normal individual only in respect to its rate and the upper limit achieved. Such a view generates the expectation that, when rate of development is controlled, as is grossly the case when groups of retardates and normals are matched with respect to mental age, there should be no difference in formal cognitive processes related to I.Q. Stated somewhat differently, this means that the familial retardate with a chronological age of 10, an I.Q. of 70, and thus a mental age of 7, would be viewed as being at the same developmental level intellectually as a child with a chronological age of 7 and an I.Q. of 100.

In contrast, according to the defect orientation, all retardates suffer from a specific physiological or cognitive defect over and above their slower general rate of cognitive development. This view generates the expectation that, even when the rate of cognitive development is controlled, as in the situation where mental ages are matched, differences in intellectual functioning which are related to I.Q. will be found. On their face, the repeated findings of differences in performance between groups of normals and retardates matched as to mental age have lent credence to the defect theory and have cast doubt on the validity of the developmental theory.

The developmental theorist's response to these frequently reported differences has been to point out that performance on any experimental task is not inexorably the product of the subject's cognitive structure alone but reflects a variety of emotional and motivational factors as well. To the developmentalist, then, it seems more reasonable to attribute differences in performance between normals and retardates of the same mental age to motivational differences which do not inhere in mental retardation but are, rather, the result of the particular histories of the retarded subjects.

It should be noted that most theories in the area of mental retardation are basically defect theories. These differ among themselves, however. A major difference involves the theoretician's effort to relate the postulated defect to some specific physiological structure. The theoretical language of some theoreticians is explicitly physiological, that of others is non-physiological, while that of others remains vague. Particular defects that have been attributed to the retarded include the following: relative impermeability of the boundaries between regions in the cognitive structure[11, 12]; primary and secondary rigidity caused by subcortical malformations, respectively[13]; inadequate neural satiation related to brain modifiability or cortical conductivity[14]; malfunctioning disinhibitory mechanisms[15]; improper development of the verbal system, resulting in a dissociation between verbal and motor systems[16, 17]; relative brevity in the persistence of the stimulus trace[18]; and impaired attention-directing mechanisms.[19]

Where the hypothesized defect is an explicit physiological one, it would appear to be a simple matter to obtain direct evidence that the defect does or does not exist. Such evidence would come from biochemical and physiological analyses as well as from pathological studies of familial retardates. A number of such studies have, of course, been carried out. Although there is an occasional report of some physical anomaly, the bulk of the evidence has indicated that the familial retardate does not suffer from any gross physiological defects. Indeed, if such evidence were readily available the defect theorist would cease relying on the more ambiguous data provided by studies of molar behavior. Failure to find direct evidence of a physiological defect in familial retardates has not deterred and should not deter theorists from postulating such defects.

In spite of the negative physiological evidence, workers such as Spitz[14] maintain that all retardates, including familial retardates, are physically defective, and that our failure to discover defects in familial retardates is due to the relatively primitive nature of our diagnostic techniques. This view is bolstered by Masland,[20] who has also noted the inadequacies of such techniques. It is perfectly legitimate for the defect theorist to assert that, although not at present observable, the physical defect that causes familial retardates to behave differently from normals of the same mental age will someday be seen. These theorists operate very much as the physicists of a not-too-distant era did when they asserted that the electron existed even though it was not directly observable. Analogously, defect theorists in the area of mental retardation undertake to validate the existence of a defect by first asserting that it should manifest itself in particular phenomena—that is, in particular behaviors of the retarded—and then devising experiments in which, if the predicted behavior is observed, the existence of the hypothesized defect is confirmed. Not only is this approach legitimate but, as noted above, it has become increasingly popular as well. A relatively comprehensive review of the literature emanating from the general defect position is now available.[21] In the following paragraphs I briefly summarize the major defect positions.

An influential defect position is that of the Russian investigator A. R. Luria,[16] whose work has now also influenced investigators in England and the United States. In the Soviet Union no distinction is made between retardates having known organic impairment and that larger group whose retardation is of unknown etiology, nor are genetic or cultural factors considered to be determinants of mental retardation. All grades of mental retardation are attributed to central-nervous-system damage believed to have occurred initially during the intrauterine period or during early childhood. Thus the diagnosis of mental retardation necessarily involves specification of a defect in some neurophysiological system; in fact, in the Soviet Union, professionals who work with the mentally retarded are called "defectologists."

Luria's interest in defective functioning appears to be an outgrowth of his more basic concern with the development of the higher cognitive processes in man. The influence of both Vygotsky and Pavlov may be seen in his work, which has been primarily concerned with the highly intricate development of the role of speech and language in regulating the child's behavior. In his comparisons between normal and retarded children, Luria has demonstrated that the behavior of retardates resembles that of chronologically younger normal children in that verbal instructions do not result in smooth regulation of motor behavior. Luria has found that retarded subjects have considerable difficulty with tasks requiring verbal mediation. Thus, Luria has inferred that the major defect in the retarded child involves an underdevelopment or a general "inertness" of the verbal system, and a dissociation of this system from the motor or action system. This dissociation is vaguely conceptualized as resulting from a disturbance in normal cortical activity.

The view that the behavior of a retardate resembles that of a chronologically younger child is, of course, consistent with the general developmental position. However, several English and American investigators[17, 22] have demonstrated that, even with mental age level controlled, retardates have more difficulty on tasks requiring verbal mediation than normal subjects have. On the other hand, other such investigations have failed to provide support for Luria's position.[23] To date, findings related to this position can best be described as equivocal.

Another major defect position is that of Herman Spitz,[14] who has extended the Köhler-Wallach[24] cortical satiation theory to the area of mental retardation. According to Spitz, all retardates suffer from inadequate neural or cortical functioning; the inadequacy is best characterized by a certain sluggishness, or less-than-normal modifiability, in the functioning of cortical cells. Thus, Spitz believes that in retardates it takes longer to induce temporary, as well as permanent, electrical, chemical, and physical changes in stimulated cortical cells, and furthermore, that once such a change is produced, it is less readily modified than in the case of normal persons.

Spitz's evidence in support of his theory has come primarily from comparisons of the performance of retardates and normals of the same chronological age on a variety of perceptual tasks—for example, figural after-effects and Necker-cube reversals. The heuristic value of Spitz's position may be seen in his recent efforts to extend his postulates beyond the visual perception area and employ them to generate specific predictions concerning the phenomena of learning transposition, generalization, and problem solving. The evidence in favor of Spitz's position is far from clear-cut, however. Spivack[25] has pointed out that Spitz's findings are in marked contrast to those of other investigators. The very nature of many of Spitz's measures—for example, a verbal report—raises the troublesome issue of how well they reflect the perceptual responses being investigated. It should be noted that, in respect to this point as well as to other criticisms, Spitz himself has become one of the most cogent critics of his own efforts.

Many of Spitz's findings could be encompassed by the general developmental position. The developmental theorist would argue that it is not surprising that one gets different results for normals and for retardates matched with respect to chronological age, since such groups are at different developmental levels (as defined by mental age). One would be tempted to say that Spitz's work has little relevance to the issue of whether familial retardates suffer from a defect over and above their slower and more limited rate of cognitive development. However, Spitz has been quite explicit in his views that the differences he obtains are not developmental phenomena but reflect a physical deficit that should manifest itself even in comparisons with normal subjects matched in mental age to the retardates.

Ellis[18] has also advanced the view that the retardate is basically different from the normal individual and that this difference is a result of central-nervous-system pathology from which all retardates suffer. Ellis views this central-nervous-system pathology as producing a short-term memory deficit which, in turn, underlies the inadequacy of much of the retardate's behavior. The theoretical model presented by Ellis includes two major constructs, stimulus trace and neural integrity.

The stimulus trace, the mechanism underlying short-term memory functions, is conceptualized as a neural event or response which varies with the intensity, duration, and meaning of the stimulus situation confronting the subject. The stimulus-trace construct is thus anchored to stimulus characteristics on the one hand and to the subject's responses to these characteristics on the other. The neural-integrity construct is conceptualized as the determinant of the nature of stimulus-trace activity, and is defined by "measures of behavioral adequacy." The typical measure of neural integrity employed by Ellis is the I.Q. Thus, a person of low I.Q. is said to suffer from a lack of neural integrity. This lack, in turn, delimits or restricts stimulus-trace activity, and such restriction results in a variety of inadequate behaviors.

In support of this theory, Ellis has noted findings from numerous experiments involving short-term retention phenomena. These include studies on serial learning, delayed-reaction tasks, fixed-interval operant behavior, electroencephalographic investigations, reaction time, and factor analyses of the WISC test (the Wechsler Intelligence Scale for Children), as well as several studies of discrimination learning in brain-damaged animals.[18] In respect to his own experimental tests, Ellis's reliance on the I.Q. as the measure of neural integrity has produced two types of comparisons: comparison of retardates and normals of the same chronological age and comparison of retardates and normals of the same mental age. In either comparison Ellis's model would predict that the retardates would be inferior on tasks involving short-term retention, due to their lower I.Q. In general, the findings obtained with groups matched as to chronological age have supported Ellis's position, while those obtained with groups matched as to mental age have not.

It should be noted that the demonstration that retardates do less well than normals of the same chronological age on tasks requiring short-term memory is a somewhat circular undertaking. It is circular to the extent that a deficit in short-term memory would influence the I.Q. score itself through its effect on certain of the intelligence subtests—for example, the digit-span test. Again, it should be emphasized that the discovery of a difference between normals and retardates of the same chronological age is just as amenable to a general developmental interpretation as to the view that all retardates suffer from central-nervous-system pathology, since the mental age of such retardates is necessarily lower than that of normal subjects in the control group.

Perhaps the oldest of the more influential defect positions is the Lewin-Kounin[11, 12] formulation that familial retardates are inherently more "rigid" than normal individuals of the same mental age. This position differs from the others discussed above in that the defect is conceptualized as inhering in a hypothesized cognitive structure without reference or reduction to any specific physiological entities. By the term *rigidity,* Lewin and Kounin were referring not to behaviors, as such, but rather to characteristics of the cognitive structure. These theorists felt that the essential defect, in retardation, was the lowered capacity for dynamic rearrangement in the "psychical system." This "stiffness" in cognitive functioning was conceptualized as being due to the relative impermeability of the boundaries between cells or regions of the cognitive structure. *Rigidity,* then, referred primarily to the nature of these boundaries, and to the resulting degree of communication or fluidity between regions.

Principal support for this position was contained in a series of experiments conducted by Kounin,[11] in which he found differences between familial retardates and normals of the same mental age on a variety of tasks involving transfer phenomena, sorting, and concept-switching. Although the Lewin-Kounin position continues to receive some support,[26] a fairly sizable amount of work[27, 28] now indicates that the differences discovered by Kounin between retardates and normals of the same mental age were due to differences in motivational variables rather than to an inherent cognitive rigidity of the retardate.

Lewin and Kounin appear to be the only defect theorists who have dealt adequately with the problem of etiology, which becomes a crucial issue in the controversy over the two theories. Their formulation was limited to familial retardates, and only such retardates were employed in Kounin's experiments. The other defect theorists have tended to argue that the distinction between familial and organic retardates is misleading, and, as a result, they have used groups of retardates of both types in their experiments. This presents an almost insurmountable problem when one attempts to evaluate the degree to which any uncovered differences in behavior support the major theoretical premise which underlies most defect approaches. This premise, clearly seen in the work of Luria, Spitz, and Ellis, is that all retardates, familials and organics alike, suffer from some specifiable defect. However, until the etiological issue is attended to in the research design, there is no way of assessing how much of the revealed difference between normals and retardates of the same mental age is a product of the gross organic pathology known to exist in the organic retardates included in the retarded group and how much is a product of the defect thought by the defect theorists to exist in all retardates.

The general developmental approach is applicable only to the familial retardate, and this approach does not speak to the issue of differences discovered between normal children and organic retardates. The developmental theorist also believes that, even when a difference in behavior is found between normals and familial retardates of the same mental age, it need not be attributed to any defect which inheres in familial mental retardation. Such differences are viewed as the possible outcome of differences in a variety of motivational factors which exist between the two groups. A sampling of the literature which lends credence to this view follows.

MOTIVATIONAL AND EMOTIONAL FACTORS

The view of those of us who believe that many of the reported differences between retardates and normals of the same mental age are a result of motivational and emotional differences which reflects differences in environmental histories does not imply that we ignore the importance of the lower intelligence per se. In some instances the personality characteristics of the retarded individual will reflect environmental factors that have little or nothing to do with intellectual endowment. For example, many of the effects of institutionalization may be constant, regardless of the person's intelligence level. In other instances we must think in terms of an interaction; that is, a person with low intellectual ability will have certain experiences and develop certain behavior patterns differing from those of a person with greater intellectual endowment. An obvious example of this is the greater amount of failure which the retardate typically experiences. What must be emphasized is the fact that the behavior pattern developed by the retardate as a result of such a history of failure may not differ in kind or ontogenesis from patterns developed by an individual of normal intellect who, because of some environmental circumstance, also experiences an inordinate amount of failure. By the same token, if the retardate can somehow be guaranteed a history of greater success, we would expect his behavior to be more normal, regardless of his intellectual level. Within this framework, I now discuss several of the personality factors which have been known to influence the performance of the retarded.

It has become increasingly clear that our understanding of the performance of the institutionalized familial retardate will be enhanced if we consider the inordinate amount of social deprivation these individuals have experienced before being placed in institutions.[29, 30] A series of recent studies[30-34] has indicated that one result of such early deprivation is a heightened motivation to interact with a supportive adult. These studies suggest that, given this heightened motivation, retardates exhibit considerable compliance with instructions when the effect of such compliance is to increase or maintain the social interaction with the adult. These findings would appear to be consistent with the often-made observation that the retarded seek attention and desire affection.[35, 36]

Recent findings suggest that the preservation so frequently noted in the behavior of the retarded is primarily a function of these motivational factors rather than a result of inherent cognitive rigidity, as suggested by Lewin[12] and Kounin.[11] Evidence is now available indicating (i) that the degree of perseveration is directly related to the degree of deprivation the individual experienced before being institutionalized,[30] and (ii) that institutionalized children of normal intellect are just as perseverative as institutionalized retardates, while noninstitutionalized retardates are no more perseverative than noninstitutionalized children of normal intellect. [31, 32]

Although there is considerable evidence that social deprivation results in a heightened motivation to interact with a supportive adult, it appears to have other effects as well. The nature of these effects is suggested in observations of fearfulness, wariness, or avoidance of strangers on the part of retardates, or of suspicion and mistrust.[36, 37] The experimental work done by Zigler and his associates on the behavior of institutionalized retarded individuals has indicated that social deprivation results in both a heightened motivation to interact with supportive adults (a positive-reaction tendency) and a wariness of doing so (a negative-reaction tendency). The construct of a negative-reaction tendency has been employed to explain certain differences between retardates and normals reported by Kounin, differences that have heretofore been attributed to the greater cognitive rigidity of retarded individuals. For instance, it has been demonstrated[38] that, once the institutionalized familial retardate's wariness has been allayed, he becomes much more responsive than the normal individual to social reinforcement. Thus, a motivational rather than a cognitive factor would seem to underlie certain rather mysterious behavioral phenomena frequently observed in familial retardates—for example, a tendency to persist longer on the second of two highly similar tasks than on the first.

Both positive- and negative-reaction tendencies have been recently investigated in a series of studies, with children of normal intellect,[39] directed at further validation of the "valence position." Stated most simply, this position asserts that the effectiveness of an adult as a reinforcing agent depends upon the valence he has for the particular child whose behavior is being reinforced. (An adult's valence for a child refers to the degree to which that adult is sought or avoided by the child.) This valence is determined by the child's history of positive and negative experiences with adults. The studies noted above have produced considerable evidence that prior positive contacts between the child and the adult increase the adult's effectiveness as a reinforcer, while negative contacts decrease it. If the experimentally manipulated negative encounters in these experiments are viewed as experimental analogs of encounters institutionalized retardates actually have experienced, then the often-reported reluctance of such children to interact with adults and their wariness of such encounters become understandable. Thus it would appear that their relatively high negative-reactive tendency motivates them toward behaviors, such as withdrawal, that reduce the quality of their performance to a level lower than that which one would expect on the basis of their intellectual capacity alone.

Another factor frequently mentioned as a determinant in the performance of the retarded is their high expectancy of failure. This failure expectancy has been viewed as an outgrowth of a lifetime characterized by confrontations with tasks with which they are intellectually ill-equipped to deal. The work of Cromwell and his colleagues[40] has lent support to the general proposition that retardates have a higher expectancy of failure than normals have, and that this results in a style of problem-solving in which the retardate is much more highly motivated to avoid failure than to achieve success. However, the results of experimental work with retardates to investigate the success-failure dimension are still somewhat inconsistent, suggesting that even such a relatively simple proposition as this one is in need of further refinement.

Recent studies[31, 33, 41] have indicated that the many failures experienced by retardates generate a cognitive style of problem-solving characterized by outer-directedness. That is, the retarded child comes to distrust his own solutions to problems and therefore seeks guides to action in the immediate environment. This outer-directedness may explain the great suggestibility so frequently observed in the retarded child. Evidence has now been presented indicating that, relative to normals of the same mental age, the retarded child is more sensitive to verbal cues from an adult, is more imitative of the behavior of adults and of his peers, and does more visual scanning. Furthermore, certain findings[31] suggest that the noninstitutionalized retardate is more outer-directed in his problem solving than the institutionalized retardate is. This makes considerable sense if one remembers that the noninstitutionalized retardate lives in an environment that is not adjusted to his intellectual shortcomings and, therefore, probably experiences more failure than the institutionalized retardate.

Another nonintellective factor important in understanding the behavior of the retarded is the retardate's motivation to obtain various types of reinforcement. The social-deprivation work discussed indicates that retardates have an extremely strong desire for attention, praise, and encouragement. Several investigators[40, 42] have suggested that, in normal development, the effectiveness of attention and praise as reinforcers diminishes with maturity and is replaced by the reinforcement inherent in the awareness that one is correct. This latter type of reinforcer appears to serve primarily as a cue for self-reinforcement.

Zigler and his associates[27, 43, 44] have argued that various experiences in the lives of the retarded cause them to care less about being correct simply for the sake of correctness than normals of the same mental age. In other words, these investigators have argued that the position of various reinforcers in the reinforcer hierarchies of normal and of retarded children of the same mental age differ.

Clearest support for the view that the retardate cares much less about being correct than the middle-class child of normal intellect does is contained in a study by Zigler and deLabry.[43] These investigators found, as Kounin[11] did, that when the only reinforcement was the information that the child was correct, retardates were poorer on a concept-switching task than middle-class normal children of the same mental age. However, when Zigler and deLabry added another condition, reward with a toy of the child's choice for concept-switching, they found that the retardates performed as well as the middle-class normal children. Since the satisfaction of giving the correct response is the incentive typically used in experimental studies, one wonders how many of the differences in performance found between retardates and normals are actually attributable to differences in capacity rather than to differences in the values such incentives may have for the two types of subjects.

Much of this work on motivational and emotional factors in the performance of the retarded is very recent. The research on several of the factors discussed is more suggestive than definitive. It is clear, however, that these factors are extremely important in determining the retardate's level of functioning. This is not to assert that these motivational factors cause familial mental retardation but to say, rather, that they lead to the retardate's behaving in a manner less effective than that dictated by his intellectual capacity. An increase in knowledge concerning motivational and emotional factors and their ontogenesis and manipulation would hold considerable promise for alleviating much of the social ineffectiveness displayed by that rather sizable group of persons who must function at a relatively low intellectual level.

SUMMARY

The heterogeneous nature of mental retardation, as well as certain common practices of workers in the area, has resulted in a variety of conceptual ambiguities. Considerable order could be brought to the area if, instead of viewing all retardates as a homogeneous group arbitrarily defined by some I.Q. score, workers would clearly distinguish between the group of retardates known to suffer from some organic defect and the larger group of retardates referred to as familial retardates. It is the etiology of familial retardation that currently constitutes the greatest mystery.

A number of authorities have emphasized the need for employing recent polygenic models of inheritance in an effort to understand the familial retardate. While appreciating the importance of environment in affecting the distribution determined by genetic inheritance, these workers have argued that familial retardates are not essentially different from individuals of greater intellect, but represent, rather, the lower portion of the intellectual curve which reflects normal intellectual variability. As emphasized by the two-group approach, retardates with known physiological or organic defect are viewed as presenting a quite different etiological problem. The familial retardate, on the other hand, is seen as a perfectly normal expression of the population gene pool, of slower and more limited intellectual development than the individual of average intellect.

This view generates the proposition that retardates and normals at the same general cognitive level—that is, of the same mental age—are similar in respect to their cognitive functioning. However, such a proposition runs headlong into findings that retardates and normals of the same mental age often differ in performance. Such findings have bolstered what is currently the most popular theoretical approach to retarded functioning—namely, the view that all retardates suffer from some specific defect which inheres in mental retardation and thus makes the retardate immutably "different" from normals, even when the general level of intellectual development is controlled. While these defect or difference approaches, as exemplified in the work of Luria, Spitz, Ellis, and Lewin and Kounin, dominate the area of mental retardation, the indirect, and therefore equivocal, nature of the evidence of these workers has generated considerable controversy.

In contrast to this approach, the general developmental position has emphasized systematic evaluation of the role of experiential, motivational, and personality factors. As a central thesis, this position asserts that performance on experimental and real-life tasks is never the single inexorable product of the retardate's cognitive structure but, rather, reflects a wide variety of relatively nonintellective factors which greatly influence the general adequacy of performance. Thus, many of the reported behavioral differences between normals and retardates of the same mental age are seen as products of motivational and experiential differences between these groups, rather than as the result of any inherent cognitive deficiency in the retardates. Factors thought to be of particular importance in the behavior of the retardate are social deprivation and the positive- and negative-reaction tendencies to which such deprivation gives rise; the high number of failure experiences and the particular approach to problem-solving which they generate; and atypical reinforcer hierarchies.

There is little question that we are witnessing a productive, exciting, and perhaps inevitably chaotic period in the history of man's concern with the problem of mental retardation. Even the disagreements that presently exist must be considered rather healthy phenomena. These disagreements will unquestionably generate new knowledge which, in the hands of practitioners, may become the vehicle through which the performance of children, regardless of intellectual level, may be improved.

REFERENCES AND NOTES

1. G. A. JERVIS, in *American Handbook of Psychiatry*, S. Arieti, Ed. (Basic Books, New York, 1959), vol. 2, pp. 1289-1313.
2. J. HIRSCH, *Science 142*, 1436 (1963).
3. I. L. GOTTESMAN, in *Handbook of Mental Deficiency*, N. R. Ellis, Ed. (McGraw-Hill, New York, 1963), pp. 253-296.
4. L. S. PENROSE, *The Biology of Mental Defect* (Sidgwick and Jackson, London, 1963).
5. C. BURT and M. HOWARD, *Brit. J. Statist. Psychol. 9*, 95 (1956).
6. ————, *ibid. 10*, 33 (1957); C. C. Hurst, in *Proc. Roy, Soc. London Ser. B 112*, 80 (1932); R. W. Pickford, *J. Psychol. 28*, 129 (1949).
7. G. ALLEN, *Amer. J. Mental Deficiency 62*, 840 (1958); C. Burt, *Amer. Psychologist 13*, 1 (1958).
8. G. E. McCLEARN, in *Psychology in the Making*, L. Postman, Ed. (Knopf, New York, 1962), pp. 144-252.
9. J. A. F. ROBERTS, *Eugenics Rev. 44*, 71 (1952).

10. E. O. Lewis, *J. Mental Sci. 79*, 298 (1933).
11. J. Kounin, *Character and Personality 9*, 251 (1941); *ibid.*, p. 273.
12. K. Lewin, *A Dynamic Theory of Personality* (McGraw-Hill, New York, 1936).
13. K. Goldstein, *Character and Personality 11*, 209 (1942-43).
14. H. H. Spitz, in *Handbook of Mental Deficiency*, N. R. Ellis, Ed. (McGraw-Hill, New York, 1963), pp. 11-40.
15. P. S. Siegel and J. G. Foshee, *J. Abnormal Soc. Psychol. 61*, 141 (1960).
16. A. R. Luria, in *Handbook of Mental Deficiency*, N. R. Ellis, Ed. (McGraw-Hill, New York, 1963), pp. 353-387.
17. N. O'Connor and B. Hermelin, *J. Abnormal Soc. Psychol. 59*, 409 (1959).
18. N. R. Ellis, in *Handbook of Mental Deficiency*, N. R. Ellis, Ed. (McGraw-Hill, New York, 1963), pp. 134-158.
19. D. Zeaman and B. J. House, *ibid.*, p. 159.
20. R. L. Masland, *Amer. J. Mental Deficiency 64*, 305 (1959).
21. E. Zigler, in *Review of Child Development Research*, M. L. Hoffman and L. W. Hoffman, Eds. (Russell Sage Foundation, New York, in press), vol. 2.
22. N. A. Milgram and H. G. Furth, *Amer. J. Mental Deficiency 67*, 733 (1963); *ibid. 70*, 849 (1966).
23. D. Balla and E. Zigler, *J. Abnormal Soc. Psychol. 69*, 664 (1964); M. Rieber, *Amer. J. Mental Deficiency 68*, 634 (1964).
24. W. Kohler and H. Wallach, *Proc. Amer. Phil. Soc. 88*, 269 (1964).
25. G. Spivack, in *Handbook of Mental Deficiency*, N. R. Ellis, Ed. (McGraw-Hill, New York, 1963), pp. 480-511.
26. M. Budoff and W. Pagel, "Learning potential and rigidity in the adolescent mentally retarded," paper presented before the Society for Research in Child Development, Minneapolis, Minn., March 1965.
27. E. Zigler, in *Readings on the Exceptional Child*, E. P. Trapp and P. Himelstein, Eds. (Appleton-Century-Crofts, New York, 1962), pp. 141-162.
28. ———, in *International Review of Research in Mental Retardation*, N. R. Ellis, Ed. (Academic Press, New York, 1966), vol. 1, pp. 77-105.
29. A. D. B. Clarke and A. M. Clarke, *Brit. J. Psychol. 45*, 197 (1954); D. Kaplun, *Proc. Amer. Ass. Mental Deficiency 40*, 68 (1935).
30. E. Zigler, *J. Abnormal Soc. Psychol. 62*, 413 (1961).
31. C. Green and E. Zigler, *Child Develop. 33*, 499 (1962).
32. E. Zigler, *J. Personality 31*, 258 (1963).
33. ———, L. Hodgden, H. Stevenson, *ibid. 26*, 106 (1958).
34. R. Shepps and E. Zigler, *Amer. J. Mental Deficiency 67*, 262 (1962); H. Stevenson and L. Fahel, *J. Personality 29*, 136 (1961); E. Zigler and J. Williams, *J. Abnormal Soc. Psychol. 66*, 197 (1963).
35. W. M. Cruickshank, *J. Clin. Psychol. 3*, 381 (1947); E. E. Doll, in *Readings on the Exceptional Child*, E. P. Trapp and P. Himelstein, Eds. (Appleton-Century-Crofts, New York, 1962), pp. 21-68.
36. E. A. Hirsh, *Amer. J. Mental Deficiency 63*, 639 (1959); B. L. Wellman, *Childhood Educ. 15*, 108 (1938).
37. M. Woodward, *Brit. J. Med. Psychol. 33*, 123 (1960).
38. P. Shallenberger and E. Zigler, *J. Abnormal Soc. Psychol. 63*, 20 (1961); E. Zigler, thesis, Univ. of Texas, Austin, 1958.
39. H. Berkowitz, E. C. Butterfield, E. Zigler, *J. Personality Soc. Psychol. 2*, 706 (1965); H. Berkowitz and E. Zigler, *ibid.*, p. 500; N. McCoy and E. Zigler, *ibid. 1*, 604 (1965).
40. R. L. Cromwell, in *Handbook of Mental Deficiency*, N. R. Ellis, Ed. (McGraw-Hill, New York, 1963), pp. 41-91.
41. J. Turnure and E. Zigler, *J. Abnormal Soc. Psychol. 69*, 427 (1964).

42. E. BELLER, *J. Genet. Psychol. 87*, 25 (1955); J. Gewirtz, *Monographs Soc. Res. Child Develop. No. 59* (1954), p. 19; G. Heathers, *J. Genet. Psychol. 87*, 37, (1955); E. Zigler, *Amer. J. Orthopsychiat. 33*, 614 (1963).
43. E. ZIGLER and J. DELABRY, *J. Abnormal Soc. Psychol. 65*, 267 (1962).
44. E. ZIGLER and E. UNELL, *Amer. J. Mental Deficiency 66*, 651 (1962).
45. I am deeply indebted to Susan Harter for her help in organizing this article and for her assistance in clarifying many of the ideas presented. Preparation of the paper was facilitated by research grant MH-06809 from the National Institutes of Mental Health and by the Gunnar Dybwad award of the National Association for Retarded Children.

18

Social Class and Mental Illness in Children: THE DIAGNOSIS OF ORGANICITY AND MENTAL RETARDATION

John F. McDermott, Jr., M.D., Saul I. Harrison, M.D.,
Jules Schrager, M.S.W., Paul Wilson, M.D.
Elizabeth Killins, M.S.W., Janet Lindy, M.A.,
Raymond W. Waggoner, Jr., M.D.

It is perhaps ironic that the sinking of the liner *Titanic* before the beginning of the First World War should have provided us with dramatic evidence that an individual's "life chances" are highly correlated with his social class position. In that catastrophe only 3 percent of the female passengers in the first class accommodations drowned. In the second class 16 percent perished, and in the third class 45 percent met their death. Thus, social class factors determined access to the "opportunity system," in this case lifeboats. Forty years later, Hollingshead and Redlich (1958) demonstrated scientifically the relationships between

Reprinted from the *Journal of the American Academy of Child Psychiatry*, Vol. VI, No. 2, April, 1967, pp. 309-320. Dr. McDermott is Associate Professor and Director of Inpatient Serivce; Dr. Harrison is Professor and Training Director; Dr. Waggoner is Instructor; Mrs. Killins is Intake Coordinator: all at the Children's Psychiatric Hospital, Department of Psychiatry, University of Michigan Medical Center, Ann Arbor, Michigan. Mr. Schrager is Director of the Department of Social Work and Mrs. Lindy is Research Associate at the University of Michigan Medical Center. Dr. Wilson is Principal Investigator, Information Processing Project, American Psychiatric Association, Washington, D.C. The authors wish to express their thanks to Miss Sue Chilman for her invaluable help in gathering the data for this study.

Presented at the Annual Meeting of the American Orthopsychiatric Association, New York, New York, March, 1965. This is one of a series of reports emerging from a long-range investigation of social class factors and mental illness in children.

social class and another aspect of the opportunity system, namely, access to treatment for mental illness. These findings have since been confirmed with respect to children (Harrison et al., 1965; Hunt, 1962). In this report we wish to consider various aspects of the relationship between the incidence of organicity and mental retardation in children and their social class membership.

Both sociological and biological predisposing factors have been implicated in the occurrence of retardation and organicity in various sectors of the population. It is easy to accept the findings that an intellectually and culturally impoverished home environment will provide a child with comparatively inadequate intellectual stimulation. Furthermore, a number of studies (Pasamanick et al., 1956; Pasamanick and Knobloch, 1961) have also demonstrated a higher incidence of prematurity and complications of pregnancy and delivery as a result of inadequate nutrition and medical (especially prenatal) care. Both of these factors seem to result in a significantly greater occurrence of disorders of brain function in the children (Pasamanick and Knobloch, 1960; Pasamanick and Lilienfeld, 1955). Socioeconomic class standing, with all of its psychological and physical ramifications, would seem to emerge as an important determinant in the incidence rates of organicity and retardation.

On the basis of these generally accepted correlations of socioeconomic status with organic brain dysfunction and mental retardation, we have undertaken to examine our own patient population as part of a series of studies exploring the association of social class and mental illness. We have attempted to determine whether our diagnostic findings follow the expectation suggested by the epidemiological pattern, and, in the case of deviation, to speculate as to the reason.

METHOD

The intake records of 853 children up to the age of fourteen, who were evaluated at the University of Michigan Children's Psychiatric Hospital from July 1, 1960 to July, 1962, were examined. These code sheets contained a variety of historical and clinical data which had been filled out by psychiatrists and social workers at the time of the children's initial evaluations. (This material had been accumulated prior to the inception of the current study.) The data were then transposed to IBM cards and run through data-processing machines. First, the children were divided into five socioeconomic class groups based on their father's occupations.[1] This factor has been found in other studies to correlate well with various other determinants of social class standing (Reiss, 1962). Two major groups of correlations were studied: (1) those between social class and the primary diagnoses of mental retardation or organic brain syndrome; (2) those between social class and clinical data usually considered contributory to making these diagnoses. These clinical data were the incidences of the following factors in each occupational class: (a) abnormalities of the mother's pregnancy with the patient; (b) complications of the patient's birth; (c) prematurity; (d) clinical signs and symptoms of organic intellectual impairment; (e) hyperactivity and reduced attention span.

RESULTS

There were no significant occupational class differences found in the incidences of the various historical and clinical factors usually thought to be associated with chronic brain syndrome and mental retardation (Fig. 1). Nevertheless, there were significant occupational class differences found between the incidences of diagnosed chronic brain syndrome and mental retardation (Fig. 2). Of particular interest was the finding that both mental retardation and chronic brain syndrome were diagnosed *less frequently* than expected in the children of unskilled or chronically unemployed parents, as compared to all other classes.[2]

We were faced, then, with two curious paradoxes. First, there are definite occupational class differences in the frequency with which we diagnose chronic brain syndrome and mental retardation, despite the fact that there are *no differences* in the frequency with which we see other historical and clinical data usually related to these diagnoses. Second, we find the smallest incidence of diagnosed chronic brain syndrome and mental retardation in our lowest occupational class, the one in which we might have anticipated finding the highest incidence of these diagnoses.

---

[1] (a) *No occupation or habitually unemployed* (N=24), combined with *Unskilled or semiskilled laborer:* employed for tasks involving either no training or very small amount of training; e.g., janitor, assembly line worker (N=284).

(b) *Skilled laborer:* employed in manual activity which requires training and experience; e.g., machinist, self-employed small farmer (N=230).

(c) *Lower white collar:* involved in a small business or in clerical or similar work which is not primarily manual and which depends on some educational or special background; e.g., policeman, sales clerk, typist (N=99).

(d) *Upper white collar:* employed in more responsible administrative white-collar position; e.g., supervisor, large-scale farmer, schoolteacher, nurse (N=96).

(e) *Professional or executive:* employment depends on professional training beyond the college level, or has important executive responsibilities, high financial status; e.g., university teacher, attorney, engineer (N=120).

[2] $P<.02$ and .01 respectively, as determined by the Chi Square Test.

INCIDENCE BY OCCUPATIONAL CLASS OF CLINICAL CHARACTERISTICS RELATABLE TO DIAGNOSES OF CHRONIC BRAIN SYNDROME AND MENTAL RETARDATION. (Data in percent)

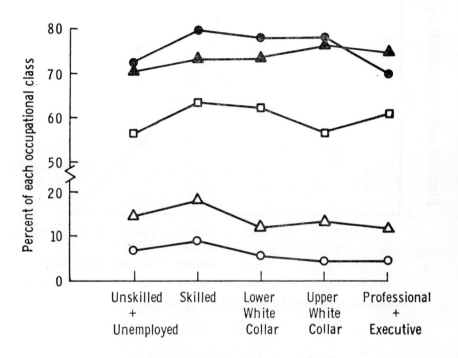

- ● Normal Pregnancy
- ▲ Uncomplicated Delivery
- △ Organic Intellectual Impairment
- ◻ Hyperactivity, Reduced Attention Span
- ○ Premature Birth (under 5 lbs. at birth)

FIGURE 1

INCIDENCE BY OCCUPATIONAL CLASS OF DIAGNOSED CHRONIC
BRAIN SYNDROME AND MENTAL RETARDATION.   (Data in percents)

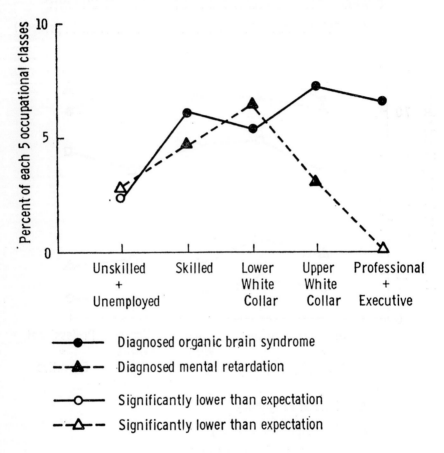

FIGURE 2

DISCUSSION

Since our findings were so clearly contrary to expectation based on
general population studies, we were led to speculate as to the cause. It
has been demonstrated before that clear-cut and significant direct relationships exist between the social level of parents and the I.Q. of their
children (President's Panel on Mental Retardation, 1962). Similarly,
cerebral dysfunction has recently been shown to be inversely related to

social class standing as well (Pasamanick and Knobloch, 1960; Pasamanick et al., 1956). Since there is a significant lack of correlation between our findings at the clinic and those broad epidemiological studies, we feel that our results are not typical and must be examined further.

Prereferral Selection Factors

The first possibility is that our findings are actual and representative of our clinic population, but differ from those broad studies cited above because of selection factors operating before referral to the clinic. It is quite probable that our clinic sees a self-selected sample, with the upper socioeconomic level having better access to medical care and a greater concern about deviation in their children (Pasamanick and Knobloch, 1961).

The question of access to our clinic, however, seems an oversimplified answer to the findings for two major reasons. The first is that, although operating as a university clinic, we find that the great majority of our patients do come from the lower socioeconomic groups. More important is that these findings are based on percentages of all the diagnoses within a particular group; that is, they are relative ones within that group, compared to other diagnoses such as psychoses, personality disorders, neuroses, and adjustment reactions.

In fact, certain selection factors should *help* make our clinic population follow expected trends more *closely*. As a psychiatric diagnostic and treatment center, the most obvious cases of severe retardation and organicity are *not* likely to reach us, being funneled more directly into specialized institutions. It is known that these most serious defects of intelligence and brain function are spread rather evenly among the social classes (President's Panel on Mental Retardation, 1962). In contrast, the mild and moderate degrees of impairment are weighed heavily at the lower end of the socioeconomic scale. These milder forms constitute a large "gray area" of cases with equivocal symptoms and signs pointing to the possible etiology of the disturbance. These youngsters often are referred as behavior and learning problems requiring thorough evaluation and careful differential diagnoses. There may be subtle problems of motor, sensory, or perceptual functioning as well as thought process, the importance of which much be flexibly interpreted along with historical factual material in terms of the total life experience of the child.

Even in those cases which are ambiguous enough to warrant psychiatric evaluation, a selection factor of a different kind may be operative, that of parental concern. As Birch (1964) points out, brain damage does not exist by itself, but in terms of its effect on personality growth. Eisenberg (1963) emphasizes that behavioral concomitants of brain damage will be determined by the social environment in which they emerge. This suggests another possible factor, namely, that the lowest socioeconomic group, although most vulnerable to brain damage, may be the least likely to *seek* professional help. We may speculate that different demands are placed on children by parents from different social classes and that perhaps the lower socioeconomic groups can tolerate a wider range of deviation in those areas of performance affected by brain dysfunction. Thus, there would be less actual conflict produced in the children, less parental concern, and, therefore, fewer referrals to the clinic initiated by the *family*.

Referral Selection Factors

The majority of our referrals are from schools, rather than directly from parents. This leads us to look for selection factors that may be operative in the larger community as well. Teachers may interpret the presence of certain symptoms differently when they occur in children from different socioeconomic classes. Behavior which may be considered cause for referral in the upper end of the socioeconomic scale may be attributed to "cultural deprivation" at the lower end. Concrete thinking and poor coordination may be considered to be cultural phenomena and shrugged off, with the attitude of "what can you expect?" This is an attitude which would permit the lower-class child to blend in with the retarded population and, thus, remain hidden to helping agencies.

Children of skilled workers, in contrast, were seen to have a higher incidence of organic brain dysfunction than the children of unskilled workers. Perhaps these children are confronted with higher expectations on the part of their teachers as well as on the part of their parents, and are more readily labeled "deviant." We have observed in a previous report that a greater interval of time is allowed to elapse between the appearance of disturbance and the eventual referral for help in the unskilled class, as compared with the skilled (McDermott et al., 1965). Thus, it is possible that what is perceived as failure of adaptation in one social group is tolerated in another; i.e., the lowest or unskilled group places less emphasis on verbal and mechanical aptitude, and the community reinforces these expectations.

Postreferral Selection Factors

We must now consider out next possibility in searching for explanations for our data—that our findings may not represent the actual state of affairs at our clinic, but are in part *apparent* findings reflecting either our own preconceptions and unwitting social class biases or factors inherent in the diagnostic process itself or both. We feel that the major value of our study lies in these considerations and their far-reaching implications for all those engaged in assessing and treating emotional and intellectual disorders in children.

First of all, it may be that we underdiagnose organicity and mental retardation in the unskilled and unemployed groups because of our own low expectations for them. Clinical assessment of intellectual concreteness, slowness, dullness, and poor mechanical ability may "fit" our *sub rosa* expectations of the lower socioeconomic group, reinforced by our interview with the parents at the time of evaluation. An "unskilled" boy, who is not much different from his "unskilled" father, does not stand out as retarded or damaged. However, the lack of mechanical skill and verbal agility in the children of parents who possess these qualities is more conspicuous to the examiner.

One of the most interesting issues raised during our investigation has been whether our findings reflect the orientation of our particular clinic. Children's Psychiatric Hospital is eclectic in practice, but psychoanalytically oriented in terms of its basic approach to understanding individual and family dynamics. We are more apt to regard a clinical sign, such as a child's hyperactivity, as a motoric expression of anxiety, rather than as a manifestation of brain damage. At some other clinics the same sign may automatically alert the examiners to the likelihood of organic brain dysfunction. Similarly, we observe distractibility at least as frequently in children who have had inadequate mothering in infancy, the time at which mother operates as a selective stimulation barrier for the child, as we do in those children with defective central nervous system screening of stimuli. We do not consider that there is a single or universal cause for a particular behavioral manifestation. If, in fact, our orientation and theories produce diagnoses "characteristic" of our outlook, and hence predictably at variance from those of other institutions, we might expect an "across-the-board" variance, that is, fewer "organic" diagnoses than the percentage expectation of the general population studies. Thus, although we have considered this factor carefully, we can only conclude that it does not serve to explain our findings, but raises an interesting issue pertinent to similar studies which may be undertaken elsewhere.

Finally, let us discuss the diagnostic process itself, proceeding from the specifics of our study to more general considerations. While certain historical information and clinical observation should not be taken as *prima facie* evidence of organicity, they should alert the examiner to this possibility when he makes his final diagnostic formulation. As noted earlier, our clinical and historical data show that our observation of certain factors, namely, those of prenatal and perinatal complications, prematurity, hyperactivity, and organic intellectual impairment, does not vary appreciably from class to class. We do note significant social class differences in the frequency with which we diagnose organic brain syndrome and mental retardation, paradoxically finding them less frequently at the lower end of the socioeconomic scale, instead of more frequently. There appears to be a difference between our clinical perceptions and our diagnostic conclusions. This observation directs our attention again to our own perception of patients. In the lower socioeconomic groups the environment often presents many more striking sociopsychological factors which must be carefully considered and weighed. For example, in a previous study we have shown a significantly higher incidence of "unstable, conflict-ridden homes" perceived by our examiners in the unskilled when compared to the skilled group (McDermott et al., 1965). We must then consider what we regard as the *relative importance* of the organic and environmental factors. In this sense, our task is similar to that of the pediatrician in the emergency room when he examines a child with chronic rheumatic heart disease and acute appendicitis. At the moment of examination, the rheumatic heart disease, while certainly not forgotten, is no longer the child's primary problem in terms of urgency. Acute appendicitis becomes the primary diagnosis and the target of the physician's main attention at the moment. In a similar fashion, the orthopsychiatric team may find environmental disorganization overshadowing the presence of a moderate degree of organic impairment in the lower-class child, resulting in a primary diagnosis other than that of organic brain syndrome. Conversely, the child who is a member of a higher socioeconomic group, with a more stable family, may be given a diagnosis of organic brain dysfunction, even where it is a condition of only mild severity, simply because this problem appears to be the most important consideration in his case at that point in time.

The necessity of focusing on the most *urgent* component of a multifaceted problem may serve to affect the ultimate diagnosis. Similarly, despite the presence of a multitude of signs and symptoms, the *utility* value of one label over another may be operative in the ultimate choice of a primary diagnosis. It may be that the lack of extreme clarity, precision, and general agreement surrounding such entities as "organic brain syndrome" and "mental retardation" provides the diagnostician with a certain amount of freedom in arriving at a final diagnosis. His perception of the *consequences* of employing a given label may advertently or inadvertently help determine his diagnosis.

The consequences of any given diagnosis may, furthermore, be partially dictated by the social class of the child. For example, the diagnosis of mental retardation may be an especially bitter pill for those in the uppermost socioeconomic group (where there were no single incidents of this diagnosis) and might have been replaced by a more palatable diagnosis, such as anxiety reaction. In other classes, perhaps the evaluator would be more concerned with the additional opportunities made available to those designated as organic or mentally retarded by the school system, for example, and be less concerned with negative parental reactions.

It would appear that diagnostic labels do more than describe; they also serve to call forth certain responses from the environment which vary from community to community. In general medicine, a diagnosis of tuberculosis or typhoid allows the physician to predict with some certainty the causative agent and the nature of the disease process inside the patient. In our work, on the other hand, the placing of a label often has less to do with etiology than with the intention and goals one has for the individual.

We are not suggesting that we, or other clinics, consistently and consciously manipulate diagnoses in order to make the diagnosis fit the hoped-for environmental response, but we do suggest that our own particular backgrounds and orientation may tend to make us err in this direction and if so, we must be aware of this. Whenever a mental health specialist finds himself diagnosing a certain entity more frequently than his colleagues, he should re-examine his approach and try to discover the reasons.

SUMMARY

The records of 853 children from Children's Psychiatric Hospital have been examined in an attempt to illuminate the relationship between social class and the diagnosis of organicity and mental retardation. More specifically, we have attempted to determine whether our diagnostic findings follow the expectation for the general population and if not, to speculate about deviant trends. We have reported two paradoxes: first, we found definite occupational class differences in the frequency with which we diagnose chronic brain syndrome and mental retardation, despite the fact that there are *no differences* in the frequency with which we see other historical and clinical data traditionally considered significant in making these diagnoses. Second, we found the smallest incidence of diagnosed chronic brain syndrome and mental retardation in our lowest occupational class, the one in which we might have anticipated finding the highest incidence of these diagnoses. Several hypotheses are considered that might account for these findings. These involve such factors as preselection of our patient population by the family and community attitudes, our own varying expectations of children from different social classes, and the impact that different diagnoses have on the communities from which the children come.

REFERENCES

BIRCH, H. G. (1964), The problem of brain damage in children. *Brain Damage in Children: The Biological and Social Aspects,* ed. H. G. Birch. Baltimore: Williams & Wilkins.

EISENBERG, L. (1963), Behavioral manifestations of cerebral damage in childhood. *Brain Damage in Children: The Biological and Social Aspects,* ed. H. G. Birch. Baltimore: Williams & Wilkins.

HARRISON, S. I., McDERMOTT, J. F., WILSON, P. T., & SCHRAGER, J. (1965), Social class and mental illness in children: choice of treatment. *Arch. Gen Psychiat.,* 13:411-417.

HOLLINGSHEAD, A. B. & REDLICH, F. C. (1958), *Social Class and Mental Illness: A Community Study.* New York: Wiley.

HUNT, R. G. (1962), Occupational status and the disposition of cases in a child guidance clinic. *Int. J. Soc. Psychiat.,* 8:199-210.

LORD, W. (1955), *A Night to Remember.* New York: Holt.

McDERMOTT, J. F., HARRISON, S. I., SCHRAGER, J., & WILSON, P. T. (1965), Social class and mental illness in children: observations of blue-collar families. *Amer. J. Orthopsychiat.,* 35:500-508.

PASAMANICK, B. & KNOBLOCH, H. (1960), Brain damage and reproductive causality. *Amer. J. Orthopsychiat.,* 30:298-305.

——— (1961), Epidemiologic studies on the complications of pregnancy and the birth process. In: *Prevention of Mental Disorders in Children,* ed. G. Caplan. New York: Basic Books, pp. 74-94.

——— LILIENFELD, A. (1956), Socioeconomic status and some precursors of neuropsychiatric disorders. *Amer. J. Orthopsychiat.,* 26:594-601.

—— LILIENFELD, A. (1955), Association of maternal and fetal factors with development of mental deficiency: I. Abnormalities in the prenatal and paranatal periods. *J. Amer. Med. Assoc.,* 159:155-160.

PRESIDENT'S PANEL ON MENTAL RETARDATION (1962), *A Proposed Program for National Action to Combat Mental Retardation.* Washington: U.S. Government Printing Office.

REISS, A. 1962), *Occupations and Social Status.* New York: Free Press of Glencoe.

WATKINS, C. & PASAMANICK, B., Eds. (1961), *Problems in Communication* [Scientific Papers and Discussions of a Regional Research Conference Held January 13-14, 1960, in New Orleans, La. under the Joint Auspices of Louisiana State Univ. School of Medicine, Dept. of Psychiatry and Neurology, and the American Psychiatric Association's Committee on Research, 1959-1960]. Washington, D.C.: American Psychiatric Association.

19

PSYCHOPATHOLOGY AND MENTAL RETARDATION

Irving Philips, M.D.

*Associate Clinical Professor of Psychiatry,
University of California School of Medicine;
Supervising Psychiatrist, Children's Service,
Langley Porter Neuropsychiatric Institute.*

A study of 227 retarded children and their families revealed that maladjustment more often than not accompanies retardation. The author points out, however, that disturbed behavior in the retarded is not due primarily to limited intellectual capacities but to delayed, disordered personality functions and disturbed interpersonal relationships with meaningful people in the environment.

Recent efforts have been made to revise the nomenclature in the field of mental retardation.[7] Mental retardation is often viewed as a discrete disease process rather than a condition of living. Diagnostic categories are often difficult to delineate. The present nomenclature in the American Psychiatric Association's *Diagnostic and Statistical Manual*[3] is outdated and outmoded and has little relevance to the present state of knowledge in the field of mental retardation.

Although mental retardation is associated with a lowered level of intellectual functioning, the mentally retarded individual usually comes to the attention of society when there is failure in social adaptation. In

Reprinted from AMERICAN JOURNAL OF PSYCHIATRY, Vol. 124: 1, July 1967, pp. 29-35. © Copyright 1967 American Psychiatric Association. Read at the 122nd annual meeting of the American Psychiatric Association, Atlantic City, N. J., May 9-13, 1966.

our society, cognitive function plays such a predominant role that the social adaptation of the retarded individual is almost always disrupted.

The retarded child is vulnerable to defects in personality development not only because of constitutional endowment but also because of his interpersonal experiences with his environment. Emotional problems are the same as those occurring in children with normal intelligence. Symptoms may be influenced by retardation but understood in relation to life experiences. If the retarded child is overwhelmed by his condition or encumbered by emotional disorder, his victimization by his conflicts may be expressed in self-depreciation, inhibition, and withdrawal or he may react in retaliation with explosive aggressive behavior that demands control and custody.

In 1958 funds were furnished by the National Institute of Mental Health to develop a program to train psychiatric personnel in the field of mental retardation at Langley Porter Neuropsychiatric Institute. Between 1958 and 1965, 227 families with a retarded child were referred to the institute for diagnostic study and evaluation. Children with mental retardation of all degrees of severity and ranging in age from nine months through adolescence were evaluated as fully as possible; psychiatric evaluation was a part of each study.

At the beginning of our program we hoped to see retarded children whose intellectual deficits were not complicated by emotional disorder. We contacted pediatric, public health, social welfare, and psychiatric facilities to request referral of children who were mentally retarded but had no emotional disorder. We did see a few such children who were making an adequate adjustment but whose parents wished help with future plans and a place to visit to discuss current problems. It was uncommon, however, to see a retarded child who presented no emotional maladjustment as part of his clinical picture. This report summarizes the work of this program as related to emotional problems of the mentally retarded. Particular difficulties occurring during the developmental years and what we have come to see as some common misconceptions concerning emotional disorder in retarded children will be discussed.

DEVELOPMENTAL PROBLEMS

The mentally retarded child is more vulnerable in all periods of his life to the development of maladaptive behavior than is the normally endowed child. He is handicapped by lowered intellect, sometimes complicated by other anomalies, that leads to a delay in and a slowed rate of personality development. Although in size and body type he may be more or less comparable to his normal "peers," his ability to cope with situations of everyday living is impaired. In addition, his disappointed family may find it difficult to regard him in the same way they would a normal child.

Society offers him fewer of the environmental supports afforded normal children. He often is placed in special schools, shunned and avoided by his peers, and excluded from much of community life. It is assumed that he can make little contribution to the society in which he lives. He is always referred to as a "child" even though he may be a young adult. The retarded child's unfavorable conception of himself is thus doubly reinforced by his family's disappointment and by society's attitudes towards him.

The retarded may be divided into two groups on the basis of etiology. Eighty-five percent are mildly retarded, with etiologies primarily involving social, cultural, and psychological factors.[13] Fifteen percent of the retarded have moderate to severe deficits associated with primarily organic etiologies such as microcephaly, mongolism, phenylketonuria, cerebral agenesis, and the like. The disorders of children in this group usually are diagnosed early in life, often at birth. The appearance of these children, complicated by various stigmata, distinguishes them from other children and they readily appear to parents, peers, and community as being different. Each of these two groups will be discussed separately in this paper, but similar emotional problems appear in both.

Moderate to Severe Retardation

The child whose retardation is diagnosed early in life often presents great difficulty to his family. The human infant is characterized by his total and long period of dependence on other persons. The interpersonal reactions of the parent with the infant may influence the child's development. The warm, tender relationship experienced by the infant with his mother may foster a sense of confidence and eventual trust in his world.

There is probably no more tragic experience for parents than to be told that their child is mentally defective. Parents faced with this disappointment may react to the child in a variety of ways, from withdrawal to guilty oversolicitude. If the parents are depressed and disappointed, inconsistent in their care, hostile and angry, inhibited and frightened, the infant may react with symptoms indicating distortions of personality development. He may view the world with a sense of distrust and suspicion, too frightened to try new tasks, or he may become angry in retaliation.

Several studies, such as those by Spitz,[11] Goldfarb,[4] and Provence and Lipton,[10] have demonstrated the effects of maternal deprivation on infant personality development. The parent who withdraws from a child may be unable to provide those experiences necessary for growth. Deprivational experiences may result in increased autoerotic play, infant depression, defects in intellectual development, delayed speech, and severe ego deficits.

During infancy various symptoms may indicate pathological personality development. These include vomiting and spitting up, frequent episodes of infection and diarrhea, head-banging, blanket- and finger-sucking, rocking, and sleep disturbances. Weaning problems are noted frequently, as well as difficulty in adjusting to changes in diet from liquid to solid foods.

During the first year of life, the moderately or severely retarded child exhibits a delay in reaching developmental landmarks and all skills, such as toilet control, locomotion, language skills, and adaptive behavior, develop late. Although he may be similar to his normal "peers" in physical size, he does not have the motor control necessary to compete with them. While other children are engaging in parallel and later in cooperative play, he has difficulty keeping up with his agemates.

When he is physically ready to play, he has outgrown in age and size those children with whom he might profitably engage in play, and the younger children find it hard to play with him. This difficulty in play may be a further crippling factor, intensifying his sense of inferiority. Self-isolation and an inhibition from attempting new or competitive tasks may result.

When he reaches school age at five years, the regular classroom may not admit him. He leaves the mainstream of community life and becomes a segregated citizen. Usually he does not enter school until the age of eight. Although there may be beneficial effects of preschool experiences for the development of social skills by retarded youngsters, the opportunities for preschool experience for most retarded children are limited or nonexistent. The child may have to remain at home and may need continuous parental supervision, further intensifying parental disappointment and causing the child to feel increasingly more isolated and unworthy.

The experience of entering school may present difficulties to the child who has had earlier problems in life. The retarded child may be more vulnerable in this situation. He may tend to consider himself different and unwanted and set himself apart from others. He may be shunned and teased by his peers, called names and taunted, be the "fall guy" for the class bully and the victim of jokes. Neighbors may forbid their children to play with him. In reaction to his inability to solve his environmental and internal conflicts, he may develop a variety of symptoms of emotional disorder. These run the gamut from simple transient behavior problems to severe neurotic, delinquent, and schizophrenic disorders.

Adolescence, beginning with the onset of puberty and the development of secondary sexual characteristics, poses a new challenge. During adolescence the conflicts inherent in earlier life experiences are reawakened with increased intensity. The added pressure of physiological changes may cause a recrudescence of dormant emotional conflicts and result in symptoms. The more complete the resolution of the developmental tasks of earlier periods of life, the less difficult the adolescent period. The retarded child who is hampered in his early development meets the pressure of adolescence additionally handicapped. The task of fulfilling his needs for identification with a group, social outlets, recreation, vocational choice, and some separation from his parents may be fraught with difficulty. Society may offer him little opportunity to achieve some solution. The result is further isolation. He may become more dependent on his parents, fearful of his own impulses, withdrawn and isolated, or react with increased aggressivity, sexual indulgence, and delinquent behavior.

Sexual development, often normal, is a cause of concern for the parent. It is necessary to help the child deal realistically with his own impulses and to offer him whatever controls are needed. If the child is confronted with parental fear, dread, disgust, and panic, he will be more frightened and also more likely to taste the forbidden fruit in a destructive and self-defeating manner. It is important to note that delinquent, perverse, and antisocial behaviors are determined not by the intellectual abilities alone but more likely by social, economic, cultural, and most of all, family attitudes.

Mild Retardation

The second group to be considered is the mildly retarded, the 85 percent whose retardation is related primarily to social, cultural, and psychological factors. This is a population generally not familiar to most professional workers, a little-studied group for whom services traditionally are minimal. Families are often broken and parents or parent surrogates are concerned largely with the harsh economic realities of staying alive or subsisting; their energies are not devoted to verbal, communication, and learning endeavors. Problems in this group are related to indifference and apathy, distrust and suspicion, sociocultural isolation, and poor and inhibited school performance.

In this group are children not diagnosed as mentally retarded at birth and who may or may not manifest slow development. They usually are diagnosed as retarded by the schools. They learn slowly, show little interest, and are poor in language and communication skills. When assigned tasks of reading, writing, and arithmetic are demanded, they fall behind. There is usually much absenteeism for repeated minor illnesses, inattention to school tasks, immaturity in school behavior and personality development, slowed language development, and low achievement test scores. They fall behind in school subjects and each term the lag behind their age group increases.

On standard achievement tests they score in the mildly retarded range and sometimes are placed in special classes. Their discouragement increases, apathy becomes more apparent, and learning is increasingly difficult. They may present a variety of behavior problems in reaction to their indifference to learning. In adolescence, they may become the school dropouts—ill prepared in either academic or vocational skills. They may become the chronic unemployable or exhibit delinquent antisocial behavior.

In this group, also, are the children with learning inhibition. Test results may indicate mild retardation but a wide scatter in performance indicates higher potential for learning. If a child does not read, his ability to perform in school is severely impeded and leads to failure in most school subjects. With the advent of the nuclear age and space exploration, there has been a great emphasis on achievement and performance and a stressing of competition.

In our clinic during the past decade there has been in increase in referrals of children with specific learning disabilities. These children often are inhibited and withdrawn and frequently present a clinical picture of a schizoid personality. They may have associated somatic problems such as eczema, asthma, malnutrition or obesity, ulcers, and frequent infectious disease.

The psychoses or the schizophrenic reactions of childhood also often appear in the 85 percent who are mildly retarded. Many centers working with these children are investigating methods of differentiating the psychotic child from the retarded child whose deficiency is due to organic causes.[1, 5, 12] This is often a difficult task.

When psychosis or mental deficiency, uncomplicated by emotional disorder, occurs as a separate entity the distinction is not as difficult.

The difficulty in distinguishing the child with severe emotional disorder from the child with mental deficiency is that psychotic reactions may occur superimposed on deficiency. The psychotic child presents a picture of retardation in that all areas of learning are affected. He is often intellectually, socially, emotionally, and developmentally retarded. Although his retardation may be functional, the clinical picture is associated with retardation.

Thus, the intellectual deficit of the retarded child may be intensified by developmental problems that may lead to conflict and result in familiar clinical patterns of emotional disorder.

COMMON MISCONCEPTIONS

There are three common misconceptions about maladaptive behavior in the retarded child. First, it is often thought that the maladaptive behavior of the retarded child is a function of his retardation rather than of his interpersonal relationships. Second, it is assumed that emotional disorder in the retarded is different in kind from that in the normal child. And third, it is thought that certain symptomatology and maladaptive behavior in a retarded child are the result of organic brain damage that produces these particular symptoms.

The constitutional endowment of any child is not the only factor determining his ability to learn and develop. The child may have ultimate limitations on his capacity to develop, but his life experiences also may interfere with the fullest development of his innate potential. It is true that organic defect resulting from injury, metabolic abnormality, congenital anomaly, infection, etc., may limit the level of functioning, but emotional disorder developing from such experiences as frustration, separation, traumatic experience, and the like, also may inhibit or distort functioning.[9]

Thus, the child who is retarded because of organic defect may also evidence emotional disorder that interferes with his maximal development. Although deficiency or disease may be a major contributing stress, the child's emotional disorder probably is not an organically inevitable concomitant of his defect but rather a function of the same kinds of processes that give rise to emotional disorder in children who have no definable disease.[2] Thus, disturbed behavior in the retarded is not primarily the result of limited intellectual capacities but is related to delayed, disordered personality functions and disturbed interpersonal relationships with meaningful people in the environment.

In addition, epidemiological studies have indicated that in 85 percent of retarded children the primary etiology of the retardation is related to psychological, social, and cultural factors. By our present means and knowledge of diagnosis no abnormalities can be found in physical or laboratory examination among the majority of these 85 percent. These mildly retarded, who come from lower economic groups living in deprived areas with poor medical care, demonstrate retarded functions as they develop rather than at birth.

A number of studies have indicated the influence of culture and family life on intellectual development. Knobloch and Pasamanick[6] reported a controlled study of infants in which they found no significant Negro-white differences in developmental quotient at birth. At three years of age, no significant differences in motor function were observed in the two groups, but significant differences were noted between the Negro and white populations in adaptive social behavior. Learning inhibition resulting from interpersonal and psychological factors may result in a lowering of the testable IQ even though evidence within the test performance indicates higher potential for learning.

The second misconception is that emotional disorder in the retarded is of a different nature than that seen in the normal child. In our experience during the past seven years we have seen in retarded children the gamut of psychopathology seen in children with normal intellectual endowment. We have seen transient, psychoneurotic, character, personality, psychophysiologic, and psychotic disorders. The following examples illustrate this.

Case 1. Mr. and Mrs. W. sought help for their 13-month-old child who was diagnosed as having Down's Syndrome. They had been to many clinics. Mrs. W. requested gastrointestinal X-rays of the youngster because he was constantly spitting up. Mr. W. reported that his wife had become more upset, suspicious, and sleepless since the birth of the child. She remarked that the boy's vomiting, often projectile in nature, took place with every feeding. He banged his head and rocked constantly in his crib; sleep patterns were reversed. At the end of a four-week study in which Mrs. W. was seen weekly for interviews, she seemed to feel better. She discussed her feelings and was relieved by the thoroughness of our examination of the child. The child's symptoms disappeared except for occasional head-banging.

Case 2. Jimmy, a three-year-old mongoloid boy, was impulsive and destructive to his schoolmates, difficult to manage at school, and almost impossible to control at home. A local nursery school was ready to expel him—something they had never done in the history of their school. The father, a former prominent athlete, maintained unrealistic expectations and felt his son would be slow but could finish high school and work in his business. He discussed with pride his son's "cute" and "all-boy" impulsivity and destructiveness.

Case 3. Billy, a six-year-old mildly retarded boy with an IQ of 68, was sullen and morose, spent most of his free time by himself, had no friends, peered off into space in school, gave little attention to his work, and consequently did not learn. In the course of our study he became quite agitated as he revealed his very active fantasy life. He presented the clinical picture of a schizoid personality.

Case 4. Helen, a 17-year-old adolescent, was socially isolated and withdrawn in her behavior. Her IQ was 68 and her school frequently reported that she could do better in her work but was withdrawn and disturbed. Her mother spent all of her free time with her, fearful that her daughter would get into trouble, that perhaps she would be attacked or be led into troublesome behavior. Helen developed phobic fears of being touched, avoided crowds, bathed frequently, and washed her hands throughout the day.

The third misconception is that certain symptomatologies and maladaptive behavior in retarded children result from organic brain damage that produces these particular symptoms. Symptoms often mentioned are hyperactivity, short attention span, distractibility, and impulsive and unexplained behavior. Although we have seen some symptoms, we have seen the same symptoms in a number of children with both low and high IQs but without demonstrable organic brain disease. We have seen these symptoms recede and disappear with psychotherapy. We have seen children described as hyperactive and destructive who are inhibited and overcontrolled in the playroom. We have seen children whose distractibility and inattentiveness could be related to interpersonal interactions occurring at particular moments. Although these children are difficult to treat, we have had some therapeutic success in working with them. The following case provides an example.

Case 5. Jim W., a youngster of ten years with a right-sided hemiplegia and convulsive episodes, was referred to our clinic by his school because of his impulsive, hyperactive behavior. Repeated intelligence tests indicated an IQ in the low 60s. He had poor concentration and gave brief and abortive attention to tasks at hand. If he was not immediately successful, he would race around the room and disregard his work. His teacher felt he could do better at school.
His parents related that he had frequent temper tantrums when frustrated and that it was impossible to reason with him. He often was involved in dangerous pursuits such as climbing out of his upper-story window and walking along the ledge or running into

the street, just avoiding passing cars. He was always a school problem and posed great difficulty to his teacher.

He was seen for weekly psychotherapeutic interviews. Initially he
was a problem to his therapist because of his hyperactivity. As therapy progressed he began to play and talk more freely about his
troubles. He began to show marked improvement in school and
home and made friends. He began to work up to his level and
learned to read, write, and do arithmetic. He obtained a job delivering papers. In the playroom, near the end of treatment, when he
was frustrated with a puzzle he reared back to throw it and smiled
at his therapist as he relaxed and said, "I know you want me to
say it and not throw it."

Such common misconceptions concerning psychopathology and mental
retardation often prevent us from looking at the retarded child as an
individual who is vulnerable to intrapersonal and interpersonal conflicts
and susceptible to our therapeutic methodologies.[8] Emotional disorder
differs little in nature in children who are retarded or who are more
favored intellectually.

SUMMARY

This paper reviews the findings of a study of 227 families in which
there was a mentally retarded child seen by the staff of the Children's
Service of the Langley Porter Neuropsychiatric Institute during the
period 1958 to 1965. The particular vulnerability of the retarded to
maladaptive behavior as well as some common misconceptions about
such behavior are discussed. Particular psychopathologies occurring in
the mentally retarded child are described.

There is a need to review the nomenclature of mental retardation to
make it more consistent with our present state of knowledge. Outmoded
concepts should be discarded and recognition of a more functional classification should be considered.

REFERENCES

1. BENDER, L.: Childhood Schizophrenia, Psychiat. Quart. 27:663-681, 1953.
2. BOATMAN, M. J., and SZUREK, S. A.: "A Clinical Study of Childhood Schizophrenia," in Jackson, D. D., ed.: The Etiology of Schizophrenia. New York: Basic
   Books, 1960: 389-440.
3. Diagnostic and Statistical Manual: Mental Disorders. Washington, D. C.: American
   Psychiatric Association, 1952.
4. GOLDFARB, W.: Variations in Adolescent Adjustment of Institutionally-Reared
   Children, Amer. J. Orthopsychiat. 17:449-457, 1947.
5. GOLDFARB, W.: Childhood Schizophrenia. Cambridge, Mass.: Commonwealth
   Fund, Harvard University Press, 1961.

6. KNOBLOCH, H., and PASAMANICK, B.: Some Thoughts on the Inheritance of Intelligence, Amer. J. Orthopsychiat. 31:454-473, 1961.
7. A Manual on Terminology and Classification in Mental Retardation, Amer. J. Ment. Defic., monograph supplement, 2nd ed., 1961.
8. PHILIPS, I.: Mental Hygiene and Mental Retardation: Implications for Planning, Ment. Hyg. 49:525-533, 1965.
9. PHILIPS, I., JEFFRESS, M., KOCH, E., and BOATMAN, M. J.: The Application of Psychiatric Clinic Services for the Retarded Child and His Family, J. Amer. Acad. Child Psychiat. 1:297-313, 1962.
10. PROVENCE, S., and LIPTON, R. C.: Infants in Institutions. New York: International Universities Press, 1962.
11. SPITZ, R. A.: Hospitalism, Psychoanal. Stud. Child. 1:54-74, 1945.
12. SZUREK, S. A.: Psychotic Episodes and Psychotic Maldevelopment, Amer. J. Orthopsychiat. 26:519-543, 1956.
13. TARJAN, G.: Research and Clinical Advances in Mental Retardation, J.A.M.A. 182:617-621, 1962.

20

THE CONTRIBUTION OF OBSTETRIC COMPLICATIONS TO THE ETIOLOGY OF BEHAVIOR DISORDERS IN CHILDHOOD

Sula Wolff, M.D.

Royal Hospital for Sick Children, Edinburgh

Rogers, Lilienfeld and Pasamanick (1955) established the fact that among children with behavior disorders a significantly greater proportion were premature or had been exposed to complications of pregnancy and delivery than among a control group of children. Since then the view has been expressed repeatedly (Stott 1962, 1965) that childhood behavior disorders in general are based on some ill-defined, congenital vulnerability to which birth injury makes a major contribution. Pasamanick's (1956) hypothesis of "a continuum of reproductive casualty" has facilitated the development of the notion that in childhood every disorder is related to every other one and that birth injury, constitutional vulnerability, social deprivation and emotional traumata, all make significant but nonspecific contributions to psychiatric morbidity.

Certain facts that emerged from the original Baltimore studies (Pasamanick *et al.* 1956, 1959) require to be emphasized. (1) The differences in frequency of perinatal complications between Negro and white sections of the population were far greater than the perinatal differences between behaviorally disturbed and nondisturbed children. (2) Although the differences between the experimental and control groups were sta-

Reprinted with permission from the JOURNAL OF CHILD PSYCHOLOGY AND PSYCHIATRY, Vol. 8, No. 1, May 1967, pp. 57-66. Copyright 1967 by Pergamon Press.

tistically significant, each type of obstetric complication occurred in an eighth or less of disturbed white children and in a third or less of disturbed Negro children. (3) It was only when obstetric complications were totalled up for each case that one or more complications were found to have occurred in a third of the white and in about two thirds of the Negro disturbed subjects. But, when this procedure of adding complications was used, no less than a quarter of the white and a half of the Negro control children had also been exposed to one or more obstetric complications. (4) The disturbed group included all children with behavior disorders who had been referred to the Division of Special Services of the Baltimore Department of Education and who were not mentally retarded. They were presumably mainly children identified as disturbed in the school setting rather than by their parents at home. When children classified as "confused, disorganized and hyperactive" were looked at separately, it was found that the difference in frequency of obstetric complications between these children and their controls was even greater than between the experimental and control groups as a whole. Even Pasamanick (1956) suggested that birth injury may contribute more to some types of behavior disorders than to others.

The present paper is a report on the frequency of obstetric complications in 100 children referred to a psychiatric department diagnosed as having reactive psychiatric disorders, and in a matched control group of non-referred children. It is part of a larger comparative study of behavior disorders and their background in Edinburgh primary school children (Wolff 1967).

THE SAMPLES

Two treatment facilities for psychiatrically disturbed children exist in Edinburgh: the Educational Child Guidance Clinic and the psychiatric department at The Royal Hospital for Sick Children. Referrals to the Child Guidance Clinic are in the main initiated by teachers; referrals to the hospital department by general practitioners and paediatricians. The latter department thus caters largely for children identified as disturbed by parents, and it is from here that the sample of referred children, the "clinic group," was drawn.

The clinic group consisted of 100 consecutive referrals of children attending primary schools within the city of Edinburgh. Excluded were children whose present I.Q. was under 80, children with diagnosed minimal brain damage (three), with schizoid personality disorder (two) and with specific reading difficulty but no behavioral problems (one). In addition four children attending schools for the maladjusted were

TABLE 1

OCCUPATIONAL CLASS

Occupational class of head of household	I	II	III	IV	V
Clinic	8	14	54	18	6
Control	8	13	51	19	9

TABLE 2

EDUCATIONAL LEVEL OF PARENTS

	Mother		Father	
	Clinic	Control	Clinic	Control
Left school before statutory school leaving age	3	7	2	—
Left school at statutory school leaving age; no other training	66	68	44	47
Left school at statutory school leaving age and completed apprenticeship	6	3	31	30
Stayed on at school at least 1 year after statutory school leaving age OR did full time non-academic course for at least one year e.g. secretarial course (Exclude incomplete nursing training)	15	15	12	13
Completed professional training other than at university, e.g. nursing, chartered accountant	3	6	2	5
At least one year of university training completed	7	1	7	5
Not known	—	—	2	—

excluded because no suitable controls were available for them, and, since mothers were to be the main informants, we excluded also children who had no mother figure (one in an institution, two with fathers only, and one with only a grandfather). Of 104 mothers asked to take part in the investigation, 100 agreed to do so.

The control group was made up by selecting from the class register of each clinic another child of the same sex and age whose father's occupation was similar to that of the clinic attender. Only three of 100 control mothers refused to co-operate and these were replaced with alternative controls who had been chosen at the same time.

Matching for sex, age and occupation of head of household was good. There were sixty-two boys and thirty-eight girls in each group. The mean age of clinic child attenders was 8.4 years (range 5.3-12.5) and of controls

TABLE 3

SIZE OF SIBSHIP OF PARENTS

| | Mother | | Father | |
Size of Sibship	Clinic	Control	Clinic	Control
1, 2 or 3	47	46	51	47
4, 5 or 6	35	31	29	35
7 +	18	23	18	18
Not known	—	--	2	—

8.3 years (range 5.3-12.5). Table 1 shows the social class distribution using the Registrar General's 1960 classification of occupations.

That matching for social class was in fact effective was confirmed by the findings that the educational levels of mothers and fathers were similar in the two groups as were the sizes of the sibships of both parents (Tables 2 and 3).

METHOD

The main method of enquiry was a focussed interview with the mother carried out by the author. It covered four areas: (1) the child's behavior within the past six months, (2) adverse events in the life of the child including an obstetric history (Appendix A), (3) adverse events in the childhood of each parent, and (4) the parents' psychiatric status.

In addition school teachers were asked to complete questionnaires for each child, and all hospital records of the child's birth and subsequent hospital attendances were examined as far as possible.

It had been hoped initially that rating scales of the severity of obstetric hazards could be based on the findings of the Perinatal Mortality Survey (Butler and Bonham, 1963; Feldstein and Butler, 1965; Feldstein, 1965). Complications of pregnancy and delivery that carried a high risk of perinatal mortality, it was thought, could legitimately be regarded as also carrying a high risk for impairment short of death. So far, however, the multivariate analysis of the data collected in the perinatal mortality survey is incomplete, so that the individual contribution of each obstetric complication to perinatal mortality is not yet known. Consequently the rating scales used in the present study had to be empirical.* (See Appendix B.)

Data analysis was done on the Chilton Atlas computer with a survey

---

* They were devised in collaboration with Dr. C. M. Drillien, Department of Child Life and Health, University of Edinburgh.

program written by Rees (1964). Differences between clinic and control groups were calculated using Kendall's rank correlation method (1948). In addition, Stuart's test allowing for the effects of matching, but applicable only to 2×2 tables, was used to test for differences in factors suggestive of an abnormal foetus, complications of pregnancy, complications of delivery and the post natal condition of the baby. (Stuart, 1957.)

(1) Place of birth

Significantly more clinic children were born in hospital than were controls. In the clinic group eighty-four children were born in hospital, four in nursing homes or homes for unmarried mothers and twelve at home. The corresponding figures in the control group were seventy-three, four and twenty-three ($\tau = 0.1364, P < 0.05$).

There was a slight but insignificant excess of first-born children in the clinic group (44 : 35). In both groups the majority of first-borns were delivered in a hospital or other institution (40 : 34). The difference between the groups is more striking for later born children. Of fifty-six in the clinic group only eight (14 per cent) were delivered at home while of sixty-five later born control children twenty-two (34 per cent) were born at home ($\tau = 0.2265, P < 0.01$). Moreover, although clinic mothers did not have significantly more subsequent children than controls, they had significantly more subsequent hospital admissions for childbirth ($\tau = 0.1938, P < 0.01$). These results are in line with the finding that clinic mothers made generally more demands on hospital services both for themselves and their children than control mothers.

(2) Sources of obstetric data

For twelve clinic and twenty-three control children born at home no information was available other than that from the mothers. In two further clinic cases and four controls no hospital records could be traced at all. In eighteen clinic and seven control cases obstetric records were incomplete. Complete records were available for the pregnancy, the birth and the infant's condition after birth in sixty-eight clinic and sixty-six control cases. Thus slightly more medical information was available for the clinic mothers. This would tend to bias the results in favor of finding more obstetric complications, at least of a minor sort, in the clinic group.

TABLE 4

MATERNAL AGE AT BIRTH OF CHILD

Maternal age	<20	20<25	25<30	30<35	35<40	40<45	45+
Clinic	8	26	35	15	11	4	1
Control	5	28	32	22	11	2	—

TABLE 5

TOTAL NUMBER OF MISCARRIAGES

	None	One	Two	Three
Clinic	63	21	14	2
Control	77	17	4	2

$\tau = -0.1582, P < 0.02$.

TABLE 6

BIRTH WEIGHT

B.W. (lb)	>3-4	>4-5	>5-6	>6-7	>7-8	>8-9	>9-10	>10
Clinic	1	4	12	23	36	13	10	1
Control	1	2	8	28	36	17	8	—

(3) *Maternal age*

Table 4 shows that maternal age at the birth of the child was similar in clinic and control groups.

(4) *Number of miscarriages*

More clinic than control mothers (nineteen compared to thirteen) had had miscarriages prior to the birth of the child studied. This is in line with the findings of Rogers *et al.* in Baltimore (1955). Subsequent miscarriages also were common in the clinic group (eighteen compared to ten). Table 5 shows the total number of miscarriages reported.

(5) *Birth weight*

Table 6 shows the distributions of birth weight in the two groups of children. They did not differ significantly.

TABLE 7

FACTORS SUGGESTIVE OF AN ABNORMAL FOETUS

Rating*	0	1	2	Not known
Clinic	84	13	2	1
Control	90	10	—	—

$\tau = -\ 0.0803$, N.S. Stuart's test for matched samples (combining the second and third columns): $z = 1.09$, N.S.

* See Appendix B.

TABLE 8

COMPLICATIONS OF PREGNANCY

Rating*	0	1	2 or more	Not known
Clinic	64	25	10	1
Control	74	13	13	—

$\tau = -\ 0.0762$, N.S. Stuart's test for matched samples (combining the second and third columns): $z = 1.26$, N.S.

* See Appendix B.

(6) *Factors suggestive of an abnormal foetus*

Although there were a few more children with complications suggestive of an abnormal foetus in the clinic group, Table 7 shows that the difference between the two groups was not significant.

(7) *Complications of pregnancy*

Again there were slightly more complications in the clinic group but the difference was not significant (Table 8). The excess was in minor complications.

(8) *Complications of delivery*

Once more there was no significant difference between the groups (Table 9).

(9) *Postnatal condition of child*

Again there was no difference between the two groups (Table 10).

TABLE 9

COMPLICATIONS OF DELIVERY

Rating*	0	1	2 or more	Not known
Clinic	76	16	7	1
Control	81	9	10	—

$\tau = -$ 0.0386, N.S. Stuart's test for matched samples (combining the second and third columns). $z = 0.67$, N.S.

* See Appendix B.

TABLE 10

POSTNATAL CONDITION OF CHILD

Condition of child*	1	2	3	Not known
Clinic	86	10	3	1
Control	87	8	5	—

$\tau = -$ 0.0019, N.S.
Stuart's test for matched samples (combining the second and third columns): $z = 0$.

* See Appendix B.

(10) Congenital abnormalities

Two clinic and two control children had minor congenital defects: overriding toes and a slight thumb deformity in the former group, very mild talipes and a small umbilical hernia in the latter. Four clinic children but no controls had severe congenital defects. Two had congenital heart disease (one coming to operation, the other attending a school for the physically handicapped); one had an imperforate anus and hypospadias necessitating numerous hospital admissions and operations; one had a bilateral hydrocoele again necessitating operation. If these abnormalities were related to the children's psychiatric disturbance, it is more likely that the stresses associated with their treatment were of etiological significance rather than that the congenital defects were pointers to some more general constitutional impairment.

DISCUSSION

These results do not contradict the findings of others that prematurity and obstetric damage can predispose children to develop behavior disorders in later life. Drillien in a comparative longitudinal study of premature and full-term babies (1964 a and b) has shown that severe prematurity (birth weight of 4½lb or less), severe complications of pregnancy and/or delivery, and severe familial stress, all make their contribution to behavior disorders in later life even when social class factors are held constant. She showed also that the most common behavior problems that are related to very severe prematurity (birth weight of 3lb or less) are overactivity and restlessness. However, the numbers of such grossly premature babies who survive must be very small indeed.

It is not surprising that, when special risk groups of children are examined, relationships between specific hazards and subsequent behavior disturbances are found which disappear when they are looked for in a more general childhood population. This merely means that the hazardous events are rare and cannot account for the majority of behavior disorders found in children. When large populations are examined, as in the Baltimore studies (Pasamanick et al. 1956, 1959), statistically significant relationships may be found between behavior disorders and traumatic antecedent events, when in fact such events are causally operative in only a minority of disturbed children.

The work of Drillien (1964 b), Pasamanick et al. (1956) and Stott (1965) suggests that perinatal factors can be causally related with any confidence to only certain types of behavior disorders in children, i.e. overactivity, restlessness and distractibility. It would not be surprising however if other behavior problems of a reactive nature, for example delinquency, followed on the social and educational failures that restless and distractible children inevitably experience.

Fraser et al. in Aberdeen (1959) compared the later development of a group of asphyxiated infants and of matched normal controls. In the asphyxiated group there were a few children with gross neurological defects which may in fact have contributed to the asphyxiated state rather than been caused by it. Many more asphyxiated children than controls had minor impairments of motor ability, perception, and perhaps impulse control (nine asphyxiated children had been knocked down in the street compared with two controls). There were, however, no other convincing differences between the groups in behavior as rated by mothers and teachers, and in intelligence.

In a recent study Ucko (1965) suggests that asphyxia at birth may result in quite specific temperamental characteristics in later life: unusual sensitivity, overreactivity to stimuli, and a tendency to become upset when customary routines are broken. The somewhat surprising feature in this study is that as many as thirty out of eighty-one boys and fifteen out of seventy-two girls, said to be reasonably representative of central London children, were described as having been "asphyxiated" at birth. Few details are given about these children's birth histories.

In the present study it has been shown that prematurity and obstetric complications do not contribute significantly to the etiology of behavior disorders in a population of psychiatrically referred primary school children from whom those few diagnosed as having constitutional disorders, had been excluded. This group of hospital attenders had on the whole been identified as in need of treatment by their parents, and not by school teachers or other outside agencies, and the ratio of boys to girls was slightly smaller than is usual for child guidance populations of this age group. The possibility exists that children identified as disturbed at school, who in Edinburgh attend an Educational Child Guidance Clinic, might include a greater excess of boys, and perhaps a greater number who had been exposed to obstetric hazards. A comparison of the two clinic populations would be of great interest.

The present findings are similar to Brandon's in the Newcastle 1000-family study (1960). He compared a group of children identified as maladjusted by Health Visitors with a group of controls, and found no difference in their obstetric histories.

The clinic group studied in the present investigation differed from the control group in that rather more children, especially more second and later born children, had been delivered in a hospital or other institution. Later born siblings of clinic children were also more often born in hospital and clinic mothers made generally more demands for hospital services for themselves and their children than did control mothers. How much this is the result of a true excess of morbidity in behaviorally disturbed children and their mothers, and how much it reflects the greater need for help and support of mothers of clinic attenders remains to be established. Despite the greater call upon medical services made by clinic mothers, the perinatal experiences of their children were no more hazardous than those of the controls.

SUMMARY

(1) The obstetric histories of 100 primary school children referred to a psychiatric department with reactive psychiatric disorders were compared with those of 100 matched controls.

(2) No significant differences were found between the two groups in maternal age, birth weight, factors suggestive of an abnormal foetus, complications of pregnancy, complications of delivery and the postnatal condition of the child.

(3) Rather more clinic than control children were born in hospital and the same was true of their later born siblings.

(4) The implications of these results are discussed. The findings do not conflict with the established predisposition to certain types of behavior disorders of very premature infants and of babies damaged at birth. The present study indicates however that children who have sustained such damage constitute only a minority of the children with behavior problems who come forward for psychiatric care.

Acknowledgements—This study is part of a larger investigation sponsored by the Mental Health Research Fund. I would like to thank the record officers of the four Edinburgh obstetric units and of other hospitals and nursing homes for giving me ready access to their case notes. I am most grateful to Dr. C. M. Drillien for helping me to devise the obstetric part of the interview schedule for use with mothers and the rating scheme for obstetric complications.

REFERENCES

BRANDON, S. (1960) *An Epidemiological Study of Maladjustment in Childhood.* M.D. Thesis, University of Durham.

BUTLER, N. R. and BONHAM, D. G. (1963) *Perinatal Mortality.* Livingstone, Edinburgh.

DRILLIEN, C. M. (1964b) The effect of obstetrical hazard on the later development of the child. In *Recent Advances in Paediatrics.* (Edited by Douglas Gairdner) Churchill, London.

FELDSTEIN, M. S. (1965) A method of evaluating perinatal mortality risk. *Br. J. prev. soc. Med. 19*, 135-139.

FELDSTEIN, M. S. and BUTLER, N. R. (1965) Analysis of factors affecting perinatal mortality. *Br. J. prev. soc. Med. 19*, 128-134.

FRASER, M. S. and WILKS, J. (1959) The residual effects of neonatal asphyxia. *J. Obstet. Gynaec. 66*, 748-752.

General Register Office (1960) *Classification of Occupations.* H.M.S.O., London.

KENDALL, M. G. (1948) *Rank Correlation Methods.* Griffin, London.

PASAMANICK, B., ROGERS, M. E. and LILIENFELD, A. M. (1956) Pregnancy experience and the development of behavior disorder in children. *Am J. Psychiat. 112*, 613-618.

PASAMANICK, B. and KNOBLOCH, H. (1959) Complications of pregnancy and neuropsychiatric disorder. *J. Obstet. Gynaec. 66*, 753-755.

REES, D. J. (1964) *Guide to a Survey Program for Atlas,* Edinburgh University Computer Unit Report No. 2.

ROGERS, M. E., LILIENFELD, A. M. and PASAMANICK, B. (1955) Prenatal and Paranatal factors in the development of childhood behavior disorders. *Acta. psychiat. scand.* Suppl. 102.

STOTT, D. H. (1962) Abnormal mothering as a cause of mental subnormality—I. A critique of some classic studies of maternal deprivation in the light of possible congenital factors. *J. Child Psychol. Psychiat. 3*, 79-91.

STOTT, D. H. (1965) Congenital indications in delinquency. *Proc. R. Soc. Med. 58*, 703-706.

STUART, A. (1957) The comparison of frequencies in matched samples. *Br. J. Stat. Psychol. 10*, 29-32.

UCKO, L. E. (1965) A comparative study of asphyxiated and non-asphyxiated boys from birth to 5 years. *Develop. Med. Child. Neurol. 7*, 643-657.

WOLFF, S. (1967) Behavioral characteristics of primary school children referred to a psychiatric department. *Br. J. Psychiat.* (In press).

APPENDIX A

Enquiry into birth history

(1) Did you have a normal pregnancy?   YES   NO   Specify ....
   Were you admitted to hospital dur-
      ing the pregnancy?   YES   NO   Specify ....
   Were you advised to go to bed at
      home during the pregnancy?   YES   NO   Specify ....
(2) Did you have a normal labor?   YES   NO   Specify ....
   Were instruments used?   YES   NO   Specify ....
(3) Was he a healthy baby?   YES   NO
(4) What was his birth weight?   ....
(5) How soon after birth did you see the   ....
   baby?   ....
   within 48 hrs?   YES   NO
(6) Where was he born?   At home   In hospital
   Name and address of hospital ....
   What was your name and address at the time? ....
   ....
   ....
(7) Maternity notes to be checked on   YES   NO

APPENDIX B

Rating scales for obstetric hazards

(1) *Factors suggestive of an abnormal foetus*
   Each of the following rated one point. Hospital admission for hyperemesis; vaginal bleeding before the 28th week; hydramnios; birth weight below 5th percentile for gestation period (i.e. 1.50-1.75 kg at = > 35 weeks, > 1.75-2.00 kg at = > 37 weeks, > 2.00-2.25 kg at = > 38 weeks, > 2.25-2.50 kg at = > 39 weeks).

(2) *Complications of pregnancy*
   Each of the following rated one point. B.W. > 2.00-2.50 kg; mild immaturity (36 < 38 weeks); mild postmaturity (42 < 44 weeks); Hb % ever < 60; hospital admission for pyelitis; cardiac disease necessitating restriction of activity; moderate essential hypertension or toxaemia (diastolic B.P. 100+ with or without albuminuria); antepostum haemorrhage (at 28 weeks +) of any kind.
   Each of the following rated two points. B.W. 2.00 kgs. or less; severe immaturity (< 36 weeks); severe postmaturity (44 weeks +); severe essential hypertension or toxaemia (diastolic B.P. 110+ with or without albuminuria).
   The following rated three points. Eclampsia diastolic B.P. 90+ and fits with no past history of epilepsy).

(3) *Complications of delivery*
   Each of the following rated one point. Total duration of 1st and 2nd stages of labor for primips. < 3hr or 48hr +, for multips. < 1½hr or 36hr +; spont. breech delivery; assisted breech with or without forceps to aftercoming head*; midcavity or high forceps for any reason other than those specified above and below*; intrapartum haemorrhage; shoulder, face or brow presentation; caesarian section.

---

* Breech extraction scores 1 point for breech delivery and another for forceps delivery = 2 points.

Each of the following rated two points. Vertex with manual rotation and forceps delivery; internal version and breech extraction; low forceps for foetal distress; prolapsed cord.

(4) *Postnatal condition of child*

The following rated zero. Good, no special resuscitation measures needed.

The following rated one point. Causing mild anxiety, but child responded well to measures of resuscitation and was well within 12hr of birth.

The following rated two points. Causing severe anxiety; child responded less quickly to measures of resuscitation or caused anxiety after 12hr.

21

BEHAVIOR PROBLEMS REVISITED:
Findings of an Anterospective Study

Stella Chess, M.D.
Associate Professor of Psychiatry,
New York University School of Medicine.

Alexander Thomas, M.D.
Professor of Psychiatry, New York University School of Medicine
and
Herbert G. Birch, M.D., Ph.D.
Research Professor of Pediatrics,
Albert Einstein College of Medicine.

A number of theoretical formulations have been advanced to explain the origin and nature of behavior problems in childhood. These have included the constitutionalist view in which the symptoms of disturbance are considered to be the direct expression of a predetermined constitutional pattern in the child, the psychoanalytic view in which disturbance is seen as the outcome of conflicts between instinctual drive seeking expression and satisfaction and repressing forces seeking to inhibit or contain them, the learning theory approach in which symptoms are viewed as conditioned maladaptive learned patterns based on conditioned reflex formations, and the culturist view in which symptoms are considered to be the more or less direct expression of sociocultural influences.

Reprinted from THE JOURNAL OF THE AMERICAN ACADEMY OF CHILD PSYCHIATRY, Vol. VI, No. 2, April, 1967, pp. 321-331. This investigation was supported by Grant MH-03614 from the National Institute of Mental Health.

A unique opportunity to investigate the genesis and evolution of behavior problems and to test the validity of these theories has presented itself during the course of our New York longitudinal study of individuality in behavioral development. In this study, in progress since 1956, 39 of the 136 children who have been followed from the earliest months of life onward by a variety of data-gathering techniques have developed behavior disturbances of various types and varying degrees of severity.

Until now, none of the numerous studies in the field has provided a body of evidence sufficient to validate one or another of the extant theoretical formulations. Aside from any other questions as to the adequacy of the data offered as evidence, the approaches have relied primarily on data gathered retrospectively. A number of recent studies, including several from our own center, have revealed significant distortions in retrospective parental reports on the early developmental histories of their children (Robbins, 1963; Wenar, 1963; Chess et al., 1966). It has become clear that retrospective data are insufficient for the study of the genesis of behavior disorders and that anterospective data gathered by longitudinal developmental studies are essential.

Previous longitudinal studies—at Berkeley (Mac Farlane et al., 1954), the Fels Institute (Kagan and Moss, 1962), Yale (Kris, 1957), and Topeka (Murphy et al., 1962)—have made certain contributions to the understanding of the evolution of behavior disorders. The possible significance of temperamental characteristics of the child in interaction with parental functioning has been indicated. A lack of correlation between the child's patterns of psychodynamic defenses and the occurrence of behavioral dysfunction has been found. Symptoms typical of various age-periods have been tabulated, their vicissitudes over time traced, and correlations among different symptoms determined. However, each of these studies has been limited either by small sample size, which has not permitted generalization of the findings, or by the absence of systematic psychiatric evaluation of the children, which has severely restricted the possibility of categorizing the behavior disturbance and of making meaningful correlations with the longitudinal behavioral data.

Our New York longitudinal study has had available, by contrast, both a total sample of substantial size and the data resulting from independent clinical psychiatric evaluation in all of the children with behavior problems. The data on the total sample include information gathered longitudinally and anterospectively at sequential age levels from early infancy onward on the nature of the child's own individual characteristics of functioning at home, in school, and in standard test situations; on parental attitudes and child care practices; on special environmental events and the child's reactions to such events; and on intellectual functioning. In addition, psychiatric evaluation has been done in each child presenting symptoms by the staff child psychiatrist. Wherever necessary, neurological examination or special testing, such as perceptual tests, have been done. Clinical follow-up of each child with a problem has also been carried out systematically.

Details of the data-gathering procedures and of the techniques of data analysis have been reported elsewhere (Chess et al., 1962; Thomas et al., 1963). Since the developmental data were gathered before the child was viewed as a problem by either the parent or the psychiatrist, they were uncontaminated by the distortions which inevitably attend retrospective histories obtained after the appearance of the behavioral disturbance. Data as to environmental influences, such as parental practices and attitudes, changes in family structure, illness and hospitalization, and the character of the school situation, were also obtained in advance of the behavioral disturbance and so were also not distorted by the fact of pathology.

The size of the sample and the nature of the data have made possible various quantitative analyses comparing children with and without behavior problems as well as individual longitudinal case studies. In all our analyses we have been concerned with tracing the ontogenesis and development of each behavioral disturbance in terms of the interaction of temperament and environment, as well as the influence of additional factors in specific cases, such as brain damage, physical abnormalities, and characteristics of intellectual functioning. *Temperament,* in our usage, refers to the behavioral style of the individual child and contains no inferences as to genetic, endocrine, somatologic or environmental etiologies. It is a phenomenological term used to describe the characteristic tempo, energy expenditure, focus, mood, and rhythmicity typifying the behaviors of the individual child, independently of their contents. We have used nine categories of reactivity within which to subsume temperamental attributes. They are activity level, rhythmicity, adaptability, approach-withdrawal, intensity of reaction, quality of mood, sensory threshold, distractibility, and persistence and attention span.[1] A child's temperamental organization, therefore, represents his characteristic mode of functioning with respect to these features of behavioral organization. It refers to the *how* rather than to the *what* or the *why* of

---

[1] See Thomas et al. (1963) for criteria of each of the nine categories and for details of the scoring method.

behavior. No implications of permanence or immutability attach to such a conception.

The prevalence rate of behavior problems in our study population approximates that found in other studies (Lapouse and Monk, 1958; Glidewell et al., 1963). The types of symptoms were typical of those usually coming to notice in preschool and early school age children of middle-class highly educated parents.

In each of the thirty-nine children with behavior problems the psychiatric assessment has been followed by a detailed culling of all the anterospective data from early infancy onward for pertinent information on temperament, environmental influences, and the sequences of symptom appearance and deevlopment. It has been possible in each case to trace the ontogenesis of the behavioral disturbances in terms of the interaction of temperament and environment. Temperament alone did not produce behavioral disturbance. Instances of children of closely similar temperamental structure to the children with behavior problems were found in the normally functioning group. Rather, it appeared that both behavioral disturbance as well as behavioral normality were the result of the interaction between the child with a given patterning of temperament and significant features of his developmental environment. Among these environmental features intrafamilial as well as extrafamilial circumstances such as school and peer group were influential. In several cases, additional special factors such as brain damage or physical abnormality were also operative in interaction with temperament and environment to produce symptoms of disturbed development.

A number of case summaries illustrating typical interactive patterns of development in children with and without behavior problems have been presented in several previous publications (Chess at al., 1963; Birch et al., 1964). At this time we would like to present some of the characteristic temperamental patterns found among the children, the environmental demands which are typically stressful for children with each of these temperamental constellations, and the parental and other environmental approaches which intensify such stressful demands to the point of symptom formation. Symptoms manifested by the children included tantrums, aggressive behavior, habit disorders, fears, learning difficulties, nonparticipation in play activities with other children, and lack of normal assertiveness.

A temperamental pattern which produced the greatest risk of behavior problem development comprises the combination of irregularity in biological functions, predominantly negative (withdrawal) responses to new stimuli, nonadaptability or slow adaptability to change, frequent negative mood, and predominantly intense reactions. As infants, children with this pattern show irregular sleep and feeding patterns, slow acceptance of new foods, prolonged adjustment periods to new routines, and frequent periods of loud crying. Their laughter, too, is characteristically loud. Mothers find them difficult to care for, and pediatricians frequently refer to them as the "difficult infants." They are not easy to feed, to put to sleep, to bathe, or to dress. New places, new activities, strange faces—all may produce initial responses of loud protest or crying. Frustration characteristically produces a violent tantrum. These children approximate 10 percent of the total study population but comprise a significantly higher proportion of the behavior problem group (Rutter et al., 1964). The stressful demands for these children are typically those of socialization, namely, the demands for alteration of spontaneous responses and patterns to conform to the rules of living of the family, the school, the peer group, etc. It is also characteristic of these children that once they do learn the rules, they function easily, consistently, and energetically.

We have found no evidence that the parents of the difficult infants are essentially different from the other parents. Nor do our studies suggest that the temperamental characteristics of the children are caused by the parents. The issue is rather that the care of these infants makes special requirements upon their parents for unusually firm, patient, consistent, and tolerant handling. Such handling is necessary if the difficult infant is to learn to adapt to new demands with a minimum of stress. If the new demand is presented inconsistently, impatiently or punitively effective change in behavior becomes stressful and even impossible. Negativism is a not infrequent outcome of such suboptimal parental functioning.

The problems of managing a difficult child not infrequently highlight a parent's individual reaction to stress. The same parents who are relaxed and consistent with an easy child may become resentful, guilty, or helpless with a difficult child, depending on their own personality structures. Other parents, by contrast, who do not feel guilty or put upon by the child's behavior may learn to enjoy the vigor, lustiness, and "stubbornness" of a difficult infant.

At the opposite end of the temperamental spectrum from the difficult infant is the child who is regular, responds positively to new stimuli (approaches), adapts quickly and easily to change, and shows a predominantly positive mood of mild or moderate intensity. These are the infants who develop regular sleep and feeding schedules easily, take to most new foods at once, smile at strangers, adapt quickly to a new school, accept most frustrations with a minimum of fuss, and learn the rules of new games quickly. They are aptly called "easy babies" and are usually a joy to their parents, pediatricians, and teachers. By contrast to the difficult infant, the easy child adapts to the demands for socialization with little or no stress and confronts his parents with few if any problems in handling. However, although these children do as a group develop significantly fewer behavior problems proportionately than do the difficult infants, their very ease of adaptability may under certain circumstances be the basis for problem behavior development. Most typically we have seen this occur when there is a severe dissonance between the expectations and demands of the intra- and extrafamilial environments. The child first adapts easily to the standards and behavioral expectations of the parent in the first few years of life. When he moves actively into functional situations outside the home, such as in peer play groups and school, stress and malfunctioning will develop if the extrafamilial standard and demands conflict sharply with the patterns learned in the home. As a typical example, the parents of one such child had a high regard for individuality of expression and disapproval of any behavior or attitude in their child which they identified as stereotypical or lacking in imagination. Self-expression was encouraged and conformity and attentiveness to rules imposed by others discouraged even when this resulted in ill manners and a disregard of the desires of others. As the child grew older she became increasingly isolated from her peer group because of continuous insistence on her own preferences. In school her progress was grossly unsatisfactory because of difficulty in listening to directions. The parents were advised to restructure their approach, to place less emphasis on individuality and instead to teach her to be responsive to the needs of others and to conform constructively in behavior in class and in activities with her peers. The parents, acutely aware of the child's growing social isolation and the potential seriousness of her educational problem, carried out this plan consistently. At follow-up, six months later, the child had adapted to the new rules easily, the conflict between standards within and without the home had become minimal, and she had become an active member of a peer group and had caught up to grade level in academic work.

It is certainly true that a severe dissonance between intra-and extrafamilial environment demands and expectations may produce stress and disturbance in psychological development for many types of youngsters, including the difficult child. In our case series, however, it has been most readily apparent as a dominant pathogenic factor in these easy children.

Another important temperamental constellation comprises the combination of negative responses of mild intensity to new stimuli with slow adaptability after repeated contact. Children with this pattern differ from the difficult infants in that their withdrawal from the new is quiet rather than loud. They also usually do not have the irregularity of function, frequent negative mood expression, and intense reactions of the difficult infants. The mildly expressed withdrawal from the new is typically seen with the first encounter with the bath, a new person, a stranger, or a new place. With the first bath the child lies still and fusses mildly, with a new food he turns his head away quietly and lets it dribble out of his mouth, with a stranger who greets him loudly he clings to his mother. If given the opportunity to re-experience new situations without pressure, such a child gradually comes to show quiet and positive interest and involvement. This characteristic sequence of response has suggested the appellation the "Slow to Warm Up" as an apt if inelegant designation for these children. A key issue in their development is whether parents and teachers allow them to make an adaptation to the new at their own tempo or insist on the immediate positive involvement which is difficult or impossible for the slow-to-warm-up children. If the adult recognizes that the slow adaptation to a new school, new peer group or new academic subject reflects the child's normal temperamental style, patient encouragement is likely. If, on the contrary, the child's slow warm-up is interpreted as timidity or lack of interest, adult impatience and pressure on the child for quick adaptation may occur. The child's reaction to this stressful pressure is typically an intensification of his withdrawal tendency. If this increased holding back in turn stimulates increased impatience and pressure on the part of the parent or teacher, a destructive child-environment interactive process will be set in motion.

In several other instances in our study population, nursery school teachers have interpreted the child's slow initial adaptation as evidence of underlying anxiety. In still another case, an elementary school teacher estimated that a child's slow initial mastery of a new accelerated academic program indicated inadequate intellectual capacity. In these cases, the longitudinal behavioral records documented a slow warm-up temperamental style and made possible the recommendation that judgment be suspended until the child could have a longer period of contact with the new situation. The subsequent successful mastery of demands of the new situation clarified the issue as one of temperamental style and not psychopathology or lack or intellectual capacity.

A contrast to the slow-to-warm-up child is the very persistent child who is most likely to experience stress not with his initial contact with a situation but during the course of his ongoing activity after the first positive adaptation has been made. His quality of persistence leads him to resist interference or attempts to divert him from an activity in which he is absorbed. If the adult interference is arbitrary and forcible, tension and frustration tend to mount quickly in these children and may reach explosive proportions.

Type-specific stress and maladaptive child-environment patterns can be identified for other temperamental patterns, such as the very distractible or highly active child, but the scope of this presentation does not permit their description.

Currently influential psychoanalytic theories of the ontogenesis of behavior problems place primary emphasis on the role of anxiety, intrapsychic conflict, and psychodynamic defenses. Our findings do not support these concepts. Our data suggest that anxiety, intrapsychic conflict, and psychodynamic defenses, when they do appear in the course of behavior problem development, are secondary phenomena which result from the stressful, maladaptive character of an unhealthy temperament-environment interaction. Once any or all of these secondary factors appear they can add a new dimension to the dynamics of the child-environment interaction and substantially influence the subsequent course of the behavior problem. It is not surprising that in retrospective studies which begin when the child already presents an extensively elaborated psychological disturbance the prominent phenomena of anxiety and conflict should be labeled as primary rather than secondary influences. Also, if the fact of temperamental individuality is not given serious attention, certain temperamental patterns, such as those of the difficult child or the child with a slow warm-up, are easily misinterpreted as the result of anxiety or as defenses against anxiety.

Our findings also challenge the validity of the currently prevalent assumption that a child's problem is a direct reaction of a one-to-one kind to unhealthy maternal influences. The slogan "To meet Johnny's mother is to understand his problem" expresses an all too frequent approach in which a study of the mother is substituted for a study of the complex factors which may have produced a child's disturbed development, of which parental influences are only one. Elsewhere we have described this unidirectional preoccupation of psychologists and psychiatrists with the pathogenic role of the mother as the "Mal de Mere" syndrome (Chess, 1964). The harm done by this preoccupation has been enormous. Innumerable mothers have been unjustly burdened with deep feelings of guilt and inadequacy as a result of being incorrectly held exclusively or even primarily responsible for their children's problems. Diagnostic procedures have tended to be restricted to a study of the mother's assumed noxious attitudes and practices, with investigations in other directions conducted in a most cursory fashion, or not at all. Treatment plans have focused on methods of changing maternal attitudes and ameliorating the effects of presumed pathogenic maternal attitudes on the child and have ignored other significant etiological factors.

Our data on the origin and development of behavior problems in children emphasize the necessity to study the child—his temperamental characteristics, neurological status, intellectual capacities, and physical handicaps. The parents should also be studied rather than given global labels such as rejecting, overprotective, anxious, etc. Parental attitudes and practices are usually selective and not global, with differentiated characteristics in different areas of the child's life and with marked variability from child to child. Parent-child interaction should be analyzed not only for parental influences on the child but just as much for the influence of the child's individual characteristics on the parent. The influence of other intra- and extrafamilial environmental factors should be estimated in relation to the interactive pattern with each specific child with his individual characteristics rather than in terms of sweeping generalizations.

Our finding that an excessively stressful maladaptive temperament-environment interaction constitutes a decisive element in the development of behavior problems suggests that treatment should emphasize the modification of the interactive process so that it is less stressful and more adaptive. This requires first of all an identification of the pertinent temperamental and environmental issues. Parents can then be armed with this knowledge in the service of modifying their interactive pattern with the child in a healthy direction. Parent guidance rather than parent treatment should be the first aim. If the parent cannot learn to understand his child and utilize this understanding effectively, it then becomes pertinent to inquire into the factors which may be responsible for such a failure of parent guidance. In our experience such failures are in a minority. Most parents do appear able to cooperate in a parent guidance program. When this is accomplished, the parent and psychiatrist can truly become allies in the treatment of the child's problem.

REFERENCES

BIRCH, H. G., THOMAS, A., & CHESS, S. (1964), Behavioral development in brain-damaged children: three case studies. *Arch. Gen. Psychiat.*, 11:596-603.
CHESS, S. (1964), Mal de Mere. *Amer. J. Orthopsychiat.*, 34:613-614.
—— HERTZIG, M., BIRCH, H. G., & THOMAS, A. (1962), Methodology of a study of adaptive functions of the preschool child. *This Journal*, 1:236-245.

—— THOMAS, A., & BIRCH, H. G. (1966), Distortions in developmental reporting made by parents of behaviorally disturbed children. *This Journal*, 5:226-234.

—— —— RUTTER, M., & BIRCH, H. G. (1963), Interaction of temperament and environment in the production of behavioral disturbances in children. *Amer. J. Psychiat.*, 120:142-148.

GLIDEWELL, J. C., DOMKE, H. R., & KANTOR, M. B. (1963), Screening in schools for behavior disorders: use of mother's report of symptoms. *J. Educ. Res.*, 56:508-515.

KAGAN, J. & MOSS, H. A. (1962), *Birth to Maturity: A Study in Psychological Development*. New York: Wiley.

KRIS, M. (1957), The use of prediction in a longitudinal study. *The Psychoanalytic Study of the Child*, 12:175-189. New York: International Universities Press.

LAPOUSE, R. & MONK, M. A. (1958), An epidemiologic study of behavior characteristics in children. *Amer. J. Pub. Hlth.*, 48:1134-1144.

MAC FARLANE, J. W., ALLEN, L., & HONZIK, M. P. (1954), *A Developmental Study of the Behavior Problems of Normal Children between Twenty-one Months and Fourteen Years* [University of California Publications in Child Development, Vol. II]. Berkeley: University of California Press.

MURPHY, L. B. ET AL. (1962), *The Widening World of Childhood*. New York: Basic Books.

ROBBINS, L. C. (1963), The accuracy of parental recall of aspects of child development and of child-rearing practices. *J. Abnorm. Soc. Psychol.*, 66:261-270.

RUTTER, M., BIRCH, H. G., THOMAS, A., & CHESS, S. (1964), Temperamental characteristics in infancy and the later development of behavioral disorders. *Brit. J. Psychiat.*, 110:651-661.

THOMAS, A., CHESS, S., BIRCH, H. G., HERTZIG, M., & KORN, S. (1963), *Behavioral Individuality in Early Childhood*. New York: New York University Press.

WENAR, C. (1963), The reliability of developmental histories: summary and evaluation of evidence. *Psychosom. Med.*, 25:505-509.

22

MASKED DEPRESSION IN CHILDREN AND ADOLESCENTS

Kurt Glaser, M.D.

Clinical Director, Rosewood State Hospital;
Associate Professor of Pediatrics; Assistant Professor of Psychiatry;
University of Maryland, School of Medicine

Depression in the adult is a well-known psychiatric condition with rather well-defined and relatively easily recognizable symptoms. In the child and adolescent, depression is often not recognized as such because it may be hidden by symptoms not readily identified with this condition. Textbooks of psychiatry and even child psychiatry give little space to the subject of depression per se, yet, when searching in different chapters, one is struck by the frequency with which signs pointing toward the existence of depression are found in cases classified under a variety of diagnoses and chapters other than depression.

Symptoms which in the adult indicate depression are not necessarily found in children with depressive reaction. Keeler[1] writes, "Depressive reactions are not commonly met within children" and in a later paragraph on the same page, "Depression in children is difficult to detect. Many of the features seen in adults, e.g. disturbances in eating and sleeping habits, psychomotor retardation, etc. are frequently absent." Toolan[2] states, "One of the reasons that suicidal attempts have been overlooked in children and adolescents is the erroneous concept that youngsters do not experience depression. It is true that they do not exhibit the signs and symptoms of adult depressive reactions but rather other symptoms."

Reprinted from AMERICAN JOURNAL OF PSYCHOTHERAPY, Vol. XXI, No. 3, pp. 565-574, July 1967. Presented at the Seventh E. A. Gutheil Memorial Conference of the Association for the Advancement of Psychotherapy, New York City, October 30, 1966.

Thus, symptoms which in the adult are usually considered diagnostic for depression—such as suicidal attempts or suicide—do not necessarily point toward the same diagnosis in children, but may be impulsive acts, indicating acute anger or rebellion[3, 4, 5] rather than chronic depression. Sleep difficulties may "resemble in manifest appearance the sleeping disorders of depressive or melancholic adults" but usually are neither the symptoms nor forerunners of depression in children.[6]

The cases discussed in this paper, some taken from the literature and others from the author's own experience, should meet two criteria. The presenting symptoms should not usually be associated with depression, yet there should be sufficient evidence that the patient's psychopathology features depressive elements. For the purpose of this presentation, depression or depressive features are understood to exist when the patient expresses feelings of inadequacy, worthlessness, low self-esteem, helplessness and hopelessness, rejection by others, isolation; yet in the eyes of the examiner or the patient's immediate environment these feelings do not correspond to the patient's actual life situation or are stronger than the patient's actual condition seems to warrant. Depression may be, but does not necessarily have to be, the underlying causative pathology or even the main psychopathologic reaction, but it must be a definite feature of the total picture of the child's disturbance.

The recognition of depressive features in the child's psychiatric make-up is important for the appropriate psychotherapeutic approach. Not only may the masking symptoms misdirect the therapist, parents, teachers, or institutional personnel in their endeavor to help the patient and instead lead them to institute damaging measures, but the depressive elements in the patient's thought process are apt to reduce further his capacity to function. Obviously, special consideration must be given to those individuals who, due to their intellectual limitations, are not able to compete with people in their immediate environment and actually are rejected by them. This will be taken up in the discussion on masked depression in the mentally retarded. Manifest behavior disturbances revealing underlying depressive reactions in children of different age levels are described below.

INFANTS AND SMALL CHILDREN

Deprivation reactions in infants and small children present themselves as developmental retardation and often affect the physical, intellectual, and emotional development of the child. Depressive elements can be operative in addition to developmental retardation. Spitz[7] first coined the term "anaclitic depression" in small children deprived of their mother's presence. He described the sequence of their reaction to separation from the mother in three phases. At first the child shows active protest and a violent emotional reaction in an apparent attempt to bring mother back. This is followed by active rejection of adults and finally by apathy, withdrawal of interest in people, and a decreased activity level.

Failure to thrive is today a well-known pediatric syndrome found in children who have suffered deprivation of stimulation and affect. Growth failure in maternal deprivation has recently been described in a book by Patton and Gardner.[8] Intellectual retardation as a result of understimulation has been widely published and researched in the past and has come recently to the foreground in an attempt at its prevention in the impoverished section of our population. Damage to personality development as a result of prolonged absence of a meaningful one-to-one relationship to a mother figure has been pointed out by the well-known publications of Goldfarb,[9] Bowlby,[10] and others. A review of the subject of maternal deprivation, including pertinent literature, was published in *Pediatrics* in 1956.[11] The existence of depressive elements in these deprived children is often not recognized, and too little attention may be given to a corrective psychiatric approach to this condition.

OLDER CHILDREN AND ADOLESCENTS

In older children *behavioral problems and delinquent behavior,* such as temper tantrums, disobedience, truancy, running away from home, may indicate depressive feelings but may not be recognized as such.[2] Keeler[1] stated that delinquent behavior was present in 7 of 11 patients studied at the Psychiatric Division of Bellevue Hospital for their reaction to the death of a parent. *Psychoneurotic reactions,* such as school phobia, can mask underlying depression,[12] and *failure to achieve in school* can be a symptom of unrecognized depression.[13, 14] A *psychophysiologic reaction* may at times be the presenting symptom in children with depressive feelings.[1]

Delinquency. Aichhorn in his book on delinquency[15] describes a seventeen-year-old shoemaker's apprentice who suddenly ran away from his job and did not return home for days. He became defiant. The boy's behavior was such that it disrupted the entire life of the family consisting of father, stepmother, five-year-old half-sister and nineteen-year-old brother who was about to enter University. The father, in desperation, wanted to send the boy to the institution for delinquents. In the interview the boy voiced a hopeless outlook on life ("It's no use"). He now revealed that at the time of his first disappearance from home he wanted to kill himself but rather ran away with the idea never to return.

In another boy, sixteen years old, who was committed to Aichhorn's institution, the presenting symptoms were vagrancy and refusal to work. The symptoms appeared shortly after the shocking accidental death of the boy's mother, and Aichhorn states in the study of the case, "perhaps the boy escaped melancholia in this way."

> *Case 1.* A twelve-year-old boy was brought to my attention because he drove and wrecked the family car while the parents were asleep. In school he had committed various mischievous acts leading to destruction of property, and he had stolen knives, among other things. He was one of three adopted boys, with one natural sister, in an economically upper class family. He was able to verbalize a great deal of hostility against his parents for their rigid control and against his sister who, he felt, was favored. He was unusually tall for his age and saw this as a source of difficulty since on the one hand he was expected to act older and on the other hand he had trouble with peers. His depression became evident at first by the content of an essay he had to write for the judge as a punishment for his unlawful driving. Later he verbalized about not liking himself and about his fears of death both during waking hours as well as in dreams. He had difficulties in going to sleep and often awoke in the middle of the night.

One may well speculate whether his driving attempts at night and his stealing and carrying knives may not have had suicidal or destructive motivation, or both. The depressive features of low self-esteem and dissatisfaction with himself were probably major contributing factors in this boy's delinquent behavior.

> *Case 2.* An eighteen-year-old girl was referred because she was keeping undesirable company and late hours; also because of drinking, promiscuous behavior, and threats of running away. She had just graduated from high school and had been accepted at a local college. Her delinquent behavior had its onset during the summer. She was an only child whose father had died when she was seven years old. Three years later her mother married a man with three children.
>
> It became evident during the first interviews that this girl was in severe conflict over her great dependency upon her mother ("I was always spoiled rotten") and her desire to be independent. She felt the mother had remarried to provide a father for her, and she blamed herself for the mother's unhappy marriage. She described herself as isolated and depressed ("nobody likes me"). The previous summer she had tried to overcome this isolation by freely giving of herself sexually. "I need affection; I don't get it at home, I try to get it from other people. Last year I looked for pity and sympathy . . . this year

I try to get close to boys—even if I know they don't like me—even if just while they are with me." To her mother she stated, "I know I am killing you slowly but surely."

It seems very likely that the depressed feelings of isolation, lack of love, and guilt led this girl to her acting-out behavior. In the course of the interviews she verbalized her desire to change her recent course of life; she dropped the idea of college (she had registered only to please her mother) and actively started to look for a job, recognizing her own lack of preparedness for any worthwhile occupation. She was restraining her behavior to correct her reputation while keeping the contact with male companions within socially acceptable limits.

These cases demonstrate delinquent behavior as the presenting symptoms, masking an underlying depression. The dynamics of the depressive reaction, different for each case, are beyond the scope of this paper.

School Phobia. Agras,[12] studying seven cases of *school phobia* (three girls and four boys· aged six to twelve) found that six of the seven children showed symptoms of depression, such as weeping for no apparent reason, and "unhappy, miserable, whining behavior." There was also a high incidence of depressive reactions among the parents of these children (termed depressive constellation by Agras).

Case 3. Acute school phobia on the second day of school was the presenting symptom of a fourteen-year-old girl in the 9th grade. After attending the first day of school without apparent difficulties, her behavior became hysterical on the second day, and a change of schools (from public school to an exclusive private day school) did not change the situation. The girl was socially active, physically attractive, and had been an average student the previous years. Her suicidal thoughts, both during waking hours and in dreams, were revealed to the therapist during the first hours of treatment; she had thought of jumping off the porch, cutting her wrists, and taking sleeping pills. She then expressed overt and covert wishes for her mother's divorce or death.

In this case we see school phobia as the presenting symptom in a child with severe intrafamily and intrapsychic conflicts, with depression very much in evidence underneath the masking symptomatology.

Learning Difficulties. School failure may be another symptom (or syndrome) masking underlying depression. Wertz,[13] in evaluating psychodynamic stresses of the eight cases he reviewed, states "the self image of these patients was uniformly poor. . . . They experienced themselves as weak and helpless with chronic feelings of inadequacy and inferiority. . . . There were identifications with the handicapped and the underdog."

Silverman *et al.* in their study on learning problems[14] present the case of eight-year-old Roy· referred for learning difficulties, aggressiveness, and hyperactivity. He was chronically fearful and preoccupied with illness and death, had experienced serious operations in both mother and father and the death of an older sister "who often fondly cared for him." Roy made statements such as: "I'd try and forget about mother and sister . . . but then I remember it in the classroom, like when I'm reading and feel sad and worried." His mother was unhappy, depressed, and unsure of herself.

In the second case report in the same paper, Jay, an eight-year-old boy, was referred because of disturbed classroom behavior and reading retardation in the presence of adequate intelligence. The school personnel described him as occasionally depressed and frequently complaining of somatic symptoms. During treatment the following observations indicated depressive features: he exaggeratedly rebuked himself, was tired and had difficulty sleeping, was preoccupied with injury, illness, and death. It is interesting to note that his mother had a "deep sense of inadequacy" and "mood swings from excitement to depression."

Both cases, referred for learning difficulties (reading disability), presented evidence of underlying depressive feelings and interestingly enough, both also showed the "depressive constellation" as described by Agras.[12]

> *Case 4.* A rapid downhill course from a good student in the 7th grade to failing marks in the 8th was the presenting symptom in a thirteen-year-old girl. She considered herself stupid, unable to keep up with her classmates, not liked by parents and siblings. The symptoms occurred at the time of her menarche· and she spent much of the interview time discussing the struggle of her changing identity from a child to an adolescent and future adult. She expressed her guilt for her mother's varicose veins, for which she felt responsible since they had occurred following her mother's pregnancies. She was overly concerned about illness and death and finally was able to express her guilt over her death wishes for members of her family. She admitted at least on one occasion to have looked for pills to kill herself.
>
> The depression, camouflaged by school failure, was not evident to her immediate environment (teacher, school counselor, parents). Her parents, very intelligent professionals, considered her happy and popular and described the family relationship as good.

> *Case 5.* School failure was the presenting problem in a very bright girl, ten and a half years old. She had had traumatic experiences in foster homes after her mother's divorce and was well aware of the current marital difficulties as well as her stepfather's behavior.

He had had psychiatric care for depressions. Her attachment to her stepfather was pathologically intense, leading during later years to overt sexual approaches. Projective tests showed feelings of inadequacy and unfulfilled dependency needs as well as depression. She wanted to be a nurse "to help children in wards who had unhappy lives." When she was fifteen, she showed delinquent behavior in addition to continued academic difficulties. She now verbalized her feelings of being unwanted as demonstrated to her by the biologic father's desertion of the family and her subsequent foster home placement. The only person by whom she felt really loved was her stepfather, which created severe incestual conflicts. She considered herself the cause of the current marital difficulties and spoke of depression and suicide. Some of her delinquent behavior gave indication of her self-destructive drive.

In this case, depressive elements and suicidal tendencies were overshadowed by the presenting symptoms of school failure, delinquency, and prominent psychosexual conflicts.

One may include in this chapter on school failure a group of older adolescents and young adults who attend college, shift their major interest from field to field, thereby losing credits for previous studies, interrupt, re-start, go part time. This faltering in the studies, the indecisiveness of choosing a career may hide the underlying lack of self-confidence and often frank depression. It also serves as a device to keep the person in the sheltered position of a student, and to avoid the responsibility of commitment toward a certain career, toward moving from the home of the parents or from the regulated dormitory set-up to face the realities of adult life.

Psychophysiologic reactions. Keeler[1] describes the case of a boy of six and a half with headaches, abdominal pains, and vomiting. He presented himself as a friendly, smiling, cooperative child, alert and playful. Extensive medical examination revealed no organic pathology. Only months later it became clear during psychiatric evaluation that the psychosomatic symptoms started shortly after he was told of his father's death, and projective tests made it quite "obvious that these surface manifestations obscured feelings of depression. . . ."

> *Case 6.* This fifteen-year-old girl had been referred because of colitis for which she had in the past been hospitalized in critical condition. Her response to medical treatment was unsatisfactory. After an initial period of blaming her parents, her friends· and the physicians who attended her for her difficulties, she changed to such statements as: "I hate myself for thinking the way about people— blaming them. Why do I always feel inferior?" She then spoke about

her inadequacies, her inability to live up to her mother's expectations, her own contribution toward her isolation from friends.

Case 7. Psychophysiologic reactions and school failure were the presenting problems of an eleven-year-old boy with an I.Q. of 125. He was an only child. He frequently missed school because of "spastic bowels" and headaches. There was considerable conflict between the parents, both in background and in personality, which was denied during the first months of treatment of the child. The mother was suffering from ulcerative colitis sufficiently severe to cause her hospitalization. The father was a health fanatic preoccupied with pills, diet, and exercise.

An earlier referral for psychiatric treatment when the child was seven had never been followed through and was almost forgotten. The presenting symptoms then had been lonesomeness, unhappiness, crying spells. Only now, when the boy was eleven, did the parents really seek help because academic failure threatened promotion to the next grade.

After some interviews the child described himself as the second smallest in class (true) and ugly (he was very attractive looking and well built). He stated, "I can't do anything right—never please father—nobody likes me." It was not tutoring or change of class or school which was needed but rather psychiatric treatment of the child to alter his self-concept, and considerable work with the parents with regard to their approach to the child and their facing up to their marital difficulties.

This last group of cases illustrates psychophysiologic reactions in children with underlying depressive features which should not be ignored or overlooked during treatment.

So far we have presented examples of masked depressive elements in the psychopathology of youngsters who were brought to the attention of the therapist for a variety of complaints such as delinquent behavior, phobias, underachievement in school, or psychosomatic symptoms. All these children were of normal or superior intelligence.

A few words may be indicated about children and adolescents with subnormal intellectual functioning.

MASKED DEPRESSION IN RETARDATES

Patients with mild to moderate degrees of mental retardation often recognize their inadequacy and the overt or covert rejection by peers and elders. Their appraisal of their position in life and the reaction of the environment to them may be realistic, but they lack the verbal tools of expressing themselves and the equipment of either correcting their inadequacies or compensating for them.

The fact that the feelings of inadequacy and rejection are often based on a realistic appraisal of the situation and the attitudes of the persons important in the patient's life presents an interesting aspect in the study of the retarded. Since often the environmental conditions and attitudes of others cannot be influenced or corrected, it becomes the very difficult task of the psychiatrist to help the retarded accept his inadequacies and the rejection by others. The feelings of inadequacy, helplessness, hopelessness, as well as rejection may find their expression in overt symptoms of depression; very often, however, these feelings produce anger against the environment, especially when superiority of siblings, schoolmates, and friends is obvious, and this anger is then expressed in acting-out behavior. This behavior may be directed against those who control the retarded (parents, teachers, or staff in the institution) and thus lead to further restrictions and more severe control and punishment which reinforce the feelings of helplessness and anger. Because of fear of punishment or inability to effectively show hostility toward the controlling persons, the retarded may direct his acts toward younger, defenseless, individuals, animals, or objects.

In the therapeutic approach it is necessary to recognize the underlying cause of the "bad behavior" and attempt to interrupt the vicious cycle. Further attempts at training and education often serve only to increase the frustration and reinforce the feelings of inadequacy. It therefore seems more appropriate to find a meaningful occupation for the retarded which allows him to experience success. Thus it is not surprising that in institutional practice it has been found for years that retardates often make very adequate attendants for other retardates who have more severe degrees of mental or physical handicap than they themselves. Such meaningful activity under proper supervision and guidance not only allows the experience of success, especially if properly recognized and rewarded by the staff, but also puts the retarded in close relationship with other people toward whom he can realistically feel superior. Unfortunately, the situation in institutions, with poorly trained, underpaid, and overworked staff, often does not disrupt the cycle of acting-out-retribution and more acting-out but rather reinforces the inappropriate behavior. Both retardates and staff experience increasing dissatisfaction, hopelessness, and helplessness.

> *Case 8.* A twenty-two-year-old girl, institutionalized for many years, had been deserted by her family and been in a foster home for some time. Her acting out consisted of homosexual promiscuity, fighting, gossiping, lying, and running away. The psychiatrist reported: "During my interviews with H. she was quite sleepy and

depressed. There was a depressive overtone to her communications while she tried to maintain a detached, noncommittal attitude. She tried to communicate that she was completely self-sufficient while feeling very helpless and dependent beneath this façade. Her long years of institutionalization gave her a certain leadership role among other girls which she used to satisfy her dependency needs by obtaining clothing and other objects from them. She explained her attempt at running away by her desire to get married to someone (anyone) while out of the institution for a few days. Her acting-out behavior had led her to be secluded in the security building of the institution some 15 times."

Case 9. A thirteen-year-old girl with WISC scores of verbal 81, performance 81 and full scale 77 was referred because her mother could not cope with her demanding attitude. The mother also complained about the girl's tics and compulsive behavior as well as sleeping and eating habits.

The natural father had died six years prior to the referral and the mother was remarried. There were two socially and scholastically successful siblings from the first marriage. During the diagnostic interviews the girl soon revealed her constant worries, her loneliness and lack of friends, her jealousy over the popularity of her sister and stated that "the kids my age act older" and "all those teenagers are dancing and talking" while she was left out.

With the recognition of the great and ever-increasing economic drain which untrained and maladjusted retardates cause upon society, habilitative programs have been increased. While the care for the retarded is certainly not the sole responsibility of the psychiatrist, he can make a major contribution. His role with this group of patients is usually different from the traditional psychotherapeutic effort on a one-to-one basis. It consists rather in the creation of a therapeutic social and occupational milieu, the training and guidance of the staff of day and residential facilities, and parent counseling. The study and proper recognition of the psychodynamic background of behavior of the retarded is thus of direct concern to the psychiatrist if he wishes to extend his services to this rather significant group of handicapped people.

SUMMARY

Behavior disturbances and psychologic reactions in children and adolescents may conceal depressive elements in the underlying psychopathology. These depressive elements are not identical with the classic disease entity of depression or with the self-limited depressive episodes known in adult psychiatry. Nevertheless, they are dynamic forces influencing the child's functioning or malfunctioning as the case may be.

In the very young child and in the mentally retarded, concealed depressive features are often not suspected. Recognition of the presence of such underlying pathology in all children, from infancy through adolescence, including those with mental handicaps, is essential for choice and direction of the therapeutic approach.

REFERENCES

1. KEELER, W. R. Children's Reactions to the Death of a Parent. In *Depression*. Hoch, P. H. and Zubin, J., Eds. Grune & Stratton, New York, 1954, p. 116.
2. TOOLAN, J. M. Suicide and Suicidal Attempts in Children and Adolescents. *Am. J. Psychiat.*, 118: 719, 1962.
3. GLASER, K. Suicide in Children and Adolescents. In *Acting Out—Theoretical and Clinical Aspects*. Abt, L. E. and Weissman, S. L., Eds. Grune & Stratton, New York, 1965, p. 87.
4. GLASER, K. Suicide—A Form of Rebellion in the Adolescent. Paper presented at the Sixth International Congress of Child Psychiatry, Edinburgh, 1966.
5. LOURIE, R. S. Clinical Studies of Attempted Suicide in Childhood. *Clin. Proc. Child Hosp.*, 22: 163, 1966.
6. FREUD, A. Normality and Pathology in Childhood. International Universities Press, New York, 1965, pp. 158-159.
7. SPITZ, R. A. and WOLF, K. M. Anaclitic Depression: An Inquiry into the Genesis of Psychiatric Conditions in Early Childhood. *Psychoanalytic Study of the Child*, Vol. 2. International Universities Press, 1946, p. 313.
8. PATTON, R. . and GARDNER, L. I. *Growth Failure in Maternal Deprivation*. C. C Thomas, Springfield, Ill., 1963.
9. GOLDFARB, W. Effects of Psychological Deprivation in Infants and Subsequent Stimulation. *Am. J. Psychiat.*, 102: 18, 1945.
10. BOWLBY, J. *Maternal Care and Mental Health*. WHO Monograph Series No. 2, 1951.
11. GLASER, K. and EISENBERG, L. Maternal Deprivation. *Pediatrics*, 18: 626, 1956.
12. AGRAS, S. The Relationship of School Phobia to Childhood Depression. *Am. J. Psychiat.*, 116: 533, 1959.
13. WERTZ, F. J. Adolescent Underachievers—Evaluating Psychodynamic and Environmental Stresses. *N. Y. State Med.*, 63: 3524, 1963.
14. SILVERMAN, J. S., FITE, M. W., and MOSHER, M. M. Clinical Findings in Reading Disability Children—Special Cases of Intellectual Inhibition. *Am. J. Orthopsychiat.*, 29: 298, 1959.
15. AICHHORN, A. *Wayward Youth*. Viking Press, New York, 1935, pp. 92 ff. and 41 ff.

23

BEHAVIOR THERAPY WITH CHILDREN:
A Broad Overview

John S. Werry, M.B., F.R.C.P.(C)
Research Child Psychiatrist, Children's Research Center,
University of Illinois (Urbana)
Assistant Professor of Psychiatry, Department of Psychology,
University of Illinois.

and

Janet P. Wollersheim, M.A.
University of Illinois (Urbana)

Behavior therapy is a term coined by Eysenck (1959) to denote a system of psychotherapy of relatively recent origin (Wolpe, 1958) which is distinguished from other types of psychotherapy by its theoretical background and its points of emphasis in the clinical area.

Unfortunately, at least three factors have militated against a positive and inquiring attitude by child psychiatrists and other child therapists toward behavior therapy. The first of these is unfamiliarity with the terminology and concepts of behavior therapy, thus making it appear much more complex than it really is. The second deterrent has been the aggressive attitude of some of the protagonists of behavior therapy who have proselytized it as the only possible approach to therapy. The third and least defensible impediment is that of a conservatism resulting perhaps from some degree of institutionalization of present techniques

Reprinted from JOURNAL OF THE AMERICAN ACADEMY OF CHILD PSYCHIATRY, Vol. VI, No. 2, April 1967, pp. 346-370. The preparation of this paper has been supported in part by a grant (MH-07346) from the National Institute of Health, U.S. Department of Health, Education and Welfare.

of therapy. The aim of this review is to acquaint child therapists with some of the concepts and techniques of behavior therapy· to offer illustrative case studies, and to indicate what the authors believe to be the pertinence of behavior therapy in the remediation of the psychopathology of childhood.

THEORETICAL CONSIDERATIONS

The theoretical framework of behavior therapy is *learning theory* which, unlike earlier systems, did not grow out of the clinical situation but rather out of rigorously controlled laboratory experiments chiefly with animals. While differences between behavior therapy and more traditional approaches are in part due to its underlying theory, some appear merely to be semantic in nature.

One major difference between behavior therapy and more traditional approaches is the emphasis of the former upon overt behavior. In their enthusiasm to make psychology a legitimate science, early twentieth-century psychologists adopted a position of rigorous empiricism. It is therefore not surprising that behavior therapists have likewise shown themselves suspicious of elegant, hypothetical constructs like that of the ego, have instead focused on more atomistic, more readily observable behaviors which in more common parlance might be described as "symptoms" or "ego functions" (Eysenck, 1959; Ullmann and Krasner, 1965). This difference is also partly attributable to the differing historical backgrounds of the two approaches: behavior therapy deriving from experimental psychology rather than from medicine. Behavior therapists, for example, do not talk about *psychopathology* but rather about *maladaptive behaviors*. Also, traditional psychotherapy has depended heavily on the medical disease model, in particular the concept of underlying unitary pathology (e.g., the unconscious conflict) producing a plethora of surface manifestations or symptoms. Experimental psychologists, on the other hand· have been interested largely in determining the functional relationships between environmental events or stimuli and organismic responses. Their interest, too, in pre-existing states within the organism has been limited, particularly since these organismic states were readily controllable in the laboratory setting.

The second major difference between behavior therapy and certain more traditional approaches is that, for the behavior therapists, maladaptive behavior (e.g., psychotic symptoms) is not seen as qualitatively different from what is arbitrarily defined as normal behavior. Both are acquired or *learned* and removed or *unlearned* in the same ways by essentially the same processes and are subject to the same general laws. The content of an individual's experience determines the specific kinds of behavior he exhibits or has learned, though organic factors may influence not only the range of potential behaviors but also the probability of certain classes of behavior being emitted and hence of becoming stabilized.

The third difference stems from behavior therapy's adherence to learning theory rather than to another theory such as that of psychoanalysis. Learning theory suggests two basic kinds of learning or conditioning (this latter term is essentially a synonym for learning). The first kind of learning, classical conditioning or *respondent learning,* was discovered by Pavlov and is probably the most familiar to child therapists. This is essentially the modification of a naturally occurring reflex arc usually involving the autonomic nervous system as effector, in which a neutral or conditioned stimulus is substituted for the natural or unconditioned stimulus. The simplest example of such learning in child psychopathology is Watson's little Albert who developed a rat phobia by being exposed to a naturally phobic stimulus, loud noise, every time he reached out to touch a white rat which had been initially an object of curiosity to the child (Watson and Rayner, 1920). The essential characteristics of this type of learning are the potency of environmental events or external stimuli in eliciting autonomic responses from a helpless and passive organism. Its pertinence to the human organism is probably paramount in all kinds of emotional reactions to external events.

The second type of learning has been emphasized by Skinner (1938) and is termed *operant conditioning.* Fundamental to the concept of the operant response is the idea, first, of choice and, second, of effecting or operating on the environment. Hence it usually involves the voluntary rather than the autonomic central nervous system. What makes the organism choose to perform one operant response rather than another in a nonnovel situation is considered to be determined by the consequences or *reinforcement* which followed the same act on previous occasions. In general, reinforcement is considered to follow the pleasure principle in which acts which are rewarded become more probable or learned, while unrewarded or punished acts become less probable or *extinguished.* The efficacy of a given reinforcer depends on several factors such as the need state of the individual (food is unlikely to be effective if the subject has just satiated himself) and, in the human, a degree of idiosyncrasy stemming from the complex uniqueness of individual experience and our capacity for symbolism.

In operant learning, particularly in a higher organism, the stimulus is much less powerful than in respondent learning since, in operant learning, the stimulus represents a sign or cue indicating the possibilities of reinforcement, of reward or punishment which the organism may elect to heed or not, according to his own particular whim or need state. Nevertheless, the stimulus in operant learning does exhibit the characteristic of *stimulus generalization* as in respondent learning. This means that there is a range of environmental events which are likely to produce a learned response. The more similar these are to those of the learning situation, the greater is the chance of the learned behavior occurring. For example, it is assumed by parents that a child who learns certain modes of conduct at his own table will behave in a similar fashion when he eats with friends.

Of practical importance in therapy is the fact that the further along the stimulus generalization gradient a particular stimulus lies (that is, the more dissimilar it is to the original), the less likely it is to evoke the learned response, and also, in the case of the respondent behavior, the weaker the response will be. Also, no matter how much practice is undertaken, learning is never perfect. Thus, on some occasions, the presentation of a stimulus will not evoke the learned response, but instead may evoke some other behavior. Further, it is possible to weaken the effect of a stimulus by presenting it in competition with another stimulus of antagonistic effects as typified by Miller's approach-avoidance conflict studies (1944). By utilizing this knowledge about the effect of the stimulus upon the response, behavior therapists can maximize the probability of occurrence of healthy behaviors and strengthen them at the expense of psychopathological alternatives.

Left to themselves, conditioned responses do not decay as a function of time or, in short, are not forgotten. They disappear in two ways. First, responses can be weakened through *extinction,* which means that the conditioned reflex is elicited without any presentation of the unconditioned stimulus, or, in the case of operant behavior, reinforcement does not follow the emission of the responses. Probably more common than extinction in the natural situation is the phenomenon of replacement or *counterconditioning* whereby the response to a given stimulus is changed to another response which is incompatible with the original one. Both extinction and counterconditioning are used extensively by behavior therapists in the treatment of already existing maladaptive responses. However, where no response exists or, in short, where the "symptom" is a sign of deficient functioning such as in the developmental type of enuresis (Barbour et al., 1963), *conditioning* is employed to develop the desired patterns of behavior.

It is possible to delineate about seven phases in behavior therapy which are, with terminological modifications, equally applicable to other forms of psychotherapy.

Problem Definition: As mentioned above, behavior therapists have an atomistic approach to problem definition with the emphasis upon discrete observable behaviors (this includes verbalizations). Although theoretically one could construct a comprehensive list of all the symptoms and then proceed systematically to eliminate them, this procedure is seldom practicable. The usual procedure is to select the symptoms which are either most distressing to the patient or to those in his social environment, or most suitable for treatment. As such, problem definition is likely to be simple and practical.

Problem Analysis: Having isolated the symptoms which are both deserving of and amenable to therapy, the therapist then attempts to determine the factors or stimuli which elicit the behavior, such as the feared situation in a phobia, and/or the factors which are perpetuating or reinforcing the problem behavior. This kind of information frequently requires some kind of observation of the child in a real-life situation such as at school or in the mother-child interaction. In respondent or emotional behavior, the therapist is likely to spend more time with stimuli; and in operant behavior, he is more likely to be concerned with determining the response-reinforcement contingencies in the child's natural environment.

Mapping Out a Plan of Therapy: From the diagnostic information gathered in the first two phases, the therapist plans his therapeutic program firm in the belief that he himself can control the patient's behavior in such a way as to maximize therapeutic effect rather than be guided by the patient himself as in play therapy or free association techniques.

Motivating the Patient for Therapy: This category requires no special description but is inserted only to indicate that though this point is seldom emphasized in papers on behavior therapy, it is no less important than in other approaches. After initial motivation, of course, the key to continued motivation lies both in the personality of the therapist and the proper structuring or *programming* of the plan of therapy.

Behavior Shaping: This is the first phase of actual treatment after initial motivation for therapy has been attained. Behavior shaping is a picturesque term which underlines the important principle of gradualism. Little by little, the therapist seeks to move the child's behavior closer to that behavior which is desired. The change is planned in gradual steps so that the behavior change can be relatively easily accomplished. Throughout treatment, the therapist assumes an active role, controlling both the stimuli and the response-reinforcement contingencies rather than waiting for an occasional *moment critique* so emphasized in other types of therapy. Because of this emphasis upon controlling environmental contingencies to alter the subject's response to stimuli, behavior therapy is as likely to be carried on in the child's own environment as in the therapist's office. Also because of the clarity and explicitness of the therapeutic program as designed by the professional behavior therapists, often it can be largely carried out by relatively unskilled persons such as the mother herself (Wahler et al., 1965; Allen and Harris, 1966), the nurse (Ayllon and Michael, 1959), nursing assistants (Wolf et al., 1964), undergraduate students (Davison, 1964, 1965), or even machines (Werry and Cohrssen, 1965).

Generalization of Behavior: Once the desired behavior has been achieved, and particularly where therapy has been carried out in the clinic rather than the child's natural setting, an active inquiry is made as to whether the behavior has *generalized* or is now manifest in all spheres of the child's natural environment where it should be. If the child is not performing the desired behavior in some situations, generalization must be produced directly by carrying therapy into other environments or by using as co-therapists persons such as parents who are with the child in many different environments.

Stabilization of Behavior: It is also necessary to determine whether the behavior has acquired some degree of stability so that it will continue to be emitted once therapy has been discontinued. Studies with animals have shown that the quickest way to achieve desired behavior is to reinforce this behavior every time it occurs or is elicited (continuous reinforcement). However, resistance to extinction can be greatly increased by then moving on to a schedule of so-called intermittent or inconsistent reinforcement (Holland and Skinner, 1961). In a large number of cases, of course, stabilization of behavior should be ensured by naturally occurring reinforcement from significant persons in the child's environment or from the improved intrapsychic state of the patient. The general plan of the behavior therapist is to arrange for continuous and immediate reinforcement of the new behavior when this behavior is being acquired. The reinforcement is then moved to an intermittent schedule which approximates that occurring in the child's natural environment.

Although the general principles of learning theory used in behavior therapy are relatively few (conditioning, counterconditioning, and extinction), the technologies of therapy or the practical methods of applying them in treatment are many. The following is a description of the major techniques used with children as reported in the literature up to the present time (July 1966). These methods have been grouped according to the principal point of focus in therapy: (1) the preceding environmental events or stimuli, (2) the response of the organism, (3) the environmental events consequent upon the response (reinforcement), and (4) the pre-existing intraorganismic state. Such a categorization is, of course, artificial since few techniques are completely pure, but it is offered in the hope that it will prove useful in the designing of individual therapeutic programs.

Stimulus Manipulation

In view of the passive-reflexive response of the organism in respondent or classical conditioning, it is not surprising that attempts to deal with psychopathological conditions which typify this kind of learning (found mostly in emotional reactions) try to overthrow the tyranny of the environmental stimulus by an attack directly on this stimulus.

Systematic Desensitization of Stimuli: This is a method which capitalizes upon the weakness of the conditioned response and its lower probability of occurrence at the extremes of the stimulus generalization gradient. It was developed by Wolpe (1958) who usually simultaneously strengthens incompatible, alternative responses (*vide infra*) such as relaxation and assertion. In our experience, the simultaneous strengthening of an incompatible alternative response is by no means necessary for success, although Rachman (1965) has shown that it is more efficient to do so. The therapist constructs a scale of stimulus situations as, for example, in the treatment for a phobia, which are arranged hierarchically according to the intensity of the emotional reaction they provoke in the patient. Wolpe and Lang (1964) have recently constructed a fear survey schedule to facilitate this process. One then proceeds to expose the patient to the weakest of the stimuli either in fact (e.g., M. C. Jones, 1924a, 1924b) or in fantasy (Wolpe, 1958). Since the emotional reaction is relatively weak, the patient can, with some encouragement from the therapist or another person such as a parent, remain in this weakly phobic situation long enough to find that nothing terrible happens to him, thus extinguishing the anxiety associated with the situation. In this way, one moves progressively up the stimulus hierarchy until ultimately the most anxiety-provoking situations can be tolerated with minimal or no anxiety.

Stimulus Attenuation: This technique is somewhat analogous to systematic desensitization and is usually used wittingly or not in combination with it. The technique relies on the interference by one stimulus with the effect of another when both are presented contemporaneously and has been used successfully by one of the authors (JSW) in the treatment of agoraphobia in an adolescent girl. The patient's mother who was very reassuring to the patient was instructed to accompany the girl on short, though ever-lengthening bus rides, thus attenuating the power of the phobic situations. Garvey and Hegrenes (1966) also used this technique in treating a case of school phobia.

Cue Conversion: This method attempts to change the sign of a stimulus in terms of its capacity to signal pleasure or pain. In general, this method has been used mostly to convert positive signals of forbidden pleasures to negative or unpleasant ones by pairing them with noxious stimuli such as electric shock, emesis, etc. With some variations' this approach has been used extensively in the treatment of alcoholism and sexual perversions in adults, although the success of the results has been somewhat dubious except perhaps in fetishism (Raymond, 1956). One problem in using this technique in the treatment of addictions and perversions revolves around the difficulty of providing an alternative prosocial outlet for the instinctual drive. There is no reason why attempts should not be made to convert negative or neutral stimuli to positive ones. Examples of this strategy have appeared recently in the treatment of homosexuality (Thorpe et al., 1964) where the appearance of a scantily dressed female photograph is the signal that the shock is about to be terminated, thus hopefully making the opposite sex a sign of relief and thus more attractive. A similar approach has been used by Lovaas et al. (1965b) in the treatment of autism where the act of moving toward an adult was the means of terminating a midly unpleasant electric shock. This procedure ultimately resulted in a significant increase in spontaneous display of affection by the children toward adults.

Obviously, the use of noxious stimuli in children presents serious ethical problems, and it really can be justified only where the condition is so severe that no other technique can reach the child or where the physical or social consequences of a given behavior are likely to be extremely serious (see Lovaas et al., 1965a, 1965b). Child therapists often make the mistake of assuming that inasmuch as society itself already punishes most of these conditions, the application of noxious stimuli is completely futile. Such a point of view fails to recognize the crucial importance of timing since punishment by society or parent is usually quite distant and the immediate consequences of the forbidden act are highly pleasurable.

Interference with Sensory Feedback: This technique has been used principally in the treatment of speech disorders such as stuttering where it seems that the patient's perception of his own speech is somehow important in the pathogenesis. Various techniques have been employed such as the shadowing technique (Cherry and Sayers, 1956) where the therapist reads and the patient repeats this back two syllables behind the reader. Under these conditions stuttering is much reduced or even absent, and in this way proper speaking habits can be strengthened. Other recent developments are the metronome method of Meyer and Mair (1963) in which the patient adjusts the cadence of his speech to a metronome rate of between 70 and 80 beats per minute. Under these conditions most patients immediately begin to speak without stuttering. One of the advantages of this particular technique is that with the development of a portable hearing aid type of metronome (Meyer and Mair, 1963) the patient can then proceed to expose himself to increasingly more anxiety-provoking talking situations, and thus carry out systematic desensitization of the anxiety component of his stuttering.

Modeling: The elegant studies by Bandura and Walters (1963) have demonstrated that children can learn a great deal simply by observing the behavior of others. Factors which facilitate the potency of the models are the consequences of the response to the model, how rewarding the model has been to the child, the competence and status of the model, and the power the model has to reward or punish the child. The experiments of Bandura and Walters indicate how some of these factors may actually be used in the therapeutic situation to enhance the potency of the therapist if he is interested in promoting identification with himself. Modeling is also likely to prove to be one of the more efficient ways of producing new patterns of complex behavior in children, particularly in younger age groups who are less amenable to verbal instruction.

Response Manipulation

Reciprocal Inhibition: In this technique, largely attributable to Wolpe (1958), the therapist strengthens responses which are incompatible with the undesirable behavior and which thus *reciprocally inhibit* the maladaptive responses (usually anxiety or withdrawal). Thus, it is essentially counterconditioning. The inhibiting responses which have been used are muscular relaxation and assertive responses (Wolpe, 1958) and pleasure associated with the gratification of various biological drives. For example, Mary Cover Jones (1924b) was able to cure a two-and-a-half-year-old boy of phobia by presentation of phobic objects while the child was eating his favorite food. The technique of reciprocal inhibition is unlikely to be successful unless it is used in conjunction with systematic desensitization since, as discussed above, the situation must be arranged such that the adaptive behavior has a higher probability of occurring than does the maladaptive behavior. Where the aim is to teach assertive responses, as, for example, in treating an overly timid child, the modeling techniques of Bandura and Walter (1963) should be helpful in initiating this type of behavior, but modeling would not likely be successful without systematic presentation of opportunities for successful display of assertion in simple situations and then in increasingly more difficult situations.

Contrived Responses: Here, a response is made to occur but in an artificial form or situation so that, if maladaptive, it can be attenuated or its normal response-reinforcement contingencies altered. Where a child simply lacks skills, he can be taught them (e.g., Quay et al., 1966). Usually this involves acting out threatening or traumatic situations in play therapy or in carefully controlled play acting (Lazarus and Abramovitz, 1962). By such means, the child can gradually develop adaptive alternative behaviors for certain situations, or extinguish maladaptive behavior or the vivid emotional components of certain traumatic memories.

Differences in the behavior therapy approach in this type of therapy are probably less than with other techniques described in this review. Nevertheless, traditional approaches have probably relied too much upon the power of verbal conceptualization or interpretation rather than on the behaviors themselves as vital instruments in extinction or conditioning processes. There probably also has been too little faith in the utility of the therapist's playing an active role in promoting and controlling the child's behavior in the therapeutic situation which is an essential component of the behavior therapy approach. The technique of emotive imagery (Lazarus and Abramovitz, 1962) illustrates some of these important differences.

Successive Approximation: This is analogous to systematic desensitization except that the emphasis is on the response rather than on the stimulus. Where the desired behavior is complex in terms of the child's ability to achieve it, or where modeling or verbal instruction are relatively ineffective because of autism or low mental age, a hierarchy of responses in terms of their closeness to the desired behavior can be constructed so that each step is relatively easily achievable, whereas the distant goal may of itself be quite inaccessible initially. Moving from readiness tasks to learning letters and thence to words is an example of the principle of successive approximation applied to the learning of reading. Successive approximation requires for its success an understanding of important principles of reinforcement (*vide infra*). However, in the example of learning to read, reinforcement factors are usually ignored since they are assumed to be intrinsic to the successful solution of the task or ubiquitous in the natural approbation which comes with progress toward a socially approved goal (see Hunt, 1965).

Negative or Massed Practice: In this technique, the symptom, usually a motor habit such as a tic, is repeated voluntarily for several periods each day. The complicated theoretical explanation (Yates, 1958) is less pertinent here than the several clinical demonstrations (Yates, 1958; H. G. Jones, 1960a; Rafi, 1962; Walton, 1961; and Agras and Marshall, 1965), of the efficacy of this treatment method especially with tics.

Reinforcement Manipulation

Here we are concerned with strengthening or weakening particular behaviors by manipulating their environmental consequences or reinforcement. These techniques are particularly relevant to operant or choice learning. It should be emphasized at this point that reinforcement depends for its success not only on its capacity to appeal to the individual child (Bijou and Baer, 1963) but also on close temporal proximity (within a few *seconds*) to the behavior which is the subject of therapeutic attention (Holland and Skinner, 1961). It is surprising how this extremely important principle of immediacy of reinforcement is so little understood and so frequently violated by child therapists and parents alike. Also important is the so-called scheduling of reinforcement as discussed above, with consistency being desirable in the early stages and deliberate inconsistency being desirable to ensure permanence in the behavior once it is achieved.

Withholding Reward: Many undesirable behaviors in children are maintained because parents or others are unwittingly reinforcing these behaviors through attention or granting the object of the undesirable behavior (e.g., Lovaas et al., 1965a; Allen and Harris, 1966). Teaching the parent or other adult figure such as the teacher who is reinforcing this kind of behavior to ignore it instead often results in its prompt extinction (Brown and Elliot, 1965). Sometimes it will be necessary to instruct or actually to demonstrate to these adults what they may have already felt they should do but which they do not carry out for a variety of personal reasons (Wahler et al., 1965).

Instituting Reward (Positive Reinforcement): In order to use this successfully, the therapist must know: (i) the type of behavior he wishes to develop in the child; (ii) how to get the child to exhibit this behavior; and (iii) what is rewarding or reinforcing to this particular child (Bijou and Baer, 1963). The first of these requires accurate problem definition before therapy is commenced. The second requires a knowledge of stimulus generalization gradients, successive approximation, and modeling techniques; and the third, a willingness to experiment with a wide variety of possible rewards, some of which, for example, candy, trinkets, etc. may require the overcoming of considerable prejudice on the part of the therapist himself and the parents of the patient.

However, in the majority of situations, the type of reinforcement to be applied will generally prove to be conditioned or symbolic such as attention or approbation from another human being. Much attention has been given in the traditional psychotherapeutic literature to the importance of the therapist-child relationship. Looked at in terms of learning theory, the importance of this lies in the reinforcing quality the therapist acquires for the child. What is lacking in the traditional approach is probably lack of emphasis on the therapist's improving his reinforcing value by using concrete rewards if necessary and in systematically using his charismatic value in reinforcing pro-social behavior. Recently, ingenious and apparently successful attempts have been made to use the peer group as an important source of reinforcement by making some kind of group reward contingent upon the amount of adaptive behavior exhibited by a deviant pupil (Patterson, 1965a). One of the important unpremeditated outcomes of this particular study was the movement of the patient from a very low to a very high status position in the peer group. In another study (Straughan et al., 1965), peer reinforcement was utilized in treating elective mutism in a fourteen-year-old boy.

Another method of applying positive reinforcement is the implementation of Premack's Principle (1959), which states that a preferred activity can be used as a reinforcement for a less popular one if the former is made contingent upon the latter. Homme and his colleagues (1963) described the use of Premack's Principle in a nursery school situation where desirable behavior such as sitting quietly in a chair and looking at the blackboard was greatly increased in frequency by instructing the children that if they sat quietly for what was initially quite a short period, they would then be permitted to get up and run around and make as much noise as they liked for a short period. An interesting feature of this particular study is that it was possible quickly to increase the time required for sitting and to decrease and eventually to omit altogether the running around time except at recess. Again, this approach, like all other applications of reinforcement, depends for its success upon the *immediate* application of the reinforcement *after* the adaptive behavior rather than application of the reinforcement at a time remote from the performance of the adaptive behavior or antecedent to it.

One final point in the application of reinforcement needs emphasizing, namely, selectivity. In certain types of behaviors such as attention-seeking, the parent is likely to reward only high intensities of this behavior (Bandura and Walters, 1963) so that a very ignored child may find that his only way of attracting attention is to scream and shout. Such intense behavior may of course produce punishment, but a very deprived child may consider even this kind of attention rewarding. What the parent should be doing, of course, is rewarding more moderate demands for attention and ignoring the intense levels.

Deprivation and Satiation: Sometimes it will prove necessary to strengthen or attenuate natural reinforcers rather than to institute reinforcers *de novo*. For example, eating in Western civilization is mostly a function of social custom rather than hunger, and the reinforcing value of food can be greatly strengthened by judicious deprivation of food (Ayllon, 1963; Wolf et al., 1964). Conversely, on occasion, the best approach to maladaptive behavior may be to weaken the reinforcer by giving the patient an overabundance of it. This is well illustrated in the treatment of a towel-hoarding patient by permitting her to hoard as much linen as she wished (Ayllon, 1963). Satiation may, on occasion, work against the therapist as can be seen in the remark of one of the pupils in a class for emotionally disturbed children who stated that he was not going to pay attention in class for a mere ten candies when he could get about a hundred in a fifteen-minute individual conditioning session after class (Quay et al., 1966).

Punishment: As used in this context, punishment is defined as the application of an aversive or noxious stimulus which may be indirect or symbolic (e.g., castigation) as well as physical (e.g., spanking). In general, though punishment obeys many of the same laws as reinforcement, particularly that of immediate contingency upon the response, its effects are somewhat more complex (Bandura and Walters, 1963). First, punishment suppresses rather than eliminates responses so that they have a tendency to reappear when the child is sure that the punishment is unlikely to occur. Second, in susceptible children, generalized inhibition may result, extending to include healthy as well as punished behaviors. Finally, what appears to be punishment may in fact, in a very deprived child, be rewarding; nor can one entirely discount the possibility of genuine masochism. Nevertheless, punishment has a definite role to play particularly in combination with reward for incompatible, adaptive, alternative behavior where it may greatly facilitate the course of therapy (Lovaas et al., 1965b; Wahler et al.' 1965) and in the cue conversion method mentioned above.

Manipulation of Intraorganismic Drive States

There is already much evidence to show that drive state greatly influences the behavior of an organism. One important effect is simply that of energizing behavior where the relationship, like most biological functions, is curvilinear. Thus, at lower levels of arousal, an increment in drive will facilitate performance, but at the higher levels performance will be impeded by an increment in drive (Duffy, 1957). More complex or less well learned functions tend to be first impaired, making primitive or chronic behaviors like psychopathological, emotional reactions more probable (Bindra, 1959; Yates, 1961). In addition to purely quantitative elements, drive also has a qualitative or directional component such as pain avoidance, restitution of homeostasis, sexual satisfaction, or reduction of cognitive dissonance (Hunt, 1965). This qualitative dimension of drive will make certain classes of behavior which in the past have successfully lowered the particular emotional tension more probable (Holland and Skinner, 1961, pp. 235-240). Hence, in behavior therapy, it may be of great advantage to manipulate both the *level* and the *type* of emotional state in order to maximize the probability of appearance of certain adaptive behaviors (e.g., Feldman and Werry, 1966). Psychopharmacological agents seem to have important quantitative effects on drive states, although the evidence for a qualitative effect is relatively unconvincing except in the case of antidepressant drugs. One of the great weaknesses of psychopharmacological studies is that drugs have been used as an end in themselves instead of as an important tool with which to facilitate the learning of new behaviors. The deliberate manipulation of drive state by pharmacotherapy in a thirteen-year-old tiqueur by Walton (1961), the use of dextroamphetamine in conjunction with the conditioning treatment of enuresis by Young and Turner (1965), and the use of drugs to induce relaxation in the successful desensitization of a three-and-a-half-year-old child by Lazarus (1960) are milestones in both behavior therapy and psychopharmacology research. Other possible ways in which drive state might be deliberately manipulated are through hypnosis, muscular relaxation, environmental structuring, food deprivation, and paying close attention to sex and personality in the selection of a therapist for individual children.

TYPES OF PROBLEMS TREATED

This section of the review is essentially nothing more than a bibliography. This is so, not only in the interests of conciseness, but also because most of the reported literature of behavior therapy to this date consists of detailed individual case studies. Child therapists who would be interested in investigating the possibilities of behavior therapy in specific conditions would gain most by reading the case studies themselves. The authors hope that some of the terminological problems will have been obviated by previous sections of the review.

In categorizing the clinical conditions, the authors have tried to strike a balance between current nosology and the symptom-oriented approach of behavior therapists.

Neurotic Symptoms

Anxiety Symptoms (phobias, fears, school phobia, etc.): Possibly because it is relatively easy to identify the eliciting stimuli, children's fears and phobias have received a great deal of attention from behavior therapists and reportedly with considerable success. The techniques employed have generally been systematic desensitization to the stimulus often with concomitant strengthening of alternative responses antagonistic to anxiety such as affectionate, feeding, and social responses. Authors who report successful cases are Mary Cover Jones (1924a, 1924b), Eysenck and Rachman (1965, pp. 209-210), and Lazarus (1960) in children with animal phobias; Lazarus and Abramovitz (1962), Kushner (1965), and Lazarus (1960) in children with specific situational anxiety such as separation anxiety, agoraphobia, etc.; Patterson (1965b), Lazarus et al. (1965), Eysenck and Rachman (1965, pp. 218-222), and Garvey and Hegrenes (1966) in children with school phobia.

Rachman and Costello (1961) offer a general theoretical review of the etiology and treatment of children's phobias from the behavior therapy point of view.

Conversion Symptoms: Because of their well-known capacity to attract positive environmental reinforcement or "secondary gain," conversion symptoms are eminently suitable to the behavior therapy approach. The principal technique used to treat conversion symptoms is withdrawal of reward for the conversion behavior and the instituting of reinforcement for pro-social alternative behavior. Harris and her colleagues (1964; Allen and Harris, 1966) were able to treat regressive crawling and severe scratching in this fashion. More traditional conversion symptoms such as blindness have as yet been treated mostly in adults (Eysenck and Rachman, 1965, pp. 93-104), though Straughan et al. (1965) treated elective mutism in a fourteen-year-old boy by using peer approval and material reinforcement.

Obsessive-Compulsive Symptoms: Published reports thus far concern only the treatment of adults, though there is no reason why the techniques used such as reciprocal inhibition should not be applied to children. As might be expected, however, the therapeutic effect in treating obsessive-compulsive symptoms has been of somewhat limited extent (Walton and Mather, 1963).

Psychophysiological Reactions

Enuresis has been the target of a large number of studies using the bed-buzzer or "conditioning" apparatus (DeLeon and Mandell, 1966; H. G. Jones, 1960b; Werry, 1966), the exact *modus operandi* of which is at the moment unclear, but is most likely reinforcement manipulation using mild punishment (Lovibond, 1963a). Cure rates have ranged from as high as 90 percent (H. G. Jones, 1960b) to as low as 30 percent (Werry and Cohrssen, 1965). Recent approaches have improved the results of therapy by simultaneous administration of drugs (Young and Turner, 1965), by the use of intermittent rather than continuous reinforcement (Lovibond, 1963b), and by a modification of the apparatus to make cessation of the punishment (i.e., the loud noise produced by the buzzer) more nearly contingent upon cessation of the act of micturition (Lovibond, 1963a).

Encopresis has yielded good results principally with the combination of successive approximation and the application of reward (Neale, 1963; Gelber and Meyer, 1965; Keehn, 1965; Peterson and London, 1965). The latter paper is remarkable in that the authors demonstrate how a cognitive or insight approach can be used *in conjunction with* the behavior therapy approach.

Wolf and his colleagues (1965) were successful in treating vomiting by withdrawing the reinforcement which usually followed the vomiting. White (1959), using successive approximation, and Hallsten (1965), using systematic desensitization and positive reinforcement, successfully treated eating problems.

Cherry and Sayers (1956) and Meyer and Mair (1963) report success in treating stuttering using stimulus feedback interference. Maclaren (1960) used auditory retraining and removal of punishment (criticism) in treating stammering, while Kerr et al. (1965) used application of reinforcement to develop vocalization in a mute child.

Walton (1961) successfully treated multiple tics in a child using the negative practice technique in combination with chemotherapy. Feldman and Werry (1966) were unsuccessful using the negative practice technique because of the development of severe anxiety, which, however, might possibly have been obviated by prior treatment with systematic desensitization techniques.

Psychotic Symptoms

To date, most published reports on behavior therapy with psychotic children have consisted of isolated experiments rather than complete treatment programs. In terms of the assumptions of behavior therapy, the principles of learning theory should apply equally to psychotic as to to normal children. This assumption is supported by the experimental studies of Ferster and DeMyer (1962), Davison (1964, 1965), Eysenck and Rachman (1965, p. 238), Hingtgen et al. (1965), Marr et al. (1966), Metz (1965), Lovaas et al. (1965a, 1965b, 1966), and Wolf et al. (1964). These findings all demonstrate how normal behavior can be increased at the expense of psychotic behavior by direct application of learning theory principles. Thus, techniques which have proved fruitful in manipulating the behavior of normal children should hold great promise for the treatment of childhood psychosis. Of particular interest in this context are the procedures aimed at developing social interaction and cooperation (Azrin and Lindsley, 1956; Allen et al., 1964; Davison, 1964, 1965).

Conduct Disorders

Williams (1959), Wahler et al. (1965), and Boardman (1962) have all successfully treated temper tantrums and other kinds of oppositional behavior by instructing parents in the manipulation of reinforcement particularly the withholding of reward. Hart et al. (1964), Bijou and Baer (1963), and Zimmerman and Zimmerman (1962) were able greatly to reduce the frequency of a wide variety of conduct problems in the school situation by similar techniques using teachers as co-therapists. Rickard and Dinoff (1965) were successful in treating rebelliousness in a summer camp by using camp counselors as therapists. Capitalizing on some experimental work by Levin and Simmons (1962a, 1962b) which demonstrated superiority of material rather than social reinforcement for conduct problem children, Schwitzgebel and Kolb (1964), Slack (1960), and Burchard and Tyler (1965) were able successfully to treat a wide variety of antisocial behavior. Quay et al. (1966) significantly improved classroom attention in conduct problem children by immediately reinforcing the desired behavior with light flashes followed by candy.

Patterson (1965a) and his coworkers (1965) successfully treated two hyperactive boys in the classroom through immediate reinforcement by an experimenter of sitting-still behavior. An untreated hyperactive child in the same classroom did not improve.

CONCLUSIONS

In this review, the authors have attempted to review behavior therapy as it has been, or might be, applied to the treatment of the psychopathology of childhood. Wherever possible, techniques, theoretical concepts, and clinical conditions have been described in familiar terms without having eliminated some of the essential differences in the new approach. Principally, behavior therapy rests upon a functional and empirical orientation, adherence to a well-formulated experimentally derived theory, and an active, systematic manipulation of patients' behavior, environmental stimuli, environmental consequences or reinforcement and even of the therapist himself. Those who, like Glover (1959), in recognizing the familiar in the new would deny any substantive difference thereto, fail to understand that a new approach may, indeed *should,* build on the foundation of existing knowledge, or to recognize that a new approach may be more heuristically cast. Nor does the new necessarily preclude the continuance of the old. A more meaningful question is to ask where the proper place for behavior therapy lies among the *therapies* of child psychopathology.

In the authors' opinion, behavior therapy is most likely to be the treatment of choice: (a) where there are discrete, easily recognizable symptoms or problem behaviors: (b) where the patient or his parent is symptom- rather than insight-oriented (Yamamoto and Goin, 1965); (c) where, because of clinical conditions or mental age, the patient is unamenable to conflict-insight-verbalization approaches (e.g., Goldfarb, 1965); (d) where child therapists are scarce since, because of its systematic and concrete nature, behavior therapy is readily able to be executed by relatively unskilled therapists with some degree of supervision (Allen and Harris, 1966; Ayllon, 1963; Brown and Elliott, 1965; Davison 1964, 1965; Wahler et al., 1965; Wolf et al., 1964).

By means of reference to a now not inconsiderable bibliography, the growing number of therapeutic successes attributable to behavior therapy have been indicated. Unfortunately, most of these reports have been by psychologists and have appeared in books (e.g., Eysenck and Rachman, 1965; Ullman and Krasner, 1965) and in scientific journals not usually read by child therapists. At the moment there is only a small number of studies which have attempted to compare behavior therapy with more traditional approaches, and the evidence for the superiority of the new technique (DeLeon and Mandell, 1966; Lang and Lazovik, 1963; Paul, 1966; Rachman, 1965; Werry and Cohrssen, 1965) seems about equaled by that which shows it to have no advantage (Cooper, 1963; Koenig and Masters, 1965; Marks and Gelder, 1965). Significantly, perhaps, Koenig and Masters showed that the *therapist* was more important than the *therapy*. Nevertheless, it would be unwise for child therapists to ignore this important development in therapy. Failure to take cognizance of developments in this area will not only lead to compartmentalization of child therapy between psychology and the other disciplines, but could also lead to an unnecessary limitation in the therapeutic spectrum offered by child psychiatric facilities. Even if behavior therapy does not prove ultimately to be superior to traditional techniques in the areas where it is most appropriate, because of its ability to utilize relatively unskilled therapists, it merits serious consideration. Further, its theoretical preciseness and its emphasis on the scientific method may open avenues to research in certain areas of psychotherapy which are presently methodologically insoluble.

Thus, behavior therapy with children, though no panacea, seems likely to bring limited but significant relief at least to certain patients presently unamenable to, or unreachable by traditional techniques and holds a potentiality for enlarging the theoretical horizons of child psychiatry.

REFERENCES

AGRAS, S. & MARSHALL, C. (1965), The application of negative practice to spasmodic torticollis. *Amer. J. Psychiat.*, 122:579-582.

ALLEN, K. E. & HARRIS, F. R. (1966), Elimination of a child's excessive scratching by training the mother in reinforcement procedures. *Behav. Res. Ther.*, 4:79-84.

—— HART, B., BUELL, J. S., HARRIS, F. R., & WOLF, M. R. (1964), Effects of social reinforcement on isolate behavior of a nursery school child. *Child Develpm.*, 35:511-518.

AYLLON, T. (1963), Intensive treatment of psychotic behavior by stimulus satiation and food reinforcement. *Behav. Res. Ther.*, 1:53-61.

—— & MICHAEL, J. (1959), The psychiatric nurse as a behavioral engineer. *J. Exp. Anal. Behav.*, 2:323-334.

AZRIN, N. H. & LINDSLEY, O. R. (1956), The reinforcement of cooperation between children. *J. Abnorm. Soc. Psychol.*, 52:100-102.

BANDURA, A. & WALTERS, R. H. (1963), *Social Learning and Personality Development*. New York: Holt, Rinehart, & Winston.

BARBOUR, R. F., BORLAND, E. M., BOYD, M. M., MILLER, A., & OPPE, T. E. (1963), Enuresis as a disorder of development. *Brit. Med. J.*, 2:787-790.

BENTLER, P. M. (1962), An infant's phobia treated with reciprocal inhibition therapy. *J. Child Psychol. Psychiat.*, 3:185-189.

BIJOU, S. W. & BAER, D. M. (1963), Some methodological contributions from a functional analysis of child development. In: *Advances in Child Development and Behavior*, ed. L. P. Lipsitt & C. S. Spiker. New York: Academic Press, Vol. I, pp. 197-231.

BINDRA, D. (1959), *Motivation: A Systematic Reinterpretation*. New York: Ronald Press, pp. 210-257.

BOARDMAN, W. K. (1962), Rusty: a brief behavior disorder. *J. Consult. Psychol.*, 26:293-297.

BROWN, P. & ELLIOT, R. (1965), Control of aggression in a nursery school class. *J. Exp. Child Psychol.*, 2:103-107.

BURCHARD, J. & TYLER, V., JR. (1965), The modification of delinquent behavior through operant conditioning. *Behav. Res. Ther.*, 2:245-250.

CHERRY, C. & SAYERS, B. (1956), Experiments upon the total inhibition of stammering by external control, and some clinical results. *J. Psychosom. Res.*, 1:233-246.

COOPER, J. E. (1963), A study of behavior therapy in thirty psychiatric patients. *Lancet*, 1:411-415.

DAVISON, G. C. (1964), A social learning therapy programme with an autistic child. *Behav. Res. Ther.*, 2:149-159.

—————— (1965), The training of undergraduates as social reinforcers for autistic children. In: *Case Studies In Behavior Modification*, ed. L. P. Ullmann & L. Krasner. New York: Holt, Rinehart, & Winston, pp. 146-148.

DeLEON, G. & MANDELL. W. (1966), A comparison of conditioning and psychotherapy in the treatment of functional enuresis. *J. Clin. Psychol.*, 22:326-330.

DUFFY, E. (1957), The psychological significance of the concept of "arousal" or "activation." *Psychol. Rev.*, 64:265-275.

EYSENCK, H. J. (1959), Learning theory and behavior therapy. *J. Ment. Sci.*, 105:61-75.

—— & RACHMAN, S. (1965), *The Causes and Cures of Neurosis: An Introduction to Modern Behavior Therapy Based on Learning Theory and the Principle of Conditioning*. San Diego: Knapp.

FELDMAN. R. & WERRY, J. S. (1966), An unsuccessful attempt to treat a tiqueur by massed practice. *Behav. Res. Ther.*, 4:111-117.

FERSTER, C. B. & DeMYER, M. K. (1962), A method for the experimental analysis of the behavior of autistic children. *Amer. J. Orthopsychiat.*, 32:89-98.

GARVEY, W. P. & HEGRENES, J. R. (1966), Desensitization techniques in the treatment of school phobia. *Amer. J. Orthopsychiat.*, 36:147-152.

GELBER, H. & MEYER, V. (1965), Behavior therapy and encopresis: the complexities involved in treatment. *Behav. Res. Ther.*, 2:227-231.

GLOVER, E. (1959), Critical note on "Wolpe's Psychotherapy." *Brit. J. Med. Psychol.*, 32:68-74.

GOLDFARB, W. (1965), Corrective socialization: a rationale for the treatment of schizophrenic children. *Canad. Psychiat. Assn. J.*, 10:481-493.

HALLSTEN, E. A., JR. (1965), Adolescent anorexia nervosa treated by desensitization. *Behav. Res. Ther.*, 3:87-91.

HARRIS, F. R., JOHNSTON, M. K., KELLEY, C. S., & WOLF, M. M. (1964), Effects of positive social reinforcement on regressed crawling of a nursery school child. *J. Educ. Psychol.*, 55:35-41.

HART, B. M., ALLEN, K. E., BUELL, J. S., HARRIS, F. R., & WOLF, M. M. (1964), Effects of social reinforcement on operant crying. *J. Exp. Child Psychol.*, 1:145-153.

HINGTGEN, J. N., SANDERS, B. J., & DeMYER, M. (1965), Shaping cooperative responses in early childhood schizophrenics. In: *Case Studies in Behavior Modification*, ed. L. P. Ullmann & L. Krasner. New York: Holt, Rinehart, & Winston, pp. 130-138.

HOLLAND, J. G. & SKINNER, B. F. (1961), *The Analysis of Behavior: A Program for Self-instruction.* New York: McGraw-Hill.

HOMME, L. E., DeBACA, P. C., DEVINE, J. V., STEINHORST, R., & RICKERT, E. J. (1963), Use of the Premack principle in controlling the behavior of nursery school children. *J. Exp. Anal. Behav.*, 6:544.

HUNT, J. McV. (1965), Intrinsic motivation and its role in psychological development. In: *Nebraska Symposium on Motivation*, ed. D. Levine. Lincoln: University of Nebraska Press, pp. 189-282.

JONES, H. G. (1960a), Continuation of Yates' treatment of a tiqueur. In: *Behavior Therapy and the Neuroses: Readings in Modern Methods of Treatment Derived from Learning Theory*, ed. H. J. Eysenck. Oxford: Pergamon, pp. 250-258.

——— (1960b), The behavioral treatment of enuresis nocturna. In: *Behavior Therapy and the Neuroses: Readings in Modern Methods of Treatment Derived from Learning Theory*, ed. H. J. Eysenck. Oxford: Pergamon, pp. 377-403.

JONES, M. C. (1924a), The elimination of children's fears. *J. Exp. Psychol.*, 7:382-390.

——— (1924b), A laboratory study of fear: the case of Peter. *Pedagog. Sem.*, 31:303-315.

KEEHN, J. D. (1965), Brief case-report: reinforcement therapy of incontinence. *Behav. Res. Ther.*, 2:239.

KERR, N., MEYERSON, L., & MICHAEL, J. (1965), A procedure for shaping vocalizations in a mute child. In: *Case Studies in Behavior Modification*, ed. L. P. Ullmann & L. Krasner. New York: Holt, Rinehart, & Winston, pp. 366-370.

KOENIG, K. P. & MASTERS, J. (1965), Experimental treatment of habitual smoking. *Behav. Res. Ther.*, 3:235-243.

KUSHNER, M. (1965), Desensitization of a post-traumatic phobia. In: *Case Studies in Behavior Modification*, ed. L. P. Ullman & L. Krasner. New York: Holt, Rinehart & Winston, pp. 193-196.

LANG, P. J. & LAZOVIK. A. (1963), Experimental desensitization of a phobia. *J. Abnorm. Soc. Psychol.*, 66:519-525.

LAZARUS, A. A. (1960), The elimination of children's phobias by deconditioning. In: *Behavior Therapy and the Neuroses: Readings in Modern Methods of Treatment Derived from Learning Theory*, ed. H. J. Eysenck. Oxford: Pergamon, pp. 114-122.

—— & ABRAMOVITZ, A. (1962), The use of "emotive imagery" in the treatment of children's phobias. *J. Ment. Sci.*, 108:191-195.

—— DAVISON, G., & POLEFKA, D. (1965), Classical and operant factors in the treatment of a school phobia. *J. Abnorm. Psychol.*, 70:225-229.

LEVIN, G. R. & SIMMONS, J. J. (1962a), Response to praise by emotionally disturbed boys. *Psychol. Rep.*, 11:10.

——— (1962b), Response to food and praise by emotionally disturbed boys. *Psychol. Rep.*, 11:539-546.

LOVAAS, O. I., BERBERICH, J. P., PERLOFF, B. F., & SCHAEFFER, B. (1966), Acquisition of imitative speech by schizophrenic children. *Science,* 151:705-707.

—— FREITAG, G., GOLD, V. J., & KASSORLA, I. C. (1965a), Experimental studies in childhood schizophrenia: analysis of self-destructive behavior. *J. Exp. Child Psychol.,* 2:67-84.

—— SCHAEFFER, B. & SIMMONS, J. Q. (1965b), Building social behavior in autistic children by use of electric shock. *J. Exp. Res. Pers.,* 1:99-109.

LOVIBOND, S. H. (1963a), The mechanism of conditioning treatment of enuresis. *Behav. Res. Ther.,* 1:3-15.

—— (1963b), Intermittent reinforcement in behavior therapy. *Behav. Res. Ther.,* 1:27-132.

MACLAREN, J. (1960), The treatment of stammering by the Cherry-Sayers method: clinical impressions. In: *Behavior Therapy and the Neuroses: Readings in Modern Methods of Treatment Derived from Learning Theory,* ed. H. J. Eysenck. Oxford: Pergamon, pp. 457-460.

MARKS, I. M. & GELDER, M. G. (1965), A controlled retrospective study of behavior therapy in phobic patients. *Brit. J. Psychiat.,* 111:561-573.

MARR, J. N., MILLER, E. R., & STRAUB, R. R. (1966), Operant conditioning of attention with a psychotic girl. *Behav. Res. Ther.,* 4:85-87.

METZ, J. R. (1965), Conditioning generalized imitation in autistic children. *J. Exp. Child Psychol.,* 2:389-399.

MEYER, V. & MAIR, J. M. M. (1963), A new technique to control stammering: a preliminary report. *Behav. Res. Ther.,* 1:251-254.

MILLER, N. E. (1944), Experimental studies of conflict. In: *Personality and the Behavior Disorders,* ed. J. McV. Hunt. New York: Ronald Press, pp. 431-465.

NEALE, D. H. (1963), Behavior therapy and encopresis in children. *Behav. Res. Ther.,* 1:139-149.

PAUL, G. L. (1966), *Insight versus Desensitization in Psychotherapy.* Stanford: Stanford University Press.

PATTERSON, G. R. (1965a), An application of conditioning techniques to the control of a hyperactive child. In: *Case Studies in Behavior Modification,* ed. L. P. Ullmann & L. Krasner. New York: Holt, Rinehart, & Winston, pp. 370-375.

—— (1965b), A learning theory approach to the treatment of the school phobic child. In: *Case Studies in Behavior Modification,* ed. L. P. Ullmann & L. Krasner. New York: Holt, Rinehart, & Winston, pp. 279-285.

—— JONES, R., WHITTIER, J. & WRIGHT, M. (1965), A behavior modification technique for the hyperactive child. *Behav. Res. Ther.* 2:217-226.

PETERSON, D. R. & LONDON, P. (1965), A role for cognition in the behavioral treatment of a child's eliminative disturbance. In: *Case Studies In Behavior Modification,* ed. L. P. Ullmann & L. Krasner. New York: Holt, Rinehart, & Winston, pp. 289-295.

PREMACK, D. (1959), Toward empirical behavior laws: I. Positive reinforcement. *Psychol. Rev.,* 66:219-233.

QUAY, H. C., WERRY, J. S., McQUEEN, M., & SPRAGUE, R. L. (1966), Remediation of the conduct problem child in the special class setting. *Except. Child,* 32:509-515.

RACHMAN, S. (1965), Studies in desensitization. I: The separate effects of relaxation and desensitization. *Behav. Res. Ther.,* 3:245-251.

—— & COSTELLO, C. G. (1961), The aetiology and treatment of children's phobias: a review. *Amer. J. Psychiat.,* 118:97-105.

RAFI, A. A. (1962), Learning theory and treatment of tics. *J. Psychosom. Res.,* 6:71-76.

RAYMOND, M. J. (1956), Case of fetishism treated by aversion therapy. *Brit. Med. J.,* 2:854-857.

RICKARD, H. C. & DINOFF, M. (1965), Shaping adaptive behavior in a therapeutic summer camp. In: *Case Studies in Behavior Modification,* ed. L. P. Ullmann & L. Krasner. New York: Holt, Rinehart, & Winston, pp. 325-328.

SCHWITZGEBEL, R. & KOLB, D. A. (1964), Inducing behavior change in adolescent delinquents. *Behav. Res. Ther.*, 1:297-304.

SKINNER, B. F. (1938), *The Behavior of Organisms: An Experimental Analysis.* New York: Appleton-Century-Crofts.

SLACK, C. W. (1960), Experimenter-subject psychotherapy: a new method of introducing intensive office treatment for unreachable cases. *Ment. Hyg.*, 44:238-256.

STRAUGHAN, J. H., POTTER, W. K., JR., & HAMILTON, S. H., JR. (1965), The behavioral treatment of an elective mute. *J. Child Psychol. Psychiat.*, 6:125-130.

THORPE, J. G., SCHMIDT, E., BROWN, P. T., & CASTELL, D. (1964), Aversion-relief therapy: a new method for general application. *Behav. Res. Ther.*, 2:71-82.

ULLMANN, L. P. & KRASNER, L., Eds. (1965), *Case Studies in Behavior Modification.* New York: Holt, Rinehart, & Winston, pp. 1-63.

WAHLER, R. G., WINKEL, G. H., PETERSON, R. F., & MORRISON, D. C. (1965), Mothers as behavior therapists for their own children. *Behav. Res. Ther.*, 3:113-124.

WALTON, D. (1961), Experimental psychology and the treatment of a tiqueur. *J. Child Psychol. Psychiat.*, 2:148-155.

—— & MATHER, M. D. (1963), The application of learning principles to the treatment of obsessive-compulsive states in the acute and chronic phases of illness. *Behav. Res. Ther.*, 1:163-174.

WATSON, J. B. & RAYNER, R. (1920), Conditioned emotional reactions. *J. Exp. Psychol,* 3:1-14.

WERRY, J. S. (1966), The conditioning treatment of enuresis. *Amer. J. Psychiat.*, 123: 226-229.

—— & COHRSSEN, J. (1965), Enuresis: an etiologic and therapeutic study. *J. Pediat.*, 67:423-431.

WHITE, J. G. (1959), The use of learning theory in the psychological treatment of children. *J. Clin. Psychol.*, 15:226-229.

WILLIAMS, C. D. (1959), The elimination of tantrum behavior by extinction procedures. *J. Abnorm. Soc. Psychol.*, 59:269.

WOLF, M., RISLEY, T., & MEES, H. (1964), Application of operant conditioning procedures to the behavior problems of an autistic child. *Behav. Res. Ther.*, 1:305-312.

—— BIRNBAUER, J. S., WILLIAMS, T., & LAWLER, J. (1965), A note on apparent extinction of the vomiting behavior of a retarded child. In: *Case Studies in Behavior Modification,* ed. L. P. Ullmann & L. Krasner. New York: Holt, Rinehart, & Winston, pp. 364-366.

WOLPE, J. (1958), *Psychotherapy by Reciprocal Inhibition.* Stanford: Stanford University Press.

—— & LANG, P. L. (1964), A fear survey schedule for use in behavior therapy. *Behav. Res. Ther.*, 2:27-30.

YAMAMOTO, J. & GOIN, M. K. (1965), On the treatment of the poor. *Amer. J. Psychiat.*, 122:267-271.

YATES, A. J. (1958), The application of learning theory to the treatment of tics. *J. Abnorm. Soc. Psychol.*, 56:175-182.

—— (1961), Abnormalities of psychomotor functions. In: *Handbook of Abnormal Psychology: An Experimental Approach,* ed. H. J. Eysenck. New York: Basic Books, pp. 52-53.

YOUNG, G. C. & TURNER, R. K. (1965), CNS stimulant drugs and conditioning treatment of nocturnal enuresis. *Behav. Res. Ther.*, 3:93-101.

ZIMMERMAN, E. H. & ZIMMERMAN, J. (1962), The alteration of behavior in a special classroom situation. *J. Exp. Anal. Behav.*, 5:59-60.

24

EMOTIONAL REACTIONS OF HANDICAPPED CHILDREN

Roger D. Freeman, M.D.

Director of Psychiatric Services, Handicapped Children's Unit,
St. Christopher Hospital for Children;
Assistant Professor of Psychiatry (Child),
Temple University School of Medicine;
Consultant, the Upsal Day School for Blind Children, Philadelphia.

INTRODUCTION

It is now well recognized that a child's emotional development, behavior, and reaction to his handicap may be more significant in determining whether he may be able to remain in the community and achieve a degree of independent functioning than the extent of the physical handicap itself. Rehabilitative procedures often require the child to subject himself to months, or even years, of unpleasant or painful experiences without the assistance of motivation and understanding as may reasonably be expected of the adult patient. Parents are becoming increasingly aware of the possible consequences of early "traumatic" experiences and ask penetrating questions of the professional worker. New technics in the modification of behavior and controversies over treatment methods and their efficacy baffle and frustrate parent and professional alike.

The present report is an attempt to communicate some general principles that may be helpful to those working with handicapped children. While much is yet unknown and it is rightly considered hazardous to

Reprinted from Rehabilitation Literature, Sept. 1967, Vol. 28, No. 9, pp. 274-281, published by National Society for Crippled Children and Adults.

fit a person into the Procrustean bed of a generalization, it is also true that much that has been established has never been put into practice.

There is an enormous literature on personality studies, normal and abnormal child development, intelligence, counseling, psychotherapy, behavior therapy, and preparation of the child for hospitalization. A review of this material is obviously beyond the scope of this discussion and will be presented elsewhere.

We shall assume that early experiences in life may have profound effects upon later functioning, that development may be affected by the attitudes of parents and society, that a person's thoughts and feelings about himself and his body are significant and merit consideration, and that the professional worker's understanding, or lack of it, may be an important variable in the outcome of the rehabilitative process.

DIAGNOSIS

In recent years emphasis has been increasing on "early diagnosis." Unfortunately, this can be a mixed blessing or an actual disservice. Unless it results in some meaningful program, it may have only academic interest and result in potentially harmful distortions in parental attitudes, expectations, and child-rearing practices. This is particularly true of a wrong diagnosis; in some instances the child's needs would be better served by providing ongoing diagnosis and parental support without firm prognostication.

In the event no diagnostic label is applied, a major task involves clarifying for the parents the reasons for uncertainty and an explanation of the process by which the diagnosis will be arrived at. Reassurance that lack of a "label" will not mean lack of a program of management is a basic requirement. Explanations may also be necessary when diagnostic terms (sometimes deliberately incorrect) must be used for administrative purposes (*e.g.,* when a "brain-damaged" child is reported as having "cerebral palsy" for purposes of state aid).

The most tragic cases of misdiagnosis are those in which the parents have been told the child has a progressive disease that will result in death. Most parents go through a gradual emotional detachment from the child, a kind of "mourning in advance," only to discover that the child does not die but may continue at an even more handicapped level for an indefinite period of time. In such a situation the parent may never be able to achieve the previous level of emotional investment, and considerable bitterness may ensue.

We have found that the vagueness of the term *emotional problem* is itself an issue that must be dealt with. Many parents misunderstand the meaning, assuming that it signifies a "mental block," unhappiness, insanity, or a neurotic type of "mental conflict," as seen in adults. In many instances the professional person uses the phrase *emotional problem* to mean a developmental deviation, which may or may not have an important environmental or "psychogenic" component in its etiology. Unless this is fully discussed, the parent may assume that he or she has been an inadequate or unworthy parent and has thereby produced the deviation in some way.

Problems in differential diagnosis are often quite complex in young handicapped children. There is little agreement as to criteria for establishing many diagnostic categories. In fact, there is dispute over whether some categories exist (as in aphasia of developmental type, minimal brain dysfunction, and developmental lags in speech). Where the developmental process is still so unpredictable, diagnostic certainty may indicate the professional's own insecurity rather than acumen.

Since many of these youngsters are nonverbal, highly dependent, immature, and anxious, hospital or office visits may be of very limited value, particularly where evaluation of behavior is indicated. Unless an older child is highly verbal, we have found it much more helpful to evaluate the child in his natural home setting, in school, or both. We have been interested in comparing impressions gained from office visits with those from the home. The differences in some cases are striking; more important, the recommendations emerging from the evaluation may be quite surprising after the home visit. Pessimistic prognoses may be altered in a positive direction as hitherto unsuspected assets are discovered. Interpretation to the family of the diagnostic impressions and recommendations is also facilitated when they feel evaluation has been performed in a situation in which the child feels most secure. In the past three years this type of home evaluation has been routine for preschool age children requiring psychiatric evaluation, where practical from the standpoint of distance.[4] Other professional workers have also used these methods (social workers, speech therapists, nurses, pediatricians, nutritionists).

AREAS OF VULNERABILITY IN THE DEVELOPMENT
OF THE HANDICAPPED CHILD

Even before the child's birth, many parents have a desire for a specific set of characteristics and sex for the child, and they may go through a more or less complicated process of choosing a name. If the child is conceived out of wedlock or at a time of marital crisis, or for any other reason is unwanted, these feelings may be complicated and exaggerated by the birth of a defective child. In particular, attempts by the mother, or sometimes even the wish, to obtain or perform an abortion may be linked up with subsequent guilt feelings surrounding the handicap.

From the time of birth the mother normally develops a sense of pride in her child, fostered by intimate contact and the attitudes of those around her, which convey the feeling that she has produced something special and worthwhile. The infant becomes a psychological extension of the parent. Prematurity may make this process much more difficult. If the handicap is obvious at birth, maternal depression and working-through of grief over the loss of the anticipated normal child make appropriate stimulation by the mother less likely. Wounded pride, feelings of guilt, and even revulsion may predominate. Anything the parents are told at this time may be crucial because of heightened vulnerability.

In the first few months, when innate reaction patterns are primary, the handicapped child may show alterations that are puzzling and even frightening to the parents. The mother's efforts to respond to the baby's cues may be partially or almost totally unsuccessful. The physician in charge of the case may not yet be able to explain this or may attribute it to a "nervous mother." Some mothers are bothered more by excessive passivity or placidity; others by restlessness and demanding behavior. Rhythmicity of certain functions may not be so readily established in the handicapped child and may further interfere with smooth mother-child interaction. Hospitalizations, illnesses, and differing professional opinions may further jeopardize an already precarious situation. While the normal child is presumably developing a sense of "basic trust" that his needs will be met, the child with developmental deviations may sense the world as chaotic, painful, unsatisfying, or capricious. It may be that this contributes to later efforts at stabilization that may be looked upon as maladaptive: withdrawal, stereotypy, ritualistic behavior, perseveration, and other forms of rigid control.

Late in the first year of life the normal mother begins to frustrate the normal child in a progressive fashion, in keeping with the increase in predictability and ability to delay gratification that the child shows. The depressed or anxious mother may not do this, or may overdo it, failing to provide the developing personality with a basic resource for coping with future tensions and developmental crises. The need for optimal frustration is no less for the handicapped than for the normal child.

Separation problems often develop at the end of the first year. The average parent deals with this by leaving the child at times, but in a way that does not produce excessive anxiety that cannot be mastered. Fear of strangers is considered normal while the infant is developing his first sense of separateness from mother. Associated medical problems of the handicapped child (*e.g.*, seizures) may prevent such separations from being undertaken by the parents, or they may feel an excessive need to avoid anything upsetting to the child. When this occurs, the child rapidly learns how to control the parents and a vicious circle is begun that leads to annoyance on the part of the parents and to ever-increasing insecurity for the child, leading to increased efforts at control of the situation and so on.

The "milestones" of motor development may be skewed in the handicapped child, producing parental concern and sometimes resulting in inappropriate "pushing" before the child is maturationally ready (as in early speech development or walking). Cues from the child that he is ready to attempt a new developmental step may be missed by the parents because of depression, overindulgence, fear of hurting the child, or a variety of other reasons. Yet these early motor activities are basic to exploration, curiosity, learning to play, and stimulation for cognitive development and for self-initiated separations from the mother. The handicap or precedures involved in the child's management may also lead to limitations of exploration and motoric expression of aggression (*e.g.*, bracing, casting). Infantile frustration and satisfaction patterns may persist beyond the usual time (such as rocking, mouthing, smelling, temper tantrums, and breath holding). The normal two-year-old is developing speech rapidly, which assists in gaining more control over impulses and action. Where speech is delayed, problems in impulse expression frequently occur. Early moves toward independence may be inhibited by some of the foregoing factors but also if the parents fear the child will hurt himself or die (*e.g.*, parents who fear death from a seizure and sleep with the child). Usually the parental anxieties are mixtures of realistic concern and their own distorted, confused concepts.

In the early preschool years the average child shows many signs of pride in his body functions and this provides an impetus or reward for practice and new successes. The handicapped child may not be so fortunate: neither he nor his parents may feel a sense of pleasure and pride. The impetus for trying new activities may be greatly reduced. "He just won't try anything and gives up so easily" is a common parental complaint. Often it is easier for child and parents to let the adult do it, rather than watch the child go through repeated and often unsuccessful attempts at mastery.

Early socialization with peers and play become increasingly important in the preschool years, but this may be a very restricted area for the handicapped child. Isolation, social anxiety, and failure to make an adequate identification as a worthwhile human being of a particular sex may ensue. Negative attitudes of parents or others may be adopted and internalized. Outbursts of poorly controlled aggression are not uncommon, especially since the child may not be presented with the consequences of his actions. Sibling rivalry problems may be difficult to deal with, since the parents often find it difficult to apply the same standards to their normal as to their handicapped children. Whereas play activities normally assist the child to master anxiety, fears, and passivity (as in receiving injections and operations) and to learn imitative patterns, much of this may be denied the handicapped. Better methods of compensating for some of these limitations need to be studied and made available to those who counsel parents.

Between the ages of three and six years, transient fears ("phobias") are quite common but usually of no pathological significance in the average child. Some handicapped children develop multiple or persistent fears. The "normal negativism" of this age may also be distorted, in the direction of either excessive compliance and passivity or truly extreme resistance in which any submission or agreement seems to be akin to unconditional surrender.

Many handicapped children of this age have marked reactions to being surpassed by their normal younger siblings. This seems to be concurrent with the dawning realization of their being different from others. When this occurs parents ask many difficult questions about how to cope with the needs of their normal children for praise without increasing feelings of inadequacy on the part of the handicapped child. The answers are rarely simple and often require an understanding of the particular family structure, feelings, and attitudes.

By the time the child reaches elementary school, less allowance is being made for the individual; he must learn to fit into situations he would rather avoid, learn and abide by group rules, and become aware of, and respect, the needs and wishes of others. Appropriate outlets for his impulses must be found and a well-established conscience should guide much of the child's behavior. This presupposes experiences with peers in which he has learned the consequences of his actions and the development of some sense of self-esteem.

Dependency, passivity, and persisting immature patterns may make socialization and peer-group acceptance of the handicapped child much more difficult, apart from the "visibility" of the handicap itself. Special educational settings may not provide the child with the social skills to deal with nonhandicapped children. Parental anxiety over school and social performance may increase the child's worries. Social anxiety, compensatory fantasies, daydreaming, "acting-out," and impulsivity may all reduce the child's ability to concentrate on learning. Problems with abstract thinking, when they occur, often become evident in the third or fourth grades and may lead to considerations of tutoring, summer school, repeating a grade, or changing schools, all of which contribute their share to social difficulties.

There should be little need here to point out that adolescence is usually a time of crisis, turmoil, rebellion, and change, as the struggle to establish a separate identity and true independence progresses. Peer-group acceptance is a necessary transition and many conflicts over social and sexual problems arise. Love objects outside the family must be found and marked changes in the body image integrated. The handicapped person, during this period, may show a greater awareness of his handicap, associated with a feeling of lack of attractiveness or physical strength, or both. Earlier, the child may have had the fantasy and wish that when grown up he would somehow become completely normal. Now, his sense of time has changed and he must adopt more realistic ideas as to his future. The adolescent who *in fact* is more dependent upon his family has a much more difficult task in becoming independent and may have more conflict over desires to remain a child and avoid the unknown terrors of maturity and responsibility. Denial of mild handicaps with compensatory acting-out, even in antisocial directions, may be seen. Refusal of habilitative measures that increase his feelings of being different may become a point over which struggles with parents and professionals occur. Parents become increasingly (and often realistically) anxious over sexual expression, marriage possibilities, and what degree of independence will be achieved.

The normal child and adolescent has probably toyed with many vocational possibilities in fantasy, at play, in part-time jobs, in school experiences, in conversations, in camp, and in other ways. Usually this leads to some choice that is in keeping with reality. The handicapped youngster may have lacked both these experiences and appropriate parental attitudes. He may have unrealistic fantasies or limited reality-testing ability, make outright denial of limitations, or he may, on the other hand, assess his limitations too pessimistically. Obviously, more needs to be considered than merely IQ.

The preceding general description has a discouraging tone. But it should not be assumed that most of these vicissitudes of normal development are inevitable for the handicapped. There is a need for much more research into the antecedents and consequences of deviant development. If one keeps in mind that the maturational forces themselves may tend to overcome developmental obstacles, a more balanced view is possible.

SOME DIFFERENCES BETWEEN THE THINKING OF
CHILDREN AND ADULTS

Some understanding of how children's thinking differs from that of adults is basic to any work with handicapped children. Inability of an adult to comprehend how he used to think and feel as a child is normal and probably adaptive. It is even a problem where fewer years intervene: How many adults can sympathize with the feelings and behavior of the adolescent? Thus, some study of what might be obvious is necessary. Treating children as though they think the way we do is common and potentially harmful, since it may lead to mistrust if not outright hostility.

In the following discussion it must be remembered that *relative* differences are being pointed out; some adult thinking still carries the childish stamp.

The young child operates largely on the basis of immediate pleasure or pain. He finds it difficult, if not impossible, to plan ahead or *choose present discomfort for a promised future relief*. He cannot easily distinguish between the pain or discomfort caused by an illness or handicap and that caused by treatment or therapy aimed at improving the problem.

Egocentrism is prominent and obvious: The world seems to resolve around him and his family. (He may state that the sun or moon follows him, because it is present both before and after a change in his location.) It takes several years before he can appreciate another's point of view, understand his effect upon another, and learn to tolerate the limitations and foibles of his parents.

Wishes, fantasies, and thoughts are readily confused with reality and actions. Things happen to us *for a reason*. The concept of a chance, fortuitous occurrence that cannot be blamed upon someone is usually not developed in the young child. Primitive morality is based upon experiences with reward and punishment, good and bad. The unpleasant consequences of a handicapping condition may, therefore, be viewed by the child as a punishment.

Children may fear the intensity of their own wishes, especially if they are socially unacceptable and directed toward the parents upon whom they must depend.

Because of dependency, limited knowledge and experience, poorly established inner controls, and a rather restricted repertoire of coping mechanisms, *regression* to previous patterns occurs much more easily than in the adult. "Trauma" (experiencing his inability to master successfully an anxiety-provoking situation) is also more common.

Sense of past and future time is not well established. Psychologically, there appears to the child to be a real possibility of being changed into someone else, "outgrowing" a handicap at maturity, "catching" a handicap, or being influenced or changed (physically or mentally) by someone else. Explanations given to the child are likely to be drawn into his current fantasies and distorted. Some repetition, at appropriate intervals, as well as inquiring as to what the child understands from the explanation, may be helpful.

More mature thought processes gradually evolve· but, in the areas of greatest emotional import, more primitive thinking tends to persist, even into adult life (as in sex, birth, and death). A child who is sophisticated in some areas of relatively conflict-free thinking may concurrently and surprisingly demonstrate less mature or even bizarre ideas in more emotionally "loaded" areas. Causal thinking matures rapidly and at ages 7 to 9 years approaches adult concepts (at least in conflict-free areas).

There is still too little appreciation of the extent and depth of a child's distorted fears and the threat he may perceive due to his small size, enforced passivity, limited experience, and poorer reality-testing. Adults often assume that a child cannot be adversely affected by medical procedures or discussions in his presence. This sometimes leads to almost unbelievable situations. Adults can sue, and often collect from, a doctor who does not inform them of the nature of the procedure to be done and its risks. Not respecting the child's needs in this regard may not be legally actionable but constitutes an "assault" in every sense of the word.

ROLE OF PLAY

We frequently lose sight of the crucial role of play in child development. Sometimes it is regarded as a regrettable waste of time or is replaced by more "constructive" activities supervised by adults. Pearson[5] has clearly outlined the need for play and warns of the increasing trend away from unsupervised play during the elementary school years. Harlow's research on primate development seems to confirm the importance of peer interactions and is reviewed by Pearson. Failure to play may contribute to continuing dependency, failure of individuation and redirecting of fantasies, excessive daydreaming, and inability to form strong emotional ties to others. This would seem to be a particular hazard for physically handicapped children. In working with parents, ways

TABLE 1

Aspects of the Handicap Relevant to Emotional Reactions

Aspect	Consequence or Example
1) Severity of physical limitation	May reduce contact with environment and adversely affect cognitive development
2) Age at onset	Congenital defects are more likely to produce diffuse personality alterations; acquired handicaps, acute disturbances
3) Duration	May affect degree of personality change or distortion
4) Course	
a) Stationary	Blindness; deafness. May be easier to cope with than when future is unknown
b) Progressive	Muscular dystrophy, degenerative diseases of many kinds. Reaction may depend upon central nervous system involvement or sparing
c) Improving	Benign hypotonia, some cases of mild brain damage and cerebral palsy
d) Episodic with periods of normality	Seizures, diabetic reactions. May be especially distressing because of extreme fluctuations
5) Appearance or "visibility"	Important in child's self-regard, social functioning, parental adaptation
6) Involvement of central nervous system	May directly impair coping mechanisms, integration, thinking, emotional control
7) Special features	
a) Weakness	Tendency towards passivity and isolation may be obstacle in development
b) Involuntary movements	Athetoid cerebral palsy, dystonia. Impairs sense of body mastery and control
c) Predictability	Seizures. Lack of predictability may lead to protective efforts that hamper development
d) How affected by stress	Many neurological, dermatologic, gastrointestinal, and allergic-respiratory conditions are exacerbated by stress; optimal frustration may not be imposed because of parental fear of worsening condition
e) Threat to life	Seizures, asthma, heart disease. Excessive degree of protection is common
f) Incontinence	Alert children may be very upset by inability to control process of elimination
8) Therapeutic measures used	Need for rest, drugs, separations from family and friends, operations, and painful procedures all may impose their own obstacles to normal development

should be found to provide for play experiences, even for the severely restricted child.

ASPECTS OF THE HANDICAP

There are certain aspects of the handicapping condition itself that may be relevant to the development of emotional disturbances in the child or parent. These are outlined in *Table 1*. Apart from these, the child's original endowment, areas for uninvolved functioning, position in the family, family stability, and nature of previous professional contacts may all play a part.

In general, factors leading to intellectual, social, and physical restrictions and limitations (whether due to the nature of the handicap, its management, or parental attitudes) tend to result in what is loosely called "emotional immaturity," passivity, dependency, poor reality-testing, poor impulse control, and, frequently, stereotyped activities such as autoerotic patterns, mannerisms, tics, and head-banging. Because the handicapped and restricted child may show these features (which seem to be more common with multiple handicaps), he is quite likely to resemble the psychotic child, who also has areas of massive immaturity, primitive fixations, and mannerisms. The differential diagnosis is often difficult. There is still controversy as to whether the psychoses associated with handicapping conditions are the "same" as childhood schizophrenia.[1] The most dramatic work on this area has been reported by Elonen and others,[2, 3] who worked with the deviant blind child. They found that the *majority* of such children who are thought to be ineducable and requiring institutional care could be sufficiently changed with intensive work to attend special or regular day schools.

INCIDENCE AND NATURE OF EMOTIONAL PROBLEMS

There is no general agreement regarding the incidence of emotional disturbance with each type of handicap. Where figures are available, they usually indicate an increased risk, at least for handicaps with early onset. Research studies are extremely difficult to perform, however. There is at present no reason to believe that a specific personality type or reaction pattern is inevitable for a child with a particular handicap. Multiple factors are undoubtedly operative. The most meaningful work, from the emotional standpoint, has been done in blindness, mental retardation, muscular dystrophy, convulsive disorders, "minimal cerebral dysfunction," cleft palate, bronchial asthma, and cystic fibrosis. There is relatively little that is helpful concerning cerebral palsy, and there are no adequate studies, in depth, on the deaf child. Many of the contributions were of a multidisciplinary nature and by no means solely to the credit of psychiatry.

GENERAL PRINCIPLES OF MANAGEMENT

This section outlines some suggestions that might be useful in the management of the handicapped child. They will not be found helpful or sufficient in every case, since there can be no substitute for adequate investigation, in depth, of an individual and his family. While it is hoped that these will be of assistance, they are not intended to replace professional consultation in the area of mental health. Some criteria for referral to a psychiatrist will be listed later.

A study of great potential significance was described by Shere and Kastenbaum.[6] They investigated mother-child interaction in a group of severely involved, nonambulatory, nonverbal cerebral palsied children. They found that the mothers, often without realizing it, fostered passivity in their children. They did not automatically know how to stimulate their children so as to provide maximum experience for cognitive development. These children lived in an environment in which they had much too little contact with objects. Physicians and others had tended to focus exclusively on physical or speech progress, so that the mothers were unaware to what extent their children depended totally upon them for object contact. It was felt that special procedures needed to be employed for the development of insight in these parents. The implications of this pilot study regarding other and less severe handicaps should be further investigated. It is probable that we often fail to provide early and meaningful direction to parents regarding stimulation, exploration, play, and appropriate play materials.

We need to understand the "working-through" process in children and parents. This applies to diagnosis and treatment. Short cuts and "one-shot" evaluations leave much to be desired because of neglect of this basic principle. Unfortunately, shortage of personnel and time are realistic factors that often prevent ideal care.

The professional worker should learn to recognize his own needs and feelings in work with a handicapped child. "Rescue fantasies" may easily develop, with the need to prove one's superiority to the parent. (It's easy when you don't have to live with the problem!) Negative feelings of anger and disgust may become a problem for both parent and worker as the child grows older. What was formerly "cute" may not evoke the same response later.

Since both child and parents have angry, frustrated feelings that they may transfer to a particular worker or institution, understanding and refraining from retaliation may be most helpful. Remember that, while parental love for their child is natural, feelings of a negative sort because of the abnormality are also natural, though unacceptable in our culture. The child's and parents' defenses against anxiety or depression need to be respected, not battered down, unless and until there is something better to offer.

Where possible, substitute outlets for a child's motoric and fantasied aggression, competitive impulses, and needs for success should be provided. Boredom, sensory and social isolation, and apathy are to be avoided, as are shame and humiliation as disciplinary or motivational technics.

While understanding ease of regression, we should do everything possible to avoid practices and procedures that are unnecessary but may force the child into a regressed position (*e.g.·* wheelchairs, bedpans, daytime use of pajamas, and unnecessary bed rest in hospitalized children).

Cooperation and compliance may be very convenient but at times may be excessive and pathological. A child who protests vehemently against a painful procedure that he does not understand is not necessarily "disturbed"; in fact he may be healthier than the "perfect patient."

Parents need to be told about the results of routine procedures that we take for granted. It is rare for a routine skull film to turn up unexpected pathology but parents and child may believe that it can determine whether something is "wrong with his brain."

Serious problems should be referred early. (*See Table 2.*)

PREPARATION FOR SURGERY OR OTHER PROCEDURES

Elective procedures should be deferred until the child and family are ready; inquiry should be made as to the stability of the home situation and other current problems. Most authorities agree that surgery is least traumatic before the age of one year and after the age of five or six. Adequate preparation involves corrections of distortions, wherever possible, as to what to expect before, during, and after the procedure and should not precede the procedure by more than a few days in most instances (for the child). Of course, the child may know that an operation is contemplated, but the *detailed* preparation should adhere to the previous stipulation. The parents need more time than this. They should have one person they can contact, rather than a "team." Mounting anxiety before a procedure, despite preparation, is often encountered and

TABLE 2

Some Criteria for Referral to a Psychiatrist

1) Suicidal threats, preoccupations, or attempts
2) Severe and persistent depression or withdrawal, out of proportion to known precipitating factors
3) Self-punitive behavior, pleasure in painful experiences, "accident proneness"
4) Severe and persistent behavioral regression without known physical cause
5) Marked resistance to habilitative measures, which cannot be modified by a flexible therapist; evidence that "psychological gain" from the handicap is producing, or adding to, such resistance
6) Severe and repeated acting-out or delinquent behavior
7) Severe separation anxiety in the school-age child; "school phobia"
8) Evidence of possible incipient psychosis: bizarre behavior, withdrawal to extreme degree, delusional or paranoid thinking, habit deterioration
9) Differential diagnostic problems. A few are:
    a) Psychosis with (or versus) mental retardation;
    b) "Bizarre behavior" in children with sensory handicaps;
    c) Deafness versus psychosis or "elective mutism";
    d) Convulsive disorder versus "conversion reaction" or "hysteria."

not necessarily a problem. Lying to the child should be avoided. The parents should also be prepared for the possibility of emotional reactions of a transient nature after surgery (*e.g.,* hostility to the parents, or clinging, demanding behavior, sleep difficulties, and other regressive patterns). Parent-child contact should be fostered by permitting rooming-in with the very young child or frequent visiting with the older child. A familiar object (doll or toy) from the home environment may help.

Preparation need not be done by the psychiatrist, psychologist, or social worker, except in special circumstances. A sensitive pediatrician, general practitioner, orthopedist (or other surgical specialist), or even a nonmedical person or parent may do the job successfully, provided the information is available to them.

PSYCHIATRIC REFERRAL

When general principles of good management fail to prevent or modify a pathological emotional reaction, referral or consultation may be in order. Depending upon the availability of a child psychiatrist with experience in this area, consultation with a knowledgeable general psychiatrist, pediatrician, or psychologist might precede this step. Consulta-

TABLE 3

Factors Conducive to Good Adjustment

1) Favorable endowment and "temperament" (hard to define or determine)
2) Stable family situation
3) Parent-child relationship predominantly positive; sense of "basic trust" established in child; parents who are sensitive but not overly intellectualizing
4) Parents and professionals working cooperatively, rather than at cross-purposes
5) Realistic information about the handicap available to child and family
6) Adequate preparation of child and parents for hospitalization and painful or complicated procedures
7) Adequate opportunities for exploration, peer contact, and play
8) Development of effective coping mechanisms to deal with anxiety
9) Minimal (but sufficient) number of professional evaluations and absence of marked differences of opinion among those who have seen the child
10) Realistic acceptance by the therapist of his own role, expectations, and needs in working with the child

tion prior to referral has certain advantages, perhaps the most significant being the avoidance of stirring false hopes or fears in the child and family. (Many parents see a psychiatric referral as indication that a new "cure" is possible, or, alternatively, that a new and crushing burden has been added to the existing handicap.) Treatment of the persistent and severe problem is in the province of the mental health professional and will not be discussed here.

The same principles applying to any referral are pertinent: Some specialists are competent and helpful, others are not. Unfortunately, most psychiatrists have not had adequate training in working with the handicapped child until relatively recently. Some criteria for referral are listed in *Table 2*.

FACTORS IN GOOD ADJUSTMENT

After so much emphasis upon problem behavior, it is appropriate to consider some factors that seem to be conducive to successful adjustment. These are listed in *Table 3*. It is true, though not always well understood, that the most competent team of professionals may be unduly pessimistic about a child's development and potential. There is, as yet, no way to predict consistently eventual "good" or "bad" adjustment. Until this goal is achieved, it is best to give every child and family a reasonable chance to maximize all areas of functioning. The factors listed, it should be stated, rarely all occur together, and successful adjustment may take place without all of them.

CONCLUSIONS

It is probable that the handicapped child, by reason of his difficult developmental process, is more vulnerable to emotional disturbances (of either developmental or acute types) than the nonhandicapped. Reliable statistics are not available, however, and it has not been possible to demonstrate a clear relationship between a particular handicap and a specific personality pattern or developmental deviation.

The amenability of emotionally disturbed handicapped children to various forms of intervention has never been adequately established. It is probably better than many have thought. Too many clinics and mental health workers have assumed a pessimistic outlook or excluded such children from services they needed. Environmental factors can be assumed to be of at least as much importance in the genesis of emotional disturbances of the handicapped as that of the nonhandicapped.

It is hoped that the recently increased interest in the handicapped child by psychiatrists and in emotional development by nonpsychiatric professionals working with such children will result in better communication and will eventually benefit children and their families.

REFERENCES

1. EATON, LOUISE, and MENOLASCINO, FRANK J. Psychotic Reactions of Childhood: A Follow-Up Study. *Am. J. Orthopsychiat.* Apr., 1967. 37:3:521-529.
2. ELONEN, ANNA S., and CAIN, ALBERT C. Diagnostic Evaluation and Treatment of Deviant Blind Children. *Am. J. Orthopsychiat.* July, 1964. 34:4:625-633.
3. ELONEN, ANNA S., and POLZIEN, MARGARET. Experimental Program for Deviant Blind Children. *New Outlook for the Blind.* Apr., 1965. 59:4:122-126.
4. FREEMAN, ROGER D. The Home Visit in Child Psychiatry: Its Usefulness in Diagnosis and Training. *J. Am. Acad. Child Psychiat.* Apr., 1967. 6:2:276-294.
5. PEARSON, GERALD H. J. The Importance of Peer Relationship in the Latency Period. *Bul.,* Philadelphia Assn. for Psychoanalysis. 16:3:109-121.
6. SHERE, EUGENIA, and KASTENBAUM, ROBERT. Mother-Child Interaction in Cerebral Palsy: Environmental and Psychosocial Obstacles to Cognitive Development. *Genet. Psychol. Monogr.* May, 1966. 73:2:255-335.

SUGGESTED READING

BAER, PAUL E. Problems in the Differential Diagnosis of Brain Damage and Childhood Schizophrenia. *Am. J. Orthopsychiat.* Oct., 1961. 31:4:728-737.

BLUMBERG, MARVIN L. Emotional and Personality Development in Neuromuscular Disorders. *A.M.A. J. Diseases of Children.* Sept., 1959. 98:3:303-310.

CAPLAN, HYMAN. The Role of Deviant Maturation in the Pathogenesis of Anxiety. *Am. J. Orthopsychiat.* Jan., 1956. 26:1:94-107.

CAPLAN, HYMAN. Some Considerations of the Body Image Concept in Child Development. *Quart. J. Child Behavior.* Oct., 1952. 4:4:382-388.

CROTHERS, BRONSON, and PAINE, RICHMOND S. *The Natural History of Cerebral Palsy.* Cambridge, Mass.: Harvard Univ. Pr., 1959.

CRUICKSHANK, WILLIAM M., ed. *Psychology of Exceptional Children and Youth.* (ed. 2) Englewood Cliffs, N. J.: Prentice-Hall, 1963.

DENHOFF, ERIC. Emotional and Psychological Background of the Neurologically Handicapped Child. *Exceptional Children.* Mar., 1961. 27:7:347-349.

FLAVELL, JOHN H. *The Developmental Psychology of Jean Piaget.* Princeton, N. J.: Van Nostrand, 1963.

FREUD, ANNA. The Role of Bodily Illness in the Mental Life of Children. *Psychoanalytic Study of the Child* (New York: Internatl. Universities Pr., 1952), 7:69-81.

GREEN, MORRIS. Care of the Child with a Long-Term, Life-Threatening Illness: Some Principles of Management. *Pediatrics.* Mar., 1967. 39:3:441-445.

MORROW, ROBERT S., and COHEN, JACOB. The Psycho-Social Factors in Muscular Dystrophy. *J. Child Psychiat.* Apr., 1954. 3:1:70-80.

PHILIPS, IRVING. Psychopathology and Mental Retardation. *Am. J. Psychiat.* July, 1967. 124:1:29-35.

PINCUS, J. H., and GLASER, G. H. The Syndrome of "Minimal Brain Damage" in Childhood. *New Eng. J. Med.* July 7, 1966. 275:1:27-35.

ROSS, ALAN O. *The Exceptional Child in the Family—Helping Parents of Exceptional Children.* New York: Grune & Stratton, 1964.

SCHECTER, MARSHALL D. The Orthopedically Handicapped Child: Emotional Reactions. *Arch. Gen. Psychiat.* Mar., 1961. 4:2:247-253.

SHAW, CHARLES R. *The Psychiatric Disorders of Childhood.* New York: Appleton-Century-Crofts, 1966.

TISZA, VERONICA B., SELVERSTONE, BETTY, ROSENBLUM, GERSHEN, and HANLON, NANCY. Psychiatric Observations of Children with Cleft Palate. *Am. J. Orthopsychiat.* Apr., 1958. 28:2:416-423.

TUREEN, LOUIS L., and WOOLSEY, ROBERT M. Some Psychiatric Aspects of Convulsive Disorders. *Missouri Med.* Feb., 1964. 61:2:91-98.

WATSON, E. JANE, and JOHNSON, ADELAIDE M. The Emotional Significance of Acquired Physical Disfigurement in Children. *Am. J. Orthopsychiat.* Jan., 1958. 28:1:85-97.

WERRY, J. S. Studies on the Hyperactive Child. IV. An Empirical Analysis of the Minimal Brain Dysfunction Syndrome. Read before the American Psychiatric Association, Detroit, May, 1967. To be published.

25

PSYCHOLOGICAL IMPLICATIONS OF CRYPTORCHISM

Leon Cytryn, M.D.

Member of the Faculty, Children's Hospital of the District of Columbia,
Assistant Professor of Pediatric Psychiatry,
George Washington University Medical School

Eileen Cytryn, M.S.W.

Psychiatric Social Worker, Deaprtment of Psychiatry,
Children's Hospital of D. C.

and

Rebecca E. Rieger, Ph.D.

Associate Chief Psychologist, Member of the Faculty,
Children's Hospital of D. C.

Cryptorchism, or undescended testicle, is a not uncommon condition. The incidence among children as given by various authors ranges between 1 to 14 percent (Robinson and Engle, 1955). Although there is a voluminous literature on the hormonal (Charny, 1960; Bernstein, 1957), pathological (Hinman, 1955; Robinson and Engle, 1954; Nelson, 1951; Lich, 1956), and fertility (Charny, 1960; Lewis, 1954) aspects of cryptorchism, there is little information on what the condition means to the affected child and his parents. Many urologists and pediatricians who

Reprinted from the JOURNAL OF THE AMERICAN ACADEMY OF CHILD PSYCHIATRY, Vol. VI, No. 2, April 1967, pp. 131-165. This study was supported in whole by Public Health Service Research Grant No. M 5992-A and Grant No. MH 05992 from the National Institute of Mental Health. Presented at the regional meeting of the American Academy of Child Psychiatry in Washington, D.C., November, 1963.

work with children with cryptorchism are convinced of the strong emotional impact of this condition upon the child and his parents. The surgical and urological literature, however, contains only scattered, brief remarks implying the possibility of a psychological disturbance in patients with this anomaly (Larson, 1957; Clarke, 1956; Bernstein, 1957; Koop, 1957). Campbell (1951) states that the reaction of the disturbed patient is characteristically one of "depression, of assumed inferiority and has sometimes led to suicide." Connolly (1959), in an excellent, comprehensive study of all aspects of cryptorchism, states that "there is no other defect which causes such a marked feeling of lack of normal virility." Blos (1960) described in detail psychiatric treatment of three children with cryptorchism and attempted to establish a definite psychological syndrome common to this condition. He lists hyperactivity, learning difficulties, and accident proneness as the most prominent features of this syndrome. The fact is stressed that cryptorchism leads to psychopathology only in a very specific matrix of family interaction involving a possessive mother and a passive, aloof father. All three boys had a distorted, vague, and incomplete body image and a bisexual sense of identity. Finally, Bell (1961) pointed out the important role of the testicles and scrotum in the emotional development of boys, especially in the area of sexual identification.

Our search through the world literature failed to reveal any systematic study describing a larger sample of children with cryptorchism and their emotional adjustment to this abnormality. It seemed therefore of interest to undertake such a study in order to explore this area further and elicit any existing trends. We were particularly interested in the nature of any existing psychological disturbances and their effect on the child's performance at home, at play, and in school. Emphasis was placed on the role of the parents and the physician in the child's adjustment. Finally, we wished to assess the impact of a corrective operation on any existing emotional difficulties.

METHODS OF PROCEDURE

The study was set up as a preliminary clinical investigation. Two groups of patients were studied. In the first (preoperative) group, a total of nineteen boys with cryptorchism were seen, usually immediately before a scheduled corrective operation, namely, orchiopexy. In the second (postoperative) group a total of eight boys were seen. All of them had undergone corrective surgery for cryptorchism at least one year before being seen in our study.

The patients were studied in 1962 and in part of 1963. They were drawn from various clinics and wards of the Children's Hospital of the District of Columbia and from the private practices of urologists and surgeons in the Washington, D.C. area. In the preoperative group, patients were seen successively as they were admitted to the hospital for surgery. The names of the postoperative group were drawn from the files of the Hospital Record Room and these children were the first sequence of patients who became available when their parents were reached by our team.

The parents in both groups were interviewed by a psychiatric social worker (E.C.) in two structured but open-ended interviews. Each interview lasted one and a half hours. Detailed information was sought as to the child's physical and mental development and his performance in school, at home, and at play. The parents were encouraged to express their feelings and ideas in regard to the child's congenital defect. The family background, the medical history, the parents' adjustment, and important events in the child's life were explored. The parents were also questioned in detail about the medical advice and guidance they had received, and the way they were able to use it.

The children in the preoperative group were seen in a psychiatric interview lasting approximately one and a half hours and later were visited daily on the ward following the operation. The children in the postoperative sample were seen only once for one and a half hours.

The interview started with a free play situation lasting about ten to fifteen minutes. Following that, the patients were encouraged to talk about themselves, their families, friends, and attitudes. Various techniques commonly used in child psychiatry were utilized, such as the three wishes, the desert island, dreams, TV stories, the Despert fables, and others. In addition, the children were confronted with a defective female doll with a missing arm and an ambulance and asked to make up a story about it. Each child was also asked to draw a man and a woman and the inside of the body. The Vocabulary of the Stanford-Binet test was also administered in order to provide a quick, rough assessment of the child's intelligence.

The *family* was assessed jointly by the child psychiatrist and the social worker and each one placed in one of four categories:

1. *No disturbance*—Cohesive family; cooperative, mature, and flexible parents, supportive of the child.
2. *Mildly disturbed*—Family cohesive, but parents less cooperative; defensive, one parent dominant, child overprotected, or raised very strictly.

3. *Moderately disturbed*—Parents in complete discord, unreasonable, immature, insufficiently supportive of the child.
4. *Very disturbed*—Chaotic family situation, marked lack of stability, complete rejection of the child by at least one parent.

The *children* were assessed jointly by the child psychiatrist and the social worker and each child placed in one of four categories according to the degree of his general emotional disturbance:

1. *No disturbance*—Age-appropriate behavior, absence of behavioral symptoms, relaxed and mature attitude, good school adjustment.
2. *Mildly disturbed*—Absence of behavioral symptoms, tense, slightly restless, somewhat anxious or depressed, immature, good school and social adjustment.
3. *Moderately disturbed*—Mild behavioral symptoms, rigid, tense, anxious and depressed, immature, poor school and social adjustment.
4. *Severely disturbed*—Severe behavioral symptoms, very restless, very anxious and depressed, poor social and school adjustment.

The children's drawings and the Stanford-Binet Vocabulary Test were evaluated by the psychologist on our team (R.R.) who was furnished with no information about the child other than his age. The figure drawings of twenty-one boys were analyzed; the drawings of the inside of the body were omitted from the present analysis. Three boys were under six years of age and their drawings were eliminated from consideration because we thought that developmental factors would obscure more dynamic aspects of the drawings. Only one boy failed to draw both the male and female figures; the single exception drew only a female. The boys ranged in age from six years and seven months to thirteen years and nine months, with a mean age of nine years and eleven months. There were eight Negro boys and thirteen whites. The drawings of fourteen boys were obtained immediately preoperatively; the remaining seven boys had had corrective operations at least one year before they were interviewed.

Analysis of the drawings used items which were open to direct observation, permitting relatively objective scoring, and items which involved more indirect, inferential judgments about self-concept, anxiety, sexual identity, and overall level of personality functioning. The objective scoring related to page placement; size; relative size of the male and female; figure drawn first; completeness of the figures; presence of secondary elaborations, shading, erasures or line breaks, and reinforce-

TABLE I

RELATIONSHIP BETWEEN THE AGE AT OPERATION & DEGREE OF EMOTIONAL DISTURBANCE

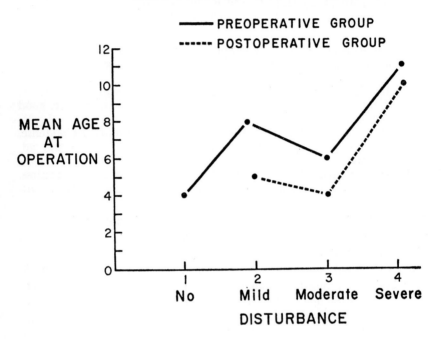

ments; and appropriate sexual differentiation between the male and female figures.

FINDINGS

General Information

Age of the Children (see Table 1). In the preoperative group, the ages of the nineteen children seen ranged from three to thirteen years. The six very disturbed children in this group had a mean age of eleven years, while the three children without emotional disturbance had a mean age of four. The ages of the children in the mildly or moderately disturbed categories clustered around the mean of eight years.

In the postoperative group, the ages of the eight children seen ranged from six to seventeen years. The age when orchiopexy was performed

TABLE II

DISTRIBUTION OF PATIENTS ACCORDING TO DEGREE OF EMOTIONAL DISTURBANCE, RACE & SOCIO-ECONOMIC STATUS

	#	Race		Socio-Economic Status	
		Negro	White	Ward Patient	Private
No Disturbance	3	1	2	1	2
Mild Disturbance	9	2	7	2	7
Moderate Disturbance	5	1	4	—	5
Severe Disturbance	10	6	4	4	6
Total	27	10	17	7	20

in this group ranged from three to fourteen years with a mean age of seven years. The four very disturbed boys in this group were operated at a mean age of ten years, and the remaining four at a mean age of five years.

Race and Socioeconomic Status (see Table 2): Of the nineteen children in the preoperative group, nine were Negro and ten were white. In the postoperative group, there were seven whites and one Negro.

There were seven ward patients in both groups, all of them Negro. The three private Negro patients were all found to be of very modest financial means, relying primarily on hospital outpatient and well-baby care.

Of the six very disturbed boys in the *preoperative* group, five were Negro, two of them private and three ward patients. Among the four very disturbed patients in the *postoperative* group only one was a Negro ward patient while the remaining three were white private patients.

Size of the Children. Nine children or 33 percent of the entire sample were strikingly undersized and looked much younger than their age. This shortness in stature has been mentioned by others in connection with cryptorchism and is generally explained on a basis of pituitary deficiency, responsible both for the failure to grow and the maldescent of the testes. The size of the children in our study, however, bore no relation to the degree of their emotional disturbance.

Heredity. Eighteen percent of the children had at least one close relative with cryptorchism. This incidence is considerably higher than is generally assumed, but again bore no relation to the degree of the emotional disturbance of the children.

Extent of Cryptorchism. There were six children in the entire sample with bilateral cryptorchism, five in the preoperative and one in the postoperative group. Three of these (50 percent) were classified as severely disturbed.

Age When Cryptorchism Was Diagnosed (see Table 3). The diagnosis of cryptorchism was made by a physician in the great majority of the children.

Of the ten very disturbed children in the entire sample, the undescended testicle was diagnosed in infancy in only two cases (20 percent). The remaining 80 percent had their condition diagnosed later in life at ages ranging from three to thirteen. This contrasts sharply with the remainder of the children in whom cryptorchism was diagnosed in infancy, in 69 percent of the cases.

While the parents' tendency to deny this readily palpable condition might account for some of the delay in diagnosis, this would not explain the failure of the physicians to make the diagnosis early, despite repeated medical examinations of the child.

The eight children in the very disturbed group whose cryptorchism was diagnosed late included six Negro patients who relied primarily on hospital outpatient and well-baby care, and one white boy who was born and reared in a rather primitive country in the Near East. The finding suggests that the physicians' failure to diagnose the condition early might be a result of inferior medical care, which precluded a thorough physical examination. Since late diagnosis was usually associated with a late operation it could coneivably play an important role in the personality development of these children.

TABLE III

RELATIONSHIP BETWEEN TIME OF DIAGNOSIS OF CRYPTORCHISM & DEGREE OF EMOTIONAL DISTURBANCE

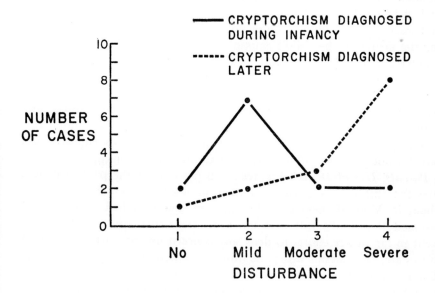

Psychological Characteristics of the Parents

Parents' Cooperation in the Study. Eight (29 percent) of the parents were very defensive and reluctant to participate in the study. However, the reluctant participants were evenly distributed among all our diagnostic categories, and the degree of denial was similarly distributed. In only one case (a postoperative child) did the parents actually refuse to participate in the study.

We interviewed only five fathers, because they proved much more reluctant than their wives to participate actively, despite our urging. Those who were seen were rather vague about details of the child's development and past life.

Parents' Guilt Feelings. Several of the parents expressed guilt feelings about the child's emotional disturbance, but only three openly assumed responsibility for the child's undescended testicle. Two of them thought that unwanted pregnancy caused the anomaly in the boy, while one recalled being hit by a chair during pregnancy and thought that this caused the testicle to be "knocked into the abdomen."

Parents' Concerns about Cryptorchism. Twelve (40 percent) of the parents voiced their concerns about the child's future. Their worries included cancer, homosexuality, transvestitism, sterility, "becoming a woman," "a sissy," "a punk," "a freak," not being able to "digest food" or just being different from other boys. These voiced parental concerns and worries were found to be of no particular significance in determining the degree of the child's emotional disturbance.

Interestingly, of the five fathers seen in our study, four linked their concerns about the child with concerns about their own adequacy in general and in the sexual area in particular. These concerns included fertility, ability to produce children of both sexes, sexual prowess, and being able to get along in life successfully. One father who himself had had cryptorchism in childhood was worried because his eight-year-old boy did not yet have pubic hair, nor had his voice changed.

Parents' Use of Denial. Eighteen (66 percent) of the parents denied that the children were aware of their undescended testicle or worried about it. Most of them told the children that they had a hernia and assumed the child's full acceptance of this explanation. One mother went so far in her efforts to deny any concern on the part of the child as to state, "He doesn't worry; he thinks everybody has only one testicle." The child of the same mother, incidentally, used denial excessively but gave it a different twist by insisting emphatically, one day before a scheduled orchiopexy, that he had two testicles in the scrotum.

Denial of the parents was found to be without correlation with the degree of emotional disturbance in the child, being present with similar frequency in all diagnostic categories.

Parents' Preparation of the Child. The high degree of denial used by the majority of the parents might explain the generally poor preoperative preparation which these boys received from their parents.

Only four (14 percent) of the parents prepared the child adequately by telling him honestly about the nature of the operation and the reason for it. About half of the remainder gave the children no explanation whatsoever, while the other half told their children that they would have a hernioplasty or, in two cases, a tonsillectomy. The information given the children included statements such as, "They will be nice to you and give you ice cream," or "They will put a rubber band around your belly," or "They will straighten your hernia," or simply, "Don't worry, we have you insured." In almost every case the degree of denial in the child paralleled the degree of denial in the

TABLE IV

RELATIONSHIP BETWEEN DEGREE OF DISTURBANCE IN FAMILIES & PATIENTS

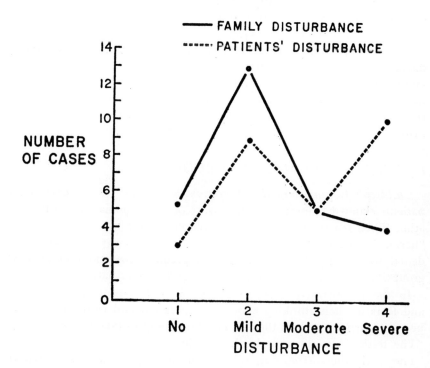

parents and the parental attitudes, but the specific information given the children by the parents did not seem decisive in the child's emotional adjustment.

Family Disturbance (see Table 4). In the first three diagnostic categories (no disturbance to moderately disturbed), the families' and the children's degree of disturbance was roughly parallel. In the severely disturbed group, however, there was a significant difference, with ten severely disturbed children and only four families so designated. Thus the children's disturbance is not simply correlated with membership in a disturbed family.

In all cases of the very disturbed children, we found a very characteristic family constellation. The mothers were usually much closer to the boys than were the fathers, assuming the primary responsibility for all aspects of the children's upbringing and discipline. They were usually very possessive of the children and either overindulgent or very strict, often with high standards. The fathers, on the other hand, were either absent or rather remote, uninvolved with the boys, and withdrawn from the mainstream of the family life. Both parents usually considered the child inadequate and immature and treated him accordingly, the fathers being more disparaging and rejecting and the mothers being overly protective. This pattern repeated itself with striking regularity in all very disturbed children and was not seen in "pure culture" in the rest of the sample. In the mildly to moderately disturbed children this pattern was usually modified, and what seemed to make the difference was the positive attitude of the father or father substitute and his interest and actual involvement with the boy.

Psychological Characteristics of the Children

Children's Coping with the Operation. Seventeen (58 percent) of the patients claimed ignorance of the nature of their anomaly and the operation. Their reactions ranged from displacement ("lump in the stomach," "hernia," "tonsils") to complete denial of any difficulty. This degree of denial was evenly distributed in both preoperative and postoperative groups, in both races and in both ward and private patients.

In the preoperative group, six boys showed considerable distortion and fears in their thinking about the operation and cryptorchism. We heard distortions such as these: "They are going to take the organ out," "The testicle was down at birth and the penis was sort of dragging," "They'll rip the stitches out," "My stomach is upside down," "I fell on a pole and this knocked my balls in," "You need testicles so you won't get bird disease."

In the postoperative group, three of the boys had quite gruesome memories of the operation: "A surgeon had blood all over him; something went wrong and he cut too deep, and blood gushed out," or, "The doctor just ripped the bandages off, and I screamed so that the dead could hear me, then they gave the boy in the next bed a blood needle a half foot long," "I was afraid before the operation. They'll jab a knife in me, and I'll be dead."

These distortions were somewhat more prevalent among the very disturbed children, but they were expressed by the less disturbed boys as well.

Psychological Description of the Children. Twelve (41 percent) of the children showed a striking combination of passivity and immaturity in their behavior.

Twenty (69 percent) were quite depressed or anxious or both when we saw them. The degree of clinical depression, in particular, was associated with other more severe behavioral symptoms.

Eleven (37 percent) of the group were very restless, either in the hospital or at home, or both.

Eighteen (66 percent) of the children had behavioral symptoms, including enuresis, encopresis, thumb sucking, fighting, stealing, sleep disturbances, fears, withdrawal, social isolation, and school difficulties. The latter was present in all of the ten very disturbed children and in several of the moderately disturbed ones.

Degree of Emotional Disturbance (see Table 2). Six (33 percent) patients in the preoperative group were classified by the authors as very disturbed and in need of psychiatric treatment. In the postoperative group, four, or 50 percent, were classified as very disturbed. The incidence of children judged in need of psychiatric treatment in the entire sample was 37 percent.

Twenty percent of the patients were classified as moderately disturbed and 33 percent were mildly disturbed.

Only three boys in the entire sample were classified as being free from emotional disturbance.

It should be stressed that our classification was based primarily on the child's performance and behavior rather than on evidence of intrapsychic pathology.

Fantasy Material. In the preoperative group, fifteen (78 percent) seemed very preoccupied with themes of aggression and annihilation. This preoccupation, however, bore no apparent relation to the degree of disturbance. Preoccupation with aggression and annihilation in the postoperative group was found in five (63 percent) of the children, and seemed to be associated with greater overall disturbance.

One might expect more concern over aggression, death, and injury in children facing an imminent operation. The same concerns in children several years after operation, however, seem more significant, especially since the mean age in the postoperative sample was eleven years, when one would expect more repression in fantasy life.

Ambulance Story. The children's responses to the mutilated doll did not seem to contribute to our diagnostic armamentarium since realistic appraisal of the missing arm, denial of it, themes of restitution (artificial arm), and statements about the finality of the crippling were found evenly distributed with no regard to the degree of emotional disturbance.

Previous Operations and Accidents. Ten (37 percent) of the children had had another operation sometime before the orchiopexy. We found this factor to have no apparent bearing on the degree of disturbance.

Seven of the children had had at least one major accident. They were evenly distributed in all of our categories. Three of the boys, all very disturbed, were reported by the parents to be careless, oblivious to dangers, and daring in their behavior.

Important Events. Eleven of the patients had experienced important events in their lives which possibly could have contributed to their emotional upheaval. One was adopted; two had younger siblings who died of a congenital disorder; the mother of two brothers died shortly before their operations; five came from broken homes; and one came from a family constantly on the move due to the father's diplomatic assignments. There was a greater preponderance (40 percent) of broken homes and instability in the lives of the very disturbed group than in those of the rest of the patients. This is not surprising since in each the father was completely or almost completely out of the picture. This in turn contributed to the typical family constellation of a dominant mother and an absent or uninvolved father which we, like Blos (1960), found to be predisposing to psychopathology in children with cryptorchism.

Attitudes toward Sex. Both the parents and the children were very reluctant to discuss sexual matters. Most of the parents emphatically denied masturbation or sexual curiosity in their children. The children generally claimed ignorance and lack of interest in the subject of sex.

Role of the Physician

In assessing the role of the physician, we had to rely on the statements of the patients and the parents, which, of course, left room for distortion. However, since this would apply to all the children in our sample, any differences found might be significant.

Physician's Preparation of the Child. Only four of all our patients reported an adequate preoperative preparation by their physician. This included an explanation of the condition and proper information about the operation, with sufficient reassurance and support. The majority (66 percent) reported not being told anything by the physician and the rest were briefly told about the operation without an age-appropriate explanation. This, however, did not seem to influence the course of the children's emotional adjustment, being found evenly distributed in all of the diagnostic categories.

Physician's Preparation of the Parents (see Table 5). Only three (30

TABLE V

PHYSICIAN'S PREPARATION OF PARENTS & DEGREE OF EMOTIONAL DISTURBANCE IN CHILDREN

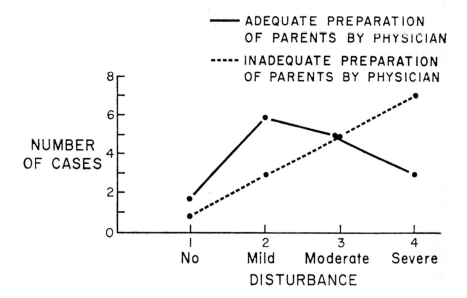

—— ADEQUATE PREPARATION OF PARENTS BY PHYSICIAN

----- INADEQUATE PREPARATION OF PARENTS BY PHYSICIAN

percent) parents of very disturbed children described an adequate pre-operative preparation by their physicians including an opportunity to voice their concerns and to ask questions. This contrasted sharply with the less disturbed group of patients where the majority of the parents (76 percent) were properly prepared by the physicians. This striking difference in parental reports, while it might be a function of denial and distortion on the part of parents of the more disturbed group, does seem significant and points to the importance of the physician's role in preventing emotional disturbances associated with cryptorchism by adequate preoperative preparation of both the parents and the patients, with the parents given priority.

Psychological Aspects of the Figure Drawings

The following results are tentative, in the absence of comparison groups and in view of the inadequate attention to the issue of rater reliability.

The most striking finding is that over half of the boys (55 percent) drew male figures with important parts missing, mainly limbs, such as arms or hands and legs or feet. A somewhat lower proportion (38 percent) left limbs off the female figures. In addition to limbs, the nose or eyes were sometimes omitted. While there was a marked tendency to omit significant parts of the body, there did not appear to be any overt indicators of anxiety specifically pertaining to the genitals. From the evidence on shading, line breaks or erasures, and line reinforcement, the genital area was essentially avoided as a site for direct anxiety indicators. A similar finding was reported in connection with a study of patients undergoing mitral heart surgery, in whose spontaneous drawings of a person there was no allusion to the nature or the site of the existing illness: only in the drawings of the inside of the body was the heart area emphasized (Meyer et al., 1961). The failure to include significant parts of the body other than the genitals (which are rarely included in test drawings) probably represents displacement and denial. Anxiety about the incomplete genitals is expressed through substitute symbolic representation. Not infrequently the feet, and somewhat less frequently the hands, serve as displacements from the genitals (Hammer, 1953) .

From the drawings an attempt was made to judge the nature of the sexual identity of the patients. Judgments were based on (a) the extent of sexual differentiation between the male and female figures; (b) the relative size of male and female figures; (c) the figure which was drawn first; and (d) the extent of concern with body integrity. Over half (52 percent) of the boys seemed to see themselves as masculine but maimed or incomplete in some significant way. This was true within both the pre- and postoperative groups. An additional 29 percent of the total group showed confusion in sexual identity. Only one boy of the twenty-one cases studied showed fairly clear-cut feminine identity, in that he was able to draw only a female figure.

Somewhat more speculative judgments from the drawings about the self-concept suggest that about 75 percent of the boys have a self-concept of inadequacy, and almost half of the boys show this to a marked degree. An additional 20 percent seem to be overcompensating, but almost all members of the group seem to represent themselves as inadequate in varying degrees. The drawings suggest that none of the group was free of anxiety and two thirds of the boys seemed to be markedly anxious.

An effort was made to assess overall ego functioning from the drawings, using a developmental approach which assumes that with increasing age there will be increasing complexity, differentiation, and attention to significant details in the drawings. Using the Goodenough norms (1926) for age-appropriate performance, one can assess a child's level of functioning in comparison with others of his own age group expressed as a ratio of "mental age" (or developmental age, in this case) to chronological age, yielding an I.Q. or D.Q. On the Goodenough tests almost two thirds of the group fall below the normal range, more than twice as many as tested below normal on the Binet Vocabulary Test which had been used as a rough estimate of intelligence. Further, 65 percent of the boys had Binet mental age estimates which were higher than those derived from the Goodenough mental age scoring.

GOODENOUGH AND BINET VOCABULARY I.Q. DISTRIBUTIONS

Estimated I.Q. Range	From Goodenough	From Binet Vocabulary
76-89	13 (62 %)	4 (24 %)
90-109	4 (19 %)	9 (53 %)
110-119	2 (9.5%)	2 (11.5%)
120-136	2 (9.5%)	2 (11.5%)
	N21	N17*

* Four boys did not take the vocabulary test.

Thus, there appears to be more disability shown in the nonverbal aspects of ego functioning where self-concept and body image are involved. With children referred to child guidance clinics, Goodenough scores have given rather poor estimates of intelligence (Thompson and Finley, 1963), probably due to the frequency of concerns over body integrity and disturbances in self-concept.

For the group as a whole, the drawings strongly support the psychiatric findings relating to anxiety over the defect, feelings of inadequacy, and disturbances in ego development and ego functioning. From the distribution of Binet Vocabulary scores, where only about one fourth of the boys fall below the normal range of intelligence, it would tentatively appear that the high incidence of reported school difficulties (about 70 percent) is not primarily on the basis of limited intellectual endowment. Boys whose self-esteem is low and whose level of anxiety is high would have difficulty investing themselves freely in the discipline of the learning process, and with each school failure their feelings of inadequacy would be reinforced in an evermore-discouraging vicious circle.

Three of our patients have been in psychotherapy for extended periods of time with one of the authors (L. C.) and their cases will be briefly described.

Case 1. This boy, four and a half years old, was extremely anxious and fearful, very immature, and concerned about hurt and injury. His mother, who was equally concerned, hovered over him anxiously at all times. The child did not give any indication of being consciously aware of his cryptorchism· despite previous medical examinations. Since the family structure was basically solid, and both parents supported the treatment process wholeheartedly, the resolution was fairly simple, despite the brief two-month psychotherapy. By giving vent to his aggressive impulses in the safety of the playroom, the child neutralized them and rendered them relatively harmless. By playing with broken objects, he was permitted to come to grips with his fears of body damage. Our reassurance about broken things being fixed, and some actual fixing, brought about a dramatic change, with diminution of anxiety and a bolder, age-appropriate attitude. He was then receptive to a realistic description of the operation, which was done on the dolls at first, and then referred directly to his own body. The boy went through the operation very well, and at the time of our last contact, some four months after the operation, the mother used the expression, "the child is transformed," so striking was his improvement in all areas of life, including home, neighborhood and kindergarten, which he attends eagerly.

Case 2. The second case treated by us preoperatively was that of a thirteen-year-old boy with a bilateral cryptorchism. He is the product of a racially mixed marriage. His father is Negro, and his mother, a German war bride. His home situation was marked by strife and both financial and emotional insecurity. The father was absent most of the time and was overtly critical and rejecting of the boy. The patient presented all the above-mentioned psychopathological features, such as depression, passivity, poor self-concept, behavioral symptoms, school difficulty, etc., in a severe degree, and had suffered three major accidents. Yet, despite his background, he was able to improve greatly over a two-month period of psychotherapy. He went through two closely spaced operations very well, and at the time of the last followup, some eight months after treatment, he seemed to have maintained his gains and continued his improvement in all areas. His greater alertness, increased self-confidence, and better effort in school were particularly impressive. In psychotherapy he was given an opportunity to talk openly about his missing testicles and to separate fact from fantasy. According to him, by the way, he became aware of his cryptorchism at the age of eight, while the medical diagnosis was not made until the age of thirteen. The child was also permitted to experiment with his aggressive feelings via the play material. He was reassured and supported by the therapist, who we think temporarily filled the role vacated by the aloof, uninterested father, while the mother derived strength from her contact with the social worker.

Case 3. The third patient, seventeen years old, had unilateral cryptorchism and was operated on at the age of fourteen. His mother was very overprotective and the father was a rather unsuccessful professional man. He constantly downgraded the boy and criticized him for characteristics which he seemed to despise in himself. The mother's attitude is best characterized by her fear of letting this seventeen-year-old boy go down to the corner store by himself. The father's attitude is best summed up in one of his remarks, "Let's face it, he just doesn't have it." The boy was very passive and depressed, looked and acted very immaturely, stuttered, and did poorly in school and social life. Despite the much longer duration of psychotherapy (almost one year), the outcome was far from excellent. There was improvement in school, and later in job performance, with some diminution of the depression. The passivity and the aloofness, however, proved to be an armor impenetrable to our efforts. At the time of our latest contact, some five months after termination of treatment, the boy was holding a job but had withdrawn from college. His social life remains limited, and he continues to be immature and still uncomfortable with people, although to a much lesser extent.

DISCUSSION

The role of an operation in a child as an activator of body-damage anxiety and fear of death has been recognized by many authorities dealing with this subject (Levy, 1945). In the event of an operation such as a tonsillectomy, the decision to operate is usually made shortly before the operation itself. The child is then confronted with an emotional trauma of relatively short duration. Before this occurs he has time to grow normally, to mature, and to develop various ways of dealing with the external world and his inner anxieties. His view of himself is unimpaired over the years by the prospect of a future operation. It is not surprising, therefore, that the majority of children undergoing a tonsillectomy recover quickly from the emotional upset caused by the operation, unless they have been showing, preoperatively, definite neurotic trends due to factors unrelated to the child's illness (Jessner et al., 1952). In fact, as pointed out by Langford (1961), Jessner et al. (1952), and Anna Freud (1952), many children actually profit from such an experience, which helps them mature and improves their self-reliance.

The situation is quite different in the cryptorchid child, however. Body-damage anxiety which occurs normally in early childhood is, in his case, constantly fed by the parents' concerns and their own anxiety. Thus, instead of parental reassurance, which helps the child to overcome these concerns, the cryptorchid child finds constant confirmation of his irrational fears in the anxious attitude of his parents. While he senses early that there is something wrong with him, he is denied the comfort of talking about it and quickly realizes that it is better kept secret.

In the normal course of emotional development, the conflict generated by the clash of the child's aggressive drives with the rules of the outside world is often linked in the child's fantasy with his fear of injury, providing the explanation for his fear. The cryptorchid child, because of the parental reinforcement of his fear of body damage and because of the mystery about the cause for parental anxiety, is likely to be particularly prone to make this connection; and if he does, we might see the beginning of a renunciation of any aggressive drives and an adoption of a passive attitude, noted in so many of our patients.

If the corrective operation is not carried out at an early stage, the trends which were described become gradually accentuated. The parents' concerns develop into an attitude containing elements of pity, rejection, fear, disappointment, and overprotection. Because of the significance ascribed to the testicles, they begin to see their son as inadequate, damaged, and defective, and in time the child himself incorporates their attitude and begins to view himself as inferior and inadequate. He is kept in the dark as to the cause for his parents' attitudes and behavior until roughly the beginning of school age, when we believe the child begins to be *fully* aware of his testicles and his cryptorchism. This realization of a vital missing part explains, but does not solve, the child's dilemma. The parents continue to deny any problems, while their disparaging or anxious attitude increases in intensity. No opportunity is afforded the child to express his feelings of loss, of object-mourning, as it were. Instead, he goes along with the attitude of the family, uses denial massively, and pretends that there is nothing the matter.

In addition, these children's body-damage anxiety may turn into a full-blown castration anxiety in the literal, rather than the commonly used symbolic sense. His early conflicts over aggressive feelings unresolved, and his manliness threatened, the cryptorchid child of school age is prone to renounce his masculinity altogether. His passivity increases and gradually pervades all areas of his life. The passive attitude in turn confirms and reinforces the parents' fears about the child's sexual inadequacy.

As the child grows older and fully realizes the significance of his loss without a forthcoming reassurance about restitution, a feeling of hopelessness begins to dominate his thinking. A more or less profound depression may result, increasing with age. Some of these features, including depression, passivity, anxiety, denial, the child's poor self-concept, his sense of damage and inadequacy, confusion over his body image and sexual identity, are dramatically illustrated in the children's drawings.

It is our belief that the most important factor, one capable of preventing permanent damage under these circumstances, is the presence of a strong, involved, interested, and supportive father. The years preceding adolescence constitute the period when sexual identity is crystallized, and a father or father substitute is needed to provide a model for identification. When such a father is available, the cryptorchid child might derive sufficient comfort and strength to go on fighting, trying to become like father despite the odds. If, however, as happened in many of our cases, the father himself is very passive and withdrawn, the child might begin to view masculinity as synonymous with passivity and renunciation of any aggressive strivings. But even during this critical preadolescent period, a psychiatric intervention may help to alleviate the damage to the child's personality, as illustrated in our second case.

Our case material suggests that if a psychotherapeutic intervention does not occur in preadolescence, then even a corrective operation will not suffice to reverse the trend in many cases, and the child might adopt passivity, depression, poor self-concept, and sometimes an ambiguous sexual identity, as a way of life, permanently woven into his character fabric. The potentially disastrous results of this particular combination of psychological traits were seen in almost all the older boys in our sample. These youngsters were confused, unhappy individuals, unsuccessful, with low self-esteem and little incentive for improvement. The third case we treated illustrates the fact that when psychotherapy in these cases is started late, the results may be disappointing.

Based on the previously mentioned considerations we can now approach several of our findings with more understanding. The greater vulnerability of the children who were operated relatively late becomes self-evident. The greater vulnerability of the Negro patients in our sample may be explained on several counts. The family situation involving a dominant mother and an absentee or uninterested father is quite prevalent, especially in the low-income Negro population, as shown in several recent sociological and anthropological studies (Frazier, 1948, 1957; Blumenfeld, 1965). Anyone who has worked in the outpatient department of a large hospital in a big city on the Eastern Seaboard might readily confirm this observation. In addition, the reliance of these low-income patients on busy clinics might have lessened their chance for a thorough medical examination which would have led to an early diagnosis and corrective operation. Finally, because of a constant personnel turnover in clinics, our low-income patients were less likely to have an interested, involved physician who could mitigate serious emotional difficulties by acting as a strong and supportive figure around whom the child and the whole family could rally and muster their strength. His main contribution would be an exhaustive, realistic explanation of the condition to both the parents and the child, and firm reassurance about its correctability.

CONCLUSIONS

We must re-emphasize the preliminary character of our study. A more definitive study would require a more rigorous methodology and include a more representative sample of patients, including children of various ages, and racial, intelligence, and socioeconomic groupings in sufficient numbers to permit statistical validation. Furthermore, our scoring criteria would have to be improved in an attempt to eliminate or at least to minimize the personal bias of the investigators. Finally, the inclusion of controls of "normal" boys and those undergoing surgery other than urogenital would add to the significance of our findings.

With all this in mind, we wish to note several trends in our study of children with undescended testicles:

1. Children with cryptorchism seem to be susceptible to emotional disturbance in far greater measure than the average population (Witmer, 1962). The disturbance starts with anxiety, restlessness, and immaturity, and, if unchecked, may develop into a character disorder with depression, passivity, poor self-concept, and confusion over body image and sexual identity.

2. In our sample, children of Negro low-income parents were more affected than white, middle-class patients.

3. The role of the physician was found to be of great importance in attempts to prevent emotional difficulties in these children.

4. A family constellation involving a dominant mother and a passive,

withdrawn or absent father was found particularly predisposing to emotional difficulties in these children.

5. An early operation during the preschool years seems most effective in avoiding future psychological troubles. An orchiopexy in early infancy, which would be ideal from an emotional standpoint, cannot be recommended because many undescended testicles descend in early childhood.

The age between one and three years is considered by most authorities (Robertson, 1958) the least opportune for hospitalization and elective surgery. The child of early school years might theoretically be best suited for a corrective operation, since he usually has more mastery over his feelings and is accessible to reasoning and factual reassurance. We learn from some histologists, however, that already at the age of six, one begins to see degenerative changes in an undescended testicle (Hinman, 1955; Robinson and Engle, 1954). Thus the period between four and six years would be the one of choice, considering all the factors involved. However, one would have to caution the surgeons about the child's emotional vulnerability at this age, and the importance of the physician's reassuring, patient, and supportive attitude.

REFERENCES

BELL, A. (1961), Some observations on the role of the scrotal sac and testicles. *J. Amer. Psychoanal. Assn.,* 9:261-286.

BERNSTEIN, K. (1957), Der derzeitige Stand der Behandlung des sogenannten Kryptorchismus. *Dtsch. med. Wschr.,* 82:1375-1377.

BLOS, P. (1960), Comments on the psychological consequences of cryptorchism: a clinical study. *The Psychoanalytic Study of the Child,* 15:395-429. New York: International Universities Press.

BLUMENFELD, R. (1965), Personal communication.

CAMPBELL, M. (1951), *Clinical Pediatric Urology.* Philadelphia: Saunders.

CHARNY, C. W. (1960), The spermatogenic potential of the undescended testis before and after treatment. *J. Urol.,* 83:697-705.

CLARKE, A. M. (1956), Undescended testis: when and why to operate. *Med. J. Austral.,* 43:222-224.

CONNOLLY, N. K. (1959), Maldescent of the testis. *Amer. Surg.,* 25:405-420.

FRAZIER, E. F. (1948), *The Negro Family in the United States.* New York: Dryden Press.

———— (1957), *The Negro in the United States.* New York: Macmillan.

FREUD, A. (1952), The role of bodily illness in the mental life of children. *The Psychoanalytic Study of the Child,* 7:69-81. New York: International Universities Press.

GOODENOUGH, F. L. (1926), *Measurement of Intelligence by Drawings,* Yonkers, N. Y.: World Book.

HAMMER, E. F. (1953), An investigation of sexual symbolism: a study of H-T-P's of eugenically sterilized subjects. *J. Proj. Tech.,* 17:401-413.

HAND, J. R. (1955), Undescended testes: report on 153 cases with evaluation of clinical findings, treatment, and results on follow-up up to thirty-three years. *Trans. Amer. Assn. Genito-Urinary Surgs.,* 47:9-50; *J. Urol.,* 75:973-989, 1956.

HINMAN, F. (1955), The implications of testicular cytology in the treatment of cryptorchidism. *Amer. J. Surg.*, 90:381-386.

JESSNER, L. ET AL. (1952), Emotional implications of tonsillectomy and adenoidectomy on
children. *The Psychoanalytic Study of the Child*, 7:126-169. New York: International Universities Press.

KOOP, C. E. (1952), Undescended testicles, differential diagnosis and management. *Med.
Clin. N. Amer.*, 36:1779-1785.

———— (1957), Observations on undescended testes: I. Significance of the empty
scrotum and indications for orchiopexy. *Arch. Surg.*, 75:891-897.

LARSON, C. P. (1957), The undescended testis. *McGill Med. J.*, 26:202-211.

LEVY, D. M. (1945), Psychic trauma of operations in children. *Amer. J. Dis. Child.*,
69:7-25.

LEWIS, L. G. (1954), Cryptorchism. *N. Y. State J. Med.*, 54:3078-3082.

LICH, R. (1956), Cryptorchidism. *Amer. Surg.*, 22:198-203.

MEYER, B. C., BLACHER, R. S., & BROWN, F. (1961), A clinical study of psychiatric and
psychological aspects of mitral surgery. *Psychosom. Med.*, 23:194-218.

NELSON, W. O. (1951), Mammalian spermatogenesis: effect of experimental cryptorchidism in the rat and non-descent of the testis in man. *Rec. Progr. Hormone Res.*,
6:29.

ROBERTSON, J. (1958), *Young Children in Hospitals*. New York: Basic Books.

ROBINSON, J. N. & ENGLE, E. T. (1954), Some observations on the cryptorchid testis.
J. Urol., 71:726-734.

———— (1955), Cryptorchism: pathogenesis and treatment. *Ped. Clin. N. Amer.*, August, 729-736.

THOMPSON, J. M. & FINLEY, C. J. (1963), The relationship between the Goodenough
Draw-a-Man test and the Stanford-Binet Form L-M in children referred for school
guidance services, *Calif. J. Educ. Res.*, 14:19-22.

WITMER, H. L. (1962), *The National Picture of Children's Emotional Disturbances.*
New York: Child Development Center.

26

THE HOME VISIT IN CHILD PSYCHIATRY: Its Usefulness in Diagnosis and Training

Roger D. Freeman, M.D.

Director of Psychiatric Services, Handicapped Children's Unit,
St. Christopher's Hospital for Children, Philadelphia, Pa.,
and Child Psychiatrist, Child Development Center, Norristown, Pa.

In the past two years I have seen sixty-six children and their families in their own homes, among them both clinic and private patients. I have been pleased with the results and now have two years of experience with incorporation of the home visit into a child psychiatry training program. This paper describes the technique we use for the home visit, certain criteria we have found helpful in the selection of cases, contraindications, results, and a discussion of its place in training.

Several trends would seem to make this presentation timely. The one-to-one relationship between child and therapist has been somewhat de-emphasized by the current interest in conjoint therapy of mother and child, family diagnosis and therapy, group therapy and group observation. The child psychiatrist is now expected, at least during his training, to learn to function in a number of situations quite different from the traditional tripartite child guidance clinic team: in schools, residential treatment centers, family service agencies, courts and pediatric inpatient and outpatient departments. He may also be asked to see children with a wide variety of complex diagnostic and therapeutic problems. With

Reprinted from the JOURNAL OF THE AMERICAN ACADEMY OF CHILD PSYCHIATRY, Vol. VI, No. 2, April, 1967, pp. 276-294. Supported in part by U.S. Children's Bureau Grant No. 416, Personnel Training Project for Handicapped Children, to St. Christopher's Hospital.

the need and demand for these diversified services increasing at a rate greatly exceeding increases in professional time available, there is pressure (at least partially justifiable) to improve our efficiency. At times, seeing a child and his family at home can help achieve this end.

REVIEW OF THE LITERATURE

Home visiting in allied fields concerned with children's problems has been carried out for many years by the general practitioner, pediatrician, visiting nurse, educator and social worker. Physicians have tended to move away from home visiting, however, as diagnostic procedures and equipment have increased in complexity, but a countertrend is recommended by O'Donnell (1965), Wilkes (1965), and Shafer (1965) for the practice of internal medicine. They describe, among other advantages, rapid insight into certain aspects of the patient's life. Social workers in the areas of public welfare and assistance, adoptions and foster home placement are generally more likely to visit the home than the psychiatric social worker from the child guidance clinic. The infrequency of clinic home visits may be due partially to supposed loss of time, but also possibly to the greater investment in individual casework.

Psychiatric home care programs for adults have been established in increasing numbers since the Amsterdam Plan was begun in 1927. The European programs include those in England (Carse et al., 1958; Mac-Millan, 1959) and Holland (Querido, 1956; Millar and Henderson, 1956; Lemkau and Crocetti, 1961). Canadian descriptions are those of Rands (1960) and Langevin et al. (1966). In the United States, a partial listing would include the Boston State Hospital Psychiatric Home Treatment Service (T. Friedman et al., 1960; Perry, 1963), the Reception Center in Philadelphia (Warner et al., 1962), a county emergency service in Maryland (Cameron, 1961), the Cleveland program for hard-to-reach adults with character disorders (Rosen, 1965), and the San Mateo County, California program described by Deutsch and Deutsch (1966). Family therapy in the home, where the identified patient is a young adult schizophrenic, is presented in detail by A. Friedman et al. (1965).

Home visiting by paramedical mental health workers for research and/or therapeutic purposes has been done by social workers, nurses and sociologists (Rowe, 1959; Morgan, 1963; Behrens and Ackerman, 1956; Henry, 1963; Levine, 1964; Egan and Robison, 1966; Rafferty and McClure, 1965). All but the first two of these reports involved families with disturbed children.

Perry (1963) states that psychiatry practiced in the home differs in many respects from that in the office or hospital: "The worker going into the home and seeing the family in interaction becomes much more acutely aware of the participation of other family members in the disturbance; it is much more difficult to locate the disturbance in the psyche of the patient when he is not all alone with you in an interview room."

The only paper describing a training program utilizing home visits is that of Schwartz, Waldron, and Tidd (1960) from the UCLA Medical Center. Adult patients considered for inpatient admission were evaluated by psychiatric residents in the home. "It is our subjective impression that the home visits have amply justified the extra time required for them from a teaching point of view."

Two surveys have been made of home visiting experiences and attitudes of psychiatrists. Brown (1962) collected information from thirty-four Boston psychiatrists (of whom three were child psychiatrists). Only 27 percent had never made a home visit; about one third made more than ten visits each year. The type of practice, rather than the psychiatrist's attitude, seemed to be the determining factor in the choice to see the patient at home. The only child psychiatrist reporting extensive home visiting experience felt that parents disliked this type of contact. Mickle (1963) reported on the results of a questionnaire sent to 266 psychiatrists in private practice in and around San Francisco (no child psychiatrists are mentioned.) Only 9 percent had never made a home visit. Reasons for the visit were the wishes of the referral source and physical incapacitation, reluctance to come to the office or marked disturbance of the patient.[1]

There are very few references to home visits in the child psychiatric literature. Occasionally a passing mention is made that the child was seen in his own home. Fraiberg and Freedman (1964) describe observation and treatment of two congenitally blind children with deviant development, one of whom was observed at home periodically and the other treated intensively by means of five home visits each week. The reasons for this arrangement are not specified but presumably they involved a greater significance of observations and interpretations to child and mother, since both handicapped children were so highly dependent upon familiar surroundings as well as the mother. Erikson (1950) mentioned that he never accepted a case without having a meal in the child's home, and described one of his experiences. Gordon (1963a, 1963b) goes to the child's home and often has a meal with the family,

---

[1] More detailed review is available in the chapter on home visits in A. Friedman et al. (1965).

both during the diagnostic and treatment phases of his work. Home observation for the purpose of cross-cultural studies of the developmental modification of aggression has been described by Pavenstedt (1965). Probably many other child analysts and psychiatrists have visited patients' homes but have not written about their experiences.

Increased interest in home visiting is apparent from a chronological tabulation of numbers of reports published: prior to 1956 only one could be found in the literature; between 1956 and 1960 there were nine; since 1960 there have been eighteen.

All of these reports were favorable. Bierer (1960) has stated, however, that psychiatric resources are better utilized in other ways.

SETTINGS

A few words are in order about the type of clinical settings in which the work described in this paper was carried out.

St. Christopher's Hospital for Children is the pediatric division of Temple University School of Medicine. The Handicapped Children's Unit provides a wide range of services: psychological testing, social service evaluation and casework, psychiatric diagnosis and treatment, nursery school, pediatric neurology, speech, audiology, physical therapy, developmental testing, and visiting nurse program. Most of the children seen have been diagnosed as having, or are suspected of having, cerebral palsy, brain damage, mental retardation, convulsive disorders, muscular dystrophy, blindness, deafness, congenital defects, or similar disorders or combinations thereof. The services related to the child's and family's emotional status are located within the Unit and are separate from those of the Child Psychiatry Clinic, which has its own staff. Clinic trainees in child psychiatry rotate through the Unit for four months of diagnostic experience (including home visits) during each of their two years of residency and carry at least two Unit cases in treatment throughout the two years. Medical students from Temple University or other medical schools may take elective work in the Unit.

The Child Development Center in Norristown is a community-based facility serving a large area adjacent to Philadelphia. Although originated by the Montgomery County Association for Physically Handicapped Children, it now accepts for evaluation all types of developmental problems, including emotional disturbances. A preschool program is operated for both diagnostic and educational purposes. Outpatient rehabilitative services are provided, including some short-term psychotherapy and counseling of parents. Long-term psychotherapy cases are referred to the local mental health clinics or to child psychiatrists in private practice.

Several private practice cases were also seen in the home, either for evaluation or in the course of therapy.

Difficulties experienced in evaluating certain children with unusually complex problems led to the development of the home visit as an aid in diagnosis.

INDICATIONS

The following are the major indications we have developed for the child psychiatric home visit. These are separated for clarity, but of course they frequently overlap.

Preschool Age

We try to see all children of preschool age at home as well as those who are older but very immature. Ease of regression in young children is well known. In a restricted hospital inpatient setting, behavior obscuring more typical functioning is quite likely, perhaps even hyperactivity or stereotyped motor patterns as described by Levy (1944).

Diane, age twenty-two months, was first seen while an inpatient because her mother described her as hyperactive and difficult to discipline. She had been admitted for investigation of possible minor seizures. The EEG was normal and no diagnosis of convulsive disorder could be made. Her behavior in the hospital was difficult to evaluate, since she was kept in a crib for part of the time and it was decided to see her and her family at home following discharge. The home was located in a slum area with one room serving as kitchen, dining room, living room, and play room for four children. The entire family slept in one room upstairs. Each of the children was noted to rock persistently, a pattern which may have been related to the extremely limited space. Diane related well and was not hyperactive during the observation in the home. The mother talked about her concern that Diane was showing symptoms similar to those which were demonstrated by her sibling who had died of a brain tumor the year before. The mother herself had reportedly suffered from petit mal spells and had been in several institutions because of unmanageable, antisocial behavior when a teenager. The father's anxiety about the "similarity in symptoms" was so great that he had been examining Diane's pupils for inequalities. Our impression was that Diane's behavior was within normal limits for her age, considering her circumstances and the degree of parental anxiety.

Inability to Evaluate or Examine the Child in the Office

Marked anxiety, fearfulness, or uncontrollable behavior may be reported by previous examiners, psychiatric or nonpsychiatric. Such reactions seem to occur in young children most often when there have been previous traumatic and repeated medical or surgical procedures. In some instances, the sight of a white coat, the characteristic odors of the hospital, or a glimpse of an examining table may set off a violent reaction.

Three-year-old Evan, the older son of a nurse, had had several operations for strabismus and bilateral hernias in the first two years of life. His mother described him as "clinging, fearful, like a frightened animal" after each operation. There were many subsequent ophthalmological examinations. He became so disturbed in office contacts that his pediatrician suspected early infantile autism, since Evan also frequently avoided cuddling and showed some withdrawn, stereotyped behavior. During her nursing work the mother had observed an older autistic child at a state hospital and became extremely anxious after the impression of autism was given to her. At home, Evan demonstrated relatively little anxiety, was able to enjoy playing games with me and his younger brother, and generally related rather well. He was seen periodically at home for over a year, during which time he began to develop useful language and has continued to improve in his relationships. Psychological evaluation was attempted, but he was so anxious in the office that he performed at a severely retarded level. At home he was able to put picture puzzles together rapidly and could identify all the letters of the alphabet. He is just beginning to adapt to new situations outside of his home.

Parental Report that the Child Is "Very Different at Home"

With young children, this is a fairly frequent report. The most important discrepancies to be assessed are those instances where mutism or lack of speech is the rule in the office.

Doris, a four-year-old girl with a three-year history of petit mal epilepsy, was referred because of "excessive sleeping" and lack of observed speech. In several years of hospital contacts, she had never said a word to anyone. No home visit had been made despite her living within three blocks of the hospital. Seen in the office with her mother or alone, she hid her face and could not be encouraged to talk or play. At home she was coy, voluble, and even provocative. She showed me around the house, describing things in well-constructed sentences. The "sleeping" seemed to be a reaction to rejection or loss of the center of attention in a very disturbed family setting. (It was not related to anticonvulsant medication.)

Laura is a seven-year-old girl with mild ataxic cerebral palsy and a history of two operations for strabismus. She was seen for evaluation by a psychologist, a speech and hearing pathologist, occupational and physical therapists, and a pediatrician, with no one eliciting a word from her. In the group setting, she was even described as "catatonic-like." A fairly severe degree of mental retardation was suggested from performance testing. At home, Laura was initially quite shy, but ignoring her and playing with her pets and siblings resulted in an outpouring of verbal material to her mother. Her productions all related clearly to her anxiety about her younger, physically normal sister who had recently surpassed her in size and physical skills, along with fears that her mother might not care for her and so abandon her. She showed a mannerism under stress or excitement of covering her mouth with her hand, probably related to her verbal withholding under other circumstances. She did indeed appear to be intellectually limited, but only to a mild degree, with associated neurotic and reactive problems. Following very limited counseling of the parents, her shyness with her peers diminished, but she still is reluctant to talk with her teacher.

Rhoda, a severely retarded, possibly psychotic three-year-old, was said by her parents to "do much more at home." A visit confirmed the child's severe retardation in all areas, but further revealed numerous bizarre habits (eating leaves and grass, stereotyped movements of the extremities), very limited relationship with others, avoidance of eye contact, and apparently unprovoked outbursts of laughing or rage. The parents grossly exaggerated her abilities. Our interpretation of the findings was facilitated by our having seen the child functioning at her best in her own home.

Severe Physical Disability

Regardless of how well motivated parents may be, there are times when it is inconsiderate to expect the child to be brought to the office. Since such a child spends the great majority of the time in the home, it is very helpful to observe him in his usual environment.

Ruth is a fourteen-year-old girl with neurofibromatosis (van Recklinghausen's disease) who had surgery several years ago for a neurofibroma which was pressing on her spinal cord. Subsequently, for reasons not completely understood, she became paralyzed from the neck down. She was not placed on a physical therapy program because the family had been assured she would be dead within a year. However, she proved this prognosis wrong and in the meantime developed severe contractures and bedsores. Seeing her in the office would have required that her special bed be moved to a special truck by means of rails from her first-floor room. At home, she was found to be depressed and upset by the bowel and bladder care administered by the mother (a nurse) and father. The parents pressed her beyond her very limited capacities (e.g., painting with a brush held between her teeth; taking "outings" in the truck despite strong feelings of embarrassment when others looked in and observed her helplessness). The reason for the psychiatric evaluation was a suspicion on the part of the parents that she might be able to do a bit more if she were "motivated." Many of Ruth's strong feelings could be indirectly ascertained by way of her very close relationship with her cat. At the same time, the tremendous emotional investment of the parents in this child was observed to have a detrimental effect upon her older brother. Psychotherapy on a regular basis was not felt to be indicated, since her adjustment and defenses seemed optimal under the circumstances, but parental counseling was provided.

Charles, a three-and-a-half-year-old boy with bright-normal intelligence, was born with osteogenesis imperfecta. He has never walked and has several "pseudo-joints" from repeated fractures. A home visit permitted observation of his role in the family. His older siblings were assigned to play with him for regular periods of time (as if it were a household chore) resulting in considerable resentment on their part. His peers were realistically dangerous because physical contact could result in another fracture (he once fractured his leg by turning around too quickly). He could hit his brother, but retaliation was obviously forbidden. This very difficult situation had apparently led to a massive denial of feeling by the parents so that they sometimes did not pay enough attention to his needs and "kidded" him so he would "not feel sorry for himself." The mother said, in his presence, that she would love him "even if he were a freak" and used terms of endearment such as "pretzel legs."

Assessment of Sibling of Referred Child

Although a particular child may be identified as the patient, it sometimes becomes obvious that others in the family have problems perhaps even of more severe degree. This may or may not be within the parents' awareness. The home visit may be quite helpful in such a case because the "nonpatient" sibling may have very strong feelings about being seen by a psychiatrist.

Audrey, age nine, suffered from an unusual form of progressive muscular dystrophy affecting females and was referred because of refusal to cooperate in physical therapy and intense sibling rivalry with thirteen-year-old Elizabeth. The latter had recently developed "dizzy spells" with periodic abdominal pain and abnormal EEG, diagnosed elsewhere as "abdominal epilepsy." The mother felt these attacks were triggered by tension induced by Audrey and her problem. Elizabeth was about to become a clinic patient also, and it was quite likely that she would be referred for psychiatric evaluation. While hospitalized for investigation of her "abdominal epilepsy," and before the diagnosis was made, Elizabeth had been told that her symptoms were "all in her mind." Her mother had had an almost unbelievable series of unfortunate medical experiences, in which her symptoms were labeled "nerves," but were found to be derived from major physical disorders. Audrey was very resistant to talking with anyone at the hospital. Seen in the home, both girls and mother provided a wealth of material helpful in understanding the normal degree of sibling rivalry and mother's concern over it. Because of her own disturbed background, the mother was unable to tolerate any expression of aggression by her children. Excessive family preoccupation with orality and pregnancy raised questions about Elizabeth's symptoms, which had begun at puberty. (Another EEG was read as normal.) Audrey's difficult behavior was of course partly due to her increasing disability and greater social awareness of its consequences, but also to envy of Elizabeth and to the mother's conflicts in dealing realistically with these problems. Two evaluations were thus performed during the same visit.

Assessment of Complex Family Situation

When relatives living in the home contribute to the child's difficulties, the parents may be aware of this possibility, but the relatives themselves are often oblivious to it. The relatives may be unwilling to come to the office or several interviews might be necessary to prepare for such an evaluation, if it could be done at all.

Debby is a three-year-old girl with frequent petit mal seizures and average intelligence who is provocative and difficult for the mother to manage. The very complex home situation was observed during a visit. The mother, who is twenty, lives in her own grandmother's house with her two children and an uncle. Because of animosity between Debby's father and his mother-in-law, who lives nearby, the latter is not permitted to see the children. Debby's mother was treated like a small child by her relatives, who criticized her openly. She was unable to set limits for Debby, and instead threatened the child in her attempts to discipline her. Although this technique seemed partly to be due to fear of hurting the little girl, the same type of maternal management was observed with Debby's brother, a toddler who had no physical difficulties.

Assessment of Difficult Differential Diagnostic Situations

Among those children of preschool age referred to us as "probably retarded and psychotic," we have identified two groups. In the clinic or hospital, both are frequently described as "bizarre."

In the home, the first group confirms the initial impression. They show no area of development close to age expectation and demonstrate bizarre mannerisms and gestures, avoidance of eye contact, and perseverative, stereotyped motor patterns (twirling, spinning, etc.). On follow-up, this group continues to show psychotic patterns.

The second group of young children appears much less bizarre or withdrawn at home, but their relationships are poorly developed. Many of these children will make eye contact only at home. A substantial number seem to improve spontaneously in relationship capacity with time, without any formal therapy, as if there might be some specific developmental lag in addition to global retardation. Thus, a very young child who had been "retarded and bizarre" in the hospital setting might, when seen a year or two later, appear more like a "typical" retarded child. Family management may also contribute to relatively poor ego development in these children, resulting in difficulty in adapting to new situations and unusual regressions under the stress of an office visit.

Assessment of Carry-over of Improvement

In the course of psychotherapy or special nursery school experience, the parents may report that the child has failed to improve at home, or has improved at home without this carrying over to the clinical setting. Where assessment of this situation is important for the decision to continue or alter management of the case, a home visit may quickly provide the necessary information.

Ellen, a four-year-old only child, was seen initially because of poor speech, uncontrollable hyperactive behavior reported at home, and a difficult differential diagnostic problem with considerations of brain damage, retardation, and borderline psychosis. The mother had had a schizophrenic reaction and was still functioning poorly. The father had been divorced by her after years of alleged gross physical abuse of her in the child's presence. Seen in the home, the mother had first been unable to organize herself sufficiently to deal with the child's behavior. She was further hampered by the need to use a cane because of a recently fractured hip. Most of her time was spent hobbling after Ellen to prevent her destroying bric-a-brac which was kept within easy reach, turning on the water, etc. The number of toys had not been limited, and the closets were full of them. No locks had been placed on doors to restrict the range of Ellen's activities. Direct suggestions were given with regard to some practical measures which could be taken to facilitate control. For several months the child attended daily a highly structured nursery school where rapid improvement took place. The mother claimed similar improvement had also occurred at home. On another visit, the home had indeed been reorganized and Ellen's behavior was significantly improved.

Some comments are also indicated regarding another situation. We have seen several children who, because of their history, were suspected of having central nervous system dysfunction, with or without EEG changes. It had been impossible to do any kind of pediatric neurological examination because of the acute disturbance of the child in the office. While the home visit was not made with this factor in mind, it was found that the home setting was conducive to observations of the child's balance, gait, gross and fine motor coordination, and presence of tremor or other abnormal movements, which were sometimes of great value to the neurologist or pediatrician.

CONTRADICTIONS

Great distance is one obvious limiting factor and must be weighed against the positive indications for the home visit.

Excessive anxiety about the visit by one or both parents may be cause to abandon the idea or work it through in advance. Paranoid parents are especially sensitive to what they may see as "spying," or they may in reality have something to hide which has never come out in previous contacts.

While we do not believe that it has impeded evaluation, seeing pre-adolescent or adolescent children, especially when more than one is present at the time of the visit, has not been as revealing as with younger children. Age-appropriate defensiveness may be heightened by the psychiatrist's presence in the home when a working relationship has not yet been developed.

Two sisters, ages eleven and thirteen, were seen at home. The younger one had occasional seizures, marked jealousy of her sister, and a very poor self-concept indicated on psychological testing. The older sister had no friends and a very low level of self-esteem. The latter's early history was complicated by a severe visual defect which was corrected later by an operation. Both parents showed flattened affect and both their families had a high incidence of emotional disturbance. Seen at home, the girls spent much of the time giggling, provoking their father, and making comments about each other. Subsequently in individual office visits, both showed much more overt psychopathology. The younger was almost completely disorganized by anxiety and told of marked fear of death and insomnia, both of which she related to her feelings about her seizures and a feeling of not being accepted by her family. The older sister was sufficiently depressed to raise the question of suicidal ruminations. I suspected that a suicide pact had been made by the two sisters, who were referred for treatment.

TECHNIQUE

No specific "technique" has been found useful in all instances. What one does changes with his increasing experience and the needs of the situation. In general, comfort and flexibility on the part of the psychiatrist foster relative comfort on the part of the family.

The home visit has sometimes been the only psychiatric contact with the family. In other cases, an office interview with the parents, or parents and child, has preceded or followed the visit. The sequence depends upon the clinical information available. It was found that some parents showed considerable anxiety if the initial contact were the home visit. This seemed to be at least partly due to fantasies that they and the child must be very "sick" for one or two psychiatrists to visit the home.

When insufficient information is available, we see the parents first, take a history, decide whether a home visit is indicated, and, if so, suggest this to them. We explain why it might be helpful to see the child at home, using, wherever possible, their own observations (e.g., that the child is very different at home). It is important to emphasize to them that a home visit is a *routine procedure* in such instances. Any questions concerning preparation of the child or children are then discussed. We emphasize our role as observers of the child in his usual environment and not as guests for whom special preparation must be made. Whenever possible, we try to arrange a time when the parents and siblings are home and the child does not miss his nap or a day of school. The parents are asked to notify us if the child appears ill on the appointed day so that we may reschedule the visit. (This has been necessary on only three occasions out of a total of eighty-five visits.)

It is essential to set aside enough time so that one need not hurry off if a longer stay seems warranted. Usually one to one and a half hours is sufficient.

I have made visits alone and some with child psychiatric trainees, medical students, visiting nurses, and social workers. I feel that a visit by more than two persons is inadvisable because it tends to make the parents, if not the child, feel overwhelmed. When there are two visitors involved, it has not been necessary to work out in advance who will take the more active role. In practice, the more experienced person may be more active at first, encouraging greater activity on the part of the other on subsequent visits.

When the visit is made with a trainee, time used in driving to the home is profitably used by reviewing the record and discussing which areas of diagnostic uncertainty might be clarified by observation. Supervision on observations made during the visit is provided on the return trip.

The approach to the child varies. Often it has been most helpful to pay little attention to the child patient initially. With a very shy child, spending some time with a pet or chatting with siblings or parents may provide a "warm-up" period. As the child's and family's comfort increases, we usually ask the child to show us his room and play areas. If the child wishes to go outside to play, we follow him, for at least part of the time. Observations are made of the neighborhood, housekeeping, appropriateness of furnishing and toys to children's ages and activities, sleeping and play arrangements, interpersonal relationships, child-patient's affect, speech, fantasy, play, interests, patterns of nonverbal communication and gesture, motor behavior, and reactions to limit setting or frustration.

Because of one's greater involvement in seeing the child at home, and perhaps because the parents are on their own territory, they usually make requests for the diagnosis, prognosis, and advice. Since it is rarely feasible to interpret findings and give recommendations during the visit, these questions need to be dealt with carefully. We explain that after the completion of the evaluation (including the nonpsychiatric parts) the team will meet to arrive at a conclusion and recommendations. As soon as possible following this meeting, a conference will be held with the parents to provide answers to their questions.

The session is terminated when it is felt that sufficient information has been obtained. No notes are taken in the home. It is a matter of personal preference whether recording is done in the car, in transit when two persons make the visit, or upon return to the office.

Fees are charged on the same basis as if the patient were seen in the clinic or office. Usually the parents are billed rather than our accepting payment while at the home. In private practice, the home visit may mean a sacrifice in income because of travel time. If the distance is great a higher fee than for an office visit may be charged, which should, of course, be discussed with the parents in advance. If one goes for dinner as part of the evaluation, considerable awkwardness may be avoided by indicating in advance that the fee will be the same as for a single office visit. Otherwise, everyone will tend to feel uncomfortable during an after-dinner chat, much as a passenger in a taxi delayed in heavy traffic might feel with the meter running.

DISCUSSION OF OBJECTIONS

The most frequently heard objection to home visits is the time factor. In some cases this may be a realistic problem, but we feel the advantages usually outweigh any disadvantages. More often the total evaluation time is decreased because several office visits are unnecessary. That other factors are involved in reluctance to make a home visit should be evident from our experience that patients living within a few blocks of the hospital or clinic are no more likely to be visited than those living at a considerable distance. The objection that parents will see the home visit as an invasion of privacy is not supported by our impressions and results. On theoretical grounds, it has been stated that the patient's or parent's *intrapsychic* reality is more important than whatever may be observed of external reality. This is not the place to discuss this in detail, but we feel that both aspects of reality are significant.

There seem to be less openly discussed reasons for reluctance to make a home visit, even where it seems clearly indicated to do so: the situation is much less structured, strategies are less clearly defined, surprises may occur, and more people may be involved simultaneously. The inexperienced, rigid or insecure psychiatrist may feel threatened under these circumstances. In the confines of his own office, the psychiatrist is apparently in better control or "one-up" (in the terminology of "One-upmanship" described by Haley [1963]), whereas the family, in strange surroundings, is "one-down." Thus, we see the problem primarily as one of role definition and security.

RESULTS

The home visit has saved us time in the completion of many evaluations, even where as much as thirty minutes of driving each way was involved. This is most dramatically demonstrated in those cases where children were nonverbal for many previous evaluations but produced considerable verbal material at home.

No family has refused the visit; on the contrary, most have welcomed it enthusiastically and expressed their appreciation. We have noticed no differences dependent upon socioeconomic group, as were reported by Morgan (1963) and Egan and Robison (1966).

As compared with their behavior in the office setting, the children seemed to be much more comfortable. Many described as "avoiding eye contact" in the hospital or clinic did not do so at home. With few exceptions, the parents have also been at least as comfortable as in the office.

Some adaptation is required on the part of the psychiatrist in developing his formulation of the dynamics of the case, since the data obtained in the two types of settings differ in quantity and quality.

While it is true that the child's or parents' more disturbed behavior in the clinical setting may be significant, it must be emphasized that we are trying to find assets as well as pathology. Sometimes therapeutic optimism may be kindled by the discovery of the child's previously hidden strengths and abilities, as has occurred a number of times with very fearful and anxious children who were diagnosed as severely retarded because of their poor performance on psychological testing.

The parents seemed to have a greater confidence in the diagnostic study which includes a home visit. This was particularly true of children with degrees of mental deficiency, whose parents tend to reinforce their own denial by their feeling that the child was not seen under the best of circumstances.

Many problems with siblings, never mentioned previously, have been observed in the home, permitting their further evaluation.

In subsequent office contacts with family members I have found my familiarity with the home and neighborhood to be a distinct asset, particularly during psychotherapy of the child.

The home visit is, in addition, a change of pace for the psychiatrist and may be a broadening and confidence-enhancing experience for a trainee.

PLACE IN TRAINING

My remarks here concern our experience with child psychiatric trainees and medical students. Pediatric residents have not yet taken part in this program.

Training in home visiting helps to provide a basis for confidence and flexibility. We have found, however, that most trainees are reluctant to go on a home visit alone until they have become familiar with the procedure. This difficulty has been circumvented by having each trainee accompany me on several home visits. From the beginning, the trainee dictates the report. With each succeeding visit he is encouraged to take a more active role. The number of visits for training purposes has averaged three in each of the two training years.

The results have been gratifying in all respects and the trainees seem to enjoy their experiences in different social and cultural milieus.

For the medical student, the home visit can provide an excellent learning experience. We believe he can obtain a better grasp of the significance of a child's problem to the total family unit, as well as aspects of the child's functioning which reflect certain family patterns. Furthermore, this experience may counterbalance tendencies in medical training to lose sight of the social and family functioning of the child, as well as counteract the stereotype of the psychiatrist as interested exclusively in intrapsychic dynamics.

SUMMARY

There have been relatively few reports in the literature which indicate the usefulness of the home visit in the psychiatric diagnosis of young children. Experience with eighty-five home visits involving sixty-six families is here summarized with regard to the clinical settings in which the work was done, indications for selection, contraindications, technique of the method, our results, and the place of home visiting in a training program. The objections to such a method of assessment are discussed briefly.

The following types of cases are among those best suited for this approach: very young and immature children; highly anxious, disturbed, and unmanageable children; those who are nonverbal in office settings but reported to talk at home; those who have had multiple medical and surgical experiences, or who have, or may have, a combination of handicaps requiring careful differential diagnosis.

The results have been highly gratifying, and we hope our report will stimulate others to embark upon similar efforts and report their experiences.

REFERENCES

BEHRENS, M. L. & ACKERMAN, N. W. (1956), The home visit as an aid in family diagnosis and therapy. *Soc. Casewk.*, 37:11-19.

BIERER, J. (1960), Past, present and future. *Int. J. Soc. Psychiat.*, 6:165-173.

BROWN, B. S. (1962), Home visiting by psychiatrists. *Arch. Gen. Psychiat.*, 7:98-107.

CAMERON, W. R. (1961), County psychiatric emergency services. *Publ. Hlth Rep.*, 76:357-360.

CARSE, J., PANTON, N. E., & WATT, A. (1958), A district mental health service: the Worthing experiment. *Lancet*, 1:39-41.

DEUTSCH, P. & DEUTSCH, R. (1966), Fighting mental illness on home ground. *Today's Hlth*, 44: (9) 21, 87-90.

EGAN, M. H. & ROBISON, O. L. (1966), Home treatment of severely disturbed children and families. *Amer. J. Orthopsychiat.*, 36:730-735.

ERIKSON, E. H. (1950), *Childhood and Society*. New York: Norton, rev. ed., 1963, pp. 53-58.

FRAIBERG, S. & FREEDMAN, D. A. (1964), Studies in the ego development of the congenitally blind child. *The Psychoanalytic Study of the Child*, 19:113-169. New York: International Universities Press.

FRIEDMAN, A. S., BOSZORMENYI-NAGY, I., JUNGREIS, J. E., LINCOLN, G., MITCHELL, H. E., SONNE, J. C., SPECK, R. V., & SPIVACK, G. (1965), *Psychotherapy for the Whole Family: Case Histories, Techniques, and Concepts of Family Therapy of Schizophrenia in the Home and Clinic*. New York: Springer.

FRIEDMAN, T. T., ROLFE, P., & PERRY, S. E. (1960), Home treatment of psychiatric patients. *Amer. J. Psychiat.*, 116:807-809.

GORDON, K. H. (1963a), Child psychiatry: how to manage children with behavior problems. *Penn. Med. J.*, 66:34-39.

———— (1963b), An approach to childhood psychosis: simultaneous treatment of mother and child. *This Journal*, 2:711-724.

HALEY, J. (1963), *Strategies of Psychotherapy*. New York: Grune & Stratton.

HENRY, J. (1963), *Culture Against Man*. New York: Random House.

LANGEVIN, H., FORTIN, J. N., & LEONARD, F. (1966), L'emploi de la thioridazine dans un service d'urgence et de traitement psychiatrique à domicile. *Can. Psychiat. Assn. J.*, 11:314-323.

LEMKAU, P. V. & CROCETTI, G. M. (1961), The Amsterdam Municipal Psychiatric Service: a psychiatric-sociological review. *Amer. J. Psychiat.*, 117:779-783.

LEVINE, R. A. (1964), Treatment in the home. *Soc. Wk.*, 9:19-28.

LEVY, D. M. (1944), On the problem of movement restraint: tics, stereotyped movements, hyperactivity. *Amer. J. Orthopsychiat.*, 14:644-671.

MACMILLAN, D. (1959), Pre-admission visitation program. *Ment. Hosp.*, 10: (3) 19.

MICKLE, J. C. (1963), Psychiatric home visits. *Arch. Gen. Psychiat.*, 9:379-383.

MILLAR, W. M. & HENDERSON, J. G. (1956), The health service in Amsterdam. *Int. J. Soc. Psychiat.*, 2:141-150.

MORGAN, R. W. (1963), The extended home visit in psychiatric research and treatment. *Psychiatry*, 26:168-175.

O'DONNELL, W. (1965), When to make unnecessary house calls. *Med. Econ.*, 42: (14)255-256, 258, 262, 264.

PAVENSTEDT, E. (1965), Observations in five Japanese homes. *This Journal*, 4:413-425.

PERRY, S. E. (1963), Home treatment and the social system of psychiatry. *Psychiatry*, 26:54-64.

QUERIDO, A. (1956), Early diagnosis and treatment services. *World Ment. Hlth,* 8:180-189.

RAFFERTY, F. T. & McCLURE, S. M. (1965), The disturbed child at home. Abst. in: *Amer. J. Orthopsychiat.,* 35:241-242.

RANDS, S. (1960), Community psychiatric services in a rural area. *Canad. J. Publ. Hlth.,* 51:404-410.

ROSEN, I. M. (1965), Encountering and treating the unmotivated character-disordered person. *Dis. Nerv. Syst.,* 26:221-224.

ROWE, R. H. (1959), The symptom in past history. In: *The Symptom as Communication in Schizophrenia,* ed. K. L. Artiss. New York: Grune & Stratton, pp. 134-171.

SCHWARTZ, D. A., WALDRON, R., & TIDD, C. W. (1960), Use of home visits for psychiatric evaluation: clinical and teaching aspects. *Arch. Gen. Psychiat.,* 3:57-65.

SHAFER, N. (1965), House calls are good investments! *Med. Econ.,* 42: (14)264, 266.

WARNER, S. L., FLEMING, B., & BULLOCK, S. (1962), The Philadelphia program for home psychiatric evaluations, precare, and involuntary hospitalization. *Amer. J. Publ. Hlth,* 52:29-38.

WILKES, E. T. (1965), Things I've learned on house calls. *Med. Econ.,* 42: (14)266, 271, 274.

27

Social Class and Mental Illness in Children:
THE QUESTION OF CHILDHOOD PSYCHOSIS

John F. McDermott, Jr., M.D.

Saul I. Harrison, M.D.

Jules Schrager, M.S.W.

Janet Lindy, M.A.

and

Elizabeth Killins, M.S.W.

Data are presented from the psychiatric evaluations of a series of children diagnosed as psychotic and divided into five groups according to social class. These data are analyzed and compared with special reference to the clinical and social questions which are raised as a result of differences among the groups.

Psychosis in adults has been described as class-related by Hollingshead and Redlich[6] who found an inverse relationship between psychosis and class status, that is, significantly greater incidence of all forms of psy-

---

Reprinted from the AMERICAN JOURNAL OF ORTHOPSYCHIATRY, Vol. 37, No. 3, April 1967, pp. 548-557. Copyright, the American Orthopsychiatric Association, Inc. Reproduced by permission. Dr. McDermott, Dr. Harrison and Miss Killens are with the Children's Psychiatric Hospital, Ann Arbor, Michigan. Mr. Schrager and Miss Lindy are with the University Hospital, University of Michigan. This is one of a series of reports emerging from a long-range investigation of social-class factors and mental illness in children. The study was conducted in the department of psychiatry, University of Michigan, Ann Arbor, Michigan. The authors wish to express their thanks to Miss Susanne Chilman for her invaluable help in gathering the data for this study.

chosis in lower socioeconomic groups. The nature of this association between social class and psychosis has been examined by other investigators. Dunham[4] discovered that although the occupation of the adult schizophrenic in the general population was typically "lower-class," the occupation of the father of the schizophrenic patient was equally distributed all along the socioeconomic continuum. He suggests on the basis of this finding, that the development of the schizophrenic condition in an individual prevents him from realizing his occupational goals; the psychiatric debility serves to determine social class, rather than social class determining the disorder. Dunham's observations and conclusions were in substantial agreement with those described in an earlier study by Morrison.[13] Here too the distribution of occupations of the fathers of schizophrenic patients were seen to be similar to the distribution of occupations of the fathers of normal individuals, and it was concluded that schizophrenia is more likely to *cause* individuals to descend the socioeconomic ladder than it is to be *fostered by* lower socioeconomic status.

The relationship between social class and psychosis in children has received less attention than this same relationship in the adult population. The inability of a psychotic child to function adequately would be expected to have little effect on his social-class standing. Although the relative socioeconomic stability of the psychotic child, in comparison to the psychotic adult, serves to simplify research aimed at investigating the relationship between social class and psychosis in children, many other problems complicate the investigation of this relationship. Differential diagnosis is often difficult; the clinical picture is so different from that of adults; so many subdivisions have been described. The term childhood psychosis has come to mean for some an umbrella that covers many diagnostic labels such as autism, symbiotic borderline states, developmental arrest, atypical children, etc. Other authors advocate considering each of these as separate and distinct entities, e.g., infantile autism should be distinguished from childhood schizophrenia.[18]

The specific issue of social class and psychosis in children has been explored intensively for this special form, designated as "early infantile autism."[8] Kanner suggests that this category of childhood psychosis is characteristically an "upper-class" phenomenon, its relationship to social class being precisely opposite to that commonly noted in adult psychosis. He described the parents of his cases as intelligent, well educated, often professionals, scientists and writers. In their "Followup Studies of Autistic Children," Kanner and Eisenberg[9] reiterate:

> Our attention was directed to the indisputable fact that the parents came from intelligent, sophisticated stock.

In a review of subsequent cases of autism in the literature, Rimland[18] found evidence which overwhelmingly supported Kanner's original report that the parents of autistic children formed a unique and highly homogeneous group in terms of intellect and personality.

Lowe[10] has reported similar patterns for parents of children diagnosed as chronic undifferentiated schizophrenia: that they are better educated and have attained higher occupational levels than parents of disturbed, nonschizophrenic children. However, Kallman[7] and Bender[2] have described schizophrenic children as coming from dramatically different kinds of families and inadequate homes.

The present study is part of a series exploring the association between social class and mental illness in children based on data obtained from our own patient population. In previous investigations of social class and mental illness in children we have found that more serious symptoms and signs of mental illness were noted more often in the lower socioeconomic groups, and that milder forms were observed more frequently in the upper groups. We now examine the most serious form of mental illness in children, psychosis, and address ourselves to the following problems: (1) Is the diagnosis of childhood psychosis in children related to social class? (2) Is the diagnosis of "borderline" psychosis in children related to social class? (3) Is the form or expression of childhood psychosis related to social class?

METHOD

The intake records of 676 children up to the age of 14, who were evaluated at the University of Michigan's Children's Psychiatric Hospital from July of 1961 to July of 1963, were examined. These code sheets contained a variety of clinical data which had been filled out by the psychiatrist at the time of the child's initial evaluation. (This material had been accumulated prior to the inception of the current study.) The data were then transposed to IBM cards and processed by computer. The children were then divided into five socioeconomic class groups based on their father's occupations.* This has been found in other

---

* (1) Unskilled or semi-skilled laborer: employed for tasks involving either no training or very small amount of training, e.g., janitor, assembly line worker (n=227); (2) skilled laborer: employed in manual activity which requires training and experience, e.g., machinist, self-employed small farmer (n=184); (3) lower white-collar: involved in a small business or in clerical or similar work which is not primarily manual and/or which depends on some educational or special background, e.g., policeman, sales clerk, typist (n=78); (4) upper white-collar: employed in more responsible administrative white-collar position, e.g. supervisor, large-scale farmer, school teacher, nurse (n=80); (5) professional or executive: employment depends on professional training beyond the college level or important executive responsibilities, high financial status, e.g. university teacher, attorney, engineer (n=107).

studies to correlate well with various other determinants of social-class standing.[15]

(1) Social class and psychosis. Childhood psychosis was operationally defined to include any of the following diagnostic entities: autistic type, symbiotic type, mixed autistic symbiotic type, and various forms of schizophrenia. The occurrence of diagnosed psychosis was tabulated within each of the five social class categories described above. The Chi-square test was employed to determine whether or not a statistically significant relationship existed between social class and the diagnosis of psychosis.

(2) Social class and borderline psychosis. The occurrence of "borderline psychosis of childhood" was tabulated within each of the social-class categories. The Chi-square test was employed to determine whether or not a statistically significant relationship existed between social class and the diagnosis of borderline psychosis.

(3) Social class and expression of psychosis. Children diagnosed as psychotic were combined with the borderline psychotic group. Both the *presence* and the *severity* of nine selected clinical signs and symptoms were examined. The primary group were: affective disturbance, disturbance of thought process, withdrawal and autism, hallucinations and delusions, and paranoid symptoms. The secondary group were: free-floating anxiety, depressive, phobic, and obsessive-compulsive symptoms. The presence and the severity of the nine selected symptoms were then examined in terms of their social-class distribution. The Chi-square test was employed to determine the interaction between social class and presence, as well as between social class and severity, of various clinical signs and symptoms.

RESULTS

Of the 676 patients evaluated, 76, or 11.2 per cent were diagnosed as psychotic. Twenty-three of the 76 were seen as frankly psychotic, and 53 as borderline psychotic. (A diagnosis of typical autistic psychosis was rare. There were only five of these children, one of professional executive parents, one upper white-collar, two skilled laborer, one unskilled laborer. Two symbiotic psychotics and two mixed autistic-symbiotic were diagnosed, split evenly at each end of the social-class scale. These numbers were not considered sufficient to draw any conclusions.) Breakdown according to age and sex (Table 1) demonstrates some differences according to social class. The usual predominance of boys was noted except in the professional executive class where there were equal numbers

TABLE 1

The Diagnosis Psychosis in Children Total N=676 (Psychotic=76)
Variables of Age and Sex

	Unskilled N=227 Psychotic=25	Skilled N=184 Psychotic=22	Lower White Collar N=78 Psychotic=9	Upper White Collar N=80 Psychotic=10	Professional-Executive N=107 Psychotic=10
Sex M:F	16:9	17:5	9:0	8:2	5:5
Age					
3- 6 years	4	6	3	0	5
7-10 years	11	6	4	4	3
11-14 years	10	10	2	6	2

of boys and girls. The children of professional executive parents tended to be seen for evaluation at earlier ages.

Contrary to hypotheses derived from our previous studies, no significant difference was found in the occurrence of diagnosed psychosis among the five social-class groups. This was true when frank psychosis was viewed separately (df=2, x^2=3.173, p=n.s.) or when psychosis and borderline psychosis were combined (df=4, x^2=0.621, p=n.s.) (Figure 1).

Neither was the presence or absence of symptoms such as withdrawal and autism, hallucinations and delusions, disturbance of thought process, affective disturbance, and paranoid thinking or behavior, or other symptoms such as depression, phobias, obsessions and compulsions, free-floating anxiety related to social class*; that is, there were no statistically significant differences in the occurrence of each of these symptoms from class to class. However, the degree of two of these factors (where the symptom or sign was rated as mild, moderate, severe, or predominant in the clinical picture) was significantly related to social class (Figures 2 and 3). "Severe or Predominant" withdrawal and autism was seen significantly more often (p=.015 one-tail test) in the professional executive group when compared to the other groups "Severe or predominant" disturbance in thought process was seen significantly more often in the

---

* It may be of interest to note how frequently these symptoms and signs were considered to be present in the psychotic children of each social class: 77 per cent of the total psychotic group demonstrated withdrawal and autism, 20 per cent severe; 32 per cent hallucinations and/or delusions, 5 per cent severe; 80 per cent disturbed thought process, 28 per cent severe; 78 per cent affective disturbance, 32 per cent severe; 43 per cent paranoid symptoms, 32 per cent severe. Of the second group of symptoms 42 per cent deprssion, 1.5 per cent severe; 18 per cent phobic symptoms, 3 per cent severe; 27 per cent obsessive-compulsive symptoms, 5 per cent severe; 62 per cent free-floating anxiety, 10 per cent severe.

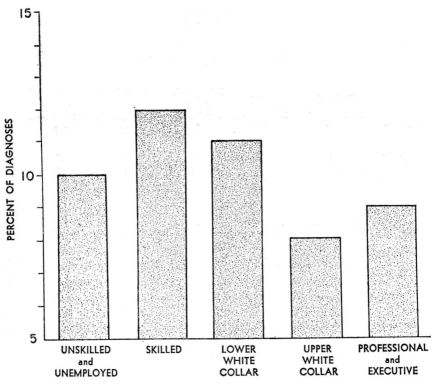

FIGURE 1. Diagnosis of psychosis in each occupational class.

children of the skilled working-class group and the professional executive group (df=3, x^2=9.498, p<.05). As illustrated graphically in Figures 2 and 3, both professional executive and skilled groups followed a similar trend.

DISCUSSION

The fact that we found no statistically significant difference in the occurrence of childhood psychosis among the various occupational classes presented a picture clearly contrary to our expectations, which were based on comparable studies of adult populations and our earlier work with children. We were stimulated to speculate as to the cause. First of all, this finding may be "actual" or "apparent." If it is actually true in the population of disturbed youngsters seen at our clinic, (and its validity is substantiated in the examination of results of other years, and providing that we see a representative sample of the population) it suggests

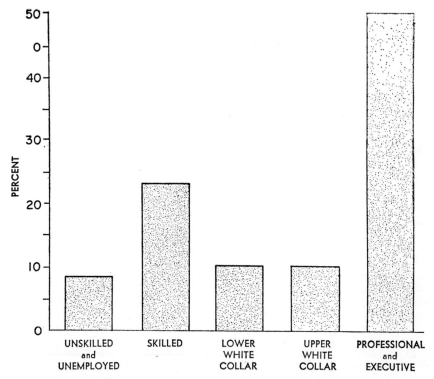

FIGURE 2. Severe withdrawal and autism in the psychotic children by class.

that social class is not as important a factor in childhood psychosis as it is in other kinds of mental illness in children. It may suggest that psychosis, like the genetically determined forms of severe mental retardation, falls in a random fashion throughout the population.[3, 16] Recognizing that correlation does not imply causation, we might, however, speculate that it would give added weight to the idea that a basic biological quality, i.e., a constitutionally determined ego defect, is operating in this particular form of mental illness, childhood psychosis, whose etiology is presently so unclear and one of the major dilemmas of child psychiatry today.

The difference in symptom expression, however, suggests that even if such a basic common factor exists, the form in which this is expressed may differ from class to class presumably due to the child's experience. The finding of severe withdrawal and autism in the professional executive group is interesting to consider further. These symptoms, when they take the form of the *diagnosis* of infantile autism, as has been noted, are

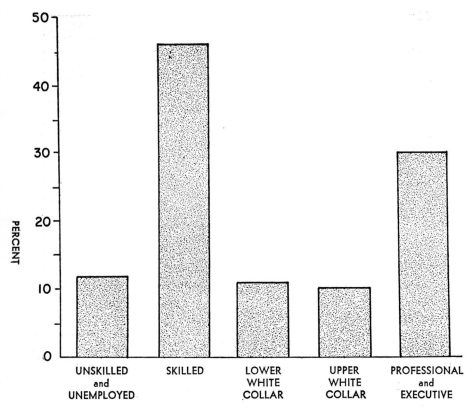

FIGURE 3. Severe disturbance of thought process seen in the psychotic children by class.

considered to be associated with predominantly educated, upper-class families. Kanner[8] was the first to describe clearly the autistic psychotic child's withdrawal from frustrating relationships with cold, interpersonally aloof parents. Extending this finding to psychosis in general, we may wonder whether the style of a particular culture or group tends to be adopted in an exaggerated form under the stress of illness and provide the form for that illness. Do the upper groups tend to isolate feelings more than others? It is felt that a characteristic of this group is to value the introspective and abstract style of thinking (versus the motoric style of the lower group) in their child-rearing practices.[17] Such intellectualization and isolation need not imply hostility so much as coldness and other parental interests outside the family, thus providing less emotional stimulation for youngsters to "learn" how to feel. Those youngsters who were vulnerable, for one reason or another, to psychosis might then tend to withdraw into solitude, the only way they have learned to behave under stress. As for thought disturbance, which seems also to be a primary affliction of upper-class psychotic children in our group, we may consider that thinking is best built on an emotional foundation, and thus may suffer a parallel fate under stress.

As for the curious finding that children of skilled working-class parents followed the same trend as those of professional executive parents, we have noted and explored more fully in a previous report[11] our observation that in many ways the children of the skilled families tend to be seen as demonstrating emotional pathology similar to children of the highest group, rather than those of their immediate social-class neighbors.

Thus far we have discussed implications of our results as if they were typical and representative of a wider general population. However, we suspect that they are not typical but "apparent." Psychosis *may* occur more often in one group than another, and in our study, for example, the finding may be a true one for the upper group, but depressed for the lower one. First of all, we must consider validity in terms of the size of our sample. Secondly, as we have noted, there is a tendency for children of the upper group who have been diagnosed as psychotic to have been seen at an earlier age than those of the lower group, thus suggesting differential problem of diagnosis from one age group to the other, assessment of "thinking" which is age appropriate varying from one group to another, etc.

"Selection" factors, which have been discussed in our previous papers[5, 11] also must be considered. The upper socioeconomic groups have better access to medical care and are said to have a greater concern about deviation in their children in such areas as withdrawal and thinking peculiarities. Our sample may be skewed by the fact that Children's Psychiatric Hospital operates an inpatient service so that many seriously ill children are referred to us for evaluation with the hope of obtaining inpatient care for them.

In addition to selection factors such as the degree and kind of parental and community concern about certain symptoms and behavior patterns in children which vary from class to class, we must look at the evaluators themselves. For example, would the observation of social withdrawal and thinking disturbance in the lower-class child be considered to be not unusual and a reflection of our low expectations for understimulated, disadvantaged children? If this were the case, it might not then be noted either by a potential source of referral or by the examiner at the clinic, allowing these children to remain unidentified as seriously mentally ill. Concreteness of thinking and difficulty conceptualizing may be considered cultural phenomena rather than psychopathology. Consider further the post-referral factors operating at the clinic itself which may influence our findings; it is possible that these findings may not actually represent an accurate picture of the children evaluated at our clinic, but reflect either our own preconceptions and unwitting social-class biases and/or factors inherent in the diagnostic process itself. This is a potential hazard for all of us in the mental health profession. There are no standard tests for mental illness such as the X-ray and blood test provide for our medical colleagues—no techniques which eliminate unwitting social-class biases. In our work the clinician himself is the diagnostic instrument.[19] It is possible that when the children of professional executive and skilled parents, who are usually a highly ambitious group, do not "make sense" to us as evaluators, we are quick to note this as psychopathology.

Finally, we wish to consider the *meaning* of the label "psychosis," which would include both the community's feeling response and subsequent service. The term is often frightening to the extent that the child may well be excluded from service in the home community. Thus the avoidance of this diagnosis by us, perhaps more in the lower group, would be understandable if the clinician feels that in many cases the label of psychosis will result in little or no treatment in the community because of the implication of severity and poor prognosis. Harrison[5] has noted that the child of the professional executive parent has twice as great a chance of being offered psychotherapy in our clinic, where ability to pay is hardly a factor, than the child whose father was an unskilled worker. Furthermore, the upper groups can buy private help for their children, but the lower groups must rely on state hospitals and mental health clinics in the community for treatment. As we know, these clinics prefer "good treatment cases," and psychosis, unfortunately, is as a rule relegated to special interest only for research purposes. Thus the diagnosis of psychosis may tend to reduce the possibility of getting help.

Where then would the sicker children be found, if we assume that the low occurrence of psychosis, particularly in the unskilled group, is artificially depressed? It is probable that many psychotic children are deliberately diagnosed and masqueraded as mentally retarded by professionals since at least in our state, it is sometimes easier to find special education for a retarded than a psychotic, especially an autistic, youngster. However in our own clinic series, psychosis is probably not confused with mental retardation or organic brain syndrome, as we found in a previous study that there were *fewer* mentally retarded youngsters diagnosed in the lower group than was expected.[12] However, in another study[11] we also reported a significantly higher incidence of diagnosed personality disorders in the unskilled group than in the other groups. Here "behavior" or acting out is implied. It has often been suggested that outwardly directed behavior is a characteristic of the lower group, whereas inwardly directed behavior is a mode of expression of the upper group who seem more disturbed in their thinking and tend to withdraw when they are psychotic.

On the other hand, we may consider the possibility that some of the individuals diagnosed as personality disorders in the lower group are masked psychotics, or latent psychotics who will later blossom into a frankly psychotic state. Bender has described pseudoschizophrenias, one of which is the pseudopsychopathic or paranoid, acting-out, aggressive antisocial type.[2] There is also the possibility that mental illness may take one form in childhood and yet another in adulthood, i.e., these youngsters appear to suffer from personality disturbances when they are children, but appear psychotic when they are adults. O'Neal and Robbins[14] found a subgroup of antisocial children who developed into schizophrenic adults.

SUMMARY

Statistical analysis of the diagnosis of psychosis in all children evaluated at the Children's Psychiatric Hospital of the University of Michigan Medical Center from July, 1961, to July, 1963, (676 patients) reveals no significant differences in the incidence of psychosis among the five social-class groups (professional, executive, upper white-collar, lower white-collar, skilled laboring-class, and unskilled laboring-class). It would appear from our studies that social class is not as important an influence in the diagnosis of psychosis in children seen at our clinic as it is in other forms of mental illness. However, the *expression* of the psychotic illness correlates with social class. Withdrawal and autism in their severe form occurred significantly more often in the professional executive group while disturbance of thinking occurred significantly more often in both professional executive and skilled working-class groups. These findings suggest the possibility that family styles and customs of child rearing may influence the expression of psychosis. Problems of methodology underlying social-class research such as case findings, biases in referral sources and evaluators alike, and hidden factors in "diagnosing" certain disorders also are considered.

REFERENCES

1. BENDER, L., and A. GRUGETT. 1956. A study of certain epidemiological factors in a group of children with childhood schizophrenia. Amer. J. Orthopsychiat. 26: 131.

2. ———. *1954*. Treatment of juvenile schizophrenia. A resume of nervous and mental diseases proceedings.
3. BIRCH, H. *1963*. Brain Damage in Children: The Biological and Social Aspects. Williams and Wilkins, Baltimore.
4. DUNHAM, H. *1964*. Social class and schizophrenia. Amer. J. Orthopsychiat. *34* (4): 634.
5. HARRISON, S. I. et al. *1965*. Social class and mental illness in children: Choice of treatment. Arch. Gen. Psychiat. *13* (Nov.).
6. HOLLINGSHEAD, A., and F. REDLICH. *1958*. Social Class and Mental Illness: A Community Study. John Wiley & Sons, Inc., New York.
7. KALLMAN, F., and B. ROTH. *1956*. Genetic aspects of pre-adolescent schizophrenia. Amer. J. Psychiat. *112*.
8. KANNER, L. *1942-43*. Autistic disturbances of affective contact. Nervous Child. *2*.
9. —— and L. EISENBERG. *1955*. Follow-up Studies of Autistic Children in The Psychopathology of Childhood. Hoch and Zubin, eds. Grune and Stratton, New York.
10. LOWE, L. *1966*. Families of Children with Early Childhood Schizophrenia. Arch. Gen. Psychiat. *14* (Jan.).
11. McDERMOTT, J., et al. *1965*. Social class and mental illness in children: Observations of children of blue collar families. Amer. J. Orthopsychiat. *35* (3): 500.
12. ———, *1965*. Social class and mental illness in children: The diagnosis of organicity in mental retardation. J. Am. Acad. Child Psychiat. (in press)
13. MORRISON, S. *1959* Principles and methods of epidemiological research and their application to psychiatric illness. J. Ment. Science. *105*. pp. 999-1011.
14. O'NEAL and ROBBINS. *1958*. The relation of childhood behavior problems to adult psychiatric states: A 30 year follow-up study of 150 subjects. Amer. J. Psychiat. *114*. pp. 961-969.
15. REISS, A., et al. *1961*. Occupations and Social Status. Free Press, New York.
16. Report of the American Medical Association Conference on Mental Retardation, Chicago 1964. Jan. 18 *1965*. J. Amer. Med. Assoc. *191*: 3. p. 243.
17. RIESSMAN, F. *1962*. The Culturally Deprived Child. Harper and Row, New York.
18. RIMLAND, B. *1964*. Infantile Autism. Appleton-Century-Crofts, Division of Meredith Publishing Company, New York.
19. SANAU, V. *1963*. The etiology and epidemiology of mental illness and problems of methodology: With special emphasis on schizophrenia. Ment. Hyg. *47* (4). pp. 607-621.

28

A FIVE TO FIFTEEN YEAR FOLLOW-UP STUDY OF INFANTILE PSYCHOSIS

Michael Rutter, M.D.

Senior Lecturer, Institute of Psychiatry and Honorary Consultant Physician, Maudsley Hospital, London

David Greenfeld, M.D.

Previous Research Assistant, Institute of Psychiatry

and

Linda Lockyer, Ph.D.

Previously Research Assistant, Institute of Psychiatry, Maudsley Hospital, London
now at Hospital for Sick Children, Toronto, Canada

I. Description of Sample

The psychoses of infancy have long been a matter of controversy. The nature of the disorders, their aetiology, relationship to adult forms of psychosis, long-term outcome and response to treatment are still areas of disagreement among clinicians. Follow-up studies should provide information relevant to some of these problems. Unfortunately, the findings of published investigations have been contradictory. To a large extent contradictions appear to be related to differences in diagnostic criteria, but the failure of many writers to describe their cases adequately has made it difficult to assess the significance of possible differences.

The problems associated with the wide variation in concepts of child

Reprinted from the British Journal of Psychiatry, Vol. 113, pp. 1169-1199. Part I is by Drs. Rutter and Lockyer. Part II (starting on page 471) is by all three authors.

psychosis and in the criteria for its diagnosis have been increased by the tendency of some writers to reject the need for diagnosis or classification (Beres, 1956; Esman, 1960; Rank, 1949; Szurek, 1956). But, as Eisenberg (1966) put it, "differential diagnosis is no academic exercise to satisfy statistical pigeon-holes, it is the very stuff of medicine." He urged that all future clinical reports should include precise specification of criteria (Eisenberg, 1957). The need for this was as evident in a recent review of the literature (Rutter, 1967) as it was in Eisenberg's review in 1957.

The first report in 1961 of the British working party on the "schizophrenic syndrome in childhood," under the chairmanship of Dr. Mildred Creak, constituted a most important step towards the goal of general agreement among psychiatrists and psychologists on the necessary diagnostic criteria for child psychosis (Creak et al., 1961). The 'nine diagnostic points' put forward by the working party were valuable in highlighting the phenomenology of child psychosis and in arousing interest in accurate diagnosis. Inevitably, there were ambiguities and inconsistencies in this first formulation of diagnostic criteria (Rutter, 1967), and a further progress report of the working party in 1964 (Creak et al., 1964) showed that some of the points had been interpreted in rather divergent ways by different clinicians. It is not yet possible to use the 'nine points' as a sufficient description of cases. Accordingly, the present paper, the first of a series reporting a five to fifteen year follow-up study of children with infantile psychosis, attempts to provide a fairly detailed description of the children and their disorders so that comparisons with other series may be possible.

METHOD

The records of the Maudsley Hospital Children's Department from 1950 to 1958, inclusive, were searched in order to select all children seen before the onset of any signs of pubescence, for whom an unequivocal diagnosis of child psychosis, schizophrenic syndrome of childhood, infantile autism, or any synonyms of these had been agreed by all Maudsley Hospital consultant psychiatrists who had seen the child. In searching for cases, the diagnosis coded on the front sheet of the records of all children attending the Department and the symptoms coded on a more detailed item sheet were used.

Sixty-three psychotic children fulfilling these criteria were identified, and for each child another child of the same sex, first attending the same Department within one year of the first attendance of the psychotic child and matching the psychotic child as closely as possible in age and

TABLE 1

Tests Used in Matching Psychotic and Control Children

Test	Psychotic Group	Control Group
Merrill-Palmer	25	16
Binet	8	28
WISC Full Scale	4	10
WISC Verbal Scale	—	1
WISC Performance Scale	3	1
Leiter	3	1
Goodenough Draw-a-Man	1	—
Vineland	9	4
Untestable	10	2
Total	63	63

measured intelligence, was selected as a control. Psychologists routinely administer an intelligence test to all children attending the Department, and at the time of the study 93 per cent of the children were in fact tested. Those not tested usually had a recent test result from the referring clinic or hospital. For each child a card, which includes details of age, IQ, and sex, is punched, and a mechanical sort of these cards was used to locate the control children. The records of the children were then examined so that children showing 'psychotic traits' or 'some psychotic features' could be excluded from both the psychotic group and the control group. This, together with the demand that there be unanimous agreement on diagnosis, resulted in the exclusion of many children who had been confidently diagnosed as psychotic by other psychiatrists, but it seemed preferable to obtain a group of children for whom there was no diagnostic doubt. The records of one additional child were found only after the study was well advanced. He was followed-up, but is excluded from all psychotic-control comparisons. The records of three possibly psychotic children could not be found.

Ideally, in matching for IQ, each pair of psychotic and control children should have been tested on the same intelligence scale, but this proved to be an impracticable demand. The tests used are shown in Table 1. The most commonly used test in the psychotic group was the Merrill-Palmer; this was also used with many of the control children, but more were tested on the Binet, a test only infrequently employed with the psychotic children. The children's IQs were not converted to standard scores because some of the tests do not have known means and standard deviations and because some of the IQs were extrapolated from scores on only a few subtests from the intelligence scale (as the children had not co-operated on the full test). Scores on the Vineland Social Maturity Scale were taken as equivalent to scores on intelligence tests. Thus the IQs must be regarded as rough approximations. Nevertheless, actual scores were used, and no account was taken of the psychologist's judgment that the child was really more (or less) intelligent than the score suggested. As will be shown in a later paper, in spite of these drawbacks and in spite of the frequent comments by the testing psychologist that the scores were unreliable or did not provide a valid measure of the child's abilities, the scores proved to be remarkably stable and also excellent predictors of the child's social and intellectual functioning five to fifteen years later.

Table 2 shows the age, sex, and IQ of the psychotic and control children. Close matching was possible, and there was no significant difference between the means or distribution of ages or IQs in the two groups. There were 49 pairs of the 63 in which the intra-pair age difference was less than twelve months, and in 30 of these the difference was six months or less; in no cases was the difference as much as two years. In 47 of the pairs the matching for IQ was within 10 points of IQ. Actual scores were available for 53 of the psychotic children and 58 of the controls. One of the psychotic children and three of the control children scored below the floor of the test on which they were matched and therefore did not receive an exact IQ. For the purposes of matching they were given the basal score on the test. Ten of the psychotic children and two of the control children did not have a score on the Vineland Social Maturity Scale and were completely untestable on any intelligence test. Examination of the findings on the untestable children who had received a Vineland score suggested that it could be assumed that untestable children had an IQ of below 50. Therefore, for the purpose of matching children on IQ this assumption was made when no score of any kind was available.

The control children were selected solely on the basis of age, sex, IQ and absence of any diagnosis involving terms such as 'with psychotic features.' Apart from this exclusion, no attempt was made to select children with any particular psychiatric disorder, and inevitably the group chosen was clinically heterogeneous. The majority (38) of the control children had some degree of mental subnormality, and very frequently retardation of speech was one of the chief complaints. At least a third had probable organic disease of the brain, and many (9) were epileptic when first seen at the hospital. Behaviourally, a third (23) presented with disorders involving socially disapproved or antisocial conduct, a

TABLE 2

Age, Sex and I.Q. of Psychotic and Control Children

Age at first attendance Maudsley Hospital	Psychotic Groups	Control Groups
2 yrs. 9 mo.-3 yrs. 11 mo........	10	7
4 yrs.-4 yrs. 11 mo..............	14	12
5 yrs.-5 yrs. 11 mo..............	10	13
6 yrs.-6 yrs. 11 mo..............	12	12
7 yrs.-7 yrs. 11 mo..............	8	6
8 yrs.-8 yrs. 11 mo..............	3	8
9 yrs.-9 yrs. 11 mo..............	4	4
10 yrs.-10 yrs. 8 mo............	2	1
Total	63	63
Mean Age .... 5 years 11 months		6 years 2 months
Sex:		
Boys	51	51
Girls	12	12
Total	63	63
Male/Female ratio	4.25:1	4.25:1
IQ:		
50 or below	27	28
51-70	18	15
71-90	12	13
91-120	6	7
Mean IQ of those testable......	62.49	60.36
Total Number Testable	53	58

quarter (15) had neurotic disorders, a few (6) showed the hyperkinetic syndrome, 8 had uncomplicated mental subnormality, and the remainder (11) had other disorders (including subacute organic reaction, enuresis and encopresis as isolated disorders, extreme clumsiness, personality disorders, and specific developmental speech disorder). In spite of the exclusion of children diagnosed as having 'psychotic features,' at follow-up, one of the control children was thought to be definitely psychotic and three others probably so.

In the initial selection of the psychotic children, the diagnoses made at the time were utilized; no attempt was made to utilize the authors' own diagnostic concepts. Nearly all the children had been seen at some time by both the late Dr. Kenneth Cameron and Dr. James Anthony. Several other psychiatrists had seen a smaller proportion of the cases, but it may be assumed that Cameron's and Anthony's criteria were most used in making the diagnosis of child psychosis. Cameron (1955 and

1958) employed Potter's criteria (1933) of "withdrawal of interest from the environment; dereistic patterns of thinking, feeling, and action; diminution or defect in emotional rapport; diminution, distortion or rigidity of affect; variation of mobility either towards increase and hypermobility, or diminution to complete immobility or to bizarre or stereotyped behavior; finally to regression," which Cameron regarded as equivalent to Despert's description (1938) of "loss of affective contact with reality . . . coincident with or determined by specific phenomena of regression and dissociation." However, as will be shown, the psychotic children differed in many ways from Potter's cases and were similar to only some of Despert's.

Anthony (1958a and b; 1962) has differentiated three types of psychosis: (1) a very early onset group which he equates with Kanner's primary infantile autism, Bender's first age group and Despert's 'no-onset' group, (2) a group in which massive regression takes place between the ages of 3 and 5 years and which includes Heller's disease, Mahler's symbiotic psychosis, Bender's second age group, Despert's 'acute-onset' type and the De Sanctis and Weygandt's dementias, and (3) a group with an onset in the middle and late years of childhood. The last group was necessarily partly eliminated, and in practice completely eliminated, from the present series by the demand that the child should first have attended the clinic before the onset of pubescence. As judged by the age of the child at the onset of the psychosis there were also very few in the second category. The great majority of the children had shown abnormalities from early infancy; thus most of the disorders could be classified with Anthony's first group of early onset psychosis.

RESULTS: DESCRIPTION OF SAMPLE

Sex

There was a marked preponderance of boys among the psychotic children (Table 2) ; the male/female ratio was 4.25:1.

Age of Onset

In over half (54 per cent) the psychotic group, the first signs of psychotic development had been apparent in early infancy with no preceding period of normal development (Table 3). In a quarter (25 per cent) there was an account of psychosis intervening after a period of apparently normal development. However, in these cases the designation of normal development depended on normal motor milestones and no history of marked early behavioral or social difficulties, plus, sometimes, an ac-

TABLE 3

AGE OF CHILDREN AT ONSET OF PSYCHOSIS

		Number of Children
Onset in Early Infancy (No period of normal development prior to onset of psychosis)		34
Onset after period of dubiously normal development		16
Onset before 24 months	10	
Onset between 24 and 30 months	5	
Onset after 30 months	1	
Onset after period of reasonably definite normal development		13
Onset before 24 months	1	
Onset between 24 and 30 months	8	
Onset between 31 and 36 months	1	
Onset between 3 and 5 years	2	
Onset between 5 and 5½ years	1	
Total		63

count of the child speaking a few words. None of these children had gained phrase speech, the history of early infancy was often inadequate, and it is probable that in most cases the psychosis had in fact begun earlier but had not been noticed by the parents.

Nevertheless in a fifth of the cases (21 per cent) there was a fairly convincing history of normal development before there were any signs of psychosis. In most cases (9) the psychosis began before the age of thirty months, but in two children psychotic development was first apparent between thirty-one and thirty-six months, and in one child development seemed normal up to the age of five years.

Behavioral Characteristics

The behavioral characteristics of the psychotic and control children are shown in Table 4. Fuller descriptions of the behavior together with case illustrations are given elsewhere (Rutter, 1966). The characteristics chosen for study were those regarded by other writers as indicating psychosis, together with a sample of some of the common behavioral disturbances associated with non-psychotic disorders. There were marked differences in the behavior of the psychotic and control children (22 of the 34 comparisons provided differences which were statistically signifi-

TABLE 4

BEHAVIORAL CHARACTERISTICS OF PSYCHOTIC AND CONTROL CHILDREN

Behavioral Characteristics	Psychotic Children	Control Children	Level of Significance
Relationships with people:			
Abnormal relationships with peers.........	63	52	.01
Autism	57	8	.001
Withdrawal	21	12	N.S.
Speech:			
Retarded development (either through delay or regression)	63	53	.01
No speech at 5 years	32	7	.001
Ever thought deaf	22	7	.01
Excessive response to sounds	12	2	.025
Echolalia	29*	19*	N.S.
Pronominal reversal	19*	8*	.001
Ritualistic and compulsive phenomena:			
Abnormal attachments	26	12	.025
Abnormal preoccupations	37	9	.001
Non-adaptability (resistance to change)....	37	10	.001
Other 'obsessional' phenomena	32	8	.001
Any of the above 4 items	57	34	.001
Any of the above 4 items in marked degree.	39	8	.001
At least 3 of the 4 items	23	4	.001
Motor Phenomena:			
Hyperkinesis	31	27	N.S.
Hypokinesis (at first attendance)	10	2	.05
Stereotyped repetitive movements (all kinds)	49	21	.001
whole body (other than rocking).........	27	5	.001
hand and finger mannerisms	19	4	.01
face, head and neck movements..........	21	13	N.S.
Poor concentration:			
Short attention span/poor persistence (at follow-up)	35	17	.01
Increased distractibility (at follow-up).....	2	12	.01
Self-injury	23	10	.025
Lack of response to painful stimuli..........	10	4	N.S.
Other Behavioral Problems:			
Feeding difficulties	23	15	N.S.
Sleeping difficulties	23	20	N.S.
Anxiety and fears	40	39	N.S.
Enuresis (after age 4 years)	44	34	N.S.
Encopresis (after age 4 years)	37	19	.01
Aggression	27	26	N.S.
Temper tantrums	49	45	N.S.
Total number of children	63	63	

* Comparison based on proportion of children with useful speech who showed the characteristic.

cant at the 5 per cent level or better), but to a large extent the differences lay in the patterning and severity of disorder. No symptom or sign
occurred solely in the psychotic children, and only two items (abnormal
relationship with other children and retarded development of speech)
occurred in all the psychotic children. The value for differential diagnosis of both items was severely limited by the finding that both were
also present in the majority of the control children (although the difference between the frequencies in the psychotic and control groups was
statistically significant).

(1) Relationships with People

Disturbed interpersonal relationships were found with nearly all the
children in both groups although they were slightly, but significantly
commoner (p<.01) with the psychotic children. What was much more
characteristic of the psychotic children was the nature of the disturbance
in relationships. Whereas most of the psychotic children (57) showed
'autism,' only a few (8) of the control children exhibited this characteristic. In fact all the psychotic children had been described as 'autistic' at
some time, but here the term is used in the more restricted sense as
applying to children who appeared markedly aloof and distant, who
showed an apparent lack of interest in people, usually manifest by persistent avoidance of eye to eye gaze, who showed little variation in facial
expression, rarely exhibited their feelings or appreciated humour and
who failed to show sympathy or empathy for other people. Actual
physical withdrawal from other people occurred in nearly a third of the
psychotic children at some time, but the incidence of withdrawal was
not significantly greater than in the control group.

(2) Speech

Retarded development of speech (shown either by delayed development from the beginning or by regression of speech development) was
characteristic of the children in both groups, although it was slightly
and significantly more frequent in the psychotic group. However, the
abnormalities in communication were much more persistent in psychotic
children; half (32) were still without speech at five years compared
with only a ninth (7) of the control group. A marked lack of response
to sounds was particularly characteristic of psychotic children; over one-
third (22) had been thought deaf at some time compared with only one-
ninth (7) of the control children. Paradoxically, although much less
common, distress in relation to sounds was also significantly more fre-

quent among the psychotic children. Echolalia occurred in over three-quarters of the speaking psychotic children, a rate twice that in the control group. Pronominal reversal, usually forming part of a more general echoing tendency, was also significantly commoner among the psychotics.

(3) Ritualistic and Compulsive Phenomena

Stereotyped activities, apparently ritualistic and compulsive in nature, often complex, and usually followed by distress if the child was prevented from carrying out the behavior, were considerably and significantly commoner among the psychotic children. These activities were subdivided into four categories (abnormal attachments, abnormal preoccupations, nonadaptability or resistance to change, and other obsessive phenomena). Of the psychotic children, 39 showed at least one of the items in marked degree compared with 8 of the control group, and 23 psychotic children exhibited at least three of the four items compared with only 4 control children.

(4) Motor Phenomena

Although marked overactivity occurred in nearly half the psychotic group it was equally common in the control group. Hypokinesis was much less frequent in both groups, but it was significantly commoner among the psychotic children than among the control children. Stereotyped repetitive movements were exhibited by twice as many psychotic as control children. Two types of stereotyped repetitive movements were particularly associated with psychosis—complex whole body movements (other than rocking) and hand and finger mannerisms.

(5) Concentration

Significantly more psychotic children showed a short attention span or poor persistence when given tasks or activities to perform, but significantly fewer had increased distractibility. Whereas among the control children, short attention span and *increased* distractibility tended to be associated, among the psychotic children short attention span was frequently associated with *decreased* distractibility.

(6) Self-injury

Over twice as many psychotic children as control children injured themselves; biting of the wrist or the back of the hand, and head banging were much the commonest forms of self-injury.

(7) Common Behavior Problems

Feeding and sleeping problems, anxiety and fears, enuresis, aggression and temper tantrums were all common among psychotic children, but these problems were equally common among the control children. Encopresis after the child's fourth birthday was significantly commoner in the psychotic group.

Cognitive Characteristics

Extreme variability in intellectual functioning was commoner in the psychotic group than in the control group (see Rutter, 1966 for details) and the variability generally followed the same pattern. The psychotic child was often untestable on verbal tasks, and when testable was at his worst on those demanding abstract thought or symbolism or sequential logic. He was at his best on tasks requiring manipulative or visuo-spatial skills, or, among verbal tests, on those requiring only immediate memory. The variability in intellectual functioning (so-called "islets of intelligence") was significantly commoner among children with continuing retardation of speech and appeared to be due to defects in the child's use and understanding of language.

Ordinal Positions and Family Size

The psychotic children came from somewhat smaller families than the control children (mean sibship size of 2.37 compared with 2.87), and in association with this there was a non-significant excess of only children among the psychotics. However, in both groups there was a significant excess of eldest children over youngest children (in a normal population the number of eldest and youngest children will necessarily be equal). When the position of the psychotic child in the sibship is re-examined in relation to the size of the sibship (Table 6), the issue appears more complicated. While there was an excess of first born (i.e. oldest) psychotic children in two-child families, this was not found in larger families. In contrast, the excess of first-born control children was only found in the larger families (Table 7). The explanation for these findings remains obscure.

Social Class

The distribution of social class (judged by the occupation of the head of the household on the Registrar-General's classification) in the control group was close to that in the general population of Greater London,

TABLE 5

ORDINAL POSITION OF PSYCHOTIC AND CONTROL CHILDREN

Ordinal Position	Psychotic Group	Control Group
Eldest	25	27
Youngest	14	14
Only	13	7
Other	11	15
Mean size of sibship	2.37	2.87

TABLE 6

POSITION IN SIBSHIP OF PSYCHOTIC CHILDREN ACCORDING TO SIZE OF SIBSHIP

Position in Sibship	1	Size of Sibship 2	3	4+	Total
1	13	18	6	1	38
2		9	6	1	16
3			4	2	6
4 or more				3	3
Total	13	27	16	7	63

TABLE 7

POSITION IN SIBSHIP OF CONTROL CHILDREN ACCORDING TO SIZE OF SIBSHIP

Position in Sibship	1	Size of Sibship 2	3	4+	Total
1	7	9	12	6	34
2		12	7	3	22
3			1	5	6
4 or more				1	1
Total	7	21	20	15	63

but there was a significant excess of social class I and a significant deficiency of social classes IV and V in the psychotic group (Table 8).

There was a tendency (which fell just short of the 5 per cent level of significance) for a greater proportion of the control children to be living otherwise than with their two natural parents (i.e. to have a 'broken

TABLE 8

Social Class (Registrar-General's Classification)

Social Class	N	Psychotics % of known	N	Controls % of known	General Population (Greater London) Heads of Households (1951) %
I	15	(23.8)	7	(11.3)	(4.6)
II	20	(31.7)	13	(21.0)	(18.9)
III	26	(41.3)	26	(42.0)	(52.8)
IV and V	2	(3.2)	16	(25.8)	(23.7)
Not known	—		1		
Total	63		63		

Proportion NOT living with their two natural parents

		Psychotics		Controls	General Population (Isle of Wight)
Not living with two natural parents	6	(9.4%)	14	(22.2%)	(13.9%)
Total	63		63		147

home'). There are no comparable figures for the general population of Greater London. However, the figure (13.9 per cent) for 9- and 10-year-old children in the Isle of Wight (Rutter *et al.*, 1966) is similar to that for the psychotic group. In so far as the differences have any significance, it is probable that there is more of an excess of 'broken homes' in the control group than there is a deficiency in the psychotic group.

Psychiatric Disorder in Parents and Sibs

Eleven parents in the psychotic group and thirteen in the control group had been under psychiatric care at some time in adult life, mostly for affective or neurotic disorders (Table 9). There was a suggestion that obsessional and phobic symptoms might have been somewhat commoner among the parents of psychotic children. None of the parents in the psychotic group had had schizophrenia.

Twice as many sibs in the control group had received psychiatric care, but the difference between the two groups fell short of statistical significance. The difference was largely accounted for by the higher rate of mental subnormality among the sibs of the control children (7 children compared with one in the psychotic group). None of the sibs of the psychotic children had received the diagnosis of psychosis, schizophrenia or autism. However, a sister of one of the children had had a disorder which had been termed 'possibly autistic.' She was an intelligent girl who had been delayed in her speech development, failed to show affec-

TABLE 9

Psychiatric Disorder in Immediate Family

	Psychotic Group	Control Group
Parents who had received psychiatric treatment	11	13
Diagnoses:		
Schizophrenia	—	1
Psychopathy	—	1
Suicide	—	1
Anxiety/depressive neurosis ..	6	9
Phobic state	2	—
Obsessional illness	1	—
Other	2	1
Sibs who had received psychiatric treatment	6	16
	(7.1%)	(13.0%)
Diagnoses:		
Mental subnormality	1	7
Neurotic disorder	2	5
Antisocial disorder	2	4
?Autistic	1	—
Total No. sibs	85	123

tion or form adequate relationships, and had a variety of obsessive manifestations in early childhood. However, unlike her brother's, the developmental difficulties proved to be transient. When seen at the age of 9 years she was a somewhat unusual personality, but appeared quite normal and certainly could not be termed psychotic or autistic. In addition, there was another child (a brother of one of the psychotic children) with a somewhat similar, although less abnormal, history, but who had not been under any psychiatric care. Both these sibs may have had a much milder disorder similar in type to that shown by their psychotic brothers. If both cases are included (and this involves a considerable stretching of the diagnostic criteria) the rate of psychosis in the sibs is still only 2.4 per cent.

'Brain Damage'

As no generally accepted criteria for 'brain damage' exist, as many proven cases of organic brain disease in childhood are unassociated with abnormalities on clinical examination of the central nervous system, and as the interpretation of findings on special tests (especially the EEG) in young children is very problematical, no precise figure can be given for the rate of 'brain damage' in this group of psychotic children. None of the children showed unequivocal abnormalities on a neurological examination when they first attended the hospital, and in only two children was there satisfactory evidence of organic brain disorder at that time. One boy had first shown signs of psychosis in infancy after an attack of meningitis at 8 months which was succeeded by the development of epilepsy. Another child also had had fits since infancy, although the psychosis appeared unrelated to any physical illness. In a further three children evidence of probable brain disease became available within a short time after first attendance at hospital. One boy was shown to have congenital syphilis with probable neural involvement, and another boy developed lead encephalopathy; the lead poisoning probably, but not definitely, preceded the onset of psychosis. A girl who had fits only up to the age of 4 years was found to have possible cortical atrophy on pneumo-encephalography.

If evidence obtained at any period up to the time the child was seen for follow-up in adolescence or early adult life is taken into account, then a larger proportion of children may be considered as probably having some form of 'brain damage' (Table 10). A strong likelihood of 'brain damage' existed in 12 children—the first two children noted above and 10 others who developed epileptic fits for the first time long after the onset of the psychosis, usually in early adolescence. In 3 children the onset of fits was associated with general regression but especially in speech. However, none of the children could be shown to have any recognized neurological disorder, although one child was found to have lead poisoning. In this boy the fits may have been due to lead intoxication caused by the pica associated with the psychosis, but at least in the others it appeared more probable that both the fits and the psychosis were due to some underlying brain pathology. Necessarily, this remains a matter for speculation rather than a proven aetiological factor.

A further 6 children probably had 'brain damage.' These included the 3 children already mentioned plus 3 others, of whom one was shown to have retinal (and probably neural) toxoplasmosis and two had persistent spike foci on electroencephalography. Another 16 children had less satisfactory evidence of brain disorder, such as uncertain abnormalities on neurological examination or on an EEG. These children may have had 'brain damage,' but the evidence was no more than suggestive and its significance might reasonably be questioned.

About half the group (29) showed no evidence of 'brain damage,' unless perceptual defects or speech abnormalities are taken into account. However, these speech and perceptual disorders may have been due to

TABLE 10
Presence of 'Brain Damage' in Psychotic Children

Strong likelihood:	12	1 epilepsy from infancy
		1 meningitis in infancy followed by onset of epilepsy
		10 onset of epilepsy long after development of psychosis
Probable	6	1 toxoplasmosis
		1 neurolues
		1 lead encephalopathy developing shortly after onset of psychosis
		2 spike focus on EEG
		1 fits in pre-school period only + possible cortical atrophy on AEG
Possible	16	4 uncertain abnormalities on neurological examination
		7 various abnormalities on EEG
		2 marked skull asymmetry
		2 dubious fits
		1 slight enlargement of temporal horn on AEG
No evidence of brain damage:	29	

AEG is air (pneumo-) Encephalogram.

developmental delays in brain maturation rather than to brain disease. Thus, in just over a quarter of the children (18 out of 63) there was evidence suggesting the probability of some organic brain disorder.

Behavioral Characteristics and IQ

Although the range of intelligence among the psychotic children was very great, the differences in intellect were associated with relatively few differences in behavioral characteristics. Compared with those of IQ 60 or above, more psychotic children with an IQ of 59 or less exhibited stereotyped repetitive movements and more were inclined to injure themselves. The retardation of speech found in all the psychotic children tended to be more profound in those who were also mentally subnormal, so that more children with an IQ below 60 were without useful speech when they first attended the Maudsley Hospital. There was also a nearly significant (critical ratio = 1.90) tendency for hyperkinesis to be more common among the psychotic children of low IQ. On the other hand the mentally subnormal psychotic children were equally likely to exhibit autism, physical withdrawal, pronominal reversal, echolalia, profound lack of response to sounds, hypokinesis, and ritualistic and compulsive

TABLE 11

BEHAVIORAL CHARACTERISTICS AND IQ IN PSYCHOTIC CHILDREN

Behavioral Characteristic	IQ below 60 No.	%	IQ 60 or above No.	%	Significance
Autism	32	(97)	25	(83)	N.S.
Physical withdrawal	10	(30)	11	(37)	N.S.
No speech (at first attendance)	22	(67)	11	(37)	.05
Pronominal reversal	8	(62)*	11	(46)*	N.S.
Echolalia	12	(92)*	17	(71)*	N.S.
Lack of response to sounds	13	(39)	9	(31)†	N.S.
Ritualistic and compulsive phenomena:					
any	31	(94)	26	(87)	N.S.
abnormal attachments	16	(48)	10	(33)	N.S.
abnormal preoccupations	19	(58)	18	(60)	N.S.
non-adaptability	20	(61)	17	(57)	N.S.
obsessive phenomena	12	(36)	20	(67)	.05
Hyperkinesis	20	(61)	11	(37)	.06
Hypokinesis	6	(18)	4	(13)	N.S.
Stereotyped repetitive movements	30	(91)	19	(63)	.025
Self-injury	17	(52)	6	(20)	.025
Total number	33		30		

* Proportion based on children with useful speech.
† Excluding one child thought to have organic deafness.

phenomena. The content of the symptoms was, of course, related to the level of intelligence. The rituals and compulsions of the more intelligent children were usually more complex and involved than those of the less intelligent. This was reflected in the rather lower incidence of obsessive phenomena (other than abnormal attachments, abnormal preoccupations, non-adaptability or resistance to change which were unrelated to IQ) among the psychotic children of IQ below 60. However, on the whole the general type of behavioral abnormalities showed little relationship to the level of intelligence. The features most characteristic of infantile psychosis were present with approximately the same frequency in children of all levels of IQ.

Comparison with Other Groups of Psychotic Children

The chief features of the present group of psychotic children were a marked preponderance of boys, an absence of psychosis in other members of the family, middle class (and especially professional) family background, marked variability in intellectual functioning, an onset of psychosis in early infancy, and a disorder with the following behavioral features: 'autistic' relationships with people, marked retardation of speech development, a lack of response to auditory stimuli, pronominal reversal and echolalia when speech developed, various ritualistic and compulsive phenomena (frequently including a striking resistance to change), stereotyped repetitive mannerisms, short attention span on given tasks together with nondistractibility, and a tendency to self-injury.

The children fulfil the 'nine points' outlined by the British Working Party (Creak et al., 1961) and there are close similarities in social, psychological and behavioral characteristics with the psychotic children described by Creak (1951, 1962, 1963a and b) and the autistic children studied by Kanner and Eisenberg (Kanner, 1943, 1943, Eisenberg and Kanner,1956; Eisenberg, 1956). The children studied by Norman (1954 and 1955), by Wolff and Chess (1965a and b), by Mittler and his colleagues (1966) and those termed autistic by Despert and Sherwin (1958) were also fairly similar. The 'atypical' children studied by Reiser and Brown (Brown, 1960 and 1963; Reiser and Brown, 1964), Annell's group of psychotic children (Annell, 1963), and the early onset 'pseudo-defective' children investigated by Bender (1947; 1955; 1959) overlap to some extent with the present group, but each probably includes many children who would not have been included here.

On the other hand, the present group of psychotic children appears different from the groups of children with a later onset such as described by Potter (1933), Bender (1947, 1955 and 1956), Piotrowski (1933 and 1937), and others. The features which differentiate early and later onset cases have been outlined in recent reviews by Eisenberg (1966) and by Rutter (1967).

Although there are many close similarities between this Maudsley group of children and the autistic children studied by Kanner and Eisenberg, a few differences should also be mentioned. There are three children in the present series in whom the psychosis did not appear until after the age of 3 years, and on these grounds they would not have been termed autistic by the Johns Hopkins workers. Two of these three children showed a profound regression of the type described by Heller, both had a very poor outcome, and although unequivocal evidence of brain disease was lacking in both, the disorders probably should be classified as Heller's disease. Other cases of regressive disorder at 3 to 5 years (not included in the present investigation) suggest that the prognosis in this group is usually bad, and the aetiology is often found to be some form of degenerative brain disease.

The disorder of the third child in whose case the onset was after the third birthday poses a more difficult problem in classification. In spite of a very late onset (age 5 years) the clinical features seemed similar to Kanner's cases of infantile autism. In addition, the outcome was rather better than most children with a regressive disorder beginning in middle childhood. The boy's development and progress up to the age of 5 years appeared entirely normal. Then during his first year at school, speech deteriorated, screaming attacks began, and he became increasingly inaccessible, autistic and withdrawn. When he attended hospital at the age of 7 years he was aloof and solitary, with no interest in people, and did not mix or play with other children. However, he would sometimes follow quite complex instructions, showed good interest in objects, and on some cognitive tests performed at or above age-level; on others he was untestable. He spoke little, apart from the repetition of phrases, and he showed pronominal reversal. His motor co-ordination was good, he was moderately overactive and he often jumped up and down screaming. In general, he appeared oblivious of external stimuli, but he stubbornly resisted all changes and insisted that everything had to be done in the way and in the order that it had been done previously.

Kanner might also have eliminated the nine children in whom the psychosis developed in the third year of the child's life after an apparently normal development up to the age of 2 years. However, in terms of family background, behavioral characteristics (and outcome) these children did not differ from the rest of the group. In the present state of knowledge there seems to be little point in classifying these children differently.

The present series also differs somewhat from the Johns Hopkins series in the frequency with which organic features were associated with psychosis. The difference may be more apparent than real in that all the children in this investigation were seen personally at follow-up, whereas Eisenberg had to rely on hospital reports in many of his cases. The difference between the two series is most marked in relation to the frequency with which fits developed during adolescence. As many of the children had only three or four fits altogether, hospital reports might well have omitted this information unless it were specifically requested. In addition, the children who developed fits tended to be of lower IQ than the others, and as fewer exhibited peaks of ability in limited areas ('islets of intelligence') some might have been excluded by Kanner and Eisenberg on the grounds of insufficient evidence of a normal intellectual potential. On the other hand, fits were reported in some of Kanner's children, and the epileptic children were indistinguishable from the rest at the time they first attended the Maudsley Hospital at about the age of 5 years. Many of the apparently brain-injured children (especially the non-epileptic) were of normal intelligence and had disorders closely similar to Kanner's classical description of infantile autism in 1943.

It is important to search for differences between disorders associated and those not associated with probable brain injury, between those disorders manifest in early infancy and those beginning after a short period of apparently normal development, between psychotic children of subnormal intelligence and those of normal intellect, and these comparisons will be made when reporting the findings at follow-up. However, in view of the generally close similarities between the children, and because of the lack of any satisfactory criteria for further subdivision, the group will be considered as a whole for most purposes. The present writers would have classified separately the two children with a Heller-type disorder, but the number is not sufficient to justify their separate consideration.

SUMMARY

In the first of a series of papers on a five to fifteen year follow-up, a group of children with infantile psychosis is described. The group consisted of the 63 children who were all those who attended the Maudsley Hospital between 1950 and 1958 inclusive, who were seen before the onset of any signs of pubescence and for whom an unequivocal diagnosis of child psychosis, schizophrenic syndrome of childhood, infantile autism or any synonyms of these had been agreed by all consultant psychiatrists at the Maudsley Hospital who had seen the child. The group is compared with a group of nonpsychotic children who attended the same hospital at the same time, and who were individually matched for age, sex, and IQ.

There was a marked preponderance of boys among the psychotic children (4.25:1). In most cases psychotic development had been evident in early infancy with no preceding period of normal development, but in a fifth of the cases there was a fairly convincing history of two to three years normal development before there were any signs of psychosis. The chief distinguishing behavioral features were autistic relationships with people, marked retardation of speech, a lack of response to auditory stimuli, pronominal reversal and echolalia when speech developed, various ritualistic and compulsive phenomena (frequently including a striking resistance to change), stereotyped repetitive mannerisms, short attention span on given tasks together with non-distractibility, and a tendency to self-injury. Extreme variability in intellectual functioning was also quite common. There was a significant excess of children from professional backgrounds, an excess of first-born children in two-child families, and not many 'broken homes.' Although several of the parents had had psychiatric treatment, none had been or were psychotic. At most, the rate of psychosis in the sibs was 2.4 per cent., but none of the sibs had a fully developed psychotic disorder. None of the children showed unequivocal abnormalities on a neurological examination when they first attended the hospital, but in a quarter evidence obtained during the follow-up period suggested the probability of some form of brain injury. Although the range of intelligence among the children was very great, the differences in intellect were associated with few differences in behavioural characteristics. It is concluded that the children are closely similar to those with infantile autism described by Kanner (1943).

Acknowledgments—We are grateful to the Consultant Psychiatrists of the Maudsley Hospital for access to their case records and for permission to see their patients. We particularly wish to acknowledge our indebtedness to Dr. James Anthony and the late Dr. Kenneth Cameron whose earlier study of psychotic children made this investigation possible. The study was supported in part by a grant from the Medical Research Council. Psychological aspects of the study formed part of a thesis submitted for a Ph.D. by Miss Lockyer.

REFERENCES

ANNELL, A. L. (1963). "The prognosis of psychotic syndromes in childhood: A follow-up study of 115 cases." *Acta psychiat. Scand., 39,* 235-297.

ANTHONY, J. (1958a). "An experimental approach to the psychopathology of childhood: Autism." *Brit. J. med. Psychol., 31,* 211-225.

ANTHONY, J. (1958b). "An aetiological approach to the diagnosis of psychosis in childhood." *Rev. Psychiat. infant., 25,* 89-96.

ANTHONY, J. (1962). "Low-grade psychosis in childhood." In: Richards, B. W. (ed.) *Proc. London Conf. Scient. Stud. ment. Def.* Vol. 2, Dagenham: May and Baker.

BENDER, L. (1947). "Childhood schizophrenia: clinical study of 100 schizophrenic children." *Amer. J. Orthopsychiat., 17,* 40-56.

———— (1955). "Twenty years of clinical research in schizophrenic children with special reference to those under six years of age." In: Caplan, G. (ed.) *Emotional Problems of Early Childhood,* pp. 503-515. London: Tavistock.

———— (1956). "Childhood schizophrenia. 2. Schizophrenia in childhood—its recognition, description and treatment." *Amer. J. Orthopsychiat., 26,* 499-506.

———— (1959). "The concept of pseudo-psychopathic schizophrenia in adolescents." *Ibid., 29,* 491-509.

BERES, D. (1956). "Ego deviation and the concept of schizophrenia." *Psychoanalyt. Stud. Child, 11,* 164-235.

BROWN, J. (1960). "Prognosis from presenting symptoms of pre-school children with atypical development." *Amer. J. Orthopsychiat., 30,* 382-390.

———— (1963). "Follow-up of children with atypical development (infantile psychosis)." *Ibid., 33,* 855-861.

CAMERON, K. (1955). "Psychosis in infancy and early childhood." *Medical Press, 234,* 3-15.

———— (1958). "A group of twenty-five psychotic children." *Rev. Psychiat. infant., 25,* 117-122.

CREAK, E. M. (1951). "Psychoses in childhood." *J. ment. Sci.*, *97*, 545-554.

———— (1962). "Juvenile psychosis and mental deficiency." In: Richards, B. W. (ed.) *Proc. London Conf. Scient. Stud. ment. Def.* Vol. 2. Dagenham: May and Baker.

———— (1963a). "Childhood psychosis: a review of 100 cases." *Brit. J. Psychiat.*, *109*, 84-89.

———— (1963b). "Schizophrenia in early childhood." *Acta paedopsychiat.*, *30*, 42-47.

———— (Chairman) (1961). "Schizophrenic syndrome in childhood." Progress report of working party. *Cerebr. Palsy Bull.*, *3*, 501-504.

———— (Chairman) (1964). "Schizophrenic syndrome in childhood." Further progress report of working party *Developmental Medicine Child. Neurol.*, *4*, 530-535.

DESPERT, J. L. (1938). "Schizophrenia in children." *Psychiat. Quart.*, *12*, 366-371.

—— and SHERWIN, A. C. (1958). "Further examination of diagnostic criteria in schizophrenic illness and psychoses in infancy and early childhood." *Amer. J. Psychiat.*, *114*, 784-790.

EISENBERG, L. (1956). "The autistic child in adolescence." *Amer. J. Psychiat.*, *112*, 607-612.

———— (1957). "The course of childhood schizophrenia." *A.M.A. Arch. Neurol. Psychiat.*, *78*, 69-83.

———— (1966). "Psychotic disorders in childhood." In: Cooke, R. E. (ed.) *Biologic Basis of Paediatric Practice*. New York: McGraw-Hill.

—— and KANNER, L. (1956). "Childhood schizophrenia." *Amer. J. Orthopsychiat.*, *26*, 556-566.

ESMAN, A. H. (1960). "Childhood psychosis and childhood schizophrenia." *Ibid.*, *30*, 391-396.

KANNER, L. (1943). "Autistic disturbances of affective contact." *Nerv. Child.* 2, 217-250.

MITTLER, P., GILLIES, S., and JUKES, E. (1966). "A follow-up report on a group of psychotic children." *J. ment. Def. Res.*, *10*, 73-83.

NORMAN, E. (1954). "Reality relationships of schizophrenic children." *Brit. J. med. Psychol.*, *27*, 126-141.

———— (1955). "Affect and withdrawal in schizophrenic children." *Ibid.*, *28*, 1-17.

PIOTROWSKI, Z. A. (1933). "The test behavior of schizophrenic children." *Amer. Ass. ment. Def. Proc.*, 57th Ann. Session, 332-347.

———— (1937). "A comparison of congenitally defective children with schizophrenic children in regard to personality structure and intelligence type." *Ibid.*, 61st Ann. Session, part 1, 78-90.

POTTER, H. W. (1933). "Schizophrenia in children." *Amer. J. Psychiat.*, *89*, 1253-1269.

RANK, B. (1949). "Adaptation of the psychoanalytic technique for the treatment of young children with atypical development." *Amer. J. Orthopsychiat.*, *19*, 130-139.

REISER, D. E., and BROWN, J. (1964). "Patterns of later development in children with infantile psychosis." *J. Amer. Acad. Child Psychiat.*, *3*, 650-667.

RUTTER, M. (1966). "Behavioral and cognitive characteristics of a series of psychotic children." In: Wing, J. K. (ed.) *Childhood Autism: Clinical, Educational and Social Aspects*. London: Pergamon Press.

———— (1967). "Psychotic disorders in early childhood." In: Coppen and Walk (eds.) *Recent Developments in Schizophrenia*. Ashford, Kent: Headley Bros.

—— YULE, W., TIZARD, J., and GRAHAM, P. (1967). "Severe reading retardation: its relationship to maladjustment, epilepsy and neurological disorders." In: *Proc. of int. Conf. Ass. for Special Education* (in press).

SZUREK, S. A. (1956). "Psychotic episodes and psychotic maldevelopment." *Amer. J. Orthopsychiat.*, *26*, 519-543.

WOLFF, S., and CHESS, S. (1965a). "A behavioral study of schizophrenic children." *Acta psychiat. Scand.*, *40*, 438-466.

—— —— (1965b). "An analysis of the language of fourteen schizophrenic children." *J. Child Psychol. Psychiat.*, *6*, 29-41.

II. Social and Behavioral Outcome

The two major follow-up studies of children suffering from infantile psychosis, that of Kanner's cases (Kanner, 1943 and 1949; Kanner and Eisenberg, 1955; Eisenberg and Kanner, 1956; Eisenberg, 1956; Kanner and Lesser, 1958) and that of psychotic children seen by Creak (1962, 1963a and b) have shown the generally poor prognosis for these children. In both studies about half the children were in full-time residential care (usually mental subnormality hospitals) at follow-up, and only 5 per cent to 17 per cent could be said to be well adjusted. Similar findings have been reported in the other published studies reviewed in Rutter, 1966a). Kanner and Eisenberg have described the course of the characteristics of aloneness or autism shown by all or nearly all children with infantile psychosis (Kanner, 1943; Kanner and Eisenberg, 1955; Eisenberg and Kanner, 1956) . Although some psychotic children emerge from their solitude to a greater or lesser extent, a lack of social perceptiveness usually remains even in adolescence or early adult life.

Unfortunately in most of the published studies only some of the children were personally examined by the authors, and there is very little information available on the developmental course of the other behavioral or cognitive attributes associated with infantile psychosis. Nor, apart from the prognostic significance of lack of useful speech by the age of 5 years, noted by Eisenberg (1956), is much known of the factors associated with a good or a bad prognosis. In addition, there have been no comparisons between the course of psychotic and non-psychotic disorders in children of the same age, sex and intelligence. It is primarily to answer these three questions that further follow-up studies are required. They are given particular consideration in the present paper, which reports a five to fifteen year follow-up study of 63 children with infantile psychosis and 63 'control' children attending the same clinic and closely matched for age, sex and IQ.

METHOD

The selection of the samples and the matching procedure, together with a description of the behavioral, cognitive, family and other characteristics of the children are provided in a companion paper (Rutter and Lockyer, 1967). All children in both the psychotic and control groups were traced and all 63 psychotic children and 61 control children were individually seen at follow-up. No detailed information was available for one control child who had emigrated to Australia, and one control child had died. All other children were examined.

In each case the child was given a neurological and psychiatric examination by D.G. and/or M.R.* using a procedure standarized as far as was compatible with the examination of children of varying age, IQ and behavioral state, many of whom showed limited co-operation. The child was also observed in an unstructured situation with other children and with adults at home, school or hospital. A detailed description of the child's past and present behavioral and social state, together with an account of illnesses and other medical information and details of the health of the rest of the family, was obtained from the parent or parent substitute, using a standard interview schedule. All behaviors to be rated were specified and categorized and each was rated on a five-point scale. A similar psychiatric interview and psychiatric history-taking procedure have been shown to be reliable in another study (Rutter and Graham, 1967; Graham and Rutter, 1967). All the children were given an individual psychological examination consisting of the WISC or WAIS, Peabody Picture-Vocabulary Scale, Schonell Graded Word Reading Test, and the Vineland Social Maturity Scale (based on an account from the parent or parent substitute).** Where appropriate, a report of the child's behavior and attainments was obtained from the school or training center attended by the child.

The mean age of the psychotic children when examined at follow-up was 15 years 7 months and the mean age of the control children was 16 years 5 months, the duration of follow-up being 9 years 8 months and 10 years 3 months respectively. The differences in age and duration of follow-up were not statistically significant. Contact with the children was maintained after follow-up, and the information on administrative placement refers to a slightly later date for the psychotic children so that the age-matching at follow-up could be more exact.

RESULTS

1. *Administrative placement*

In both groups over a third of the children were in long-stay hospitals at follow-up, and the proportion of psychotic children in long-term care was only slightly higher than the proportion of control children (44 per cent compared with 36 per cent or 52 per cent compared with

---

* All the psychotic children were examined by M.R. including 7 also seen by D.G. 27 of the control children were seen by M.R. and D.G., and 34 control children were examined by D.G. alone. The ratings of children seen by M.R. or D.G. alone were reviewed by both together to ensure comparability of standards.

** Two children were tested by M.R. All other children were tested by L.L. (see Lockyer and Rutter, 1967 for details).

TABLE 1

PLACEMENT AT FOLLOW-UP (TOTAL GROUP)

	Psychotic	Controls
Employed	2	14
Ordinary School	3	7
Special School	11	6
Village Trust	3	—
Training Centre	7	10
Home, not employed	9	2
Long-stay hospital	28	22
Total Children	63	61

TABLE 2

PLACEMENT AT FOLLOW-UP (CHILDREN AGED 16 YEARS OR OVER)

	Psychotic	Controls
Employed	2	12
Ordinary School	1	—
Special School	1	3
Village Trust	3	—
Senior training centre	4	6
Home, not employed	7	1
Long-stay hospital	20	14
Total Children	38	36

39 per cent among those who had passed their sixteenth birthday). However, there was a larger difference between the groups with regard to the proportion in paid employment (Tables 1 and 2). Of the 38 psychotic children aged 16 years or over only two had paid jobs, compared with 12 out of 36 control children. A few other psychotic children were doing some kind of potentially remunerative work—one girl did unpaid typing and duplicating at home, a boy helped in his father's shop, and three children did various jobs while living in a Village Trust. It appears that some of these and some others would have been capable of employment, at least in a sheltered setting, had adequate training facilities been available.

Five psychotic children attended an Industrial Rehabilitation Unit, but the Units are not really designed to aid handicapped school leavers who have never been in employment, and attendance proved to be of

TABLE 3

Social Adjustment at Follow-up

Adjustment	Psychotics No.	%	Controls No.	%
Normal	1 }	9 (14)	7 }	20 (33)
Good	8 }		13 }	
Fair	16	(25)	19	(31)
Poor	8	(13)	7	(11)
Very poor	30	(48)	15	(25)
	63		61	

x^2 (for trends) = 9.37, p < .01

limited value. One of these five children obtained a job following attendance at an I.R.U. course, but the other four were told that there were no suitable jobs for them, poor concentration and poor work habits being cited as reasons. Nevertheless, one boy was later found a job by his parents through their contacting local factories. More recently (after the comparison given in Table 2 was made) one more of the five who went to an I.R.U. has also obtained regular work. This boy had attended an ordinary school and then a senior training center.

2. Overall social adjustment

Adjustment at follow-up was assessed in terms of the child's general level of social competence at that time. A rating of 'good' was made when the child was leading a normal or near-normal social life and was functioning satisfactorily at school or at work. Adjustment was termed 'fair' if the child was making social and educational progress in spite of significant, even marked, abnormalities in behavior or interpersonal relationships. 'Poor' was rated when the child was severely handicapped and unable to lead an independent life, but where there was still some measure of social adjustment and it was felt that some potential for social progress remained. Adjustment was rated 'very poor' when the children were unable to lead any kind of independent existence.

As shown in Table 3 there was a marked and highly significant difference in the social adjustment of the two groups at follow-up. Twice as many control children as psychotic children were rated as well adjusted and half as many were poorly adjusted. Nine of the psychotic children (14 per cent) had a good adjustment, but all but one of these still showed some oddities of personality. A quarter showed a fair adjustment. In five

of the 16 children rated 'fair' only a persisting and isolated major handicap prevented a higher rating. Two children remained without any
useful speech, although nearly normal in all other respects. Two other
children were chiefly handicapped by poor speech and limited intelligence, and the fifth child by a lack of education and by a preoccupation with fantasy. Some of these children and some of the 8 children
(13 per cent of the total psychotic group) who were rated 'poor' were
still making a little progress and might reach a better level of adjustment when older, but nearly half the group (18 per cent) were very
poorly adjusted and showed no indication that they were capable of any
kind of independent life.

3. Schooling

A high proportion of the psychotic children had had very little schooling. Twenty-one never attended school and a further six had less than
six months schooling in all. An additional four children attended school
in one of the hospital units for psychotic children but did not attend
any school outside hospital, and four more attended school for periods
lasting between 6 and 24 months. Thus, less than half the children (28
out of 63) had as much as two years' regular schooling.

Many of the children who had not been to school were mentally subnormal (sometimes severely so) as well as psychotic, but the relationship
between IQ level and schooling was not very close. As well as several
children scoring between 50 and 70 on IQ tests who did not go to
school, there were five children whose IQ was at least 70 who had less
than two years' schooling (two had had no schooling). Two of these five
children had considerable behaviour problems which would have made
schooling difficult (although children as seriously disturbed have attended school quite successsfully). However, two children (IQ 78 and
85) had been regarded as ineducable in early childhood, and in spite of
becoming easily manageable and eager to learn neither was admitted to
school. One of these two children has just recently started school at 12
years, after the follow-up assessment was made, but the other boy was
excluded from school at 6 years and never re-admitted. His father
taught him to read (his reading when assessed at follow-up was at a well
above average level) but his knowledge of arithmetic and other subjects
remained rudimentary through lack of instruction.

The educational progress of the children is dealt with more fully elsewhere (Rutter, 1967; Lockyer and Rutter, in preparation). However,
it should be noted here that the educational achievements of the psy-

chotic children and the control children were closely similar. About a quarter (15 psychotic children and 17 control children) were reading at an 8-year level and better at follow-up. Nevertheless, in both groups most of the children's educational achievements were well below that expected on the basis of their age and measured IQ. There were a few striking exceptions, and the number of 'O' levels was roughly appropriate for the IQ distribution (Rutter and Lockyer, 1967). Only one of the 63 psychotic children has passed the 'O' level examinations. One other child has not yet reached the appropriate age for the examination but is expected to pass in at least one or two subjects. An additional psychotic child followed-up but not included in the psychotic-control comparisons (because his records were not found until after the matching had been completed) has also passed in one 'O' level subject. Thus it seems likely that, at most, only 3 (5 per cent) of the 64 psychotic children seen between 1950 and 1958 will obtain 'O' levels.

4. Treatment

Most of the psychotic children who were seen at the Maudsley Hospital received their main treatment elsewhere. The treatments employed were extremely heterogeneous and included prolonged courses of daily psychoanalytic psychotherapy, short-term or supportive psychotherapy of various kinds, a variety of drugs, E.C.T. (1 case), insulin coma (1 case), leucotomy (1 case), family counselling, periods of in-patient care in various units for psychotic children, speech therapy, and retraining techniques. In addition, several children received various unorthodox treatments from unrecognized medical therapists and some received little beyond routine long-term institutional care. The study was not designed to evaluate the effects of different forms of treatment, but an attempt was made to relate the outcome to the type of treatment used. The analysis was greatly complicated by the fact that during the course of the follow-up period several therapeutic procedures had been employed with most children. The isolated cases who had E.C.T., insulin coma or leucotomy were either not improved or worse after the treatment. Otherwise all forms of treatment seemed to have much the same rate of success and failure. Thus there was no predictable relationship between the form of treatment and the type of outcome. The only exception was the effect of schooling (see below). However, it should be emphasized that the study was in no sense a therapeutic trial, so that these findings must be regarded with considerable caution.

TABLE 4

Course of Individual Behavioral Characteristics
in Psychotic Group

Characteristic	Loss of Characteristic	Improved	No change	Worse	Development of behavior during follow-up	Not known
Autism	9	24	16	6	0	2
Withdrawal	15	2	1	1	2	—
Disturbed relations:						
Peers	1	35	22	4	1	—
Parents	7	27	15	7	1	5
Speech retardation	9	15	31	6	1	—
Morbid attachments	7	5	4	1	9	—
Morbid preoccupations	9	11	4	3	10	—
Non-adaptability	11	8	3	2	11	2
Obsessive phenomena	8	6	6	3	7	2
Stereotyped mannerisms	13	16	12	3	5	—
Aggression	20	6	2	2	7	—
Anxiety or Fears	19	7	8	4	2	—
Self-injury	7	2	6	1	7	—

5. *Developmental course of individual behavioral characteristics*
(a) *"Autism"*

All the psychotic children had marked difficulties in relationships with other people in early and middle childhood, those with other children being almost always worse than those with adults. In about a quarter to a third of the psychotic group the abnormalities in relationships remained much the same as the child grew older, but more often there had been a considerable improvement by the time of adolescence. Even so, only one child had fully normal peer relationships at follow-up, and only 7 had fully normal relationships with adults.

In nearly all the psychotic children the abnormality in inter-personal relationships was 'autistic' in type (as defined in Rutter and Lockyer, 1967). In over half the psychotic group the 'autism' became less marked during the follow-up period, and in 9 cases the children could no longer be termed 'autistic' at follow-up. In view of the generally held view that the speech and intellectual difficulties are secondary to 'autistic' withdrawal it is important to note that the loss of "autism" was not necessarily associated with improvement in other handicaps, and it was not associated with any marked improvement in intellectual functioning. In fact the IQ rose in only 4 cases and fell in 5. One of the children who ceased to be autistic was normal at follow-up, another one had a 'good' adjustment, five had a 'fair' adjustment and two a 'poor' adjustment. None had a 'very poor' adjustment.

Five children whose 'autism' improved became somewhat outgoing and jovial in personality (although shallow and lacking empathy). Much more characteristically they remained very reserved, lacked warmth, had little social "know-how" and seemed unaware of the feelings of others. This lack of empathy or social perceptiveness sometimes led the children to make outrageous or tactless remarks—usually accurate but embarrassing observations of the type common in the normal young child. For example, an intelligent 17-year-old girl commented "what a *very* ugly baby" when introduced to the newly produced offspring of a friend of the family. Typically this remark was made without any sense of mischief—just lack of appreciation that this was an inappropriate remark for such an occasion and an unawareness that the comment might prove hurtful to the other person. Similarly other children would often inform mere acquaintances of intimate details of whatever happened to interest them at the time without realizing that it might not be socially acceptable to do so (for example one girl had a phase of informing people whenever she menstruated, and a boy liked to tell everyone exactly what his father earned and what everything in the house cost). In the same way the children usually could not discern when they were being teased or when a remark was made in jest, so that they recounted 'tall' stories without realizing that they were not true.

Socially embarrassing behavior probably developed in the same way. For example, an intelligent adolescent boy came down completely nude when his parents were giving a party, in order to ask where his pajamas were. Similarly, an adolescent on a picnic with some family friends stood up and urinated in full view of the company—again a lack of understanding of how other people felt and how they would react to his behavior.

(b) *Physical withdrawal*

Actual physical withdrawal from people was not particularly common in psychotic children at any age (present in a third of the group), but when it occurred it was nearly always a feature of early childhood. Only 5 of the 63 psychotic children showed physical withdrawal at follow-up.

(c) *Speech*

About half (31) the psychotic group showed neither improvement nor deterioration in speech, and altogether 29 were without useful speech at the time of follow-up. Seven children were rated as having worse speech at follow-up than at first hospital attendance, but in only four of these children was there a *marked* change. In three of the four the deterioration in speech was associated with the onset of epileptic fits in adolescence.

For example, 'A' was a boy whose first symptoms were nocturnal screaming attacks and rocking at about age 15 months. His development was particularly retarded with regard to relationships and to speech, there being no recognizable words until nearly 3 years. About age 4 years he became increasingly autistic and fearful, and when seen at the Maudsley Hospital at age 8 years he was severely autistic. He had a habit of playing with plasticine which he made into small balls and placed in neat symmetrical rows. His speech was of normal complexity and he had a good vocabulary. However, he talked to himself all the time, tended to speak in song and often echoed words and phrases. He was manneristic, mildly overactive, and extremely fearful and anxious. His IQ was 65. At the age of 15 years he was admitted to a mental subnormality hospital, at which time he was markedly echolalic but talked constantly. The next year he began rocking vigorously all day long and spoke less. Aged 19 he had a grand mal fit and also became more overactive. Nearly a year later there was one more fit. When seen at follow-up, aged 21 years, he was rather detached, spoke only occasional single words, would follow few instructions and rocked a great deal. His SQ was 28 and his WAIS Performance scale IQ was 46.

At the other end of the spectrum there were several children without any speech when first seen at hospital who developed useful speech during the follow-up period. Eisenberg (1956) found only one child in the Johns Hopkins series who developed speech after the age of 5 years, and stated that the prognosis was very bad for the child without useful speech at that age. In contrast, of the 32 children without speech at 5 years in the present investigation no fewer than 7 subsequently gained speech—one at 5½ years, one at 6 years, one at 7 years, two at 8 years, and two at 11 years. However, the child's IQ made a big difference to the prognosis. Of the 22 children without speech at 5 years, and with an initial IQ of 59 or less, only two gained speech. Only one of the two (a boy of IQ 56) made much use of his speech, and apart from this boy none was receiving schooling. Three-quarters of these non-speaking children with an IQ below 60 were in long-stay hospitals at follow-up and their adjustment was mainly very poor. There were 10 children without speech at 5 years whose initial IQ was at least 60. In two children the IQ (65) was based on only a very few subtests, and both later repeatedly scored in the idiot range of intelligence; neither gained speech and both were in mental subnormality hospitals at follow-up. However, of the 8 children with an initial IQ of 60 or above, but without speech at 5 years, 5 subsequently gained speech and 4 ceased to be 'autistic.' The poor outcome in children without speech at 5 years seemed to be related as much to their low IQ as to any factor more specifically related to speech.

The pattern of speech development in the children who improved was fairly consistent. In infancy and very early childhood the child not only did not speak but also appeared relatively unresponsive to sounds of all kinds. He did not respond when called by name, appeared not to understand what was said to him, and sometimes was regarded as deaf. Babbling was often reported as diminished in quantity, but the vocalizations had a normal tone quality. Response to sounds was always first to improve; the child gradually paid more attention to what was said to him, became able to follow instructions and to understand the speech of others. Vocalizations then became more frequent and more meaningful and occasionally there was a phase in which the child spoke in a meaningful way, but in which his language was largely idiosyncratic. Generally the child's speech gradually improved in quantity, quality and complexity, but in some cases speech seems to have developed in large steps with the sudden appearance of formed sentences, giving the impression that the child could have spoken earlier if he had been motivated to do so. In the early stages of speech development, and sometimes for much longer, extending into later childhood and adolescence, much of the speech was echolalic, with persisting pronominal reversal. Of the children who gained useful speech, three-quarters were echolalic, and over half showed persisting confusion of 'I' and 'you.' The echoing was both immediate and delayed—the children tended to echo what was said to them and would also repeat out of context stereotyped phrases they had heard from other people or from the television.

About two-fifths of the children who developed speech had some articulation difficulties for a while, but in the majority these were merely consonant omissions and substitutions of the type commonly found in association with immature or infantile speech. However, five children had more marked and persistent articulation difficulties, sometimes associated with a lack of facility in tongue movement.

Ten of the 63 psychotic children achieved a normal level of speech development, 4 of these had abnormalities of delivery, as did 7 other children. Some had a monotonous flat delivery with little lability, change of emphasis or emotional expression. In others, speech was staccato and lacking in cadence and inflections. The overall effect was often a kind of 'mechanical' speech like that given to visitors from other planets in children's television programs.

Finally, as speech improved, not only were there often abnormalities in delivery but also there were abnormalities in the child's use of speech. Frequently there was a formality of language and a lack of ease in the use of words leading to a pedantic way of putting things. Often, too, the children tended to converse mainly by a series of obsessive questions related to the child's particular preoccupation at that time. Most handicapping was the continuing difficulty with abstract concepts. The children tended to give over-literal and concrete answers to questions, scored poorly on the comprehension sub-test of the Wechsler scales, and had difficulty with school subjects that involved more than rote memory. It was particularly striking that some of the children who had been markedly delayed in their speech development in early childhood became verbally very fluent, and in adolescence their intellectual skills were largely verbal and mathematical. This pattern was confined to a small sub-group of intelligent, clumsy, psychotic children (Rutter, 1966b). In spite of their verbal fluency they continued to have difficulty with abstract concepts and logical argument.

As noted above, there were a few children who improved markedly in all respects except that they remained entirely without useful speech. These were all children who had been profoundly unresponsive to sounds and had often been regarded as deaf for prolonged periods.

For example, 'B' was a girl of 5 years when first seen at the Maudsley Hospital. She had been markedly autistic from early infancy, was profoundly unresponsive to sounds, and had been diagnosed as severely deaf by an audiologist at a London teaching hospital. Her motor development was fairly normal, but she was entirely without speech. She appeared uninterested in people and did not play with other children at all. She was anxious, grossly hyperkinetic, constantly cleaning, dressing and undressing herself. She resisted changes of any kind, and had a curious way of walking with her hands out in front of her as if she were blind. There were frequent episodes of aggression and destruction. Her co-operation on psychological testing was very poor, but she passed several items on the Merrill-Palmer at just below her age level and her IQ was estimated to be about 65. She was an in-patient for a year and was then transferred to a school for deaf children. Two years later it became apparent that she was not deaf and she was transferred to a hospital unit for psychotic children and then at the age of 12 years to a residential school. She gradually improved in her behavior and relationships, but continued to do things according to fixed routines and had little expression of emotion. She was seen at follow-up when she was aged 17 years. She was still entirely without speech and her understanding of speech remained limited. Apart from lack of speech her chief problem was inertia and under-activity. She was friendly, sought the company of people, and was particularly attached to the house-mother at the school. There were several children with whom she associated, but she had no particular friends. Things continued to be done according to a routine, and changes caused her to be upset, although less than previously. She was able to perform all the necessary household chores and was self-sufficient. There were a few fears, and she tended to get in a temper if teased. At interview she was friendly and co-operated, but was strikingly lacking in spontaneity or emotional response. Her WAIS IQ on the performance scale was 49.

(d) Ritualistic and compulsive behavior

Most of the psychotic children tended to become more adaptable and malleable as they grew older, and *marked* protest at environmental change was less common at follow-up. However, although resistance to change, abnormal preoccupations, morbid attachments or collections and other obsessive phenomena tended to diminish somewhat by adolescence, in only a minority of the children had the characteristic gone altogether. Furthermore, in a substantial minority of the psychotic group these characteristics developed for the first time during the follow-up period (see Table 4)—usually about the age of 6 or 7 years. As might be expected there was also a tendency for ritualistic and compulsive phenomena to become more complex as the children grew older. In most cases, although obsessive characteristics often increased in middle childhood, there was usually a diminution again in adolescence.

(e) Aggression and self-injury

Many younger psychotic children were aggressive, and a few were admitted to hospital in middle childhood primarily because of a concern over possible (never actual) injury to brothers or sisters. Aggression towards a parent was also a concern in a few psychotic children about the age of 11 or 12 years. The problem at that time was usually related to the children becoming bigger, with a consequence that childish aggression was more difficult to control, rather than to any significant increase in the frequency or severity of aggressive behavior. Aggression was really serious in only two of the older children; both were fairly intelligent girls who were admitted to hospital in early adolescence because of aggressive behavior. One of these girls had severely frightened her mother by threatening behavior but had not actually hurt anyone. The other girl had attacked other hospital patients and is still in a maximum security hospital. In both children the aggression diminished after a year or so and neither is aggressive now.

A tendency to self-injury often diminished as the children grew older, but just as often it increased in the early teens and it was a severe problem in a few adolescents. Self-injury, together with other symptoms, sometimes got worse about the time of puberty only to improve again in later adolescence.

(f) Sexual difficulties

At the time of follow-up no psychotic children had yet shown any mature heterosexual interests, and there were very few sexual difficulties of any kind. A few of the older children were beginning to show some interest in the opposite sex, but many appeared to have no interest.

Three children exhibited childish sexual difficulties when they were first seen (masturbating other children and taking off their trousers to examine their genitals) but none of these three children had sexual problems at follow-up when adolescent. Two other adolescents (both in long-term institutional care) showed sexual problems at the time of follow-up—one masturbated in public and the other boy caused difficulties by homosexual advances to other patients.

(g) Delusions and hallucinations

Several adolescent children continued to have childish fantasies, but all distinguished between reality and make-believe and no child was thought to have delusions. A few children behaved in an odd manner which gave rise to the suspicion that they were having hallucinatory experiences, but in none was there convincing evidence of hallucinations, and no child with speech described sensations or happenings which were hallucinatory.

(h) Hyperkinesis

Marked hyperkinesis was a common feature of both the psychotic and non-psychotic disorders and it followed a similar developmental sequence in both groups. Usually the severe overactivity shown in early and middle childhood was gradually replaced during middle and later childhood by a mixture of over- and underactivity and finally by an inert under-activity in which the children appeared markedly lacking in any

TABLE 5

ACTIVITY LEVEL: INITIAL AND FOLLOW-UP (PSYCHOTIC CHILDREN)
(Children aged 13 years or more at follow-up)
Activity Level at Follow-up

		Hyperkinetic	Hypokinetic	Mixed	Normal	Total
Initial Activity Level	Hyperkinetic	3	13	4	4	24
	Hypokinetic	0	2	1	3	6
	Mixed	0	1	0	0	1
	Normal	2	5	0	12	19
	Total	5	21	5	19	50

TABLE 6

ACTIVITY LEVEL: INITIAL AND FOLLOW-UP (CONTROL CHILDREN)
(Children aged 13 years or more at follow-up)
Activity Level at Follow-up

		Hyperkinetic	Hypokinetic	Mixed	Normal	Total
Initial Activity Level	Hyperkinetic	3	10	0	6	19
	Hypokinetic	0	0	0	1	1
	Mixed	0	0	0	1	1
	Normal	5	7	0	19	31
	Total	8	17	0	27	52

drive or impetus to do anything. They tended just to sit unless constantly prodded to continue with their tasks. However, when they did move they moved at a normal pace—thus it was an underactivity rather than any slowing of movement. This underactivity, lack of drive and lack of initiative was perhaps the most prominent of all the problems of the adolescent psychotic children and was often the chief factor preventing employment.

Of 24 psychotic children hyperkinetic at the time of first hospital attendance and aged at least 13 years at follow-up, 13 had become hypokinetic and 4 were in a state varying between hyperkinesis and hypokinesis. Of 19 children originally normokinetic only 5 were hypokinetic at follow-up. A similar trend was seen in the control group, where 10 children out of the 19 originally hyperkinetic had become hypokinetic at follow-up, in comparison with 7 out of the 31 initially normokinetic children. The sequence of hyperkinesis to hypokinesis is even more marked if only those children markedly hypokinetic at follow-up are considered. Pooling both groups, there were 19 children markedly hypokinetic at follow-up, and of these 13 had been hyperkinetic initially.

(i) *Epileptic fits*

Of the 63 psychotic children, 10 developed fits for the first time during the follow-up period, many years after the onset of psychosis. Fits began at 6-7 years in two children, 11-13 years in four children and at 16-19 years in another four children. None of these 10 children exhibited neurological abnormalities when first seen, but it was noteworthy that these children were mostly mentally subnormal as well as psychotic; 8 had an IQ below 60 when tested on first referral to hospital. One of the two more intelligent children regressed in speech, intelligence, and behavior at about the time fits began, but the other child has continued to do well and is making good progress in school. Altogether, in 3 of the 10 children who developed fits the onset of fits was associated with a marked deterioration in speech.

All the fits were major in type, and in all cases the fits were relatively infrequent so that most of the 10 children had only four or five attacks in all.

Nearly as many control children (7) also developed fits during the follow-up period, and again this was more frequent among the control children of low intelligence.

(j) *Other behavior*

In general, most children became more adaptable and were easier to deal with after adolescence, although the children were sometimes temporarily more disturbed during early adolescence. Of all the symptoms, anxiety, fears, eating and sleep disturbances improved most markedly, and in the majority of cases these symptoms were a real problem only during infancy and early childhood. However, as with other behaviors, occasionally they increased in severity, and in a very few cases they appeared for the first time in middle or late childhood.

4. *General course of psychotic disorder*

Although there was a variability in the child's progress at different times, with plateaus, peaks and troughs, it was quite rare to see marked remissions and relapses as in adult psychotic illnesses. From middle childhood onwards the course was usually fairly regular (apart from an occasional disturbance about the time of puberty), with a continuation of the improvement or deterioration evident by then. Nevertheless, there were some exceptions. The late deterioration associated with the onset of fits has already been mentioned. In addition there were two or three children who regressed long after the onset of psychosis and who had never had any fits.

One of these was 'C,' who was first seen at the age of 4 years and in whom the psychosis appeared to have a somewhat later onset than usual. Some behavior difficulties were apparent from age 1 year, but these became more marked when he was 2½ years. He became quieter, talked less and developed numerous fears. His relationships were autistic, there were various obsessive rituals and preoccupations and he had a habit of smelling objects. There was some echolalic phrase speech, he was considerably hyperkinetic and showed some aggression towards other children. His IQ on the Merrill-Palmer was 59. At 6 years he started school, and at the age of 9 years his WISC IQ was 52. Up to then his speech and interpersonal relationships were improving and behavior difficulties had diminished. Then, about the age of 10 years he became noisy and excitable and a year later quiet and underactive. He lost interest in things and showed increasing obsessive questioning and touching. He was readmitted to hospital at 12 years, being then isolated, ritualistic, manneristic, and echolalic; phases of withdrawal alternated with restlessness and aggressive behavior. He was untestable on the WISC. A year later he was transferred to a mental subnormality hospital. At 16 years his IQ on the Binet was 38. On follow-up at age 17 years, he was detached, emotionally flat, remarkably hypokinetic, manneristic and with only a little echolalic speech. His Vineland SQ was 28 and his WAIS Performance IQ was 39.

If marked improvement was to occur it was usually evident by the age of 6 or 7 years, but occasionally important changes took place later, such as in 'D,' a boy who first began to talk at the age of 11 years. He first attended the Maudsley Hospital at 5 years, having failed to develop speech and having shown 'autistic' withdrawal from early infancy. He showed a marked lack of response to sounds and had been thought deaf. Paradoxically he also appeared distressed by loud noises and put his hands to his ears. He had a habit of touching people's eyes and had periods of special attachments and preoccupations (e.g. collecting cans). His IQ on the Merrill-Palmer test was 85. About the age of 6 years he became more restless and overactive and was constantly in trouble for meddling with things (playing with petrol pumps, flooding a farm by turning on all the taps, etc.) and he had a phase of constantly opening doors. He attended a training center from age 7 years and started being treated by an 'osteopath' shortly after that. There was a gradual improvement from about that time; he became more responsive to sounds, would follow instructions, made better relationships with people and ceased to have any behavior problems. When seen at follow-up, aged nearly 11 years, he was still at a training center, without any abnormalities of behavior but still without any speech. He was bright, alert, observant, friendly and responsive and communicated remarkably well by gesture. There was no trace of autism, although he was still without friends of his own age. In the next year he began to have intensive speech therapy and started at school. When seen again at 12 years he was talking, using sentences and had a fair vocabulary. Although still considerably retarded in speech he was making rapid progress.

5. *Factors related to outcome*

There were four main variables which showed important associations with outcome in the psychotic group. These were IQ, speech, severity of disorder, and amount of schooling. The IQ was chiefly of value in distinguishing the children with a 'poor' or 'very poor' social adjustment at follow-up, whereas the other variables were more useful in differentiating those with a 'good' adjustment from those with a 'fair' adjustment. Among the major variables which were *not* related to outcome were the sex of the child (although there was a slight tendency for girls not to fall into either the 'good' or 'very poor' adjustment groups), the presence or absence of a period of normal development prior to the onset of psychosis, evidence of brain injury, and the family situation. Children in whom there was evidence suggesting the probable presence of brain injury made as much (or as little) progress as children in whom there was no evidence of brain injury. However, there was a slight (but non-significant) tendency for children who developed fits in adolescence to fall more frequently into the 'very poor' adjustment group at follow-up.

Unfortunately it was possible to consider only limited aspects of the family situation in relation to prognosis. Neither a history of mental illness in a parent nor the presence of a 'broken home' (i.e. the child *not* living with his natural parents) bore any relation to outcome. However, parental attitudes and behavior towards the child were not measured, and it may be that these would have been found to be of prognostic value. It should also be noted that the majority of the children were cared for in residential schools or in long-stay hospitals so that there was only a limited opportunity for the family characteristics to impinge on the child.

Of all the items related to outcome, the most important was the child's response to IQ testing. Of the 63 psychotic children, 19 were completely untestable on any IQ test even after several sessions and the use of several different tests of cognitive function. Of these 19 untestable children, 18 were very poorly adjusted at follow-up, thus constituting over half (60 per cent) of the 'very poor' adjustment group. The association between no scorable response to an IQ test and social outcome is statistically significant (e.g. critical ratio for difference between proportions 'poor' versus 'very poor' = 3.05, p<.01). The only untestable child to have a better outcome was also the only untestable child to have a Vineland social quotient of over 60.

There was a significant trend (among the testable children) for a higher IQ (or SQ) score when first seen at the Maudsley Hospital to be associated with a better social adjustment at follow-up, the range extending from a mean IQ of 45 for the 'very poor' adjustment group to a mean IQ of 83 for the 'good' adjustment group. The difference in mean IQ between the 'good' and 'fair' adjustment groups was not significant, and the difference between the 'fair' and 'poor' and the 'poor' and 'very poor' groups fell just short of significance (t = 1.82 and 1.79 respectively, p<.10), but the difference between the 'fair' and the 'very poor' groups was highly significant (t = 6.3, p<.01).

A sharper differentiation was possible when the initial IQs were split into those above and those below 60. Whereas the great majority of the 'poor' group (75 per cent) and the 'very poor' group (83 per cent) had an IQ below 60, only one child in the 'fair' group (6 per cent) and no child in the 'good' adjustment group had an IQ as low as that. Thus the IQ very sharply differentiated between the children with either 'poor' or 'very poor' adjustment and those with 'good' or 'fair' adjustment (critical ratio = 3.68 comparing 'fair' and 'poor' groups, p<.001).

A lack of response to sounds so profound that at some time it had been suspected that the child was deaf, and a lack of useful speech by age 5 years, were both of prognostic significance. There is a moderately strong association between these two variables, and it is probable that both are measures of the severity of language disorder. Whereas IQ was the most efficient predictor of poor outcome, the speech variables more effectively distinguished between children with a 'good' adjustment at follow-up and those with a 'fair' or worse outcome. No child in the 'good' adjustment group had shown a profound lack of response to sounds, compared with between a quarter and a half the children in the other groups

TABLE 7

FACTORS RELATED TO SOCIAL ADJUSTMENT AT FOLLOW-UP

Item	Social Adjustment at Follow-up							
	Good		Fair		Poor		Very poor	
	No.	%*	No.	%*	No.	%*	No.	%*
Sex: proportion of girls	0	(0)	6	(38)	3	(38)	3	(10)
Parental mental illness or 'broken home'...	3	(33)	4	(25)	1	(13)	8	(27)
Normal Development prior to onset								
psychosis: Definite	1	(11)	5	(31)	1	(13)	6	(20)
Possible	2	(22)	4	(25)	3	(38)	7	(23)
Probable 'brain damage'	3	(33)	3	(18)	2	(25)	10	(33)
Late onset of fits	1	(11)	0	(0)	1	(13)	7	(23)
IQ less than 60	0	(0)	1	(6)	6	(75)	25	(83)
Untestable	0	(0)	1	(6)	0	(0)	18	(60)
Mean IQ (of those testable)	83		74		59		45	
At least 2 years' schooling	9	(100)	10	(63)	3	(38)	6	(20)
Marked lack of response to sounds	0	(0)	8	(50)	2	(25)	14	(47)
Useful speech at 5 years	9	(100)	9	(56)	5	(63)	8	(27)
Retardation of speech at least moderate...	4	(44)†	7	(78)†	4	(80)†	6	(75)†
Echolalia	4	(44)†	8	(89)†	4	(80)†	7	(88)†
Autism: moderately severe	3	(33)	10	(63)	8	(100)	26	(87)
any	7	(78)	13	(81)	8	(100)	29	(97)
Withdrawal: moderately severe	2	(22)	5	(31)	3	(38)	6	(20)
any	2	(22)	6	(38)	3	(38)	8	(27)
Disturbed relationship: peers:								
moderately severe	6	(67)	14	(88)	8	(100)	29	(97)
any	9	(100)	16	(100)	8	(100)	30	(100)
Rituals or compulsions: moderately severe..	2	(22)	9	(56)	4	(50)	15	(50)
any	5	(56)	13	(81)	8	(100)	25	(83)
Hyperactivity: moderately severe	2	(22)	3	(18)	4	(50)	13	(43)
any	4	(44)	10	(63)	6	(75)	21	(70)
Mannerisms: moderately severe	1	(11)	6	(38)	3	(38)	18	(60)
any	6	(67)	7	(44)	5	(63)	26	(87)
Aggression: moderately severe	4	(44)	10	(63)	5	(63)	11	(37)
any	5	(56)	13	(81)	8	(100)	23	(77)
Anxiety: moderately severe	1	(11)	4	(25)	3	(38)	7	(23)
any	5	(56)	9	(56)	5	(63)	17	(57)
Eating disorder: moderately severe	1	(11)	5	(31)	2	(25)	10	(33)
any	2	(22)	8	(50)	5	(63)	15	(50)
Sleeping disorder: moderately severe	0	(0)	3	(18)	4	(50)	4	(13)
any	2	(22)	7	(44)	4	(50)	10	(33)
Mean Symptom Score	14		24		28		25	
Total number of children	9		16		8		30	

* The % figures refer to the proportion of children in each social adjustment category having the item in question (listed on the left-hand side of the table).
† % of children with some speech.

(the difference between the 'good' and 'fair' groups is statistically significant, C.R. = 2.57; p<.02). Similarly the difference between the 'good' and 'fair' groups with regard to the proportion lacking useful speech at 5 years was also statistically significant (C.R. = 2.34, p<.02). Although there is a fairly close association between IQ and level of speech development, it is unlikely that IQ differences can account for these findings, as the difference in IQ between the 'good' and 'fair' groups was small and not statistically significant. Furthermore, the association between IQ and speech was most marked in the under 50 IQ group, which was unrepresented in either the 'good' or 'fair' adjustment groups. On the other hand, the nearly significant difference (C.R. = 1.90, p<.06) between the 'poor' and 'very poor' groups with regard to the proportion without useful speech at 5 years is more likely to be merely a reflection of the demonstrated IQ difference between these two groups.

With all the major symptoms, there was a tendency for the symptom to be less frequently exhibited and less severely exhibited in the group of children with 'good' adjustment at follow-up. None of the differences between the groups concerning individual symptoms were statistically significant, and apart from the lack of response to sounds and the presence or absence of speech at 5 years already mentioned no one symptom appeared to be more related to outcome than the others. However, summating the major symptom ratings (each symptom was rated on a 5-point scale) to obtain a total symptom score, the difference between mean total score of the 'good' adjustment group (14) and the 'fair' adjustment group (24) was statistically significant (t = 3.4, p<.01).

The amount of schooling experienced by the child was the only other item related to outcome. All the children in the 'good' outcome group had attended school for at least two years compared with only 63 per cent of the 'fair' group, 38 per cent of the 'poor' group, and 20 per cent of the 'very poor' group. In view of the association between a child's IQ and the likelihood of his receiving schooling, this association must be regarded with caution. However, as already noted, several intelligent children did not attend school for as long as two years, and the IQ difference between the 'good' and 'fair' adjustment groups was small and not significant. Thus it appears that schooling probably did have some effect on the child's social adjustment in adolescence and early adult life—at least in so far as it influenced the likelihood of the child having a 'good' rather than a 'fair' outcome.

DISCUSSION

The overall outcome of infantile psychosis in the present study of

Maudsley Hospital cases was closely similar to that found in the follow-up of Kanner's cases (Eisenberg, 1956) and of Creak's cases (Creak, 1962; 1963a and b). Only a minority of psychotic children reach a good level of social adjustment by the time of adolescence, and very few enter paid employment. About half remain incapable of any kind of independent existence and most of these are cared for in mental subnormality hospitals.

Although the generally poor prognosis for children with infantile psychosis has been amply demonstrated, there are also grounds for a limited optimism. In particular, it was notable that there were some psychotic children who made substantial progress. The progress made must be regarded as a minimal estimate of what progress *can* be made, since the provision of education and treatment was often very inadequate, and there was evidence that the amount of schooling received by the child influenced his later social adjustment (as well as his educational attainments).

A quarter of the psychotic group were able to read at an 8-year level or better. It was especially striking that the scholastic attainments of the psychotic children were as good as those of a control group of children of similar age, sex and IQ, but with non-psychotic disorders of emotions or behavior. Few psychotic children progressed as well as might have been expected on the basis of their IQ level, but nevertheless two boys achieved 'O' levels and another boy is expected to do so. It should also be noted that two of these three children had been regarded as mentally defective when young (although this was not confirmed by psychological testing at the Maudsley Hospital). It must be emphasized, however, that in spite of comparable scholastic progress of psychotic and control children, the overall social adjustment of the psychotic group was considerably worse, and very few psychotic children were in paid work. In part this was related to the continuing behavior problems of the psychotic child—in particular his inactivity, inertia, poor concentration and poor work habits, but to a considerable extent the rather disappointing work record of the psychotic group may be attributed to the grave deficiency of training facilities for the handicapped school leaver. Of course, it remains an open question how far the inertia and poor work habits of the psychotic child can be overcome by a suitable training program.

Less than half the group of psychotic children received as much as two years' schooling, and many received no schooling whatsoever. It is probable that some of those who did not attend school were so severely handicapped that it would be unreasonable to expect appreciable scholastic progress. On the other hand, among those who did not have schooling there were several children within the normal range of intelligence and with only mild behavior difficulties. There can be no doubt that these children should have received education. But, also, most workers would accept that even markedly retarded children should receive a substantial trial period at school before it is concluded that they cannot benefit from the usual educational measures. This was rarely available for the children in the present study. In addition, it has been previously demonstrated that the quality of care provided for even the severely subnormal child makes a considerable difference to his social and intellectual progress (Tizard, 1965).

It has been shown that the amount of schooling received by the psychotic child is related to the level of his social adjustment when he reaches adolescence. In part his association may be merely a function of the relationship between a child's IQ and the likelihood of his receiving schooling. On the other hand, several intelligent children did not go to school, and the main effect of schooling seemed to lie in the differentiation of the 'good' and 'fair' adjustment groups—groups which did not differ significantly in mean IQ. Further indirect evidence in favor of the beneficial effects of schooling is provided by comparison of the present study with that reported by Eisenberg (1956). The two studies are closely comparable in nearly all respects, the one important exception being that, whereas the children in Eisenberg's investigation who were not speaking at 5 years had a very poor outcome, in the present study there were several examples of children who gained speech after 5 years and made fair progress. In all cases the late acquisition of speech occurred at a time when the child was receiving good schooling and/or speech therapy, and it appears likely that the somewhat better results in this respect in the present study may be due to better schooling.

It was found that the psychiatric and psychological assessment of young psychotic children can provide data of considerable prognostic importance. Of all the items, the child's response to IQ testing is probably the most important. The child who is untestable (provided that he is tested by a psychologist experienced in the testing of psychotic children, that several sessions have been given to testing and that suitable tests have been used) has a very poor prognosis, and the child with an IQ below 60 is also unlikely to have a good outcome. Unfortunately, the relationship between IQ and outcome was not reported in either the Eisenberg study or the Creak study, the two investigations which concerned children most comparable to those in the present series. However, three other studies which include cases of infantile psychosis provide some support for the present findings. Mittler, Gillies, and Jukes (1966) found that no psychotic child with an IQ below 50 or untestable on admission to the Smith Hospital later attended any school within the educational system. Brown (1960), in a follow-up study of 'atypical' children, found that 'little appropriate use of toys' (an item which probably reflected a low IQ) was the variable most strongly associated with a poor outcome. In a follow-up study of a heterogenous group of psychotic children, Annell (1963) found that stereotypes and an IQ below 80 were indicators of poor prognosis.

The prognostic significance of the severity of language disturbance has been mentioned by several writers. Eisenberg (1956) found that children without useful speech at 5 years had a much worse outcome than those with useful speech at that age, and Creak (1962) commented on the bad prognosis associated with a prolonged failure in speech development. Brown (1960) found that when atypical children 'excluded stimuli,' especially acoustic stimuli, the prognosis was poor. This item appears comparable to the item 'profound lack of response to sounds' which was related to a poor outcome in the present study. Brown (1960) also found that children who remained without speech after the age of 3 years did less well than other children. In the same study, children with a severe disorder did less well than those with a milder disorder. Accordingly, other studies, although not always comparable in methods or diagnostic criteria, provide support for the finding that the most important prognostic factors are the child's response to IQ testing, his response to sounds, his level of speech at 5 years, the overall severity of the psychosis and, probably, the amount of schooling he receives.

The findings are also relevant to a consideration of the nature of infantile psychosis. The high frequency with which the psychotic children developed fits during adolescence strongly suggests the importance of 'organic' neurological factors. It should be noted that none of these children had any abnormality on a neurological examination when first seen at the Maudsley Hospital. The development of fits was particularly common among the children whose IQ was below 50 or 60. It is well known that many mentally subnormal children become epileptic, and indeed the control children (in whom overt brain damage was common) developed fits almost as frequently as did the psychotic children. Thus the development of fits does not differentiate the psychotic child from the child with severe subnormality or with brain 'damage,' but it clearly distinguishes him from the child with a psychogenic disorder.

Severe hyperkinesis was found to be a symptom with a particularly characteristic developmental course. Children *hyper*kinetic in early childhood frequently became *hypo*kinetic in adolescence. Hyperkinesis is known to be common among children who are mentally subnormal, and it is much more frequent in boys than girls (Birch, 1964). These facts, together with the fairly consistent progression from hyperkinesis to hypo-kinesis, suggest that this behavioral feature is linked with physiological rather than psychological variables—perhaps with some aspect of brain maturation.

It has often been thought that the psychotic child's intellectual and speech difficulties are secondary to his autistic withdrawal—that he *can* speak and function efficiently but doesn't because of profoundly impaired interpersonal relationships. However, it was found that when the children ceased to be autistic they did not necessarily show improvement in other handicaps; in particular, they did not show any marked improvement in intellectual functioning. Also, there were several children who, in spite of great improvement in behavior and in social relationships, still remained without speech. Therefore it seems improbable that the psychotic child's handicaps are due mainly to social withdrawal.

The importance of IQ and speech development in relation to prognosis suggests that cognitive and language defects may also be basic in the development of infantile psychosis. Stronger evidence in favor of a basic language defect is provided by the patterns of cognitive functions in psychotic children. This issue has been briefly considered in previous papers (Rutter, 1965, 1966b) but will be more fully discussed in papers to be published on the psychological findings in this group of children with infantile psychosis.

SUMMARY

The 63 children with infantile psychosis who attended the Maudsley Hospital between 1950 and 1958 were individually matched for age, sex, IQ and year of attendance with a control group of children with non-psychotic disorders of emotions or behavior. Both groups were re-examined by the authors in 1963-64 and given individual psychiatric, neurological, social and psychological assessments. The social outcome at follow-up of the psychotic children was significantly worse than that of the control children, especially with regard to the proportion in paid employment. The developmental course of autism, speech, ritualistic and compulsive behavior, aggression and self-injury, hyperkinesis and other behavioral characteristics of the psychotic children are described. The general course of infantile psychosis is outlined and it is noted that 10 of the 63 psychotic children developed fits in adolescence. Children who were untestable on any IQ test or had an IQ below 60 had a poor outcome. A severe disorder, and particularly a severe retardation of language development as shown by a profound lack of response to sounds and lack of useful speech at 5 years were also indicators of a less than good prognosis. The amount of schooling received by the psychotic child was related to the level of his social adjustment at adolescence. The often inadequate treatment and education provided is noted and it is suggested that there are grounds for a limited optimism that with better facilities somewhat better results might be obtained

Acknowledgments—We are most grateful to the many physicians who allowed us to see their patients and to the many schools, training centres and other institutions which gave us every co-operation. The study was supported in part by a grant from the Medical Research Council. Psychological aspects of the study formed part of a thesis submitted for a Ph.D. by Miss Lockyer.

REFERENCES

ANNELL, A. L. (1963). "The prognosis of psychotic syndromes in children: a follow-up study of 115 cases." *Acta psychiat. Scand., 39,* 235-297.

BIRCH, H. G. (ed.) (1964). *Brain Damage in Children: the Biological and Social Aspects.* Baltimore: Williams & Wilkins.

BROWN, J. L. (1960). "Prognosis from presenting symptoms of pre-school children with atypical development." *Amer. J. Orthopsychiatry, 30,* 382-390.

CREAK, M. (1962). "Juvenile psychosis and mental deficiency." In: Richards, B. W. (ed.) *Proc. London Conf. Scient. Stud. ment. Def.,* Vol. 2. Dagenham: May & Baker.

———— (1963a). "Schizophrenia in early childhood." *Acta paedopsychiat., 30,* 42-47.

———— (1963b). "Childhood psychosis: a review of 100 cases." *Brit. J. Psychiat., 109,* 84-89.

EISENBERG, L. (1956). "The autistic child in adolescence." *Amer. J. Psychiat., 112,* 607-612.

—— and KANNER, L. (1956). "Early infantile autism, 1943-55." *Amer. J. Orthopsychiat., 26,* 556-566.

GRAHAM, P. J., and RUTTER, M. L. (1968). "The reliability and validity of the psychiatric assessment of the child: II. interview with parents." *Brit. J. Psychiat., 114.* (In the press.)

KANNER, L. (1943). "Autistic disturbances of affective contact." *Nerv. Child., 2,* 217-250.

———— (1949). "Problems of nosology and psychodynamics of early infantile autism." *Amer. J. Orthopsychiat., 19,* 416-426.

—— and EISENBERG, L. (1955). "Notes on the follow-up studies of autistic children." In: Hoch, P. H., and Zubin, J. (eds.) *Psychopathology of Childhood.* New York: Grune and Stratton.

—— and LESSER, L. I. (1958). "Early infantile autism." *Ped. Clin. N. America, 5,* 711-730.

LOCKYER, L., and RUTTER, M. (1967). "A five to fifteen year follow-up study of infantile psychosis. III. Psychological and educational outcome." (In preparation.)

MITTLER, P., GILLIES, S., and JUKES, E. (1966). "Prognosis in psychotic children: report of a follow-up study." *J. ment. Def. Res., 10,* 73-83.

RUTTER, M. L. (1965). "The influence of organic and emotional factors on the origins, nature and outcome of childhood psychosis." *Develop. Med. Child. Neurol., 7,* 518-528.

———— (1966a). "Prognosis: psychotic children in adolescence and early adult life." In: Wing, J. K. (ed.) *Childhood Autism: Clinical, Educational and Social Aspects.* London: Pergamon Press.

RUTTER, M. L. (1966b). "Behavioral and cognitive characteristics of a series of psychotic children." In: Wing, J. K. (ed.) *Childhood Autism: Clinical, Educational and Social Aspects.* London: Pergamon Press.

———— (1967). "Schooling and the 'autistic' child." *Special Education, 16,* 19-24.

RUTTER, M. L., and GRAHAM, P. J. (1968). "The reliability and validity of the psychiatric assessment of the child. I. Interview with the child." *Brit. J. Psychiat., 114.* (In the press.)

—— and LOCKYER, L. (1967). "A five to fifteen year follow-up study of infantile psychosis. I. Description of sample." *Brit. J. Psychiat., 113,* 1169-1182.

TIZARD, J. (1965). *Community Services for the Mentally Handicapped.* London: Oxford University Press.

29

EARLY CHARACTERISTICS OF MONOZYGOTIC TWINS DISCORDANT FOR SCHIZOPHRENIA

James R. Stabenau, M.D.
National Institute of Mental Health, Bethesda, Md.
and
William Pollin, M.D.
National Institute of Mental Health, Bethesda, Md.

In the attempt to understand why schizophrenic symptoms appear in one individual and not in another, major investigative efforts have been directed toward: (1) assessing the genetic component which controls the cellular and physiological characteristics of the central nervous system, thereby influencing what is called temperament, nervous disposition, personality, or mind; (2) assessing the environmental experiential factors which temper the degree of development and expression of the personality; or (3) the complex interaction of endowment and environment.

The study of pairs of monozygotic twins, when one twin has developed schizophrenic symptomatology and the other has not, has the unique research power of controlling for the genetic differences which occur between siblings and randomly selected individuals. Differences in environmental experience from the intra-uterine period through the onset of illness are therefore highlighted in these pairs.

Characteristics of an infant at birth, the classically designated time for the "beginning" of life, already encompass the effects of intra-uterine

Reprinted from Archives of General Psychiatry, Vol. 17, December 1967, pp. 723-734.

experience. What might be considered the "inherited-genetic" temperament or personality (tense/placid, active/quiet, irritable/calm) is already a product of a nature and nurture interplay. Monozygotic twins with presumed identical genetic makeup, as estimated by blood-group typing and fingerprint pattern similarity, show many physical similarities at birth. However, based on differences in intra-uterine nutritive experience and positioning, there are differences in size and degree of maturity within most pairs. Further differences, such as the ease of the birth process and subsequent secondary effects of relative immaturity, may lead to a variety of physiologic changes which differ significantly in the two twins, and may have substantial consequences. One example would be brief periods of anoxia or hypoglycemia in one twin. These may subsequently lead to differences in level of activity, and hence differences in what is seen as neonatal "personality." Thus, two individuals of similar genetic potential will be seen to possess different characteristics shortly after birth, and upon first presentation to their parents and the world.

Of major interest is the effect these early differences have upon the parents, how the parents react to these "different," "identical" twins, and how the parents' different reactions to each twin serve to reinforce or influence their subsequent behavior patterns.

With the importance of detailed knowledge of the degree of neonatal maturity and early experience in mind as determinants in personality development, this report will consider early characteristics of monozygotic twins discordant for schizophrenia, based on 86 cases reported in the world literature, and the case material from the National Institute of Mental Health (NIMH) study of schizophrenia in monozygotic twins.

METHODS

Fourteen pairs of monozygotic twins discordant for schizophrenia, along with their parents, were intensively studied at the National Institutes of Health (NIH). Detailed descriptions of the study and the methodology have been reported.[1, 2] Identical blood-group types for each member of a twin pair, along with similarity of fingerprints and anthropometric characteristics, served as presumptive evidence of monozygosity. A panel of two independent psychiatric consultants interviewed each twin separately. Their diagnostic impressions, coupled with detailed hospital records of the schizophrenic (S) index cases, were employed to decide on the presence and character of the schizophrenic symptoms for all twins. In this sample each index twin had been hospitalized for schizophrenic symptoms and was felt to have evidence for the classifica-

TABLE 1

CASE REPORTS, MONOZYGOTIC TWINS DISCORDANT FOR SCHIZOPHRENIA

Investigator	Year	Country	No. Cases	Sex M	Sex F	Sampling* Method	Zygosity†
Grillmayr	1929	Austria	1		1	CR	No
Burkhardt	1929	Germany	1		1	CR	Yes
Wigers	1934	Norway	1	1		CR	Yes
Kasanin	1934	US	1	1		CR	No
Reed	1935	Canada	1		1	CR	No
Kallmann	1948	US	1		1	CR	No
Kallmann	1953	US	1		1	CR	No
Hobson	1964	US	1		1	CR	Yes
Total single case reports			8	2	6		
Rosanoff	1934	US	9	7	2	RH	No
Essen-Möller	1941	Sweden	6	3	3	CA	Yes
Slater	1953	UK	15	8	7	RH & CA	Yes
Kurihara	1959	Japan	26	8	18	R	Yes
Tienari	1963	Finland	16	16	0	BR	Yes
Kringlen	1964	Norway	6	6	0	RH & CA	Yes
Pollin, Stabenau	1966	US	14	4	10	R	Yes
Total cases			100	54	46		

* Resident hospital population (RH), consecutive hospital admission (CA), birth registry (BR), referral (R), case report (CR).
† Zygosity was determined by blood type and/or fingerprints.

tion as schizophrenic. In each of the 14 pairs the co-twin had neither been hospitalized for psychiatric problems, nor did the diagnostic panel feel there was evidence indicating a past or current schizophrenic reactive pattern. In order to locate pairs with such clear discordance of symptoms, a nonrandom and nonsequential sample of "volunteer" families would necessarily be produced. There are, however, studies from Sweden, the United Kingdom, Finland, and Norway of consecutive and more random samples of discordant monozygotic twin pairs.[3-6] Studies by Essen-Möller and Slater contain evidence on diagnosis and zygosity which is relatively satisfactory, but early life history material in their case reports is sparse and lacking in detail.[3, 4] Studies by Tienari and Kringlen, of male subjects only, have case history details which cover the birth and early personality characteristics of the twins, along with clear evidence for the consideration of diagnosis and zygosity.[5, 6] In addition, there are single case reports[7-14] and other studies of twin series.[1, 2, 15, 16]

A summary analysis was made for the material covering birth, neonatal, childhood, and pre-illness environmental experience from 100 pairs of monozygotic twins discordant for schizophrenia from our series and those reported in the world literature. The cases included were those in which zygosity, diagnosis, and discordance for schizophrenia were reasonably established. Table 1 lists the investigators, their countries, the number of cases, sampling method, and whether zygosity was determined by blood and/or fingerprints. The reports for these 100 pairs were reviewed for variables that appeared to distinguish the twins, which the parents used to differentiate or delineate early differences between the twins, or which the twins used in describing consistent differences between themselves. Twenty-six items were selected as those most often used by the case report authors to differentiate one subject from his co-twin by intrapair co-twin comparison. For the NIH sample verbatim quotes from tape-recorded interviews with both twins and their parents were used to designate a trait that distinguished one twin of a given pair from the other. Only when it was clearly described as a characteristic for one twin and not the other was a trait considered for the twin pair. Two problems frequently encountered in reviewing the published case reports were: investigators directed attention to certain variables with which others did not concern themselves; and investigators used different words to describe what appeared to have been the same variable. Where possible, the original author's description of the trait was used to judge its presence in the case material of another investigator.

RESULTS

The tabulation of the 26 characteristics is shown in Table 2. For each item, the number of twins is listed for whom the item clearly differentiated one twin from the other, index or control, by intrapair co-twin comparison. The items are ranked according to the ratio I/C and C/I for the schizophrenic indexes (I) and nonschizophrenic co-twin controls (C).

Characteristic of the pre-illness index twin were nine behavioral traits: submissive; sensitive; serious-worrier; obedient-gentle; dependent; well-behaved; quiet-shy; stubborn; and neurotic as a child; and six physical traits: having had a central nervous system illness as a child; any birth complication; neonatal asphyxia; weaker; shorter; and lighter at birth. The criterion employed here was that the designated trait was present for the index twins by a ratio of 2:1 or greater. Conversely, six traits: more intelligent; better at school; the spokesman; outgoing-lively; the leader; and married while co-twin remained unmarried, characterized

TABLE 2

MONOZYGOTIC TWINS DISCORDANT FOR SCHIZOPHRENIA:
EARLY CHARACTERISTICS*

Item	Other Studies I†	Other Studies C‡	NIMH Study I	NIMH Study C	Total I	Total C	Ratio (I/C)
Neurotic as child	11	1	5	0	16	1	16.0
Submissive	27	2	10	2	37	4	9.3
Sensitive	26	3	12	2	38	5	7.6
Serious-worrier	10	2	12	2	22	4	5.5
Obedient-gentle	21	2	10	4	31	6	5.2
CNS illness as child	12	2	5	2	17	4	4.3
Birth complication (any)	18	5	6	1	24	6	4.0
Asphyxia at birth	8	3	4	0	12	3	4.0
Dependent	2	0	10	3	12	3	4.0
Well-behaved	9	0	7	5	16	5	3.2
Quiet-shy	16	4	9	4	25	8	3.1
Stubborn	14	4	6	3	20	7	2.9
Weaker	16	10	11	1	27	11	2.5
Shorter	27	16	13	1	40	17	2.4
Lighter at birth	29	18	12	2	41	20	2.1
Slower development (walking)	3	1	6	4	9	5	1.8
Somatic illness as child	9	9	9	5	18	14	1.3
Second-born	27	29	10	4	37	33	1.1
Fiery	9	5	5	9	14	14	1.0
							Ratio (C/I)
Athletic	0	4	5	3	5	7	1.4
Leader	9	21	5	9	14	30	2.1
Outgoing-lively	8	26	5	9	13	35	2.7
Spokesman	4	11	3	11	7	22	3.1
Better at school	6	18	2	11	8	29	3.6
More intelligent	2	7	2	9	4	16	4.0
Married, co-twin not married	1	21	0	5	1	26	26.0

N pairs = 100.
* Number of twins clearly differentiated by intrapair co-twin comparison.
† Schizophrenic index twin (I).
‡ Nonschizophrenic monozygotic co-twin (C).

the controls. Five items: slower in development; somatic illness as a child; second-born; fiery disposition; and athletic did not serve as early characteristics which differentiated schizophrenic monozygotic twins from their nonschizophrenic co-twins to the described degree.

A graphic demonstration of the differential pattern in these early characteristics for the schizophrenic twins as compared to their non-schizophrenic co-twin controls was made by arranging the items accord-

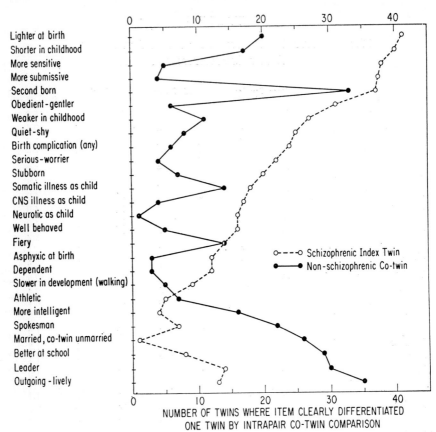

Differentiating characteristics of monozygotic twins discordant for schizophrenia (100 pairs).

ing to frequency of description for the index and then the controls (Figure).

The methodology employed in the NIMH Twin Study, ie, using family members to mutually evaluate and react to each other's historical account; family and community sources; and objective photography and written records, has given us considerable confidence in the data. It does remain, however, that a core of irreducible doubt regarding validity of the findings which is associated with any retrospective study still exists. The case material from the non-NIMH cases did vary with respect to the number of family members seen and the detail of information obtained. Nevertheless, the same trends that appear in the overall sample are found to a degree in each of the subsamples from such culturally different areas as Japan, the Scandinavian countries, the United Kingdom, and the United States of America.[2-6, 16] However, individual items discriminating between S and non-S co-twins, such as the association of lower weight at birth and subsequent development of schizophrenia, were not found to be equally present in all subsamples. Since the twins studied lived during a time span covering nearly 100 years and the reports issued from investigators of clearly hereditary to clearly environmental investigational bias, we feel with some confidence that these data are not primarily artifactual in nature, but do represent early underlying premorbid characteristics for schizophrenic twins.

COMMENT

We would like to construct a representative description of the life course of pairs of twins raised by their biological parents in intact family settings.

Using the NIMH series life history material which is available in sufficient detail and which is quite consistent with the accumulated world case literature, a tentative theoretical formulation might be made as to the phase-by-phase difference in personality development and life experience for pairs of monozygotic twins who become discordant for schizophrenia. The formulation will be divided into life periods during which major differences in life experience for the twins seemed most evident.

Fetal Intra-uterine Development.—Studies have shown that relative differences in intra-uterine nutritive environment (i.e., placental placement, anastomoses between placentas of the fetuses, cord embarrassment, and relative disadvantageous fetal positioning) may lead at birth to one of a monozygotic twin pair weighing less and being less mature or fully developed as compared to his co-twin.[17-19] Twins who share a common chorion, and especially those few also sharing a common amnion, are most likely to be born with excessive differences in maturity or development.

Material was available in 69 of the 100 case report pairs giving an indication which twin was lighter at birth or whether the twin weight was equal. For the schizophrenic index twins, 41 of 61 were lighter than their nonschizophrenic co-twins at birth ($P < 0.01$). Thus a statistically significant relationship between relative fetal maturity, as measured by birth weight, and the development of schizophrenia within discordant monozygotic twin pairs is apparent. The following will consider the possible intervening stages of development between birth and adulthood for such twins.

Birth Process.—More often the heavier of the twins is born first. The second, lighter one, is more often likely to experience periods of anoxic cyanosis during delivery or respiratory distress after delivery as a consequence of immaturity. The lighter, less mature twin, relative to his co-twin, often feeds less well, may display a lag in development, and may be seen as, and in fact often is, the weaker and slower of the two.[20-21] In contrast, the heavier twin, even when near or below the "premature" weight threshold, tends to be seen as the "healthy normal" twin, and indeed, does not require as extensive neonatal care, is less likely to have respiratory embarrassment, and does not teeter on the very brink of survival as often as his co-twin.

Early Biologic Differences (First Three Months).—Early in the first week or two, the mother often finds that the heavier twin nurses well and sleeps better, while the lighter twin (premature or near premature) is a feeding problem. His "natural" loss of weight following delivery places him in an even more precarious state. He usually cries more readily and is less easily calmed down or satisfied.

Graham et al, in a study of 81 infants suffering from transient periods of neonatal anoxia and 265 nonanoxic controls, found significant increases in pain threshold, irritability, and tension, and decreases in measures of maturation and visual capacity.[22] The syndrome of the dysmature infant may encompass neonatal anoxia[23] and hypoglycemia.[24] Recent analysis of the NIMH series of twins has shown that the adult protein-bound iodine value appears to be in part determined by the degree of maturity at birth, as measured by the birthweight.[20] Thus another variable to consider is the relative thyrometabolic state at birth, as it may directly influence the development of the central nervous system and indirectly influence subsequent somatic growth and intellectual development.

It does not seem to be just the biologic differences, but the feelings elicited in the parents that begin to shape the parent-child interaction. This excerpt and the following are from verbatim typescripts of the recorded first contact with the family, a group interview of the parents and both twins by the two NIMH investigators. The mother from family 9 stated,

> Actually when I think back, it's been all his life, even from the time he (index) was brought home from the hospital—hasn't had quite the placid disposition that (control) has. For a long time

(index) was lighter than (control)—not much but 7 or 8 lb until they were 13 or 14.

The mother from family 4 stated, regarding the period just after birth, "At first (index) was smaller and I think I fed her at first with an eye dropper." The same mother, commenting on the period from 6 to 12 months of age, stated,

> (Index) was more of a feeding problem than (control)—wouldn't swallow. She (index) would hold it in her mouth—would hold the food in her mouth—and I had that checked and there was nothing organically wrong. . . . Well, I think (control) always remained the heavier and a little taller—now I imagine they are about equal.

The mother from family 3 stated,

> During that spell there she (index) was a really small baby and she wouldn't eat the way you wanted her to—she would fall asleep all the time and you would have to keep waking her up and at certain times it got to be really bad and you really cried tears while you were feeding her. . . . I was worried about her (index). I always thought if a child didn't eat they were sick. I was concerned about her health because I felt that if she didn't get this food, that it really would make her ill.

Early Parent-Child Interaction (3 to 6 Months).—Thus, characteristic differences between monozygotic twins may be established in utero and during the birth process. Though present from birth, these differences primarily differentiate the parental response to each twin during the first six months. Moss, in a study of 30 firstborn children and their mothers by means of direct observation during the first three months of life, concluded that,

> . . . the state of the infant affects the quantity and quality of maternal behavior and thus in turn would seem to influence the course of future social learning.[25]

Knobloch, in a large-scale study of infants and mothers, has shown that the number of tense mothers increased with the degree of neurologic disturbance in the infant.[26] Many of the low birthweight twins are in actual peril of death. It has been shown that for some parents, reaction to the impending loss of a child modified their relation to that child; what followed was infantilization of the child, leading to overdependence on the parents.[27]

The very fact that one twin is slightly more vigorous and responsive than the other may lead to an unconscious splitting of ambivalent feelings toward the pregnancy, with the resultant direction of feelings of warmth and acceptance being directed toward the heavier, more "capable/healthy" infant, and a thinly repressed hostility and rejection toward the lighter, "weak" part of the pregnancy.

The mother from family 18 stated,

> I didn't think they'd live. They looked so tiny. . . . People said, "Oh, you're going to smother them." They used to whimper just a little weak whimper, not a real lusty cry like most babies, and I wanted them so badly—*one* baby anyway, or the two if it was going to be twins.

The mother from family 10 stated, "One of them (index) was fussy and worried and the other one going around doing everything (control)."

Thomas et al, in their studies of behavior, individuality, and early childhood, cite two cases in which mothers of twins showed differences in initial and subsequent patterning of reactivity.[28] In each family the mother started with the same general maternal attitude toward the two infants, but developed increasingly dissimilar affective bonds and responses to them as they grew older. Bayley and Schaefer report from the Berkeley Growth Study that, although they were unable to show consistent stability of maternal or child behavior over time, several correlations between the two were established.[29] Loving mothers had happier sons (at age 3), while the controlling, hostile mothers had excitable, unhappy sons. In adolescence, girls who are maladjusted (rated as gloomy, unhappy, sullen, and hostile) more often have mothers who are hostilely controlling, that is, punitive, irritable, controlling, isolating, and who make excessive contact with their daughters. Although no twins were reported studied, they note for two brothers separately studied that maternal behavior was markedly different toward each; it was never recognized by the blind raters that the mother was the same person. An additional feature for some families in the NIMH series was that during the early neonatal period the father was either psychologically or physically unavailable to the mother. Where relative intramarital dissatisfaction existed (that is, father felt mother was not strong enough under the load, or mother felt father was not providing the family enough of himself), the mother appeared to have been left with an inner sense of ineffectual rage that was directed away from the husband and was displaced toward the "weak, ineffective, helpless" twin. Seemingly the thought "I need you, husband" was transformed and directed toward the weak and helpless child as "You need me." This appeared to have further led to the development of a different parent/child relation for each twin.

Emergence of Individual Personality (Second Year).—While during the first six months early differences between the twins are of a more *biologic* nature, by age 12 to 24 months parents find differences in *behavioral* characteristics of the twins. The lighter at birth often appeared the fussier, more troublesome, more fragile, and more helpless. Studies of prematurity suggest some of this relates to maturational processes. Shirley has reported a behavior syndrome which characterizes prematurely-born children as showing: irascibleness, stubbornness, negativism, shyness, and overdependence on the mother.[30] The author states:

> Indications are that in family relations prematures differ from their siblings in being more jealous, less good to the siblings, and making more demands for attention, showing off and in being dependent and less self-reliant as they grow older. In general, prematures seem to try to preserve their status as over-protected and over cared-for members of the family group.

The parent may feel the need to do something special for the weaker twin, and thus have a different set of expectations for that child which will be perceived by that twin as being different from those for his heavier, stronger, healthier sibling. This may reinforce a feeling that for him there is something especially hazardous in the world about him. The feelings of internal disequilibrium, as experienced in the initial physiologic imbalance associated with the periods of respiratory distress and difficulty in assimilating food which characterized his first few hours of neonatal existence, may be projected onto the outside world to a greater degree during this period. Thus the environment might take on the appearance of a hostile, threatening, disorganized world. Characteristically at this age, for the pre-schizophrenic index twin, there has appeared a phase of worriedness and fearfulness. None of the nonschizophrenic co-twins in the NIMH series had been described in these terms.

From the study of families of normal monozygotic twins, not all twins with birth weight differences are reacted to in the above manner. As our sample of control families is too small, and as yet not optimally matched to the above sample, it would be premature to discuss this issue at this time.

During the twins' first few years, the parents in the discordant group often described finding little satisfaction in each other. There was frequently a lack of complementarity and support for each other which did not allow a full degree of communication and expression of affect between them. This is in contrast to the findings for normal families,[31] and is similar to the pattern that Caplan describes for parents when the crisis of premature birth was disruptive to the developing family.[32] A split between the parents may readily be perceived by the already sensitized, fearful youngster; i.e., one good and one bad parent, not too dissimilar from the parents' view of the twins. Incorporation and internalization of this split by the sensitive twin may add to his sense of internal confusion and faulty identity formation. Index from family 14 stated, "I had the fear if my mother should leave father where would it leave me."

Individuation Vs Dependence (Second to Sixth Year).—The heavier, stronger twin often begins to walk first, talk with more facility, and be capable of earlier mastery of complex coordinated tasks. Overall, there is an *expansion of differentiation* most noted in motoric mastery. On the other hand, the lighter twin, as a result of a relative developmental lag, is seen as less independent, less competent, and less secure, and therefore makes fewer attempts at ego-stretching experiences for fear of failure. A phase of ego restriction may then be seen to begin for him, though he often may have a more advanced verbal capacity than his co-twin.[33]

The details of the mutual interplay between biological competence of the child, the evoked parental response, and the child's response to the subsequent parental attitude is exceedingly complex and not within the proper scope of this paper. However, Levy and Kanner describe an aspect of this behavior ("maternal" overprotection) as excessive contact, treatment of the child as a baby for an inappropriate length of time (infantilization), and prevention of social maturation, that is, the mother not letting the child grow up.[34, 35] Subsequently, with little encouragement for exploration, the child clings to the mother for dependent support. The maternal reaction may take the form of either overindulgence or maternal domination. Harper, in discussing the special problem of the premature, speculates,

> A certain amount of the handling of the prematurely born is not related directly to the physical or physiologic hazards of low birthweight, but rather is an indirect result of the mother's apprehension and of her tendency to insulate him from the normal hazards of life.[36]

Sontag reports, from experience at the Fels Institute on mental growth and personality development, that:

From years 3 to 6 it would appear that the learning of broad patterns of behavior in relation to parents is of primary importance in establishing a foundation for later interaction with the environment. The child who is emotionally dependent upon his parents during these years would appear to be establishing a mode of behavior which is not conducive to the "learning to learn" during this time. However, if the child is learning to meet some of his needs, through appropriate aggressive behavior, competitiveness or individual problem-solving, it would appear that he is laying groundwork for the kind of motivation characterized in need for achievement which may operate as a motive in learning experiences.[37]

Not all parents respond to initially premature children in this manner. Gifford, in a longitudinal direct study of a pair of normal premature monozygotic twins, notes,

The smaller twin's relative 'immaturity' in birth weight but not in gestational age, followed by a maturational lag in motor coordination, might be interpreted as a constitutional basis for the advantageous ego characteristic of social responsiveness, which has proved to have enduring qualities. In contrast, the larger twin's maturational lead in motor development which might be related to the character traits of perseverence, self-sufficiency, became a disadvantage in the early part of the second year, when she showed some depression and regressive imitation of her twin. But this disadvantage was temporary and she has retained her superiority in motor skill and co-ordination.[33]

Social Competence and Self-Esteem (Sixth Year to Adolescence).—The more socially competent, heavier twin turns to peers, and his sense of identity and self-image improves as overt signs of confidence appear in the attainment of better school grades as compared to his co-twin, and in significant and continued peer relations. The heavier twin at birth usually is the longer and continues to be slightly taller in adulthood.[38] For normal twins, Shields has documented a significant positive direct relationship between height and IQ.[39] Other studies have shown that in twins of disparate birth weights, the low-weight twins have significantly lower IQ and impaired performances as compared to their heavier monozygotic co-twins.[40-42] Large-scale longitudinal studies of prematures by Wiener et al, have revealed "Premature twins are psychologically impaired," and "The degree of impairment increases with decreasing birth weight." Further,

Perceptive motor disturbances, flaws in comprehension and abstract reasoning, perseveration trends, poor gross motor development, immature speech and impaired IQ significantly identified low birth-weight children.[43]

DeHirsch et al report,

> Prematurely born children whose IQ fell within the average range of intelligence did less well than maturely born peers on a large battery of tests administered at kindergarten age. While they showed some indication of a "catching up" during the years between kindergarten and end of second grade, significant lags persisted well onto the eighth year of life.[44]

Lane and Albee, in a study of schizophrenics, their siblings, and normals, have shown that schizophrenics during childhood scored significantly lower in IQ than their own siblings, as well as normal nonschizophrenic children.[45] This evidence may demonstrate that the defect in intellectual functioning in schizophrenia (perhaps secondary to disturbances in attention and perception related to faulty object relations, subtle central nervous system dysfunction, or both) occurs in a period before the onset of overt symptomatology of adult schizophrenia. On the other hand, it may indicate that such a reduced function may play a contributory part in the process leading to the subsequent development of schizophrenia.

During this period, from 6 to adolescence, first major separation of twins in school or in summertime activities becomes an issue, and often points up the dependence of the lighter twin upon the heavier. Following the early period of worry and self-doubt and the first experience of less efficacy, there is an intensified dependence upon the co-twin which precedes, but also overlaps, the heavier twin's turning to "others." Thus, as the heavier twin turns to others for expansion of ego by identification with them, that is, leaving the twinship, the lighter clings dependently to the twinship, restricting attempts to relate to others.

Separation (Adulthood).—In late adolescence and early adulthood there are periods of separation of long duration for the twins. Here there often is a collapse of the dependency of the lighter on the heavier twin as the heavier moves toward individuality, i.e., becomes the one to dress differently, have different friends than his co-twin, and as he begins a stable heterosexual relationship. As noted in the case material (Table 2), in 26 instances where the schizophrenic index had not married, his co-twin had married.

The lighter twin often responds by withdrawal and makes abortive attempts to duplicate the co-twin's success through inappropriate choices of friends, situations, etc., resulting in failure and suggesting that the lighter twin has begun a lifelong repetition-compulsion of being in the inferior position. Another psychodynamic view is that a unique co-twin transference is manifest in that all significant figures are heretofore reacted to as being "more successful, more competent," leaving the index with an intensified feeling of low self-esteem and reduced efficacy. The index in family 7 stated: "I was more or less the black sheep or something," while the index in family 8 said, "I was skinny when I was little, I was the typical 90 lb weakling." The role of efficacy in the development of schizophrenia has been poignantly described by White.[46]

Further, the heavier twin's successes and pride in his accomplishments act to reinforce the feeling of inadequacy in the lower birth weight index. In many pairs, a move of the family home or the loss of a significant family figure during this period has led to an accentuation of insecurity in that the customarily taken-for-granted minor, but supportive, relationships are in one fell swoop removed from the lighter, less secure twin. The heavier recoups, however, by leaving his twin and relating more to peers, accentuating a sense of loneliness and despair in the lighter twin. Often, disorganization, withdrawal, and schizophrenic symptomatology develop in the lighter birth weight twin at just this time, i.e., when the heavier, more differentiated twin is making a sudden spurt in the development of an individual identity and the establishment of heterosexual and genital level of personality organization. In a retrospective study, Prout and White have reported personality trait differences similar to those noted in this report between schizophrenic and nonschizophrenic siblings. Independence and rebelliousness characterized the control adolescent sibling, while the preschizophrenic adolescent was often dependent, scared, quiet, and unsociable. Further, though both schizophrenic and nonschizophrenic individuals underwent personality change during the adolescent period, for the healthy siblings the change was in a positive direction, toward increased responsibility, while for the preschizophrenic there was more self-involvement, sensitization, and seriousness.[47] Planansky, in a careful review of the character structure of nonschizophrenic monozygotic co-twins as reported in the literature, concluded that typical schizophrenia can be paired with all types, including schizoid, neurotic, and nonpathologic personality patterns.[48]

Thus, by late adolescence distinctions between the preschizophrenic monozygotic twin and his sibling have developed through the interplay of early nongenetic biologic, parental attitudinal, interactional, social, and environmental experimental differences. The review of monozygotic twins discordant for schizophrenia has produced an aggregate of descriptive terms describing early characteristics which seem to differentiate the schizophrenic from the nonschizophrenic co-twin. Other studies of retrospective nature provide similar differentiating features which characterize the preschizophrenic; but, as in our review, the data must be considered to bear the imprint of the bias of recall at a time when the

pathology already exists.[49, 50] Pollack et al reduced the source of error
from investigator bias by blindly analyzing characteristics for 33 schizophrenics and their nonschizophrenic siblings.[51] They found,

> The schizophrenic patients were more irritable and more shy than
> their siblings from as early as the 2- to 5-year period. They were
> rated higher on chronic worrying or unhappiness; they were more
> shy and dependent, had more neurotic traits and conduct problems,
> and they were more often rated as non-affectionate during the 5 to
> 12 year period. The patients in the group performed less well in
> school than their siblings and had more difficulty relating to their
> peers.

A study from the Judge Baker Center in Boston suggests that these
findings differentiating schizophrenic from nonschizophrenic siblings, as
reported in the numerous different retrospective investigations of families of schizophrenics, have validity. Child guidance center records for
children who later became schizophrenic, and records from matched
control children who were nonschizophrenic in adulthood, were reliably
judged and compared blindly. The pre-schizophrenics were found to be
preoccupied, self-conscious, embarrassed, insecure, tense, or worried,
and more often they related feelings of being overcome with anxiety,
vulnerability, defenselessness, isolation, being unloved, and unable to
communicate with others.[52] A current prospective investigation by Mednick and associates has compared 25 children, born to schizophrenic
mothers and raised by them, to 25 children matched in age and sex,
who at the average age of 19 months were separated and reared apart
from their psychotic mothers. They found the former children significantly different from the latter in being more shy, withdrawn, and un-
engaged as judged independently by their school teachers.[53]

While the description of the preschizophrenic state has been more
sharply characterized, the exact nature of possible causes and their interplay is only beginning. It appears from the material in this report that
differences in early biologic maturity relate to differences in competence,
which in turn appear related to the development of schizophrenic symptomatology.

Studies by Bender, Goldfarb, and Vorster suggest that for childhood
schizophrenia, and perhaps for a subgroup of adult schizophrenics,
subtle impairment of the central nervous system may be of significant
etiologic importance.[54-56]

However, as indicated in this report as well as in the work of Wynne,
Lidz, Bowen, Jackson, and Laing, it is the understanding of the interplay between innate capacities of the child and environmental, familial,

and social forces that may best explain the development of schizophrenia in one child and not another.[57-61] Thus, the yield from these current investigative efforts may be in designating more clearly the variables which describe the population in which high risk for schizophrenia exists, and in which a prospective longitudinal lifetime study of such individuals may lead to the more complete understanding of causal relationships.

REFERENCES

1. Pollin, W.; Stabenau, J.; and Tupin, J.: Family Studies With Identical Twins Discordant for Schizophrenia, *Psychiatry* 28:60-78, 1965.
2. Pollin, W., et al: Life History Differences in Identical Twins Discordant for Schizophrenia, *Amer. J. Orthopsychiat.* 36:492-509, 1966.
3. Essen-Moller, E.: Psychiatrische Untersuchungen an einer Serie von Zwillingen, *Acta Psychiat. Scand.*, vol. 16 (suppl. 23), 1941.
4. Slater, E.: *Psychotic and Neurotic Illnesses in Twins,* London: Her Majesty's Stationery Office, 1953.
5. Tienari, P.: Psychiatric Illnesses in Identical Twins, *Acta Psychiat. Scand., 39* (suppl. 171), 1963.
6. Kringlen, E.: Schizophrenia in Male Monozygotic Twins, *Acta Psychiat. Scand.,* vol. 40 (suppl. 178), 1964.
7. Grillmayr, W., and Kohlmann, T.: Diskordante Psychiatrische Bilder bei einem eineiigen Zwillingspaar, *Wien Z Nervenheilk* 2:441-460, 1929.
8. Burkhardt, H.: Uber ein Diskordantes eineiigees Zwillingsparr, *Z Neurol. Psychiat.* 121:B77-282, 1929.
9. Wigers, F.: Ein Eineiiges, Bezüglich Schizophrenie Diskordantes Zwillingspaar, *Acta Psychiat. Neurol.* 9:541-556, 1934.
10. Kasanin, J.: A Case of Schizophrenia in Only One of Identical Twins, *Amer. J. Psychiat.* 91:21-28, 1934.
11. Reed, G.: Uniovular Twins: Schizophrenia and Tuberculosis, *Canad. Med. Assoc. J.* 32:180-182, 1935.
12. Kallmann, F. J.: "Heredity and Constitution in Relation to the Treatment of Mental Disorders," in Hoch, P. (ed.): *Failures in Psychiatric Treatment,* New York: Grune and Stratton, Inc., 1948.
13. Kallmann, F. J.: *Heredity in Health and Mental Disorder,* New York: W. W. Norton and Co., Inc., 1953.
14. Hobson, J. A.: Identical Twins Discordant for Schizophrenia, *J. Nerv. Ment. Dis.* 138:432-442, 1964.
15. Rosanoff, A., et al: The Etiology of So-Called Schizophrenic Psychosis, With Special Reference to Their Occurrence in Twins, *Amer. J. Psychiat.* 91:247-286, 1934.
16. Kurihara, M.: A Study of Schizophrenia by the Twin Method, *Psychiat. Neurol. Jap.* 61:1721-1741, 1959.
17. Price, D.: Primary Biases in Twin Studies: A Review of Prenatal and Natal Difference-Producing Factors in Monozygotic Pairs, *Amer. J. Hum. Genet.* 2:293, 1950.
18. Morison, J.: Congenital Malformations in One of Monozygotic Twins, *Arch. Dis. Child* 24:214-218, 1949.
19. Sydow, G., and Rinne, A.: Very Unequal "Identical" Twins, *Acta Paediat. 47:* 163-171, 1958.
20. Stabenau, J., and Pollin, W.: Maturity at Birth and Adult Protein Bound Iodine, *Nature* 215:996-997 (Aug. 26) 1967.

21. STABENAU, J.; POLLIN, W.; and MOSHER, L.: A Study of Monozygotic Twins Discordant for Schizophrenia: Some Biologic Variables, *Arch. Gen. Psychiat.*, to be published.

22. GRAHAM, F.; MATARAZZO, R.; and CALDWELL, B.: Behavioral Differences Between Normal and Traumatized New Borns: I. The Test Procedures: II. Standardization, Reliability and Validity, *Psychol. Monogr. 70:*20-21, 1956.

23. CLEMETSON, C.: The Difference in Birthweight of Human Twins and Twin Blood Studies: I. Oxygen Analysis of Umbilical Cord Blood, *J. Obstet. Gynaec. Brit. Comm. 63:*1-8, 1956.

24. CORNBLATH, M.; JOASSIN, G.; and WEISSKOPE, B.: Hypoglycemia in the Newborn, *Pediat. Clin. N. Amer. 13:*905-920, 1966.

25. MOSS, H.: Sex, Age and State as Determinants of Mother-Infant Interaction, *Merrill-Palmer Quart. 13:*19-36, 1967.

26. KNOBLOCH, H.: The Developmental Behavioral Approach to the Neurological Examination in Infancy, *Child Develop. 33:*181-198, 1962.

27. GREEN, M., and SOLNIT, A.: Reactions to the Threatened Loss of a Child: A Vulnerable Child Syndrome, *Pediatrics 34:*58-66, 1964.

28. THOMAS, A., et al: "Behavior Individuality in Early Childhood," in Haimowitz, M., and Haimowitz, N. (eds.): *Human Development,* New York: Thomas Y. Crowell Co., 1966.

29. BAYLEY, N., and SCHAEFER, E.: "Maternal Behavior and Personality Development: Data From the Birth and Growth Study," in *Psychiatric Research Reports of the American Psychiatric Association,* No. 13, 1960.

30. SHIRLEY M.: A Behavior Syndrome Characterizing Prematurely Born Children, *Child Develop. 10:*115-128, 1939.

31. STABENAU, J., et al: A Comparative Study of Families of Schizophrenics, Delinquents and Normals, *Psychiatry 28:*45-59, 1965.

32. CAPLAN, G.: Patterns of Parental Response to the Crisis of Premature Birth, *Psychiatry 23:*365-374, 1960.

33. GIFFORD, S., et al: Differences in Individual Development Within a Pair of Identical Twins, *Int. J. Psychoanal. 47:*261-268, 1966.

34. LEVY, D. M.: *Maternal Overprotection,* New York: Columbia University Press, 1943.

35. KANNER, L.: *Child Psychiatry,* Springfield, Ill.: Charles C Thomas, Publisher, 1957.

36. HARPER, P.: "Comments on the Prevention of Prematurity," in *Fifth Conference on Physiology of Prematurity,* New York: Macy Foundation, 1961, pp. 218-221.

37. SONTAG, L.; BAKER, C.; and NELSON, V.: Mental Growth and Personality Development: A Longitudinal Study, *Monogr. Soc. Res. Child Develop. 23* (2):1-143, 1958.

38. TANNER, J.: *Growth at Adolescence,* Oxford: Blackwell Scientific Publications, 1962.

39. SHIELDS, J.: *Monozygotic Twins Brought Up Apart and Brought Up Together,* London: Oxford University Press, 1962.

40. BABSON, S.. et al: Growth and Development of Twins of Dissimilar Size at Birth, *Pediatrics 33:*327-333, 1964.

41. DRILLIEN, C.: The Incidence of Mental and Physical Handicaps of School-Age Children of Very Low Birthweight, *Pediatrics 27:*452-464, 1961.

42. CHURCHILL, J.: The Relationship Between Intelligence and Birthweight in Twins, *Neurology 15:*341-347, 1965.

43. WIENER, G., et al: Correlates of Low Birth Weight: Psychological Status at Six to Seven Years of Age, *Pediatrics 35:*434-444, 1965.

44. DeHIRSCH, K.; JANSKY, J.; and LANGFORD, W. S.: Comparisons Between Prematurely and Maturely Born Children at Three Age Levels, *Amer. J. Orthopsychiat. 36:*616-628, 1966.

45. LANE, E., and ALBEE, G.: Early Childhood Intellectual Differences Between Schizophrenic Adults and Their Siblings, *J. Abnorm. Soc. Psychol. 68:*193-195, 1964.

46. WHITE, R.: "Ego and Reality in Psychoanalytic Theory, A Proposal Regarding Independent Ego Energies," in *Psychological Issues*, New York: International Universities Press, 1963, vol. 3, No. 3.

47. PROUT, C., and WHITE, M.: The Schizophrenic's Sibling, *J. Nerv. Ment. Dis. 123:* 162-170, 1956.

48. PLANANSKY, K.: Schizoidness in Twins, *Acta Genet. Med. Roma 15:*151-166, 1966.

49. LU, Y.: Mother-Child Role Relations in Schizophrenia: A Comparison of Schizophrenic Patients With Non-Schizophrenic Siblings, *Psychiatry 24:*133-142, 1961.

50. McGHIE, A.: A Comparative Study of the Mother-Child Relationship in Schizophrenia, *Brit. J. Med. Psychol. 34:*195-221, 1961.

51. POLLACK, M., et al: Childhood Development Patterns of Hospitalized Adult Schizophrenic and Non-Schizophrenic Patients and Their Siblings, *Amer. J. Orthopsychiat. 36:*510-517, 1966.

52. FLEMING, P.: Emotional Antecedents of Schizophrenia: Inner Experiences of Children and Adolescents Who Were Later Hospitalized for Schizophrenia, read before the Conference on Life History Research in Psychopathology, New York, May 12, 1967.

53. MEDNICK, S., and SCHULSINGER, F.: A Pre-Schizophrenic Sample, *Acta Psychiat. Scand 40:* (suppl. 180)135-146, 1964.

54. BENDER, L.: "Twenty Years of Clinical Research on Schizophrenic Children With Special Reference to Those Under Six Years of Age," in Caplan, G. (ed.): *Emotional Problems of Early Childhood*, New York: Basic Books, 1955.

55. GOLDFARB, W.: *Childhood Schizophrenia*, Cambridge: Harvard University Press, 1961.

56. VORSTER, D.: An Investigation Into the Part Played by Organic Factors in Childhood Schizophrenia, *J. Ment. Sci. 106:*494-522, 1960.

57. WYNNE, L., et al: Pseudo-Mutuality in the Family Relations of Schizophrenics, *Psychiatry 21:*205-220, 1958.

58. LIDZ, T., et al: Intrafamilial Environment of the Schizophrenic Patient: VI. The Transmission of Irrationality, *Arch. Neurol. Psychiat. 79:*305-316, 1958.

59. BOWEN, M.: "A Family Concept of Schizophrenia," in Jackson, D. D. (ed.): *The Etiology of Schizophrenia*, New York: Basic Books, 1960.

60. JACKSON, D.: *The Etiology of Schizophrenia*, New York: Basic Books, Inc., 1960.

61. LAING, R., and ESTERSON, A.: *Sanity, Madness and the Family*, London: Tavistock Publications Ltd., 1964.

30

PERCEPTUAL AND MOTOR DISCRIMINATION IN PSYCHOTIC AND NORMAL CHILDREN

Beate Hermelin
and
N. O'Connor

Institute of Psychiatry, Maudsley Hospital, London

A. INTRODUCTION

Describing the syndrome of childhood psychosis, clinicians have emphasized the apparent inability of affected children to structure and make appropriate use of sensory stimuli. Experimental results have supported this view, showing that such children have greater difficulties than either normal or subnormal controls in solving discrimination problems (see Hermelin and O'Connor[6] and Gillies[3]). On the other hand, the relatively good motor abilities of such children have been noted[4, 11] and experimental results have suggested that tasks in which motor performance predominates are easier learned by them than are tasks with strong visual components.[5, 6] This seems to suggest differential impairment of input compared with output mechanisms. While visual discrimination may require the integration of sensory input, organization of output might be more important in the learning of motor habits.

Experiments with animals, such as those of Warren,[14, 15] suggest that position learning may not depend on the same pattern of abilities required by visual discrimination tasks. There also exist interspecies differ-

Reprinted from THE JOURNAL OF GENETIC PSYCHOLOGY, 1967, *110*, pp. 117-125. Copyright, 1967, by The Journal Press.

ences in the facility with which different discrimination problems are solved. Rats and cats learn position discrimination faster than object discrimination.[1, 10, 13] For subnormal human subjects, House and Zeaman[7] and Zeaman and House[16] found that position discrimination was easier to learn than either color or shape discrimination tasks. In the following experiment normal and psychotic children of like mental age were compared for their ability to solve length discrimination and position discrimination problems.

As normal children were thought to be more efficient in the processing of visual information than were psychotics, the former might be expected to achieve a better level of performance than the latter on a length discrimination task. On the other hand, this same characteristic of the normals—i.e., the awareness of visually presented length differences— might make it more difficult for the latter than for the psychotics to ignore the negative length dimension in position learning. Such a result has been reported by Warren[12] for monkeys.

A further prediction was that in a series of stimuli varying in length, the longest and shortest ones would be selected more often than the two middle-sized ones; and correspondingly in position discrimination, the extreme right or left positions might differ in ease of position learning from the two middle ones.

B. SUBJECTS

The subjects were 32 psychotic and 32 normal children. The psychotics were selected in accordance with the presence of behavioral items listed on a check list developed by Creak *et al.*[2] No attempt was made to establish subcategories, so that according to a definition, such as Rimland's,[11] autistic as well as schizophrenic children were included. The selection was made on the basis of observable behavior only, as historical and neurological information proved unreliable. The psychotics had a mean chronological age of 11 years, ranging from 6 to 15 years. For the purpose of the present experiment, matching with a normal group was carried out on the basis of time scores obtained on the Seguin form board. The scores of the psychotics on this perceptual motor intelligence test ranged from 17 seconds to 40 seconds, with a mean of 27 seconds. The mean score of the normals was 29 seconds, with a range from 17 seconds to 45 seconds. The normal children had a mean chronological age of 4 years, 4 months ranging from 3 years, 3 months to 5 years, 1 month. They attended a day nursery, while the psychotics were all institutional.

C. EXPERIMENT 1

1. Procedure

The material consisted of four upturned aluminum boxes, 1 inch high and 1.5 inches wide. They differed in length from each other by a constant amount of 1 inch, ranging from 6 inches to 3 inches. They were placed on a table in a line, with a distance of 4 inches between any two. For the visual discrimination task, a piece of candy was placed under a box of a particular length, independent of its position in the series which was varied from trial to trial. For the position discrimination a piece of candy was placed under a box in a particular position, independent of length which varied from trial to trial. There were four tasks. In the first of these either the selection of the extreme right hand or left hand stimulus was rewarded for alternate subjects. For the second, the half left or half right position was rewarded for alternate subjects. These were the two position discrimination tasks. In the length discrimination tasks the rewarded responses were those to the longest or shortest of the boxes, and the second longest or second shortest. Thus in addition to comparing the subjects on position and length discrimination, the relative difficulty of selecting either the extremes or the middle of a series in respect to length and position was investigated. The position of the stimuli in the length discrimination, or the lengths of the stimuli in the position discrimination, were varied over 48 trials by using twice all possible combinations of digits one to four.

Subjects were tested individually. Each had to learn one of the four tasks in a session lasting approximately 20 minutes. The eight subgroups of eight subjects were matched for chronological age within the normal and psychotic subgroups, and all groups were matched for Seguin time scores. For a first trial a piece of candy was placed under the correct stimulus in full view of the subject, who was asked to find it. A screen was interposed between each of the 48 subsequent trials, while the stimuli were rearranged. No correction for incorrect responses was allowed. Between trial intervals were of approximately five seconds duration, and no verbal instructions or comments were given.

2. Results

The data used for analysis were the number of errors made out of a possible total of 48. An analysis of variance compared psychotics with normals on position and length discrimination scores for the middle or end stimuli of the series. This showed that normals performed better than psychotics on all tasks ($p = .05$). The predicted groups-by-conditions interaction was not found, as both groups performed significantly better $(p = .001)$ on the position discrimination than on the length discrimination tasks. A significant interaction $(p = .05)$ between serial position and conditions demonstrated that, while the serial position of the correct stimulus made significant difference in length discrimination, this was not the case in position learning. Subsequent t-tests showed that for both groups length discrimination was not significantly more difficult than was position discrimination, provided the correct stimulus was either the longest or the shortest in the series. If, however, the correct response consisted of selecting either the second longest or second shortest, the tasks became significantly more difficult.

D. EXPERIMENT 2

In the first experiment each task represented a positive dimension— i.e., length or position—and correspondingly one negative one—i.e., position and length. The results showed the relatively greater ease in learning the position discrimination while ignoring length, as compared with learning to select a stimulus according to length while ignoring its position. This was the case for normals as well as psychotics, and the predicted groups-by-conditions interaction had not been found. An interpretation of the results would thus have to be made in developmental rather than in clinical terms. In this experiment responding to position, while ignoring length, seemed to have been easier than ignoring position and responding to length. The same result had been reported by Warren[13] for cats. On the other hand, monkeys with prior experience of object discrimination showed the reverse pattern, and learned an object discrimination with varying positions more easily than a position discrimination with varying objects.[12] Both monkeys and cats had performed better on position discrimination with two identical than with two different varying objects.

In order to investigate whether length variation had any distracting effect for children in learning a position habit, a second experiment was carried out using four aluminum boxes of identical length. They were 1 inch high, 2 inches wide, and 4 inches long. If size differences had been completely ignored in the previous position discrimination task, no difference in scores would be expected whether boxes of varying length or of identical length were used. If, on the other hand, the dimension of varying length had been appreciated, using the same length boxes for a position discrimination task should be easier and result in improved performance.

1. *Procedure*

The same 64 children as in the first experiment acted as subjects. Those who had been presented previously with the length discrimination test now had to learn a position habit, while those who had been learning a position discrimination were now required to solve a length discrimination problem. As previously, subjects responded either to the end or middle stimuli of the series: i.e., shortest and longest and extreme left or right, or second shortest and second longest and half left or half right. If either positive or negative transfer accounted for any resulting change in performance, then both groups should be equally affected, as all subjects had already been presented with one previous task.

If the scores obtained by subjects who did the position discrimination task with boxes of different length were the same as the scores of those who did the task with boxes of the same length, then the subjects, operationally speaking, might be said to have treated the two kinds of boxes as equivalent. When we consider the length discrimination tasks, there were no differences in the material presented in the first and the second experiment. Under these circumstances, if the two groups obtained similar scores it would provide a check on the initial matching of the groups.

2. *Results*

The data for analysis were again the total number of errors out of a possible 48. Analyses of variance resulted as previously in a significant conditions-by-serial-place interaction. Response to the two middle-sized stimuli was significantly more difficult than response to the largest or smallest, or to any of the position tasks. The main effect between the groups was not significant in the analysis; as compared with the previous experiment psychotics had somewhat higher and the normals somewhat lower scores.

There are no significant differences when the results of the two experiments are compared by analysis of variance. Subjects perform similarly whether presented with length discrimination before or after a position discrimination. Likewise there is no difference in performance of position discrimination, whether this follows or precedes a length discrimination task. Scores on position learning with stimuli of the same or differing length do not differ significantly.

There were only six children out of the 64, three normal and three psychotic, who did not learn the position habit to a criterion of 10 consecutive correct responses. On the other hand, 20 psychotics and 15 normals failed to reach this criterion in the length discrimination tasks. While it had been established that length differences did not detract from the learning of position discrimination, the question whether position habits might interfere with the learning of a length discrimination remained to be answered. The responses of the 35 subjects who had failed to learn the length discrimination were therefore analyzed for alternative response patterns. There was no marked tendency in either group to persist with position responses to one particular stimulus. Sixty-six per cent of the responses by the psychotics and 71 per cent of those of the normals were changed after one trial, and 92 per cent and 94 per cent, respectively, after three trials. Thus in the length discrimination tasks long runs to any one particular position scarcely occur at all.

Of those who did not solve the length discrimination problem, the 20 psychotics gave a total of 960 responses and the 15 normals a total of 720. An analysis of variance tested whether the same number of responses had been directed to the extreme right and left position and the two middle position stimuli. This showed that both groups made significantly more responses to the two stimuli in the middle position than to the two on the extreme right and extreme left.

E. DISCUSSION

It had been predicted that normal and psychotic children would differ in the ease with which they learned discrimination habits, according to whether this learning depended on the relative predominance of either input or output capacity. While it was realized that both processes were represented in the two conditions used, length discrimination was thought to depend mainly on the analysis of input data. Position discrimination is essentially the learning of a motor habit, and this can be thought of as the organization of movement or output. Because of the apparent interception of many psychotic children on the one hand and their relatively intact motor capacity on the other, it was predicted that normals would be better than psychotics in learning a length discrimination, while the reverse might be the case in position discrimination learning. This prediction would result in a groups-by-conditions interaction in an analysis of variance, which in fact was not present in the results. Normals as well as psychotics found it easier to learn the position than the length discrimination, and the difference in scores between those conditions was the same for both groups. Therefore an interpretation of the results must be thought of in developmental rather than in clinical terms. The organization of motor movements and the analysis of kinesthetic feedback may be prior to their interaction with visual input data. This may be so for animals and young children as well as for those with impaired cognitive functions. This interpretation is supported by the finding that, while irrelevant input in the form of variation in length did not interfere with the learning of a position discrimination, position response tendencies hindered the learning of a length discrimination.

Warren[12] found that monkeys learned fastest when the task was the discrimination of two different objects remaining in the same position throughout learning. This is in agreement with Miller's[9] results in humans, that discrimination is made easier by increasing the number of dimensions that differentiate stimuli. The monkeys also learned easily to discriminate two identical objects according to position. On the other hand, they made significantly more errors when position problems had to be solved with two different, randomly varied objects. For cats[13] position learning with two identical objects was easier than with two different ones, whether these were varied randomly or remained in the same position throughout. The cats seem to have been distracted by the irrelevant dimension of object difference. All these results suggest that the animals perceived the difference between objects during position learning. No such indication is given by the results of the present experiment, in which there was no difference in position learning scores in a task using identical stimuli and one where the stimuli varied in length.

Turning to the length discrimination problem, those subjects who do solve the tasks do so in fewer trials if the correct stimulus is either the longest or shortest of the series. An explanation for this may be given in terms of Inhelder and Piaget,[8] describing an experiment where children are presented with a collection of sticks of different length. The longest of these is placed in front of the child and he is asked to draw the one that comes next in length, then the next, and so on to the shortest of the series. Children who were able to do this were yet unable to use the sticks themselves rather than draw them, to produce such a series. Inhelder and Piaget explain these results by pointing out that the actual seriation involves the element of reversibility, while serialization in the drawing does not. In making the drawing, the child only has to make a single comparison: i.e., each line has to be shorter than the one preceding it. On the other hand, in actually ordering the elements, each one except the tallest and the shortest is shorter than some and longer than other sticks. Thus a simultaneous comparison has to be made, where a certain element is both shorter than the ones already in the series and longer than those that remain to be ordered. The required operation thus becomes multidirectional or reversible. This interpretation applies directly to the authors' findings. The shortest and longest of the boxes are shorter or longer than all the three remaining ones and a unidirectional comparison is all that is needed. Each of the two boxes of intermediate length on the other hand is longer than some and shorter than others and a multidirectional comparison is needed to solve the problem. The difference between the performance on the two types of length discrimination tasks—i.e., intermediate and extreme lengths—is therefore explicable in terms of cognitive stages of development.

Position discrimination is equally easy whether the correct response has to be directed toward the extreme right and left, or the half right and half left stimulus. The apparently high error score of the psychotics in one of the position learning tasks is due to the extremely bad performance of one subject. However, those subjects who could not learn a length discrimination directed their responses more often toward the middle than toward the end position stimuli.

We are not aware of any other psychological experiment in which the behavior of psychotic and normal children could be understood in terms of mechanisms applying to both groups. It is sometimes assumed that the behavior of psychotic children may be so bizarre that it is difficult or impossible to perceive structure and consistency in it. In the present study the results obtained from these children were neither quantitively nor qualitively much different from those of a group of younger normals. It is thus suggested that an interpretation of the results be sought in cognitive developmental terms.

F. SUMMARY

Normal and psychotic children of like mental age were compared for their ability to learn position and length discrimination problems. Position learning was further investigated by using identical as well as differing stimuli. It was found that all subjects learned position discrimination faster than length discrimination, and that there was no difference in position learning according to whether identical or different stimuli were used. While length discrimination was easier when the shortest or the longest of four boxes was the rewarded stimulus, the middle positions rather than the extreme right or left were easiest in position learning. The results are explained in cognitive development terms.

REFERENCES

1. BITTERMAN, M. E., TAYLOR, D. W., & ELAN, C. E. Simultaneous and successive discriminations under identical stimulating conditions. *Amer. J. Psychol.*, 1955, *68*, 237-248.

2. CREAK, M., *et al.* Schizophrenic syndrome in children. Lancet, 1961, *2*, 818.
3. GILLIES, S. Discrimination learning in psychotic children and subnormal controls. Paper to the Annual Conference of the British Psychological Society. *Psychol. Bull.*, 1965, *18*, 59.
4. GOLDFARB, W. Childhood Schizophrenia. Cambridge, Mass.: Harvard Univ. Press, 1961.
5. HERMELIN, B., & O'CONNOR, N. Cross modal transfer in normal, subnormal and autistic children. *Neuropsychologica*, 1964, *2*, 229-235.
6. ————. Visual imperception in psychotic children. *Brit. J. Psychol.*, 1965, in press.
7. HOUSE, B. J., & ZEAMAN, D. Position discrimination and reversal in low grade retardates. *J. Comp. & Physiol. Psychol.*, 1959, *52*, 564-565.
8. INHELDER, B., & PIAGET, J. The Early Growth of Logic in the Child: Classification and Seriation. London: Routledge & Kegan Paul, 1964.
9. MILLER, G. S. The magical number seven, plus or minus two: Some limits on a capacity for processing information. *Psychol. Rev.*, 1956, *63*, 81-97.
10. NORTH, A. J., MALLER, O., & HUGHES, C. Conditional discrimination and stimulus patterning. *J. Comp. & Physiol. Psychol.*, 1958, *51*, 711-715.
11. RIMLAND, B. Infantile Autism: The Syndrome and Its Implication for a Neural Theory of Behaviour. London: Methuen, 1965.
12. WARREN, J. M. Solution of object and positional discrimination in rhesus monkeys. *J. Comp. & Physiol. Psychol.*, 1959, *52*, 92-93.
13. ————. Stimulus preservation in discrimination learning in cats. *J. Genet. Psychol.*, 1959, *52*, 99-101.
14. ————. Solution of sign-differentiated objects and positional discrimination by rhesus monkeys. *J. Genet. Psychol.*, 1960, *96*, 365.
15. ————. Individual differences in discrimination learning of cats. *J. Genet. Psychol.*, 1961, *98*, 89-93.
16. ZEAMAN, D., & HOUSE, B. J. The role of attention in retardate discriminating learning. In N. Ellis (Ed.), *Handbook of Mental Deficiency*. New York: McGraw-Hill, 1963.

31

PSYCHOSES OF CHILDHOOD: A Five Year Follow-up Study of Experiences in a Mental Retardation Clinic

Frank J. Menolascino, M.D.

and

Louise Eaton, M.D.

Nebraska Psychiatric Institute
University of Nebraska College of Medicine

Many young children who become psychotic function as if mentally retarded. Recognition of this group of children has aroused interest concerning the psychoses of childhood among a wide range of professional workers.

The purpose of this study is to follow the course of growth and development of a group of 32 psychotic children who were previously reported (Menolascino, 1956b). This is a five year follow-up report which is part of a long-range study of this group. Our aim is to gain better understanding of these disorders with a view to further clarification of diagnosis and treatment expectations. As background for this presentation, other follow-up studies in the literature are summarized.

Follow-up studies on children previously diagnosed as psychotic are limited in number compared to descriptive and theoretical contributions

Reprinted from the AMERICAN JOURNAL OF MENTAL DEFIENCY, Vol. 72, No. 3, November, 1967, pp. 370-380. This investigation was supported by research grant No. HD-00370 from the National Institute of Child Health and Human Development and Project No. 405 from the Children's Bureau, H. E. W.

in the literature. Further, these studies are difficult to evaluate due to inexactness of diagnostic criteria, variations in definitions of treatment, and differences in evaluating improvement (Eisenberg, 1957; Ward, 1963). Most of the literature refers to childhood schizophrenia and endeavors to clarify its etiology and its relationship, if any, to early infantile autism and/or to adult forms of schizophrenia (Bender, 1955; Ward, 1963). Longitudinal studies on children who have schizophrenia-like psychoses superimposed on, or accompanying, chronic brain syndromes are essentially lacking.

Eisenberg (1957) and Robinson (1961) reviewed the historical development of concepts concerning childhood psychosis from De Sanctis (1906), who implied his impression of the course of the disorder from the name he gave it: dementia praecocissima. Bradley (1941) reviewed the literature through 1940 and concluded that the prognosis of childhood schizophrenia appeared uniformly poor. In 1943 Lourie, Pacella, and Piotrowski reported a series of 20 children who were considered to be schizophrenic by Potter's (1933) criteria. After 4-11 years, three developed signs of organic pathology. Of the remaining 17 cases, 4 achieved "normal" adjustments, 5 made borderline to fair adjustments, 3 developed typical adult schizophrenia, and 5 failed to show any change or deteriorated. No recoveries or remissions could be correlated with any type of treatment.

Reports during the 1940's and 1950's were in agreement that an appreciable percentage of remissions of childhood schizophrenia occurred despite differences in definitions of the terms involved. After careful review of this topic, Eisenberg (1957) concluded that about 25 per cent could be expected to attain a moderately good social adjustment during adolescence, about 33 per cent deteriorated and required continuous institutionalization, and the remaining 42 per cent fluctuated about a marginal level. Kanner and Eisenberg (1955) called attention to speech development in relation to prognosis. In their series of 19 who were mute at age 4, 18 remained severely withdrawn and unable to attend public school 12 years later.

Reiser and Brown (1964) reported follow-up on 125 children diagnosed in pre-school years as having atypical development (infantile psychosis). Ages on follow-up ranged from 9 to 22 years. Of those over 10 years, 36 per cent were receiving schooling through normal channels and approximately 23 per cent were in schools for the retarded. They reported fifty-nine per cent were absorbing enough formal learning to compete in society and that treatment may act as a catalyst in accelerating ego by their parents.

In 1965, Rutter reported a follow-up study of 63 pre-pubescent children diagnosed as child psychosis or one of its synonyms at Maudsley Hospital. Of the 63 psychotic children, 34 had evidence which strongly suggested organic brain disease. Thirty had marked speech problems, ranging from 5 with receptive aphasia, through 14 with mixed aphasic patterns, and 11 had abnormalities of speech production thought to be central in origin. He called attention to misdiagnosis regarding this group. He felt that intelligence testing even in mute psychotic children at age five is a good predictor of their performance ten years later. He noted high correlation between low intelligence and absence of speech at age five and feels that intelligence testing is a better prognostic guide than presence or absence of useful speech at five years. He stated that the child's emotional relationships may be fundamental in determining whether or not he is able to overcome his handicaps and adds that the child's placement and education received were important determinants of treatment results.

Bennett and Klein (1966) recently reviewed a thirty year follow-up of a group of 14 cases of childhood schizophrenia initially reported by Potter (1933). By 1966 only one of this group had been able to maintain himself outside a hospital setting, and seven were severely deteriorated. They stated the present clinical pictures observed in this group could not be differentiated from those of other adult schizophrenic patients with deterioration in the same hospitals.

Havelkova (1966) reported a group of 71 psychotic children where 42 have received psychiatric care and 29 were not treated. Her preliminary report indicated positive correlations between early treatment of the mildly to moderately ill child and subsequent school adjustment; however, she reported very poor outcome in a subgroup she describes as remaining autistic after the age of 5 or 6. An unexpected finding was that most of the psychotic children did not fulfill expectations in the intellectual area, including those who had shown promising early potential. There was a trend toward a relative decrease in intellectual functions in later years. This trend was less marked in the children who were intensively treated in the pre-school age. This is the first study of this type of which we are aware where a control series has been developed, follow-up is being done regularly, and which apparently includes a broad spectrum of types of psychotic children.

METHOD AND SAMPLE

This group of 32 psychotic children was selected from a group of 616 children examined in the Mental Retardation Clinical Evaluation Unit since 1958. These children were under eight years at the time of initial evaluation and referred from a variety of sources. Each child had been suspected of being mentally retarded. The initial sample involved 22 boys and 10 girls, whose average age was 4 years, 8 months.

The multidisciplinary team approach to this group of psychotic children, the initial evaluation procedures, and results have been described in a previous publication (Menolascino, 1956b). The three diagnostic categories used in both studies and their requirements are: (1) Chronic Brain Syndrome with Psychosis, after Ingram (1963) and Kucera (1961); (2) Childhood Schizophrenia, after Creak (1963), and Despert and Sherwin (1958); and (3) Early Infantile Autism, after Kanner (1943) and Rimland (1964).

Five year follow-up was obtained on 29 of the original group of 32 children. The follow-up evaluation consisted of an interim history, physical, neurological and laboratory studies as indicated, behavioral observations, and psychological tests.

In each case, the treatment decision was the consensus of our multidisciplinary team. The degree of emotional disturbance of the child and the parental cooperation dictated the type of treatment offered rather than presence or absence of specific clinical findings (e.g. positive neurological signs).

In this study, *intensive treatment* is defined as an initial period of hospitalization during which additional observations were made and therapy was begun for the child and his parents. Treatment for the child included play therapy a minimum of three times a week, milieu therapy through psychiatric nursing and other child care personnel, psychopharmacological adjuncts and other medical management if indicated, plus special education and speech therapy as prescribed. The most frequent pattern for parents involved individual weekly therapy, followed by other sessions as a couple or in a group. When this type of therapy for child and parents was followed by daypatient care or outpatient therapy as prescribed, the total period is described as "intensive."

Those patients described as having *moderate treatment* were seen once a week on an outpatient basis, or after a brief period of intensive treatment were seen at less frequent intervals primarily for follow-up and general medical management.

Those described as receiving *no treatment* received the same evaluative procedures as the two treatment groups but were seen by us for follow-up only.

Follow-up results are presented for each of the three diagnostic categories (as in our earlier report), with recognition that this sample is too small for definitive conclusions even if diagnostic criteria were clear.

I. *Chronic Brain Syndrome with Psychosis* (22 Cases)

Our most interesting observations concern this group classified as chronic brain syndrome with psychosis. Etiologies range from unknown to known causes, and include the presence of multiple factors interacting. Degree of neurological impairment was noted to range from minimal cerebral dysfunction to massive cerebral damage involving multiple areas. Twenty-two of the twenty-four children of this original subgroup have been followed for the five year period.

Four of the psychotic brain damaged children received *no treatment*. Each of these cases involved a situation wherein we felt we could be of no further service. Four cases were seen for *moderate treatment*. None of these was considered a case for intensive psychotherapy. Counseling for the parents and pharmacological therapy for the child were the chief modes of treatment. Table I presents the present status and changes noted during the five years for these eight patients.

Of the children who received no therapy, two children remained at home during the follow-up period. One of these showed essentially no changes in neurological status, language development, degree of intellectual retardation, or general behavior. Behavior was the only sphere registering detectable change in the other child. Improved affect was noted. The child who was placed in a foster-home had appeared the least damaged of this group in the original study. On five year follow-up his performance on psychological tests improved, placing him in the borderline range of intelligence. The child who had appeared most damaged in the initial study was placed in a home for the retarded. He appeared more severely retarded at this time than before; no changes were noted in his other spheres of functioning.

In the group of four children who received moderate treatment, three developed seizure phenomena and the electroencephalogram of one changed from normal in 1959, through "abnormal" in 1960 and 1961, to "abnormal spike and wave originating from the left cerebral hemisphere" in 1965. The electro-encephalograms of the two who developed clinically detectable seizures during this time had been reported as abnormal with focal spikes at the time of the initial study (one with multiple foci, the other had a right anterior temporal focus). All four of these children had initially been considered severely retarded intellec-

TABLE I
CHRONIC BRAIN SYNDROME WITH PSYCHOSIS
Cases with no treatment (4).
Cases with moderate treatment (4)

			Present Status			
Sex	Treatment	Residence	Neurological Changes	Language Development	Intellectual Retardation	Behavior
F	No therapy	Home	.....	Minimal	Severe	Primitive
M	No therapy	Fosterhome	.....	Normal	Borderline ↑	Normal
F	No therapy	Home	.....	Moderate	Moderate	Immature Affect ↑
M*	No therapy	Home for retarded	.....	None	Severe ↓	Autistic
F	Moderate treatment	Home for retarded	S	None	Severe	Autistic
F	Moderate treatment	Home	.....	Minimal	Severe	Primitive Restless Autistic
M	Moderate treatment	Home	S	None ↓	Severe	Hyperacti͘ Infantile Autistic
M	Moderate treatment	Home for retarded	EEG, S	Minimal	Severe ↓	Primitive Restless

N=22 (This section: 8 of 22) Two of original series lost to follow-up.
↑=Improvement recorded during five years.
↓=Poorer function noted.
EEG=Electroencephalographic changes.
S=Seizures.
*=Initial diagnosis "childhood schizophrenia," changed to chronic brain syndrome with psychosis.

tually. During the follow-up period two remained at home and two were placed in homes for the retarded. The other changes noted in this group were that one of the two was placed in a home for the retarded became more severely retarded in his intellectual performance and one child who remained at home who had previously had essentially no language development lost what little he had. Both of these youngsters were among those who developed seizure activity during this period and both were on anticonvulsant therapy at the time of follow-up evaluation.

Of the fourteen cases of chronic brain syndrome with psychosis who had intensive treatment, five did not complete the recommended treatment program and were either removed from treatment or were terminated because of lack of parental cooperation; thus, the intensive treatment period was six months or less for the five children. Table 2 indicates the present status and changes during the follow-up period of this group.

From Table II one notes immediately that four of the five children had some neurological findings at the time of the initial evaluation. Three of the four had an increase in these findings (quantitatively or qualitatively) on five year follow-up. All of these children were placed in residential settings: four in a home for the retarded, one in a state psychiatric hospital. The child in this group who had originally tested highest on intelligence tests and tests of language development is one of

TABLE II
CHRONIC BRAIN SYNDROME WITH PSYCHOSIS
Cases with Incompleted Intensive Therapy (5)

| Sex | Treatment | Residence | Present Status | | | |
			Neurological Changes	Language Development	Intellectual Retardation	Behavior
M*	Intensive—W	Home for retarded	.....	Minimal	Severe ↓	Non-psychotic "A loner"
M*	Intensive—T	Home for retarded	+ ↓	None	Severe ↓	No affect Passively cooperative
F*	Intensive—T	Home for retarded	+ ↓	Moderate ↓	Moderate ↓	Unpredictably available "A loner"
M*	Intensive—T	State Hospital	+	None	Severe ↓	Infantile Autistic
M*	Intensive—T	Home for retarded	+ ↓	None	Severe ↑	Non-psychotic Has friends Residual posturing

N=22 (This section 5 of 22).
↑=Improvement recorded during five years.
↓=Poorer function noted.
W=Withdrawn from therapy.
T=Therapy terminated by staff.
+=Neurological changes.
+↓=Increased neurological findings.
*=Initial diagnosis "childhood schizophrenia," changed to chronic brain syndrome with psychosis.

those who showed increased neurological findings on follow-up as well as poorer language development and increased intellectual retardation. The only improvement noted was in one boy who had progressed to a non-psychotic condition (despite residual posturing); while his degree of retardation was still described as severe, improvement was noted. The child who went to the psychiatric hospital developed no neurological nor further behavioral changes but showed intellectual retardation comparable to all but one of those living in homes for the retarded.

The remaining nine children had long-term *intensive treatment*. One, who has an associated central language disorder, is showing limited and slow improvement. A second child, whose initial level of mental retardation was described as mild, continues to function at about the same level. The other seven, whose intensive treatment ranged from a minimum of seven months to a maximum of five years, show no improvement or a lower level of over-all behavioral performance. Table III reviews the individual results.

On five year follow-up three of the nine children who received intensive therapy still live at home; four are in homes for the retarded, and two are in a psychiatric hospital. The following changes were noted in the three children who remained at home: development of seizures occurred in one; electro-encephalographic changes plus febrile seizures

TABLE III

CHRONIC BRAIN SYNDROME WITH PSYCHOSIS

Cases with Intensive Therapy (9)

Sex	Treatment	Residence	Present Status				
			Neurological Changes	Language Development	Intellectual Retardation	Behavior
M*	Intensive	Home	S	Moderate (Articulation defect)	Mild	Immature Non-critical
M*	Intensive	Home	EEG, (S)	Severe	Scattered ↓	Hyperactive Impulsive Affect ↑
M*	Intensive	State Hospital	+	Minimal	Severe ↓	Autistic "Anxious"
M	Intensive	Home for retarded	.....	None	Severe	Primitive Autistic
M*	Intensive	Home for retarded	EEG	Moderate	Moderate ↓	Affectionate Unpredictable Residual mannerisms
M	Intensive	Home	.....	Moderate	Scattered ↑	Immature Friendly
M*	Intensive	State Hospital	.....	None	Severe	Primitive Autistic
F*	Intensive	Home for retarded	+	None	Severe ↓	Non-psychotic Primitive
M	Intensive	Home for retarded	.....	Minimal	Moderate ↓	Good affect ↑ Primitive Residual mannerisms

N=22 (This section 9 of 22).
↑=Improvement recorded during five years.
↓=Poorer function noted.
+=Neurological changes.
EEG=Electroencephalographic changes.
S=Seizures; (S)=seizures with fever only.
*=Initial diagnosis "childhood schizophrenia," changed to chronic brain syndrome with psychosis.

and poorer intellectual test performance occurred in the second child, who despite these findings has developed improved affect; the third child shows slight improvement in language development and in intellectual test performance. Of the four in homes for the retarded, two developed increased neurological findings and a third developed an abnormal electroencephalogram. Two of these children showed some improvement in language development, one combined with increased affect, despite somewhat poorer performance on intellectual testing. Both of the two children who reside in a psychiatric hospital have continued the same "autistic" behavioral patterns. One of these children has developed neurological changes. He was originally described as having generalized hyperextensibility, clumsiness, sluggish pupils, a dolichocephalic skull, and short attention span. Two years later he was described as hypotonic, poorly coordinated, and hyperkinetic in behavior. On five year followup, he had developed a marked body tremor, vomiting, and was receiving general medical and neurological re-evaluation. While autistic, he now

TABLE IV

CHILDHOOD SCHIZOPHRENIA (5)

Sex	Treatment	Residence	Present Status			
			Neurological Changes	Language Development	Intellectual Retardation	Behavior
M	Intensive	State Hospital	.....	Minimal ↑	Severe ↓	Withdrawn
M	Intensive	State Hospital	.....	Minimal ↑	Severe ↓	Withdrawn
M	Intensive	State Hospital	.....	Minimal ↑	Severe, except islands ↓	Withdrawn
F	Intensive	Home	.....	Moderate ↑	Borderline ↑	Affect ↑ Immature
F	Intensive	Home	.....	None	Severe	Primitive Autistic

↑=Improvement recorded during five years.
↓=Poorer function noted.

appears chronically anxious and functions less successfully in intellectual assessment. The other child shows essentially no changes in the recorded spheres.

II. *Childhood Schizophrenia* (Five Cases)

The group designated as childhood schizophrenia appeared to be somewhat more homogeneous on follow-up.

Three of these children, despite intensive treatment, showed little response and have been patients in a state hospital for three years or more. None of these was thought to be more than mildly mentally retarded at initial evaluation. All three function at a severely retarded level now, though one exhibits islands of intact functioning. Language has shown slight progress in these youngsters, but is still an area of severe handicap.

Two youngsters remain at home: one has shown a moderate response to therapy and is now in a special education program; the other remains severely mentally retarded and has no language. Among factors leading to different therapeutic results in these two cases are differences in severity of psychopathology in the parents, parental motivation toward treatment, possible cultural influences, dissimilar early developmental patterns, and differences in innate potential of the two children as measured by psychological and developmental tests. These factors were all weighed in favor of the youngster who has shown progress.

At best, treatment response would have to be described as poor in this diagnostic group. Despite apparent clinical similarities in these cases diagnosed as childhood schizophrenia which suggest it may be a unitary diagnostic entity, we maintain some reservations. We also feel that other

TABLE V

EARLY INFANTILE AUTISM

Sex	Treatment	Residence	Present Status			
			Neurological Changes	Language Development	Intellectual Retardation	Behavior
M*	Moderate	Home	Focal seizures	None	Severe	Autistic
F	Intensive	Home	.....	Moderate	Mild	Immature Affect ↑

↑=Improvement recorded during five years.
↓=Poorer function noted.
*=Initial diagnosis "early infantile autism," changed to chronic brain syndrome with psychosis.

factors besides language development, psychological test performance, family dimensions, and type and intensity of treatment will have to be studied and perhaps correlated with these, before one can begin to predict which cases will respond to treatment in the under eight age group.

III. Early Infantile Autism (Two Cases)

The two cases of early infantile autism showed divergent pictures on follow-up. The first child developed neurological signs and now has seizures (electroencephalogram is consistent with a focal seizure disorder). Language has not developed; he remains severely retarded. Our impression at this time is that his autism was secondary to unrecognized neurological damage, compounded by parental rejection during infancy when he was apathetic and nonreactive. The other child in this diagnostic category improved in affective availability and made general behavioral and adaptive progress. Speech and language were established and intellectual functioning was close to age level at last examination.

Retrospectively, we feel that the only similarities in these two cases stemmed from behavioral pictures which were much alike at an early age and which were described by the diagnostic phrase, early infantile autism. The neurological disorder in the first child became apparent with the passage of time, making clearer the underlying impairments which are unresponsive to traditional forms of psychotherapeutic intervention.

DISCUSSION

Since our follow-up revealed no correlation between treatment and prognosis in this sample of psychotic children, it is pertinent to review and examine some of the specific diagnostic and treatment problems found in this study. We must stress that our sample of psychotic children was first referred as suspected mentally retarded. This probably biases our sample as compared to samples of psychotic children reported from other clinical settings. However, it should be noted that Kanner's initial report of eleven children with early infantile autism had also been weighted with children initially referred as possible mental retardates (Kanner, 1943).

Language development has been regarded by some workers (Eisenberg & Kanner, 1955) as the most reliable prognostic indicator in childhood psychoses. Our initial sample was heavily weighted with severely handicapped children as to speech and language developmental levels (81%). Progress in these children has been minimal (see Tables). We observed that those who showed the least language retardation on initial examination showed the least mental retardation. This was a fairly consistent relationship on follow-up.

In our total group of children, those who initially tested in the mildly retarded and low normal ranges respectively continue to perform at approximately the same levels at this time. Seven of the eight who originally tested in the moderately retarded group are now functioning in the severely retarded range. Scattered psychological test findings suggestive of higher potential were found initially in five children who had severe language retardation; now all five function in the severely retarded range.

Our impression is that psychological tests are of limited value as prognostic indicators in young psychotic children because of difficulties in obtaining adequate examinations. There were 19 children in our original sample whose psychological test performance was considered inadequate for prognostic use (seven, essentially untestable; and 12 with marked motor-performance discrepancies suggesting possible higher potential). In follow-up evaluation, none of these 19 children has improved in test performance despite some overall improvement in cooperation in the testing situation. This is in contrast to a report by Rutter (1966, p. 521) who states: "The IQ at 5 years, even in mute psychotic children, proved to be a remarkably good predictor of their performance 10 years later." We concur in part, however, for this proved true in five year follow-up of the small part of our sample for whom "adequate" testing could be obtained.

We noted that initial psychological test results need to be carefully evaluated when considering a child's "potential." Too often marked discrepancies between verbal and motor performance (or certain types of intratest scatter) are interpreted as meaning the child has much more ability than he demonstrates without regard for some special handicap which may be interfering with his performance. This can lead to false optimism during the initial interpretation of findings to parents and to subsequent increased frustration when treatment does not produce the anticipated rise in performance.

In our study 12 cases underwent change in formal diagnosis from childhood schizophrenia to chronic brain syndrome with psychosis, as did one case of early infantile autism. This underscores the striking similarities among the clinical pictures of these childhood psychoses. Change in diagnosis was primarily a result of increased neurological findings, which appears to be in part a function of time.

This emphasizes the necessity of careful and thorough neurological examinations in young psychotic children to detect associated handicaps as early as possible. It also suggests the clinician be more cautious in disregarding "soft neurological signs" since these may be the forerunners of more definitive signs of neurological damage as the child develops. Too often these have been viewed as residuals of "old" central nervous system dysfunction or damage, rather than prodromal manifestations of underlying neurological disturbance.

Our follow-up study suggests that chronic brain syndrome with psychosis in childhood is more common than has generally been recognized. Pollack (1966) made this point strongly in his presentation entitled "Mental Subnormality and 'Childhood Schizophrenia'." He also questioned the discreteness of the other diagnostic categories used in our study. Most of these psychotic youngsters, whom we have diagnosed as chronic brain syndrome with psychosis, might have been diagnosed as early infantile autism, childhood schizophrenia, or mental deficiency with psychosis depending on the individual clinician's orientation. Unfortunately, differential diagnosis is not yet sufficiently precise for reliable comparison of cases among different investigators.

It is significant that nine of the 22 children who were diagnosed as having chronic brain syndrome with psychosis had changes in neurological status during the follow-up period. In three cases, questionable or minor neurological findings at initial evaluation became clear-cut neurological signs. Three additional cases developed neurological signs or symptoms. Without change on neurological examination, three other youngsters have developed electroencephalographic findings consistent with cerebral dysfunction. Two of these have developed seizures which are controlled with medication; the other is seizure free except with elevated temperature.

This would suggest need for increased caution in the interpretation of the meaning of minor, minimal, or "soft" neurological signs. It would appear that they may be early signs or harbingers of what may become more marked disability as the child develops in a substantial percentage of children rather than signs to be disregarded or ignored as symptoms of a previous insult, having only historical interest. Reconsideration of this aspect in diagnosis and treatment seems imperative.

We found no correlation between treatment and response in our sample of psychotic children. Despite the therapeutic nihilism this might imply, we continue to believe that psychotherapy and other treatment modalities should be tried whenever possible. As a result of critical review of therapy with these children, another useful observation was made during this study: while the lack of flexibility and limited adaptive patterns present in some of these children represent a therapeutic problem (and limitation), it has an unexpected dividend. Five of these youngsters showed such prompt improvement following removal from their stressful interpersonal environment that it was evident that environmental manipulation was the key to improvement rather than the other modes of therapy. Return of the child to the stressful environment reprecipitated the psychosis. This finding has therapeutic and placement implications which should be borne in mind for some of these children. This, the most optimistic observation made in this study, underscores the need for creative and experimental approaches to therapy for these children.

Our original selection of diagnostic categories was based on what seemed to us to be the clearest definitions of the psychoses in childhood. The progress of our cases and of those in the literature causes us to question the discreteness of these diagnostic categories. We believe a schizophrenia-like psychosis can occur at any age superimposed on a wide variety of underlying psychophysiological adaptations with the child's basic intellectual endowment ranging from superior to retarded, either with or without the presence of neurological handicap. We think that early infantile autism is not a unitary diagnostic category but is a clinical syndrome described by Kanner (1943) which results from a variety of etiological factors (Menolascino, (1965a). We doubt that most such cases can be differentiated from childhood schizophrenia except in age of onset. Similarly, we raise serious questions as to the unitary nature of childhood schizophrenia. In our experience, schizophrenia-like psychoses superimposed on underlying chronic brain syndromes (from any of a number of causes with varying degrees of cerebral dysfunction and/or damage) are more common than either early infantile autism or childhood schizophrenia.

Our follow-up study results suggest that it is hazardous to employ diagnostic "labels" in the psychotic reactions of childhood without full recognition of the multiplicity of factors (both intrinsic and experimental) which can initiate their onset. Difficulties in differential diagnosis of these disorders are compounded by similarities of the initial clinical examination findings at which time the disorganizing effects of a psychotic process in childhood may produce symptoms indistinguishable from some of those of chronic brain syndrome with psychosis. We do not mean to minimize the need for research concerning etiological factors in the psychoses of childhood. It is our intent, rather, to emphasize the multiplicity of factors which influence the outcome of each case regardless of primary etiology. This approach may also serve to help explain some of the observed differences in response to treatment in cases which appear similar clinically. Such considerations suggest the need for further descriptive delineation of the psychotic reactions in childhood and underscore the need for recognition of different therapeutic and long term management expectations depending on the many factors involved.

SUMMARY

A brief review of the literature concerning follow-up studies on children with childhood psychosis is presented. A five year progress report of 29 cases from our previously reported series of 32 is detailed.

Specific diagnosis beyond "psychosis" was an unstable characteristic of this group. Attention is called to changes in neurological status in 42 per cent of the children diagnosed as chronic brain syndrome with psychosis during the five year follow-up. Caution in the use of psychological testing in prognosis in the very young psychotic child is suggested. Optimism due to "islands of intact functioning" has not proved justified on five year follow-up; however, children who tested highest five years ago continue to do so. Speech development appears highly significant in prognosis; however, further study of the correlation of this with intelligence testing is needed. At this time there appears to be no correlation between treatment and prognosis in this sample of psychotic young children.

REFERENCES

BENDER, L. Twenty years of clinical research on schizophrenic children, with special reference to those under six years of age. In G. Caplan (ed.), *Emotional problems of early childhood.* New York: Basic Books, 1955. Pp. 503-515.

BENNETT, S., & KLEIN, H. Childhood schizophrenia: 30 years later. *Amer. J. Psychiat.,* 1966, 122, 1121-1124.

BRADLEY, C. *Schizophrenia in childhood.* New York: Macmillan, 1941.

CREAK, M. Childhood psychosis: a review of 100 cases. *Brit. J. Psychiat.,* 1963, 109, 84-89.

DE SANCTIS, S. Sopra Alcune Varietá Della Demenza Precoce. *Riv. Sper. Freniat.,* 1906, 32, 141-165.

DESPERT, J. L., & SHERWIN, A. C. Further examination of diagnostic criteria in schizophrenic illness and psychoses of infancy and early childhood. *Amer. J. Psychiat.,* 1958, 114, 784-790.

EISENBERG, L. The course of childhood schizophrenia. *Arch. Neurol. Psychiat.,* 1957, 78, 69-83.

HAVELKOVA, M. Follow-up study of 71 psychotic children, treated and untreated. Personal communication. Summary of paper presented to Fourth World Psychiatry Congress, Madrid, September, 1966.

INGRAM, T. Chronic brain syndromes in childhood other than cerebral palsy, epilepsy, and mental defect. In W. Bax & R. MacKeith (eds.), *Minimal cerebral dysfunction.* London: William Heineman, Ltd., 1963. Pp. 10-17.

KANNER, L. Autistic disturbances of affective contact. *Nerv. Child.,* 1943, 2, 217-250.

KANNER, L., & EISENBERG, L. Notes on the follow-up studies of autistic children. In P. H. Hoch and J. Zubin (eds.), *Psychopathology of childhood, Vol. 44.* New York: Grune & Stratton, 1955. Pp. 227-239.

KUCERA, O. KOLEKTIV. *Psychopathologické projery pri lehkych detskych encefalopatiích (Psychopathologic manifestations in children with mild encephalopathy).* Prague: Statni Zdravotnicke Naklodetelství, 1961. Pp. 235-247 (pages cited are in English).

LOURIE, R. S., PACELLA, B. L., & PIOTROWSKI, Z. A. Studies on the prognosis in schizophrenic-like psychoses in children. *Amer. J. Psychiat.,* 1943, 99, 542-552.

MENOLASCINO, F. J. Autistic reactions in early childhood: Differential diagnostic considerations. *J. child Psychol., Psychiat.,* 1965, 6, 203-218. (a)

MENOLASCINO, F. J. Psychoses of childhood: Experiences of a mental retardation pilot project. *Amer. J. ment. Defic.,* 1965, 70, 83-92. (b)

POLLACK, M. Mental subnormality and "childhood schizophrenia." Paper read at conf. on Psychopathology of Mental Develop., Amer. Psychol. Assn., Feb., 1966, New York City.

POTTER, H. W. Schizophrenia in children. *Amer. J. Psychiat.,* 1933, 12, 1253-1270.

REISER, D. E., & BROWN, J. L. Patterns of later development in children with infantile psychosis. *J. Amer. Acad. child Psychiat.,* 1964, 2, 460-483.

RIMLAND, B. *Infantile autism.* New York: Meredith, 1964.

ROBINSON, J. F. The psychoses of early childhood. *Amer. J. Orthopsychiat.,* 1961, 31, 536-550.

RUTTER, M. The influence of organic and emotional factors on the origins, nature and outcome of childhood psychosis. *Develop. Med. Child Neurol.,* 1965, 7, 518-528.

WARD, T. F. The course of childhood schizophrenia. *Dis. Nerv. Syst.,* 1963, 24, 211-220.

32

FAILURE TO THRIVE IN THE "NEGLECTED" CHILD

Dexter M. Bullard, Jr., M.D.

Instructor in Psychiatry, Harvard Medical School

Helen H. Glaser, M.D.

Clinical Assistant Professor of Pediatrics,
Stanford University Medical School

Margaret C. Heagarty, M.D.

Instructor of Pediatrics, Harvard Medical School

and

Elizabeth C. Pivchik, M.S.W.

Assistant Case Work Supervisor,
The Children's Hospital Medical Center, Boston

Children who fail to thrive without obvious physical cause
present the physician and the hospital with a baffling, time-
consuming, and often unrewarding period of diagnostic
study. Case reports here demonstrate the descriptive in-
adequacy of the term "neglect" in relation to them. Re-
quired refinements in conceptualization and in the col-
lection of clinical data are indicated.

Reprinted from the AMERICAN JOURNAL OF ORTHOPSYCHIATRY, Vol. 37, No. 4, July 1967, pp. 680-690. Copyright, the American Orthopsychiatric Association, Inc. Reproduced by Permission. The authors also wish to acknowledge the support and guidance of Dr. George Gardner, Dr. Charles Janeway, Dr. Joel J. Alpert, and Elizabeth Maginnis and the assistance of Nancy Smith and Susan Bush. This study was supported in part by grants from the William F. Milton Fund of Harvard University and the U.S. Children's Bureau Grant #12 HS-118.

Failure to thrive, a syndrome of infancy and early childhood, is characterized by growth failure, signs of severe malnutrition, and variable degrees of developmental retardation. The true incidence of this disorder is not known, but its more severe form accounts for three or more admissions per month to the Boston Children's Hospital Medical Center. Of these hospitalized patients, about two out of three are found to have organic disease. Congenital heart disease, central nervous system defects, and other congenital anomalies account for the majority of the established diagnoses. The remaining third of the patients do not demonstrate organic pathology, and the cause of their disorder remains uncertain. It is this group of children that concerns us here.

THE FAILURE-TO-THRIVE SYNDROME

Hospital records for all children with failure to thrive admitted from January 1958 to June 1965 were reviewed. Of 151 children, 50 had no primary organic illness. Examination of the clinical features of these 50 cases revealed a number of consistent characteristics. The disorder usually had its onset in early infancy and progressed steadily until 6-to-12 months of age, when one or more hospitalizations occurred. The clinical signs and symptoms that distinguished this syndrome were: failure to grow and gain weight, developmental "slowness," occasional vomiting and/or diarrhea, and frequent feeding difficulties. As the disorder progressed, weakness, tiredness, and irritability were often noted. Progressive weight loss and extreme emaciation were the factors that most commonly precipitated admission to the hospital.

The past histories of these 50 children revealed essentially uncomplicated gestations and births. Nontraumatic medical disease between birth and hospitalization was limited to respiratory infections. Chronic disease occurred in a substantial number of siblings of these patients. Nineteen of the 50 families were afflicted with disorders such as asthma, retardation, and congenital heart disease, including five siblings with evidence of failure to thrive.

On admission to the hospital, the children were emaciated, malnourished, and below the third percentile for weight (a criterion for selection). Sixty per cent were also below the third percentile for height.[12] Ten per cent had healed or healing fractures and contusions. The children's social behavior was often described as "apprehensive," "frightened," "apathetic," or "withdrawn." These children all showed mild to severe retardation of gross and fine motor development, but a striking absence of other physical findings.

The results of one and often two or three hospitalizations were generally unrewarding. A vast array of radiologic and laboratory examinations was negative except for retardation of bone age in 23 of 27 roentgenographic examinations of the long bones. Loss of weight during hospitalization occurred in one-third of the group, but there were individual examples of striking improvement. Clinic follow-up after hospitalization was frequently inconstant, and the responsibility for the patient was often shifted to other sources of medical care.

RESULTS OF A FOLLOW-UP

A follow-up study of 41 patients from 8 months to 9 years after hospitalization revealed a high frequency of pathological sequelae. A continuation of growth failure was evident in one-third of the patients. Six of the 41 children had intelligence quotients below 80 on psychometric testing and appeared clinically retarded to both pediatric and child psychiatric examiners. An equal number of children demonstrated moderate to severe emotional disorders, including one instance of psychosis. Thirty-five per cent showed no evidence of physical, mental, or emotional disorder, demonstrating the potential reversibility of failure to thrive. A not unexpected finding was the fact that the families of the children who did not show sequelae were relatively stable. In summary, more than one-half of the follow-up group showed evidence either of continued growth failure, emotional disorder, mental retardation, or some combination of these.

Thus, the failure-to-thrive syndrome constitutes a disorder of some magnitude, even in the absence of organic etiology. The initial acute phase of the condition represents a severe and sometimes life-threatening situation for the child and a significant emotional and financial drain on the family's resources. This phase also represents a considerable and unrewarding investment of hospital care. Even more unfortunate is the high frequency of pathologic sequelae in these children during the chronic phase of the disorder.

DEFINING "NEGLECT"

After the early intensive diagnostic study of failure to thrive, the inability to find an organic basis usually leads the physician to look for social or psychological causes. Indeed, in recent years a number of case reports have appeared linking failure to thrive with a variety of social and psychological conditions. Of these conditions the one most widely recognized is parental neglect.

In some instances there is no doubt about the fact of neglect. Social casework interview and review of the social history reveal clear evidence of parental uninterest. Visits to the home, interviews with neighbors, and additional history gathered from the child's family further support the clinical conviction that the child is indeed "neglected," as the term has been legally defined. Contributing to the weight of evidence are parents who show signs of instability as evidenced by severe marital strife, erratic living habits, inability to maintain employment or provide financial support for the care of the children. Alcoholism may be implicated, as well as a history of entanglements with the law. Often the mother herself will describe a lack of feeling for the child, will admit leaving the child for long periods of time unattended or with strangers, or otherwise demonstrate inability to provide for the child's basic material needs. In such cases decision-making is not difficult for the care-taking agency, as the following case example demonstrates.

> Alice C. was admitted to The Children's Hospital Medical Center at 4½ months of age because of failure to gain weight. Weighing 5 pounds, 15 ounces at birth, she weighed 8 pounds on admission, well below the third percentile. Her mother initially denied feeding problems and had taken Alice to a local physician, who diagnosed a urinary tract infection. The neighbors feared she had leukemia. On admission Alice was markedly emaciated, had a severe diaper rash over her buttocks and genitalia, but showed no other positive findings on physical examination. Results of a number of laboratory studies were within normal limits, and the case was referred to the social worker.
>
> The social service interview revealed a chronically unstable home situation. The parents, married only 2 years, were separated because of the father's drinking. There were 8 moves during this time and one eviction because of nonpayment of rent. The family history revealed that the mother was raised in a foster home, married to escape it, and resented her 2 children, the patient and a 1½-year-old brother. She was openly abusive to the boy during the interview. Discussion with the state Society for Prevention of Cruelty to Children revealed frequent complaints from neighbors, who described drinking parties and unfed children.
>
> A court hearing was scheduled. The patient was taken home from the hospital against advice, and the judge recommended further investigation of the home. Visits by the Visiting Nurse Association documented that the home was unsanitary; the children were unclean, unfed, and in danger of being burned by an unsafe stove. The mother then left the patient with a neighbor and moved to a nearby city. At this point Alice was placed in a foster home by the state Division of Child Guardianship.

Here evidence of the parent's neglect was not difficult to obtain and fell well within the state law on child neglect. For such children, early removal from the parents results in considerable improvement in their condition, provided that the new home is a satisfactory one. The possibility of such a favorable outcome was demonstrated in 2 of our follow-up patients, who were seen 3 years after hospitalization. These children, in foster homes, were developing normally and showed no evidence of growth retardation, emotional or mental disorder.

However, a substantial number, 58 per cent, of children in our study at no time revealed evidence of parental neglect. Two major reasons for difficulty in establishing such a social diagnosis are: (1) contradictory or inadequate data-gathering by physicians or care-taking agencies, and (2) absence of clear-cut criteria for assessment of the severity of the disorder, the role of social and environmental factors, and prediction of its outcome. Two case examples serve to demonstrate these two problems.

> Linda S. was first seen at Children's Hospital Medical Center at the age of 2 years, referred by the City Health Department because of cessation of growth and weight loss over the previous 6 months despite adequate food intake by report. The history described a normal pregnancy and delivery and a normal feeding history. Physical examination revealed a severely malnourished child of 18 pounds, with a diaper rash. During the next 6 months the diaper rash responded to treatment, but the child continued to lose weight. A variety of radiologic and laboratory studies were unrevealing, and the social service department was asked to evaluate the family situation.
>
> The family consisted of the father, age 22; mother, age 21; a son, age 4 years; the patient, age 2 years 7 months; and a son, age 11 months. The father worked in a respected firm and was continuing his studies in order to improve his opportunity for promotion.
>
> The patient's mother was one of 2 children with a sister 4 years younger. Mother herself had been underweight, asthmatic, and anemic until Linda was born. The mother was told by her physician that she was at this time in better health than she had ever been and was indeed of normal weight without evidence of chronic illness. The social worker described her as "an attractive young woman, soft spoken, articulate, and able to give pertinent information after some initial anxiety."
>
> In reviewing Linda's growth and development, the mother stated that she did not know she was pregnant with Linda until her fourth month, when she was being fitted for a diaphragm. Pregnancy was without complications. Labor was 12 hours in duration, and the

mother said she had no labor pains during that period. She reported that while Linda was in the hospital, several of the nurses told her that Linda was an unusual baby, that she cried only when she was picked up to be fed and seemed comfortable only when she was lying in a bassinet with no one touching her. Mother described Linda's left foot as being reversed when she was born, with the toes pointing backward and the heel to the front. (Review of the hospital record of the neonatal examination revealed no evidence of this deformity.) At home Linda showed the same reaction the nurses reported in the hospital. She cried all the harder if mother picked her up to comfort or to feed her and seemed content only when she was left alone in her crib. In infancy the mother noted that Linda slept 12 to 15 hours a day, resisting feeding when she was awakened but at other times having an insatiable appetite. She described Linda as not thriving as well as her older brother, and feared she was allergic. She crawled at 7 months and at that time began to bang her head when she was approached by her brother or her parents. At 12 months her foot showed no deformity or difficulty on walking. A few weeks prior to admission Linda did not sleep for 5 days, staying in her bed, moaning softly. Mother said when the family tried to comfort her following a head-banging episode, she seemed not to hear their soothing words and would not respond to being held or patted. Mother said she felt lost and did not know what to do to make Linda happy. She said that Linda's speech consisted only of occasional single words.

During the home visit, the social worker observed the boys playing together while Linda stood silently watching them. Occasionally when one child approached her, Linda looked distressed, cried softly, and looked at her mother without saying a word. When mother stopped the child from teasing Linda, she remained standing near her mother without touching her. When Mrs. S. was asked to pick her up, Linda sat stiffly in her lap without expression. Mother said Linda had never reached out to her to be held or picked up.

In describing the mother-child relationship in the home, the social worker noted that Mrs. S. did not seem to be affected by the striking absence of an affectionate relationship between herself and her daughter. At least outwardly, mother did not express appropriate distress about Linda's pathetically unhappy demeanor and the behavior that Mrs. S. described. When it was pointed out that there was some disturbance in Linda's way of relating to people, Mrs. S. said she was afraid Linda was mentally ill, and had avoided asking about this because she did not want an answer. Following these interviews the patient was returned to the out-patient department and then admitted to the hospital.

On admission, Linda was examined by 2 resident physicians and a medical student. The initial diagnoses considered were malabsorption syndrome or other digestive defects. In the hospital, study of the patient included 43 laboratory examinations. Positive findings were restricted to initial electrolyte abnormalities that were due to dehydration. All studies were normal on second examination. Following the social worker's review of the case with the medical staff, the patient was seen in psychiatric consultation. It was felt that she presented a picture of failure to thrive on the basis of emotional deprivation. The psychiatrist felt that her ultimate prognosis depended to a considerable degree on her mother's willingness to undertake psychotherapy. He advised that active follow-up with the patient be maintained for several years after her discharge.

The patient was hospitalized for one month and 6 days during which time she gained more than 7 pounds. She became "an outgoing little girl who was playful on the ward, cooperative, and happy." She began to talk, feed herself, and play with other patients. Before discharge it was noted, "Child to be discharged home, recognizing that mother has not recognized the cause of Linda's trouble and is not willing to be under psychiatric care."

Linda was discharged at age 2 years 8 months, to be followed on a weekly basis in the Child Development Clinic. In the next 6 weeks, despite careful follow-up, she lost 2 pounds. At the end of 6 weeks, rehospitalization was recommended but was refused. Following this visit the mother telephoned the case worker to say that the parents were not planning further visits to Children's Hospital. They had contacted a private physician in their community who allegedly had told the family that Linda was allergic to dairy products and had a little sugar in her blood. The parents saw no need for further social service work and felt that when the child's medical condition was corrected she would improve emotionally. Three weeks later a telephone call to the patient's mother revealed that Linda had been more active since she had been taking her allergy shots 4 times a week. The doctor "felt she had a touch of diabetes and needed to be on a special diet." Mother saw no further need for continued care or help.

(These comments are a bland recording of what was an intensely emotional and disturbing situation in which this family rejected all attempts of the physician to interview them, arrange for examination, or plan for other medical care. During this period Linda again became a mute, withdrawn child, showing a limp and unresisting accommodation to being held. She lost facial expressiveness and appeared completely untouched by the people around her.)

Four months, later, we subsequently learned, the patient, then 3 years one month of age, was admitted to another hospital weighing 12 pounds—6 pounds less than when we had first seen her. On admission she was lifeless and very near death. Her mother stated that she had been taking Linda to a private physician where she was being treated for allergy and diabetes.

On admission mother was noted to be pleasant, quiet, and shy. A home visit was made by a worker new to the case, who noted that the family lived in a neat, clean project apartment, and wrote, "We feel there is no neglect on the part of the parents for this child." During hospitalization Linda responded well to care and attention. She was described as "extremely affectionate" and "quite spoiled with all the attention that was given her." During hospitalization Mrs. S.'s visits became less frequent, and upon discharge Mr. S. had not seen his daughter for 3 weeks. During the mother's visits she did not stay long with her daughter and "dreamed a lot out of the window and left for short intervals frequently." The record stated "Linda is not an autistic child. She is able to express warmth and appreciation. During play sessions with a play worker, she learned how to do simple weaving, play simple card games, and relate well to the play worker and head nurse." The patient remained in the hospital for 4 weeks, improved markedly, gained 13 pounds, and weighed 25 pounds at discharge. On discharge both parents were seen by the chief of service, but they refused offers of follow-up help or treatment, and were extremely hostile toward him when he advised continued contact. They neither called for further appointments nor kept appointments that were made for them.

Linda illustrates vividly a tragic end-result of our deficiencies in gathering accurate and reliable data of sufficient amount for protective intervention. In this child's initial workup in the out-patient department, the mother was viewed as a benign influence on the child's development. Only after exhaustive study and a continual decline in the child's condition was the social environment recognized as a possible cause of the disorder. Early in the course of the patient's second hospitalization a different social worker was even more emphatic about the parents' adequacy to care for Linda. Such statements, incorporated in the medical record, compound the difficulties in intervention. This family's frequent changes of medical resources served to protect them from continued medical surveillance, and further prevented adequate data collection. What is more, the family's own apparent search for an adequate explanation of the child's condition, albeit only in the direction of an organic cause, testified to a kind of interest in the child's welfare.

Further, this case illustrates the difficulty in assessing the contribution of the parents to a child's failure to thrive. In this instance the good appearance of the home, the healthy condition of the siblings, and the family's search for medical care, all tended to conceal the basic life-threatening disturbance in the nurturance of this child. The usual criteria for assessing "neglect" were insufficient to establish it as a primary factor in this case. As a result, Linda illness progressed for 2 years without resolution, interrupted only temporarily when death seemed imminent. It is likely that this child has already suffered irreversible sequelae.

A second case will demonstrate other problems in defining "neglect," assessing the severity of the failure-to-thrive syndrome, and predicting its outcome at the present state of our knowledge of this disorder.

> Susan L., first seen at our clinic at 4 months of age, developed difficulties during the first few weeks of life. The subsequent history of her illness revealed a failure to gain weight, and episodes of vomiting, which became regular during the first several months of her life. During this period she became restless and irritable. Signs of malnutrition became more pronounced, and she was admitted to Children's Hospital. At that time extensive laboratory investigations were undertaken without significant findings. The child gained weight rapidly during her hospitalization. Investigation of the family setting yielded valuable information. The patient had a 4½-year-old brother whose mental retardation led to considerable conflict between the parents and anguish in the mother. All of her attempts to place this hyperactive, aggressive child in an institution had failed. A prominent difficulty with this retarded boy was his nocturnal restlessness, which had led this overconcerned mother to lose sleep and develop marked chronic fatigue.

> During the hospitalization of Susan the parents were interviewed. The father was found to be a quiet, sensible, hard-working person. The mother was found to have a severe characterologic disorder. Her symptoms concerned her own inability to cope with the demands of her children, unrealistic expectations of her husband, and many dramatic neurasthenic complaints. In psychiatric interviews (even when rested and relatively free of any immediate concern about her retarded child), she demonstrated hyperactivity, overtalkativeness, and extreme anxiety. Her thoughts shifted rapidly from topic to topic, her feelings varied quickly from anger to a forced gaiety, and thence to emotions clearly depressive in nature. Her history and reports from outside sources confirmed the impression that hers was a long-standing condition without marked change in the past several years. Though not readily falling into a single diagnostic category, the impression was of severe and chronic disorder of character in which depressive, compensatory euphoric, and hysterical elements were prominent.

> Following the baby's discharge from the hospital, the family was seen in the clinic over a 6-month period. During this time numerous observations were made of Mrs. L.'s method of feeding Susan. Each feeding followed a characteristic pattern. In her hyperactive attention to the feeding process Mrs. L. rarely left the bottle in Susan's mouth for more than a minute. She constantly and vigorously jiggled and patted the baby to encourage her to eat. The results were always

the same. After 5 minutes of jostling and intermittent feeding, Susan vomited or regurgitated whatever she had taken. This was followed by irritation in Mrs. L. and a further increase in activity with further vomiting. This had been the pattern since birth, and Mrs. L. had become angry and discouraged with herself and her baby.

During the first several months following hospitalization, Mrs. L. formed a strong dependent tie to the clinic, coming regularly for her appointments and calling frequently at times of stress, particularly in regard to her uncontrolled retarded child. Susan, however, continued to do poorly and gained only small amounts of weight.

As the months passed and Susan grew to be 10 months old, she began to vomit less frequently. At this time she also seemed less disturbed by the mother's excessive physical stimulation. After a 2 months absence from the clinic because of a family move, Susan was found to have gained markedly in weight and height and to have made considerable progress in motor development. At the time of her last visit she was 11 months old and in the twenty-fifth percentile for height and weight. She showed no retardation on the Infant Catell scale and was a lively, alert, and smiling baby. During this period the mother showed no change in attitude toward us or her behavior toward Susan except pleasure in her improvement. The hyperactive and jostling behavior continued, although now Susan could sit up and hold the bottle helrself.

This case illustrates another aspect of the difficulty in establishing the precise role of the parent in the child's failure to thrive. On first inspection of this family's situation and the mother's personality it was easy to implicate her character pathology as the reason for the child's failure to thrive. In a broad sense, the term "maternal deprivation," as defined by Ainsworth to include a distortion of mother-child interaction,[1] could have been used to describe this mother-child relationship and to raise the question of "neglect." The inadequacy of these terms is demonstrated by the specificity of the difficulty as it related to the child's failure to thrive and to the reversibility of the disorder. The principal cause of the child's failure to thrive was not just the mother's character disorder but also physical overstimulation due to jostling and patting during feeding. The principal reason for improvement was not just the supportive relationship of the clinic or her social worker or doctor, but the child's increasing immunity to jostling and ability to fend for herself.

When one tries to apply the term "neglect" to this case, one immediately faces the problem of definition. This mother did not "neglect" her child in the common-sense understanding of the word. Yet, the manner of her care had serious and immediate consequences for the child's development, and no one could predict with certainty the final outcome of this case. Had this child not improved, intervention might well have been necessary. Such intervention would have to have been justified by a vastly wider definition of "neglect." As failure to thrive of undiagnosed etiology frequently poses this problem, this is a matter of some concern.

Turning to a psychological perspective, one can link failure to thrive to the concept of "maternal deprivation," as elaborated by Bowlby in 1951.[4] Case reports of children who fail to thrive in the absence of organic pathology have shown that their condition can be related to maternal deprivation.[10, 3] The term "masked deprivation" has been used to describe a group of children who demonstrated a type of retarded development that previously had been associated with institutional care.[11] The condition was "masked" by the presence of parental figures in the home. Similar descriptions of children who failed to thrive were reported as examples of "environmental retardation."[6] All of these studies have associated failure to thrive with aspects of maternal care that go beyond food and shelter and involve the quality of the mothering process and the nature of the mother-child relationship.

Several studies have sought to define more specifically a disorder in the mothering or parental figures that is related to failure to thrive. Parental role reversal was implicated in growth and development failure of one group of children.[2] In another group of reported cases, failure to thrive was associated with a disorder in the mother's "claiming behavior."[7] These mothers suffered from an inability to establish an appropriate nurturing relationship to the child, or could not "claim" the child, as a result of early difficulties with their own mothers. "Mothering breakdown" and "the failing to thrive mother" are other terms used to describe some failing or disorder in the mothering figure.[8] These studies demonstrated in a number of instances that parental psychopathology as expressed in a disorder of the mother-child relationship may be followed by failure to thrive on the child's part and that a range of parental psychopathology may be implicated.

Both from a theoretical and practical point of view, the study of maternal or parental psychopathology has advanced considerably our understanding of the failure-to-thrive syndrome. The quality as well as quantity of "mothering" has been implicated in the etiology of failure of growth and development in infancy, thereby adding a substantial dimension to earlier studies, which focused on the presence or absence of a "mothering" figure. As a consequence, a much expanded area of study has been opened to investigators in this field.

But significant limitations remain in our understanding of the nature of parental psychopathology and its relationship to infant growth failure. As Prugh has pointed out, each case requires individual diagnostic study to elicit the exact nature of the disorder.[11] Current concepts are applicable in some cases and not in others.

A major limitation of our knowledge at present has to do with the extent of the syndrome's reversibility. In our follow-up study more than one-third of the patients showed no obvious ill effects of the disorder at the time of their follow-up examination. Of course, the ultimate outcome is as yet not known; but at the time of reexamination, the direction of the child's development was toward improvement. Even severe cases of failure to thrive with a demonstrably poor environment may enjoy a favorable outcome. The following case will illustrate this.

> Mary A. was admitted to Children's Hospital at the age of 6 months with both growth and developmental retardation, signs of emaciation, and a weight and height below the third percentile. She had also had 2 fractures, one said to be from falling accidentally from the changing table. Interviews at the time of hospitalization and subsequent to it suggested a depressive disorder in the mother and a resulting incapacity to care adequately for her child. Following hospitalization, the child was cared for in her home under supervision by the local physician and case worker with the state Society for Prevention of Cruelty to Children.

> At the follow-up almost 6 years later both parents gave a history substantiating the earlier impressions of a disorder in the mother, characterized by depressive feelings, temper outbursts, and an inability to provide proper care and supervision for their children. On examination at age 6 years 4 months, however, Mary showed no evidence of growth retardation, mental retaardation, or emotional disorder. At this time the family was intact and had adequate financial support. The mother showed no evidence of mental disorder or incapacity to care for her home or her children.

In this case, the child's striking improvement does not rule out the possibility of some reduction in what otherwise would have been her optimal level of the intellectual achievement or emotional stability. Nevertheless the course of her disorder was changed and the improvement was marked. At the time of first hospitalization, however, this outcome could not have been predicted with any degree of certainty, using study techniques now at our disposal.

Another limitation is particularly relevant to the failure-to-thrive syndrome. A deficiency exists in our understanding of the critical elements constituting deprivation at different developmental stages. The case of Susan L. illustrates this point. Her mother's characterologic disorder will certainly influence Susan's emotional development. Yet, the essential ingredient relating to the failure to thrive was Mrs. L.'s mealtime overstimulation of the child at a given developmental phase, one which was characterized by a high level of oral need and a low level of motor skills in the area of self-defense. When Susan reached a more advanced stage of development, she appeared to be less vulnerable to her mother's behavior. To make the mother's psychopathology relevant to failure to thrive requires a knowledge of its specific impact on the child at each stage of development.

A final limitation is that we do not know what role the child's behavior plays in the development of this disorder. Recent studies of temperament have documented the range of normal differences in children as well as the persistence of these differences through infancy and childhood.[13] The "overactive" or "colicky" baby even without other difficulties often produces considerable stress in the mother. Similar strains are noted clinically in mothers of babies who resist or show little interest initially in feeding.[5] It is easy to see the child as a helpless victim and the parent as carrying total responsibility for the infant's nurturance. While this is essentially true, the contribution of temperament and the infant's response to nurturance are important variables that will influence the development of any pathology. In fact, it has been suggested that a specific kind of irritating behavior on the part of the child may be responsible for provoking physical attack from abusing parents.[9]

These limitations in our terms "neglect" and "maternal deprivation" are due chiefly to the subtlety of the condition and to lack of knowledge about the mechanisms that operate to produce this disorder. The term "neglect" will have to be defined more broadly, and lose its accusatory connotation, if it is to be used more successfully in the failure-to-thrive syndrome. Otherwise "neglect" should be replaced by a more accurate and less pejorative word. The term "maternal deprivation" when applied to failure to thrive should be used more specifically and should refer to possible inadequacies in feeding, holding, and other specific care-taking activities of the mother. It should be qualified by consideration of the age and developmental level of the child at a time of the acute phase of the disorder. Further, an attempt should be made to describe the duration of the deprivation. The relation of these variables to ultimate outcome then could better be evaluated.

In more practical terms, what new directions should be undertaken in our studies of this syndrome? First, the feeding process in these children should be studied directly to determine patterns of mother-child interaction. Both the mother's behavior and the child's response to feeding should be recorded qualitatively and quantitatively. Only in so doing can we begin to understand what transpires between the mother and infant that leads to lack of growth. Secondly, the actual food intake-utilization pattern must be established more carefully to ascertain the role of food assimilation in these infants. Finally, observation of the child in the home setting during feeding and other activities will be necessary to establish the actual character of the child's care and feeding. The home setting is as important a focus as the hospital in the diagnostic study of this condition.

SUMMARY

Failure to thrive in infancy and early childhood, when of nonorganic etiology, is a serious disorder of growth and development frequently requiring admission to the hospital. In its acute phase it significantly compromises the health and sometimes endangers the life of the child. It causes prolonged family stress and results in a diagnostically un-rewarding and a financially burdensome hospitalization. Follow-up study reveals significant residual sequelae in growth failure, mental retardation, and emotional disorder.

Investigations of social and psychological aspects of this syndrome have led to demonstrations of parental neglect and variable forms of "maternal deprivation." Our study of a group of 50 children with this syndrome demonstrates the inadequacy of the word "neglected," as it is commonly understood, to describe most children with this disorder. Similarly, the term "maternal deprivation," useful as an orienting concept, nonetheless lacks specificity in denoting the mechanisms that operate to produce the failure-to-thrive syndrome.

The concept of maternal deprivation needs to be elaborated to take into account reversibility, developmental stages, and the relationship between physical and emotional nutrients in infancy. Several avenues of investigation are indicated and include direct and systematic observation of the mother-child feeding and nonfeeding interaction patterns in relation to careful study of actual nutritional intake. Direct observation and evaluation of the child and parents in the home setting are important if we are to sharpen our tools for differential diagnosis of dysfunction in the family of the child with failure to thrive.

REFERENCES

1. Ainsworth, M. D. 1962. The effects of maternal deprivation: A review of findings and controversy in the context of research strategy. In Deprivation of Maternal Care: A Reassessment of Its Effects. Public Health Papers No. 14, World Health Organization, Geneva, Switzerland.

2. BARBERO, G. J., M. C. MORRIS, and M. T. REFORD. *1963*. Malidentification of mother-baby-father relationships expressed in infant failure to thrive. *In* The Neglected Battered Child Syndrome: Role Reversal in Parents. Child Welfare League of America, Inc., New York.

3. BLODGETT, F. M. *1963*. Growth Retardation Related to Maternal Deprivation. *In* Modern Perspectives in Child Development. A. J. Solnit and S. A. Provence, eds. International Press, New York.

4. BOWLBY, J. *1952*. Maternal Care and Mental Health. 2nd ed. Monograph Series, No. 2. World Health Organization, Geneva, Switzerland.

5. BRAZELTON, T. B. *1961*. Psychophysiologic reactions in the neonate. J. of Pediatrics. *58:* 508-512.

6. COLEMAN, R., and S. A. PROVENCE. *1957*. Developmental retardation (hospitalism) in infants living in families. Pediatrics. *19:* 285-292.

7. ELMER, E. *1960*. Failure to thrive—role of the mother. Pediatrics. *25:* 717-725.

8. LEONARD, M. F., J. P. RHYMES, and A. J. SOLNIT. *1966*. Failure to thrive in infants. Amer. J. of Diseases of Children. *3:* 600-612.

9. MILOWE, F. D., and R. S. LOURIE. *1964*. The child's role in the battered child syndrome (abstract). J. of Pediatrics. *65:* 1079.

10. PATTON, R. G., and L. I. GARDNER. *1963*. Growth Failure in Maternal Deprivation. Charles C Thomas, Springfield, Illinois.

11. PRUGH, D. C., and R. G. HARLOW. *1962*. "Masked deprivation" in infants and young children. *In* Deprivation of Medical Care: A Reassessment of Its Effects. Public Health Papers, No. 14. World Health Organization, Geneva, Switzerland.

12. STUART, H. C. *1958*. Growth charts as cited in Pediatric Methods and Standards. Fred H. Harvie, ed. Lea and Febiger, Philadelphia.

13. THOMAS, A., S. CHESS, and H. G. BIRCH, et al. *1963*. Behavioral Individuality in Early Childhood. New York University Press. New York.

33

DEVELOPMENTAL CHARACTERISTICS OF ABUSED CHILDREN

Elizabeth Elmer, M.S.S.

and

Grace S. Gregg, M.D.

Department of Pediatrics, University of Pittsburgh School of Medicine, and Children's Hospital of Pittsburgh

Two questions of importance to the pediatrician and the community are how physical abuse affects the subsequent development of young children and whether active intervention is demonstrably helpful in management. Although abuse has been widely assumed to be harmful beyond the immediate physical effects, to date there has been a paucity of definitive studies to document this belief. This paper will describe the developmental characteristics of a group of abused children when they were admitted to Children's Hospital of Pittsburgh and when they were evaluated some years later; the results of intervention will also be assessed. This is the only known study of abuse which was based on examinations of the children as well as interviews of the caretakers; the study was retrospective in nature.

SELECTION OF STUDY GROUP

Silverman,[1] followed by others, described multiple skeletal injuries as a strong indicator of abuse; this condition, in fact, led to the coining of

Reprinted from PEDIATRICS, Vol. 40, No. 4, Part I, October 1967, pp. 596-602. The original version of this paper was presented by G.S.G. to the Child Development Section of the American Academy of Pediatrics, Chicago, Illinois, October 1966. The paper is based on the study "Neglected and Abused Children and Their Families, Phase I: The Fifty Families Study," which was supported by Public Health Service, Grant No. MH-00880 from the National Institute of Mental Health.

the phrase, "the battered child."[2] Most such patients are too young to propel themselves into danger, hence the belief that the child care practices of adult family members must be questioned in relation to the children's extensive bone damage.

The criteria for selection of the children were:

1. multiple bone injuries in various stages of healing, as determined by x-ray survey of the skeleton;

2. absence of clinical disease which might account for the injuries; and

3. a history of assault or gross neglect, or absence of history to satisfactorily explain the injuries.

Over a period of 13 years (from 1949 to 1962), a total of 50 children who satisfied these criteria were admitted to Children's Hospital of Pittsburgh, but many were not identified at the time as possibly abused. Eventually, when the significance of this type of injury became more clear, a group of Children's Hospital staff decided to study the children to assess their development subsequent to injury and hospital treatment. The research staff was composed of two social workers, a pediatrician, a psychologist, a psychiatrist, and a radiologist. The project was called "Neglected and Abused Children and Their Families, Phase I: The Fifty Families Study."[3]

All the families were located; however, 19 of the 50 children were not available for study (Table 1). Three children had expired in the hospital from intracranial trauma, and another was brought to the Emergency Room dead from malnutrition a few months after discharge from the hospital. We discovered that four other children had died within a few months after discharge from the hospital—two of them allegedly at the hands of their mothers, and both women were indicted for murder. We could not learn the cause of death of the remaining two. In addition, we found that five children had been admitted to state institutions for the retarded. It is not possible to state whether their severe retardation preceded or followed their injuries. Thus, 13 of the total group (26%) were either institutionalized or deceased. Six other patients could not be studied because their famiiles, for various reasons, refused to participate. We were able to study 33 children, two of whom were siblings added to the original group because of a history of physical abuse.

METHODS OF STUDY

Data concerning the children on admission to the hospital were obtained by review of their medical charts. Unfortunately, little attempt had been made to estimate the children's precise developmental levels, although some were functioning as if severely retarded. We also reviewed pertinent past medical history from other sources. Social service reports were studied, but this type of material was sparse because of the tendency in the past to treat only the presenting medical problem with little recognition of possible family pathology.

In 1963 the children were reevaluated. The length of time since hospital treatment varied from 1 year and 5 months to 10 years. For the majority, more than 5 years had elapsed since the identification of their bone injuries.

Two structured interviews with each mother yielded data about the child's health and development and a history of the family emphasizing child care practices. Each mother also responded to two standardized questionnaires, the Parental Attitude Research Instrument of Schaefer and Bell[4] and the Srole Anomie Scale.[5] Social and legal agencies provided important collateral data.

Each child came to the hospital for a series of out-patient procedures consisting of pediatric, psychiatric, audiometric, and psychological evaluations and a skeletal survey. The Columbia Mental Maturity Scale was used to determine gross intellectual functioning and the Rorschach Test was administered to children old enough to respond. Some very young children failed to respond to either test and were later retested in their own communities by means of either the Form L-M of the Stanford-Binet Intelligence Test or the Wechsler Intelligence Scale for Children. For the final estimate of intellectual functioning of the older children, school records were considered along with the results of formal testing in the hospital. It was not possible to administer psychological tests to other members of the family, although this would have been helpful in understanding the children's performance.

The schools provided reports of classroom behavior in relation to peers and authority figures. The psychologist and the psychiatrist of the research staff assessed the children's general emotional health as reflected in the psychological protocols and observed during the interviews. Speech problems were noted by both clinicians.

Upon the completion of all examinations and interviews, the current functioning of each child was assessed. The original design had purposely excluded any attempt to determine the circumstances of the children's old injuries because we had assumed abuse as the only cause. However, as the cases were reconstructed, this assumption proved erroneous and it became necessary to consider other possible etiological factors such as traumatic delivery and accidents. Consideration of family history, reports from legal and social agencies, and clinical observations at the time of reevaluation led to a consensus that the injuries of four children had

TABLE 1

FIFTY CHILDREN WITH MULTIPLE SKELETAL INJURIES:
AVAILABILITY FOR REEVALUATION

Children	Number	Total
Available for study		33
original group	31	
sibling* with history of abuse		
obtained in interview	2	
Not available for study		19
deceased	8	
institutionalized	5	
families refused to participate	6	
Total		52

* The two siblings had never been admitted to Children's Hospital of Pittsburgh but were admitted to the study because of our interest in families who abuse more than one child.

been accidental while those of seven children could not be satisfactorily explained. We did not attempt to determine the etiology of injuries in the children who could not be seen in follow-up study. The following results pertain to the 20 children who were: (1) treated in Children's Hospital, (2) reevaluated some years later, and (3) unanimously judged abused. Although the number is small, meaningful patterns emerged in both the admission and the follow-up data, suggesting possible guidelines for diagnosis and management and productive areas for future study.

RESULTS

Most of the 20 families lived in urban Pittsburgh or small neighboring communities, their socioeconomic status was low, and their stated religion was Protestant; 13 were Caucasian and 7 were Negro. The families who refused to participate appeared to be of a slightly higher social class than those who consented; otherwise there was no discernible difference. Nor was there any apparent difference between the children studied and those not studied, with the exception that most of the deceased children were under 5 months of age at the time of hospital admission. Ten children were male and 10 were female. With one exception, all were under 40 months of age (with a range of 3 to 39 months) at the time of treatment for bone injuries, and the majority were brought to the hospital development and integration.

Only one condition pertained to all the children at time of admission; this was the presence of multiple skeletal injuries incurred at various times. Metabolic, endocrine, hemorrhagic, and other skeletal diseases were excluded by appropriate laboratory studies, and there were no major congenital anomalies. More than half the entire study population were under the 3rd percentile in weight and some were extremely malnourished. Six of those with failure to thrive* also had signs of central nervous system damage—two clearly secondary to subdural hematoma, the rest of uncertain etiology.

We have separated the children into two groups according to medical history at time of admission. The first group, 11 children, had been healthy newborns of normal weight without history of serious illness. Nine were in the normal range for height and weight and only two showed signs of growth failure. Their median age was 13 months.

The second group consisted of nine children with significant past medical histories. Six children had birth weights ranging from 1,644 to 2,381 gm (3 lb, 10 oz to 5 lb, 4 oz); the majority had weighed over 2,041 gm (4 lb, 8 oz). Four premature infants had apparently done well, but two had been ill during the neonatal period. The other three children were normal according to birth weight and neonatal course, but each had a history of serious disease. One child had convulsions of unknown etiology, one had vague symptoms of brain damage, and one had herpes encephalitis. All nine children might have been predisposed to failure to thrive, and all showed signs of severe growth failure upon admission to the hospital with bone injuries. Their median age was 25 months.

In both groups, the parents presented the children with two sharply contrasting types of complaint, those suggesting recent injury (such as "fell out of bed" or "won't move his leg") and those suggesting long-standing organic disease rather than trauma (for example, gastrointestinal disorders or malnutrition). The type of complaint appeared important because it either drew attention in a clear-cut way to the child's injuries or diverted attention elsewhere in an ambiguous manner. Table 2 shows the distribution of the two groups of children by type of complaint and physical development.

When all 20 children were grouped according to race, we found that the majority of those with both ambiguous complaints and failure to thrive were Caucasian; only one child with both characteristics was Negro (Table 3). The distribution of prematurity by race was also of interest: one of the seven Negro children was premature, an approxima-

---

* Failure to thrive is defined as height and weight below the 3rd percentile for age and sex.

TABLE 2

TYPE OF PRESENTING COMPLAINT OF 20 ABUSED CHILDREN ACCORDING TO
HEALTH HISTORY AND PHYSICAL DEVELOPMENT AT TIME OF ADMISSION

Health History	Complaint Suggesting Recent Injury	Complaint Suggesting Organic Disease
Benign		
normal growth on admission	7	2
retarded growth on admission	0	2
Significant		
normal growth on admission	0	0
retarded growth on admission	2	7
Total	9	11

tion of the 16% prematurity rate among non-whites in this geographic area.[6] Five of the 13 white children were premature, a proportion much greater than the expected rate of 7% among whites in this area.

When the children were reevaluated in 1963, we learned that they had had no serious acute or chronic illness since treatment for bone injuries. There was no evidence of congenital anomalies unsuspected at time of hospital admission, and no metabolic, endocrine, hemorrhagic, or skeletal diseases had appeared, thus confirming the radiologist's diagnosis of multiple skeletal trauma. Two premature and three full-term infants continued to have signs of central nervous system damage. All 20 had normal hearing despite the probability of past blows about the head.

Of the first group (11 children with benign medical histories at time of admission), 9 were in the normal range of physical growth (3rd to 97th percentile in height and weight for age and sex) and only 2 were below normal. Four of the 11 scored below 80 on intelligence tests and thus were functioning in the range of mental retardation. Emotional disturbance was present in three children and over half of the group had speech problems.

Of the second group (nine children with significant histories prior to bone injuries), three, all premature, were below the 3rd percentile in height and weight according to Drillien's standardization for premature development;[7] but, two of the three were reevaluated within 1½ years of the time of admission, permitting little time for catchup growth to occur.[8] Two other premature infants were disproportionately obese. The remaining four children were normal in height and weight. Mental retardation characterized all but three of the nine, and emotional disturb-

TABLE 3

20 Abused Children Classified by Race: Physical Development and Type of Complaint at Time of Hospital Admission

Finding	Negro	Caucasian
Failure to thrive and ambiguous complaint	1	8
Failure to thrive or ambiguous complaint	1	3
Neither failure to thrive nor ambiguous complaint	5	2
	—	—
Total	7	13

TABLE 4

Developmental Characteristics at Time of Reevaluation of 20 Abused Children, Classified by Medical History at Time of Admission

Characteristics	Benign History	Positive History
Physical development		
normal or above	9	6
below normal	2	3
Intellectual functioning		
normal	7	3
below normal	4	6
Emotional health		
normal	7	5
poor	4	4
Speech		
normal	7	4
poor	4	5
Physical Defect		
not present	8	5
present	3	4

ance and speech problems occurred frequently. (See Table 4 for distribution of developmental characteristics in both groups.)

Eight of all 20 children were diagnosed as emotionally disturbed—four were seen as mildly, two as moderately, and two as severely disturbed.

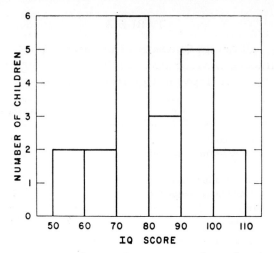

FIG. 1. Distribution of I.Q. scores of 20 abused
children at time of reevaluation.

The I.Q. scores of the 20 children ranged from 52 to 103; 50% fell below 80. Figure 1 shows that, while none was severely retarded,† neither was there a single child of high average intelligence.

Seven of the 20 children had physical defects clearly related to their old injuries; most of them represented handicaps of some magnitude. For example, one child had undergone an eye enucleation and wore a prosthesis, and another wore long leg braces because of lower motor neurone involvement secondary to injury of the spinal cord. Examples of cosmetic defects were a deformity of the skull resulting from bilateral craniotomy for subdural hematoma and plastic repair of a damaged lip.

When the children were considered by race, the seven Negro children were found to have a lower proportion of growth retardation and emotional disturbance than the others. None of the Negro children had physical defects related to trauma. The proportion of speech problems and mental retardation was about the same in the two groups.

At the time of reevaluation 10 children either were living in substitute homes or had had prolonged periods in an institution. Seven of these had had symptoms of growth failure at the time of hospital treatment, and all seven had fully recovered physically. In contrast, of the 10 who were still living in their original homes, six either remained below normal

_____

† By the time of reevaluation, however, 5 of the original 50 were in state institutions for the retarded.

or had fallen below the 3rd percentile in physical growth. The effect of environmental improvement on intellectual functioning could not be determined precisely because of the absence of appropriate measures at the time of hospitalization. However, of the 10 with major environmental improvement, seven were functioning in the normal range of intelligence; of the 10 still in the original homes, only 3 had normal I.Q. tests.

COMMENT

Only two of the 20 children were normal in all areas considered, thus confirming the speculation that severe physical abuse is predictive of unusual difficulties in development. However, only one condition clearly resulted from abuse alone: the physical defects of one third of the children.

Growth failure appeared to be reversible; gross measurements at the time of reevaluation gave no indication that many children had failed to thrive as infants. The other deficiencies which were present could have been the result of factors other than abuse. Prematurity[9] and maternal deprivation[10] strongly influence development; social class affects development, probably through child care practices.[11]

Children with growth failure and ambiguous complaint at the time of hospital admission appeared to have suffered prolonged neglect in addition to abuse; this was borne out by their older age. In contrast, those with normal growth and complaints suggesting recent injury did not appear to have been neglected, a speculation supported by their younger age. When reevaluated, the latter showed more positive development in all respects, and the only two normal children were in this group.

The fact that most of the children with the constellation of ambiguous complaint, growth failure, and older age were Caucasian and only one was Negro suggests that prolonged neglect more frequently accompanies the abuse of Caucasian children than Negro children. The idea that abused Negro children may receive better daily care than their Caucasian counterparts was supported by the finding that upon reevaluation the only two normal children were Negro. Another interesting aspect of the racial distribution was the skew in expected proportion of prematurity. It is possible that the birth of a premature infant may be more stressful for Caucasian than Negro parents, thus encouraging a greater degree of deviance in child care. Furthermore, the Negro mother is likely to have the support of a larger extended family to help in the care of the prematurely born infant.

The passage of time and the increasing ability of the children to escape from abuse probably accounted for a certain amount of recovery. A more active effort on their behalf was the attempt of authoritative agencies to improve the children's environments following abuse. As previously noted, the environment, whether changed or not, appeared to be a powerful factor in the ability of the children to achieve their growth potential. An improved environment has also been shown to substantially benefit intellectual functioning,[12] and our results may suggest similar findings. However, 50% of the abused study group were mentally retarded upon reevaluation despite improved environments and recovery from growth failure. Many had suffered at a vulnerable age from trauma, irreversible nervous system damage, starvation, maternal deprivation, or distorted parent-child interaction. Any one of these experiences could have precluded normal intelligence.

As limited as the children appeared on reevaluation, later reports show that some are having increasing trouble as they approach adolescence. At least five will probably become public charges because of mental retardation or serious emotional disturbances, and several others may be able to remain in the community only if kept in a sheltered environment. Only a few of the children give promise of becoming self-sufficient adults.

The pertinence of these findings for other, less severely traumatized children is an important question that requires further study. It should be noted, however, that extensive injuries at different times do not in themselves indicate abuse. (Four of the original children, not discussed here, also had multiple bone injuries but were judged not abused.) Also, at present we have no way of identifying the abused children who escape physical injury; therefore, it is impossible to track the development of such a group of children for comparison purposes.

The serious outcome for so large a proportion of the original study children makes it imperative to recognize abuse as early as possible. The differential diagnosis of any very young child with an injury should include the possibility of abuse; it should also be considered in the older child with ambiguous organic complaint who shows signs of growth failure. To rule out the possibility of unsuspected trauma, skeletal survey ought to be a part of the routine medical evaluation in either situation.

CONCLUSIONS

The account of these patients documents the necessity for critical attention to the entire environment, including cultural factors believed to be especially important in the care and development of the injured child. It further documents the necessity for early intervention when abuse is suspected. Drastic management by removal from the home, the only method of intervention referred to in this paper, is indicated when the caretaker cannot respond to milder measures designed to improve his relations with the infant. Other methods such as home helps, intensive psychotherapy, or day care for the infant should be carefully tried if the child is considered safe from further assault. Of course, ongoing evaluation should be part of any attempt at intervention.

REFERENCES

1. SILVERMAN, F. N.: The roentgen manifestations of unrecognized skeletal trauma in infants. Amer. J. Roentgen., 69:413, 1953.
2. KEMPE, C. H., SILVERMAN, F. N., STEELE, B. F., DROEGEMUELLER, W., and SILVER, H. K.: The battered-child syndrome. J.A.M.A., 181:17, 1962.
3. ELMER, E.: Children in Jeopardy. University of Pittsburgh Press, in press.
4. SCHAEFER, E. S., and BELL, R. Q.: Development of a parental attitude research instrument. Child. Develop., 29:339, 1958.
5. SROLE, L.: Social integration and certain corollaries: An exploratory study. Amer. Sociol. Rev., 21:709, 1956.
6. Vital Statistics of the United States, 1962, Vol. 1: Natality. Washington, D.C.: U.S. Department of Health, Education and Welfare, 1964.
7. DRILLIEN, C. M.: The Growth and Development of the Prematurely Born Infant. Baltimore: The Williams and Wilkins Co., Appendix 11A and 11B, pp. 327-336, 1964.
8. PRADER, A., TANNER, J. S., and VON HARNACK, G. A.: Catch-up growth following illness or starvation. J. Pediat., 62:646, 1963.
9. WIENER, G., RIDER, R. V., OPPEL, W. C., FISCHER, L. K., and HARPER, P. A.: Correlates of low birth weight: Psychological status at six to seven years of age. Pediatrics, 35:434, 1965.
10. AINSWORTH, M. D. S.: Further research into the effects of maternal deprivation. In Bowlby, J.: Child Care and the Growth of Love, edited by M. Fry. Baltimore, Maryland: Penguin Books, 1965.
11. LESSER, G., FIFER, G., and CLARK, D. H.: Mental abilities of children from different social-class and cultural groups. Monographs of the Society for Research in Child Development. Vol. 30, No. 4. Chicago: University of Chicago Press, 1965.
12. SKEELS, H. M.: Adult status of children with contrasting early life experiences. Monographs of the Society for Research in Child Development. Vol. 31, No. 3. Chicago: University of Chicago Press, 1966.